Nunn and Lumb's Applied Respiratory Physiology

Nunn and Lumb's Applied Respiratory Physiology

NINTH EDITION

Andrew Lumb MB BS FRCA

Consultant Anaesthetist,
St James's University Hospital,
Leeds, UK
Honorary Clinical Associate Professor,
University of Leeds,
Leeds, UK

Caroline Thomas BSc MBChB MRCS(Ed) FRCA

Consultant Anaesthetist,
St James's University Hospital,
Leeds, UK
Honorary Senior Clinical Lecturer,
University of Leeds,
Leeds, UK

For additional online content visit ExpertConsult.com

ELSEVIER

Elsevier

ISBN: 978-0-7020-7908-5
Ink ISBN: 978-0-7020-7934-4
eBook ISBN: 978-0-7020-7933-7

Content Strategist: Jeremy Bowes
Content Development Specialist: Nani Clansey
Project Manager: Julie Taylor
Design: Amy Buxton
Illustration Manager: Teresa McBryan
Marketing Manager: Michele Milano

Printed in Great Britain

Last digit is the print number: 9 8 7 6 5 4

Working together
to grow libraries in
developing countries

www.elsevier.com • www.bookaid.org

To Lorraine, Emma and Jenny (AL)
and
Simon, Martha and Ted (CT)

Foreword

It is truly an honor to be asked to write the Foreword to this newest edition of the landmark text in Respiratory Physiology. For 50 years this has been the acknowledged source for education and reference for physicians, scientists and students whose clinical practice and curiosity involve the respiratory system. The first edition of the pioneering text *Nunn's Applied Respiratory Physiology* was published in 1969 with Dr. John Nunn as the Editor. After the 4th edition, the torch was passed to Dr. Andrew Lumb who maintained the excellent standards and expanded the focus through the 5th to 8th editions. Now with this 9th edition, the text has become Nunn and Lumb's Applied Physiology and Dr. Lumb has shared the authorship with Dr. Caroline Thomas.

I have been told that an efficient method of teaching is to: "Say what you're going to say, say it, and then repeat what you said". The Authors follow this scheme using Key Points at the beginning of each chapter then following at the end with an online Summary to reinforce the educational material. Also, they have maintained the use of a large number of clear and memorable figures and diagrams. I believe their frequent use of electrical or hydrostatic models to explain the underlying physiology is one of the elements that makes this text so useful to learners.

The Editors have continued the logical progression of this text, refined in previous editions, beginning with Part 1 on Basic Principles and then building on this foundation to develop Part 2 on Applied Physiology and finally to extend to Part 3 on The Physiology of Pulmonary Disease. Part 1 explains respiration starting with the relevant anatomy and progressing through lung mechanics, pulmonary circulation and gas exchange to cellular respiration. The final chapter deals with the non-respiratory functions of the lungs. Part 2 then discusses several specific clinical conditions such as pregnancy, paediatrics, sleep, extremes of barometric pressure, anaesthesia and air pollution. A very well written and useful addition to the is 9th edition is Chapter 15 on Obesity. Obesity has become an epidemic in the developed world and the ventilatory management of obese patients during minimally invasive surgery is currently a significant clinical issue. Part 3 on the Physiology of Pulmonary Disease presents chapters on a range of very important clinical topics from ventilatory failure to pulmonary surgery. Of particular note are the up-to-date chapters on acute lung injury and respiratory support. This is a rapidly evolving area and recent developments are presented clearly and concisely.

I find Respiratory Physiology a difficult topic. I tell students that if the answer is simple, you don't understand the question. Yet in the practice of Anaesthesia we are forced to make important decisions on how to manage the airway, gas exchange and respiratory mechanics of diverse individual patients on a daily basis. This text helps walk us through many of these complex clinical decisions. I would like to thank and congratulate Drs. Lumb and Thomas for their excellent work.

Peter Slinger
Professor of Anesthesia , University of Toronto

Preface to the Ninth Edition

Over the past five decades *Nunn's Applied Respiratory Physiology* has developed into a renowned textbook on respiration, providing both physiologists and clinicians with a unique fusion of underlying principles and their applications. After writing four editions, Dr John Nunn retired in 1991, and a new author was required. As Dr Nunn's final research fellow in the Clinical Research Centre in Harrow, AL was honoured to be chosen as his successor. AL has now also completed four editions and has chosen a successor to lead the project into the future whilst maintaining the fundamental ethos of the book. As practising clinicians with a fascination for physiology, the authors of the ninth edition have again focussed on combining a clear, logical and comprehensive account of basic respiratory physiology with a wide range of applications, both physiological and clinical. This approach acknowledges the popularity of the book amongst doctors from many medical specialities, but also provides greater insight into the applications of respiratory physiology to readers with a scientific background. The clinical chapters of Part 3 are not intended to be comprehensive reviews of the pulmonary diseases considered, but rather to provide a detailed description of physiological changes, accompanied by a brief account of the clinical features and treatment of the disease.

In this edition, the number of references provided has been reduced by around a third in recognition of the ease with which online searches may now be performed. References retained are either historical or seminal papers, or recent high-quality publications. Key references are identified by bold type in the reference list following each chapter. These highlighted references either provide outstanding recent reviews of their subject or describe research that has made a significant impact on the topic under consideration.

Advances in respiratory physiology since the last edition are too numerous to mention individually. Appreciation of the impact of air quality on the lungs continues to develop, and there is increasing awareness of the global health burden of pollution. Chapter 20 has been updated in recognition of this and the publication of new worldwide guidelines on pollution levels. The harmful effects of hyperoxia are becoming more accepted in clinical practice, and the physiological mechanisms of these are described in Chapter 25. There is much recent literature on this topic, exemplified by the U-shaped curve of oxygen levels and mortality in critical care patients (see Fig. 25.6). The optimal strategy for artificial ventilation in healthy lungs, for example, during anaesthesia, remains disputed; the section in Chapter 21 has been updated to reflect the physiological effects of these strategies, for example, the recent focus on driving pressure as the potentially damaging component. The role of intraoperative ventilation strategy in the prevention of postoperative pulmonary complications is becoming more clear.

In keeping with its increasing worldwide prevalence, the effects of severe obesity on the respiratory system are now brought together into a new chapter for this edition. Chapter 15 covers the predictable aspects of obesity on respiration, such as the effect of the mass of the chest wall and abdomen on lung mechanics and lung volumes. Less predictable topics include the effects of obesity hormones on respiratory control. The chapter also covers the impact of childhood obesity on lung development, which may lead to lung dysanapsis in which airway and gas exchange tissues grow disproportionately.

For this edition the book is printed with a larger page format to improve the clarity of the figures and tables, and remains available in both print and electronic format. This allows readers wishing to dip into the book access to chapter summaries or individual chapters. For those who own a print copy, online access is automatically available. This content includes additional chapters and self-assessment material, useful for students approaching exams and, new for this edition, a series of 24 mini-lectures by AL to enhance the information provided in print.

We wish to thank the many people who have helped with the preparation of the book at Elsevier and our colleagues who have assisted our acquisition of knowledge in subjects not so close to our own areas of expertise. We are indebted to Professor Peter Slinger for his kind words in the Foreword and would like to thank Drs B. Oliver, J. Black, K. McKay and P. Johnson for permission to use the images in Figure 28.3. Last, but by no means least, we thank our families for their continuing encouragement and for tolerating preoccupied and reclusive parents/spouses for so long. AL's daughter Jenny, when aged 5, often enquired about his activities in the study, until one evening she nicely summarized the years of work by confidently stating that 'if you don't breathe, you die'. So what were the other 423 pages about?

Andrew Lumb and Caroline Thomas
Leeds 2019

Contents

Videos Table of Contents

PART I

Basic Principles

Functional Anatomy of the Respiratory Tract

KEY POINTS

- In addition to conducting air to and from the lungs, the nose, mouth and pharynx have other important functions including speech, swallowing and airway protection.
- Starting at the trachea, the airway divides about 23 times, terminating in an estimated 30 000 pulmonary acini, each containing more than 10 000 alveoli.

- The alveolar wall is ideally designed to provide the minimal physical barrier to gas transfer, whilst also being structurally strong enough to resist the large mechanical forces applied to the lung.

This chapter is not a comprehensive account of respiratory anatomy but concentrates on those aspects that are most relevant to an understanding of function. The respiratory muscles are covered in Chapter 5.

Mouth, Nose and Pharynx

Breathing is normally possible through either the nose or the mouth, the two alternative air passages converging in the oropharynx. Nasal breathing is the norm and has two major advantages over mouth breathing: filtration of particulate matter by the vibrissae hairs and better humidification of inspired gas. Humidification by the nose is highly efficient because the nasal septum and turbinates increase the surface area of mucosa available for evaporation and produce turbulent flow, increasing contact between the mucosa and air. However, the nose may offer more resistance to airflow than the mouth, particularly when obstructed by polyps, adenoids or congestion of the nasal mucosa. Nasal resistance may make oral breathing obligatory, and many children and adults breathe only or partly through their mouths at rest. With increasing levels of exercise in normal adults, the respiratory minute volume increases, and at a level of around 35 L.min^{-1} the oral airway comes into play. Deflection of gas into either the nasal or the oral route is under voluntary control and accomplished with the soft palate, tongue and lips. These functions are best considered in relation to a midline sagittal section (Fig. 1.1).

Figure 1.1, *A*, shows the normal position for nose breathing: the mouth is closed by occlusion of the lips, and the tongue is lying against the hard palate. The soft palate is clear of the posterior pharyngeal wall. Figure 1.1, *B*, shows forced mouth breathing, for instance when blowing through the mouth without pinching the nose. The soft palate becomes rigid and is arched upwards and backwards by contraction of tensor and levator palati to lie against a band of the superior constrictor of the pharynx known as Passavant's ridge, which, together with the soft palate, forms the palatopharyngeal sphincter. Note also that the orifices of the pharyngotympanic (Eustachian) tubes lie above the palatopharyngeal sphincter and can be inflated by the subject only when the nose is pinched. As the mouth pressure is raised, this tends to force the soft palate against the posterior pharyngeal wall to act as a valve. The combined palatopharyngeal sphincter and valvular action of the soft palate is very strong and can easily withstand mouth pressures in excess of 10 kPa (100 cmH$_2$O).

Figure 1.1, *C*, shows the occlusion of the respiratory tract during a Valsalva manoeuvre. The airway is occluded at many sites: the lips are closed, the tongue is in contact with the hard palate anteriorly, the palatopharyngeal sphincter is tightly closed, the epiglottis is in contact with the posterior pharyngeal wall, and the vocal folds are closed, becoming visible in the midline in the figure.

During swallowing the nasopharynx is occluded by contraction of both tensor and levator palati. The larynx is elevated 2 to 3 cm by contraction of the infrahyoid muscles, stylopharyngeus and palatopharyngeus, coming to lie under the epiglottis. In addition, the aryepiglottic folds are approximated, causing total occlusion of the entrance to the larynx. This extremely effective protection of the larynx is

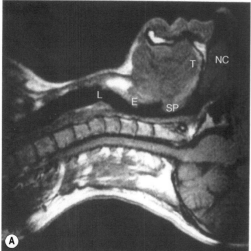

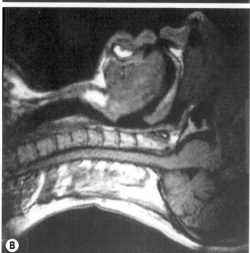

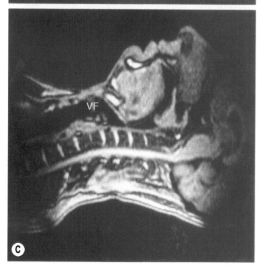

• **Fig. 1.1** Magnetic resonance imaging scans showing median sagittal sections of the pharynx in a normal subject. **(A)** Normal nasal breathing with the oral airway occluded by lips and tongue. **(B)** Deliberate oral breathing with the nasal airway occluded by elevation and backwards movement of the soft palate. **(C)** A Valsalva manoeuvre in which the subject deliberately tries to exhale against a closed airway. Data acquisition for scans **(A)** and **(B)** took 45 s, so anatomical differences between inspiration and expiration will not be visible. I am indebted to Professor M. Bellamy for being the subject. *E,* Epiglottis; *L,* larynx; *NC,* nasal cavity; *SP,* soft palate; *T,* tongue; *VF,* vocal fold.

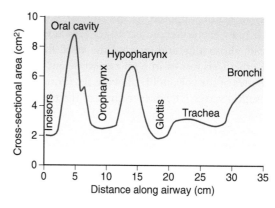

• **Fig. 1.2** Normal acoustic reflectometry pattern of airway cross-sectional area during mouth breathing.

capable of withstanding pharyngeal pressures as high as 80 kPa (800 cmH$_2$O), which may be generated during swallowing.

Upper airway cross-sectional areas can be estimated from conventional radiographs, magnetic resonance imaging (MRI) as in Figure 1.1 or acoustic pharyngometry. In the latter technique, a single sound pulse with a duration of 100 μs is generated within the apparatus and passes along the airway of the subject. Recording of the timing and frequency of sound waves reflected back from the airway allows calculation of the cross-sectional area, which is then presented as a function of the distance travelled along the airway (Fig. 1.2). Acoustic pharyngometry measurements correlate well with MRI scans of the airway, and the technique is now sufficiently developed for use in clinical situations such as estimating airway size in patients with sleep-disordered breathing (Chapter 14).[1]

The Larynx

The larynx evolved in the lungfish for the protection of the airway during such activities as feeding and perfusion of the gills with water. Although protection of the airway remains important, the larynx now has many other functions, all involving some degree of laryngeal occlusion.

Speech

Phonation, the laryngeal component of speech, requires a combination of changes in position, tension and mass of the vocal folds (cords). Rotation of the arytenoid cartilages by the posterior cricoarytenoid muscles opens the vocal folds, while contraction of the lateral cricoarytenoid and oblique arytenoid muscles opposes this. With the vocal folds almost closed, the respiratory muscles generate a positive pressure of 5 to 35 cmH$_2$O, which may then be released by slight opening of the vocal folds to produce sound waves. The cricothyroid muscle tilts the cricoid and arytenoid cartilages backwards and also moves them posteriorly in relation to the thyroid cartilage. This produces up to 50% elongation and therefore tensioning of the vocal folds, an action opposed by the thyroarytenoid muscles, which draw the arytenoid cartilages forwards towards the thyroid, shortening and relaxing the vocal folds. Tensioning of the folds results in both transverse and longitudinal resonance of the vocal fold, allowing the formation of complex sound waves. The deeper fibres of the thyroarytenoids comprise the vocales muscles, which exert fine control over the pitch of the voice by creating slight variations in both the tension and mass of the vocal folds. A more dramatic example of the effect of vocal fold mass on voice production occurs with inflammation of the laryngeal mucosa and the resulting hoarse voice or complete inability to phonate.

Effort Closure

Tighter occlusion of the larynx, known as effort closure, is required for making expulsive efforts. It is also needed to lock the thoracic cage, securing the origin of the muscles of the upper arm arising from the rib cage, thus increasing the power which can be transmitted to the arm. In addition to simple apposition of the vocal folds described previously, the aryepiglottic muscles and their continuation, the oblique and transverse arytenoids, act as a powerful sphincter capable of closing the inlet of the larynx by bringing the aryepiglottic folds tightly together. The full process enables the larynx to withstand the highest pressures which can be generated in the thorax, usually at least 12 kPa (120 cmH$_2$O) and often more. Sudden release of the obstruction is essential for effective coughing (page 46), when the linear velocity of air through the larynx is said to approach the speed of sound.

Laryngeal muscles are involved in controlling airway resistance, particularly during expiration, and this aspect of vocal fold function is described in Chapter 5.

The Tracheobronchial Tree

An accurate and complete model of the branching pattern of the human bronchial tree remains elusive, although several different models have been described. The most useful and widely accepted approach remains that of Weibel,[2] who numbered successive generations of air passages from the trachea (generation 0) down to alveolar sacs (generation 23). This 'regular dichotomy' model assumes that each bronchus regularly divides into two approximately equal size daughter bronchi. As a rough approximation it may therefore be assumed that the number of passages in each generation is double that in the previous generation, and the number of air passages in each generation is approximately indicated by the number 2 raised to the power of the generation number. This formula indicates one trachea, two main bronchi, four lobar bronchi, 16 segmental bronchi and so on. However, this mathematical relationship is unlikely to be true in practice, where bronchus length is variable, pairs of daughter bronchi are often unequal in size, and trifurcations may occur.

Work using computed tomography to reconstruct, in three dimensions, the branching pattern of the airways has shown that a regular dichotomy system does occur for at least the first six generations.[3] Beyond this point, the same study demonstrated trifurcation of some bronchi and airways that terminated at generation 8. Table 1.1 traces the characteristics of progressive generations of airways in the respiratory tract.

Trachea (Generation 0)

The adult trachea has a mean diameter of 1.8 cm and length of 11 cm. Anteriorly it comprises a row of U-shaped cartilages which are joined posteriorly by a fibrous membrane incorporating the trachealis muscle (Fig. 1.3). The part of the trachea in the neck is not subjected to intrathoracic pressure changes, but it is very vulnerable to pressures arising in the neck due, for example, to tumours or haematoma formation. An external pressure of the order of 4 kPa (40 cmH$_2$O) is sufficient to occlude the trachea. Within the chest, the trachea can be compressed by raised intrathoracic pressure during, for example, a cough, when the decreased diameter increases the linear velocity of gas flow, and therefore the efficiency of removal of secretions (page 47).

Main, Lobar and Segmental Bronchi (Generations 1–4)

The trachea bifurcates asymmetrically, and the right bronchus is wider and makes a smaller angle with the long axis of the trachea. Foreign bodies therefore tend to enter the right bronchus in preference to the left. Main, lobar and segmental bronchi have firm cartilaginous support in their walls that is U-shaped in the main bronchi, but in the form of irregularly shaped and helical plates lower down, with bronchial muscle between. Bronchi in this group (down to generation 4) are sufficiently regular to be individually named (Fig. 1.4). The total cross-sectional area of the respiratory tract is minimal at the third generation (Fig. 1.5).

These bronchi are subjected to the full effect of changes in intrathoracic pressure and will collapse when the intrathoracic pressure exceeds the intraluminar pressure by around 5 kPa (50 cmH$_2$O). This occurs in the larger bronchi during a forced expiration, limiting peak expiratory flow rate (see Fig. 3.7).

Small Bronchi (Generations 5–11)

The small bronchi extend through about seven generations, with their diameter progressively falling from 3.5 to 1 mm. Down to the level of the smallest true bronchi, air passages lie in close proximity to branches of the pulmonary artery in a sheath containing pulmonary lymphatics, which can be distended with oedema fluid, giving rise to the characteristic 'cuffing' responsible for the earliest radiographic changes in pulmonary oedema. Because these air passages are not directly attached to the lung parenchyma, they are not subject

TABLE 1.1   Structural Characteristics of the Air Passages

		Generation	Number	Mean Diameter (mm)	Area Supplied	Cartilage	Muscle	Nutrition	Emplacement	Epithelium
Trachea		0	1	18	Both lungs	U-shaped	Links open end of cartilage			Columnar ciliated epithelium
Main bronchi	Conducting airways	1	2	12	Individual lungs			From the bronchial circulation	Within connective tissue sheath alongside arterial vessels	
Lobar bronchi		2→3	4→8	8→5	Lobes	Irregular shape	Helical bands			
Segmental bronchi		4	16	4	Segments					
Small bronchi		5→11	32→2000	3→1	Secondary lobules					
Bronchioles Terminal bronchioles	Acinar airways	12→14	4000→16 000	1→0.7			Strong helical muscle bands			Cuboidal
Respiratory bronchioles		15→18	32 000→260 000	0.4	Pulmonary acinus	Absent	Muscle bands between alveoli	From the pulmonary circulation	Embedded directly in the lung parenchyma	Cuboidal to flat between alveoli
Alveolar ducts		19→22	520 000→4 000 000	0.3			Thin bands in alveolar septa		Form the lung parenchyma	Alveolar epithelium
Alveolar sacs		23	8 000 000	0.2						

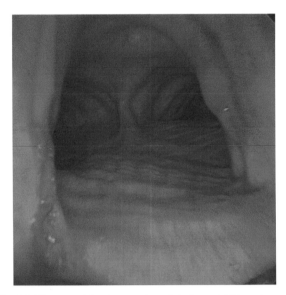

• **Fig. 1.3** The normal trachea as viewed during a rigid bronchoscopy (page 399). The ridges of the cartilage rings are seen anteriorly, and the longitudinal fibres of the trachealis muscle are seen posteriorly, dividing at the carina and continuing down both right and left main bronchi. The less acute angle of the right main bronchus from the trachea can be seen, with its lumen clearly visible, illustrating why inhaled objects preferentially enter the right lung.

to direct traction and rely for their patency on cartilage within their walls and on the transmural pressure gradient, which is normally positive from lumen to intrathoracic space. In the normal subject this pressure gradient is seldom reversed and, even during a forced expiration, the intraluminar pressure in the small bronchi rapidly rises to more than 80% of the alveolar pressure, which is more than the extramural (intrathoracic) pressure.

Bronchioles (Generations 12–14)

An important change occurs at about the 11th generation, where the internal diameter is around 1 mm. Cartilage disappears from the airway wall below this level and

ceases to be a factor in maintaining patency. However, beyond this level the air passages are directly embedded in the lung parenchyma, the elastic recoil of which holds the air passages open like the guy ropes of a tent. Therefore the calibre of the airways beyond the 11th generation is mainly influenced by lung volume because the forces holding their lumina open are stronger at higher lung volumes. The converse of this factor causes airway closure at reduced lung volume (see Chapter 3). In succeeding generations, the number of bronchioles increases far more rapidly than the calibre diminishes (Table 1.1). Therefore the total cross-sectional area increases until, in the terminal bronchioles, it is about 100 times the area at the level of the large bronchi (Fig. 1.5). Thus the flow resistance of these smaller air passages (<2 mm diameter) is negligible under normal conditions. However, the resistance of the bronchioles can increase to very high values when their strong helical muscular bands are contracted by the mechanisms described in Chapters 3 and 28. Down to the terminal bronchiole the air passages are referred to as conducting airways, which derive their nutrition from the bronchial circulation and are thus influenced by systemic arterial blood gas levels. Beyond this point the smaller air passages are referred to as acinar airways and rely upon the pulmonary circulation for their metabolic needs.

Respiratory Bronchioles (Generations 15–18)

Down to the smallest bronchioles, the functions of the air passages are solely conduction and humidification. Beyond this point there is a gradual transition from conduction to gas exchange. In the four generations of respiratory bronchioles there is a gradual increase in the number of alveoli in their walls. Like the bronchioles, the respiratory bronchioles are embedded in lung parenchyma; however, they have a well-defined muscle layer with bands which loop over the opening of the alveolar ducts and the mouths of the mural alveoli. There is no significant change in the

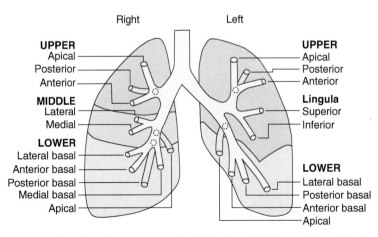

• **Fig. 1.4** Lobes and bronchopulmonary segments of the lungs. *Red,* upper lobes; *blue,* lower lobes; *green,* right middle lobe. The 19 major lung segments are labelled.

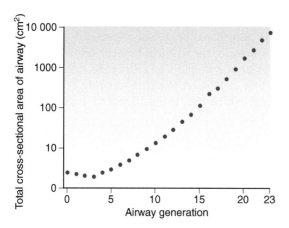

• **Fig. 1.5** The total cross-sectional area of the air passages at different generations of the airways. Note that the minimum cross-sectional area is at generation 3 (lobar to segmental bronchi). The total cross-sectional area becomes very large in the smaller air passages, approaching a square metre in the alveolar ducts.

calibre of advancing generations of respiratory bronchioles (~0.4 mm diameter).

Alveolar Ducts (Generations 19–22)

Alveolar ducts arise from the terminal respiratory bronchiole, from which they differ by having no walls other than the mouths of mural alveoli (~20 in number). The alveolar septa comprise a series of rings forming the walls of the alveolar ducts and containing smooth muscle. Approximately 35% of the alveolar gas resides in the alveolar ducts and the alveoli that arise directly from them.

Alveolar Sacs (Generation 23)

The last generation of the air passages differs from alveolar ducts solely because they are blind. It is estimated that about 17 alveoli arise from each alveolar sac and account for about half of the total number of alveoli.

Pulmonary Acinus

This is defined as the region of lung supplied by a first-order respiratory bronchiole, and includes the respiratory bronchioles, alveolar ducts and alveolar sacs distal to a single terminal bronchiole (Fig. 1.6). This represents the aforementioned generations 15 to 23, but in practice the number of generations within a single acinus is quite variable, being between six and 12 divisions beyond the terminal bronchiole. A human lung contains about 30 000 acini, each with a diameter of around 3.5 mm and containing in excess of 10 000 alveoli. A single pulmonary acinus is probably the equivalent of the alveolus when it is considered from a functional standpoint, as gas movement within the acinus when breathing at rest is by diffusion rather than tidal ventilation. Acinar morphometry therefore becomes crucial,[4] in particular the path length between the start of

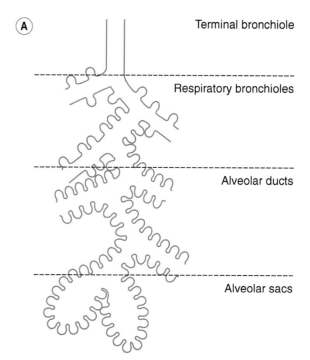

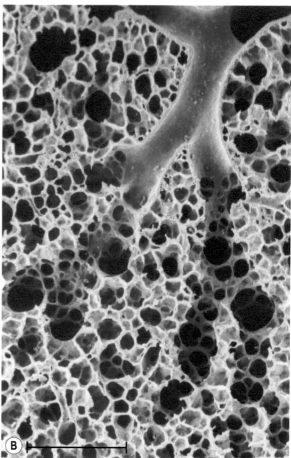

• **Fig. 1.6** **(A)** Schematic diagram of a single pulmonary acinus showing four generations between the terminal bronchiole and the alveolar sacs. The average number of generations in the human lung is eight, but may be as many as 12. **(B)** Section of rabbit lung showing respiratory bronchioles leading to alveolar ducts and sacs. Human alveoli would be considerably larger. Scale bar = 0.5 mm. (Photograph kindly supplied by Professor E. R. Weibel.)

the acinus and the most distal alveolus, which in humans is between 5 and 12 mm.

Respiratory Epithelium

Before inspired air reaches the alveoli it must be 'conditioned', that is, warmed and humidified, and airborne particles, pathogens and irritant chemicals removed. These tasks are undertaken by the respiratory epithelium and its overlying layer of airway lining fluid, and are described in Chapter 11. To facilitate these functions the respiratory epithelium contains numerous cell types.

Ciliated Epithelial Cells[5]

These are the most abundant cell type in the respiratory epithelium. In the nose, pharynx and larger airways the epithelial cells are pseudostratified, gradually changing to a single layer of columnar cells in bronchi, cuboidal cells in bronchioles and finally thinning further to merge with the type I alveolar epithelial cells (see later). They are differentiated from either basal or secretory cells (see later) and are characterized by the presence of around 300 cilia per cell (page 165). The ratio of secretory to ciliated cells in the airway decreases in more distal airways from about equal in the trachea to almost three-quarters ciliated in the bronchioles.

Goblet Cells

These are present at a density of approximately 6000 per mm² (in the trachea) and are responsible for producing the thick layer of mucus that lines all but the smallest conducting airways (page 165).

Airway Glands[6]

Submucosal glands occur predominantly in the trachea and larger bronchi, diminishing in both size and numbers in more distal airways. The glands consist of a series of branching ducts, ending with a single terminal duct opening into the airway and contain both serous cells and mucous cells, with serous cells occurring in the gland acinus, whereas mucous cells are found closer to the collecting duct. The serous cells have the highest levels of membrane-bound cystic fibrosis transmembrane conductance regulator in the lung (Chapter 28).

Basal Cells

These cells lie underneath the columnar cells, giving rise to the pseudostratified appearance, and are absent in the bronchioles and beyond. They are the stem cells responsible for producing new epithelial and goblet cells.

Mast Cells

The lungs contain numerous mast cells which are located underneath the epithelial cells of the airways and in the alveolar septa. Some also lie free in the lumen of the airways and may be recovered by bronchial lavage. Their important role in bronchoconstriction is described in Chapter 28.

Club Cells (Formerly Clara Cells)

These nonciliated bronchiolar epithelial cells are found in the mucosa of the terminal bronchioles, where they may be the precursor of epithelial cells in the absence of basal cells. They are metabolically active, secreting a club cell secretory protein which has antioxidant and immune-modulatory functions.[7]

Neuroepithelial Cells

These cells are found throughout the bronchial tree but occur in larger numbers in the terminal bronchioles. They may be found individually or in clusters as neuroepithelial bodies, and are of uncertain function in the adult lung. Present in foetal lung tissue in a greater number, they may have a role in controlling lung development. Similar cells elsewhere in the body secrete a variety of amines and peptides such as calcitonin, gastrin-releasing peptide, calcitonin gene-related peptide and serotonin.

The Alveoli

The mean total number of alveoli has been estimated as 400 million, but ranges from about 270 to 790 million, correlating with the height of the subject and total lung volume.[8] The size of the alveoli is dependent on lung volume, but at functional residual capacity (FRC) they are larger in the upper part of the lung because of gravity. At total lung capacity this situation reverses, and there are estimated to be 32 alveoli per mm³ at the lung apices compared with 21 at the lung bases.[9] At FRC the mean diameter of a single alveolus is 0.2 mm, and the total surface area of the alveoli is around 130 m².

The Alveolar Septa

The septa are under tension generated partly by collagen and elastin fibres, but more by surface tension at the air–fluid interface (page 14). They are therefore generally flat, making the alveoli polyhedral rather than spherical. The septa are perforated by small fenestrations known as the pores of Kohn (Fig. 1.7), which provide collateral ventilation between alveoli. Collateral ventilation also occurs between small bronchioles and neighbouring alveoli (Lambert channels) and through interbronchiolar pathways of Martin, and is more pronounced in patients with emphysema (page 332) and in some other species of mammal (page 310).

On one side of the alveolar wall the capillary endothelium and the alveolar epithelium are closely apposed, with almost no interstitial space, such that the total thickness from gas to blood is around 0.3 μm (Figs 1.8 and 1.9).[10] This may be considered the 'active' side of the capillary, and gas exchange must be more efficient on this side. The other side of the capillary, which may be considered the 'service' side, is usually more than 1- to 2-μm thick, and contains a recognizable interstitial space containing elastin and collagen fibres, nerve endings and occasional migrant

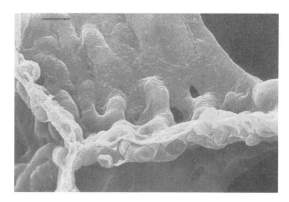

• **Fig. 1.7** Scanning electron micrograph of the junction of three alveolar septa which are shown in both surface view and section view showing the polyhedral structure. Two pores of Kohn are seen to the right of centre. Red blood cells are seen in the cut ends of the capillaries. Scale bar = 10 μm. (From Weibel ER. *The Pathway for Oxygen*. Cambridge, Mass.: Harvard University Press; 1984. With permission. © Harvard University Press.)

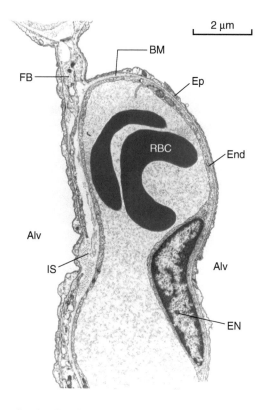

• **Fig. 1.8** Details of the interstitial space, the capillary endothelium and the alveolar epithelium. Thickening of the interstitial space is confined to the left of the capillary (the service side), whereas the total alveolar/capillary membrane remains thin on the right (the active side), except where it is thickened by the endothelial nucleus. *Alv*, Alveolus; *BM*, basement membrane; *EN*, endothelial nucleus; *End*, endothelium; *Ep*, epithelium; *FB*, fibroblast process; *IS*, interstitial space; *RBC*, red blood cell. (Electron micrograph kindly supplied by Professor E. R. Weibel.)

polymorphs and macrophages. The distinction between the two sides of the capillary has considerable pathophysiological significance, as the active side tends to be spared in the accumulation of both oedema fluid and fibrous tissue (Chapter 29).

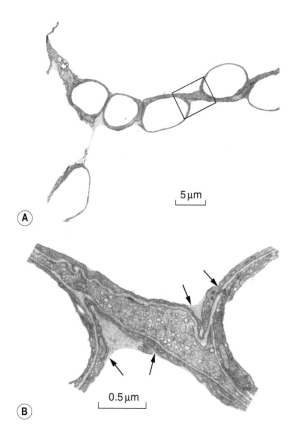

• **Fig. 1.9 (A)** Transmission electron micrograph of alveolar septum with lung inflated to 40% of total lung capacity. The section in the box is enlarged in **(B)** to show alveolar lining fluid, which has pooled in two concavities of the alveolar epithelium and has also spanned the pore of Kohn in **(A)**. There is a thin film of osmiophilic material *(arrows)*, probably surfactant, at the interface between air and the alveolar lining fluid. (From reference 10 by permission of the authors and the editors of *Journal of Applied Physiology*.)

The Fibre Scaffold[11]

The connective tissue scaffold which forms the lung structure has three interconnected types of fibre:

1. Axial spiral fibres running from the hilum along the length of the airways
2. Peripheral fibres originating in the visceral pleura and spreading inwards into the lung tissue
3. Septal fibres, a network of which forms a basket-like structure[12] of alveolar septa, through which are threaded the pulmonary capillaries, which are themselves a network

As a result, capillaries pass repeatedly from one side of the fibre scaffold to the other (Fig. 1.7), the fibre always residing on the thick (or service) side of the capillary, allowing the other side to bulge into the lumen of the alveolus. The left side of the capillary in Figure 1.8 is the side with the fibres. Structural integrity of the whole fibre scaffold is believed to be maintained by the individual fibres being under tension, referred to as a *tensegrity structure*,[11] such that when any fibres are damaged, the alveolar septum disintegrates and adjacent alveoli change shape, ultimately leading to emphysema.

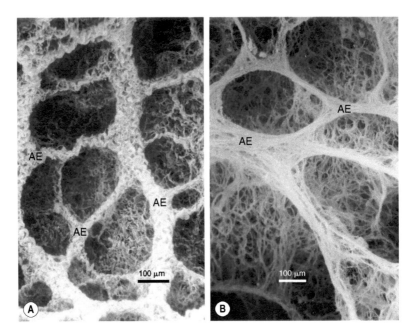

• **Fig. 1.10** Electron micrographs of the collagen fibre network of rat lung at low lung volume **(A)** and when fully inflated **(B)**.[12] Note the folded, zigzag shape of the collagen at low lung volume in **(A)**. (Photograph from Professor Ohtani. Reproduced by permission of *Archives of Histology and Cytology*.)

How the shape of this complex structure changes with breathing remains uncertain.[13] Increasing lung volume may be achieved by increasing the size of alveolar ducts, expanding alveoli or recruiting previously collapsed alveoli. All three undoubtedly contribute, as lung volume increases approximately fivefold from residual volume to total lung capacity (page 22). Recent work using a new imaging technique demonstrated only small changes in alveolar size at different lung volumes, but a large change in alveolar numbers, indicating recruitment as the main mechanism for increasing lung volume.[8,13] Change in alveolar size is facilitated by the molecular structures of both the elastin and collagen that make up the fibre scaffold, with the collagen forming helices or zigzags at lower lung volumes (Fig. 1.10).[12]

At the cellular level, the scaffolding for the alveolar septa is provided by the basement membrane, which provides the blood–gas barrier with enough strength to withstand the enormous forces applied to lung tissue.[14] At the centre of the basement membrane is a layer of type IV collagen, the lamina densa, which is around 50 nm thick and made up of many layers of a diamond-shaped matrix of collagen molecules. On each side of the lamina densa the collagen layer is attached to the alveolar or endothelial cells by a series of proteins collectively known as laminins, of which seven subtypes are now known. The laminins are more than simple structural molecules, having complex interactions with membrane proteins and the intracellular cytoskeleton to help regulate cell shape, permeability and so on. These aspects of the function of the basement membrane are important. Increases in the capillary transmural pressure gradient greater than around 3 kPa (30 cmH$_2$O) may cause disruption of

endothelium and/or epithelium, whereas the basement membrane tends to remain intact, sometimes as the only remaining separation between blood and gas.

Alveolar Cell Types

Capillary Endothelial Cells

These cells are continuous with the endothelium of the general circulation and, in the pulmonary capillary bed, have a thickness of only 0.1 μm, except where expanded to contain nuclei (Fig. 1.8). Electron microscopy shows the flat parts of the cytoplasm are devoid of all organelles except for small vacuoles (caveolae or plasmalemmal vesicles) which may open onto the basement membrane or the lumen of the capillary or be entirely contained within the cytoplasm (Fig. 1.9). The endothelial cells abut one another at fairly loose junctions of the order of 5 nm wide. These junctions permit the passage of quite large molecules, and the pulmonary lymph contains albumin at about half the concentration as that found in plasma. Macrophages pass freely through these junctions under normal conditions, and polymorphs can also pass in response to chemotaxis (page 353).

Alveolar Epithelial Cells: Type I[15]

These cells line the alveoli and exist as a thin sheet of around 0.1 μm in thickness, except where expanded to contain nuclei. Like the endothelium, the flat part of the cytoplasm is devoid of organelles, except for small vacuoles. Epithelial cells each cover several capillaries and are joined into a continuous sheet by tight junctions with a gap of around 1 nm. These junctions may be seen as narrow lines snaking across the septa in Figure 1.7. The tightness of these junctions is crucial for preventing the escape of large molecules, such as albumin, into the alveoli, thus preserving the oncotic pressure gradient essential for the avoidance of pulmonary oedema (page 340). Nevertheless, these junctions permit the free passage of macrophages, and polymorphs may also pass in response to a chemotactic stimulus. Figure 1.9 shows the type I cell covered with a film of alveolar lining fluid. Type I cells are end cells and do not divide in vivo.

Alveolar Epithelial Cells: Type II

These are the stem cells from which type I cells arise.[16] They do not function as gas exchange membranes and are rounded in shape and situated at the junction of septa. They have large nuclei and microvilli (Fig. 1.11). The cytoplasm contains characteristic striated osmiophilic organelles that contain stored surfactant (page 16). Type II cells are also involved in pulmonary defence mechanisms in that they may secrete cytokines and contribute to pulmonary inflammation. They are resistant to oxygen toxicity, tending to replace type I cells after prolonged exposure to high concentrations of oxygen.

Alveolar Macrophages

The lung is richly endowed with these phagocytes which pass freely from the circulation, through the interstitial space and thence through the gaps between alveolar epithelial cells

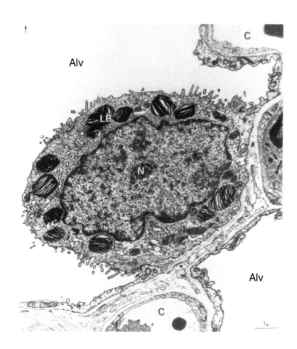

• **Fig. 1.11** Electron micrograph of a type II alveolar epithelial cell of a dog. Note the large nucleus, the microvilli and the osmiophilic lamellar bodies thought to release surfactant. Alv, alveolus; C, capillary; LB, lamellar bodies; N, nucleus. (From reference 17 by permission of Professor E. R. Weibel and the editors of *Physiological Reviews*.)

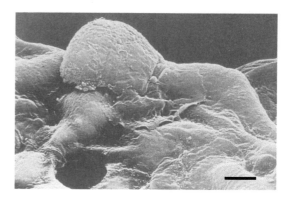

• **Fig. 1.12** Scanning electron micrograph of an alveolar macrophage advancing to the right over epithelial type I cells. Scale bar = 3 μm. (From Weibel ER. *The Pathway for Oxygen*. Cambridge, Mass.: Harvard University Press; 1984. With permission. © Harvard University Press.)

to lie on their surface within the alveolar lining fluid (Fig. 1.12).[18] They are remarkable for their ability to live and function outside the body. Macrophages form the major component of host defence within the alveoli, being active in combating infection and scavenging foreign bodies such as small dust particles. They contain a variety of destructive enzymes but are also capable of generating reactive oxygen species (Chapter 25). These are highly effective bactericidal agents, but their presence in lung tissue may rebound to damage the host. Dead macrophages release the enzyme trypsin, which may cause tissue damage in patients who are deficient in the protein α_1-antitrypsin.

The Pulmonary Vasculature

Pulmonary Arteries

Although the pulmonary circulation carries about the same flow as the systemic circulation, the arterial pressure and the vascular resistance are normally only one-sixth as great. The media of the pulmonary arteries is about half as thick as in systemic arteries of corresponding size. In the larger vessels it consists mainly of elastic tissue, but in the smaller vessels it is mainly muscular, the transition is in vessels of around 1 mm diameter. Pulmonary arteries lie close to the corresponding airways in connective tissue sheaths. Table 1.2 shows a scheme for consideration of the branching of the pulmonary arterial tree. This may be compared with Weibel's scheme for the airways (Table 1.1).

Pulmonary Arterioles

The transition to arterioles occurs at an internal diameter of 100 μm. These vessels differ radically from their counterparts in the systemic circulation and are virtually devoid of muscular tissue. There is a thin media of elastic tissue separated from the blood by endothelium. Structurally there is no real difference between pulmonary arterioles and venules.

TABLE 1.2	Dimensions of the Branches of the Human Pulmonary Artery		
Orders	Numbers	Mean Diameter (mm)	Cumulative Volume (mL)
17	1	30	64
16	3	15	81
15	8	8.1	85
14	20	5.8	96
13	66	3.7	108
12	203	2.1	116
11	675	1.3	122
10	2300	0.85	128
9	5900	0.53	132
8	18 000	0.35	136
7	53 000	0.22	138
6	160 000	0.14	141
5	470 000	0.086	142
4	1 400 000	0.054	144
3	4 200 000	0.034	145
2	13 000 000	0.021	146
1	300 000 000	0.013	151

In contrast to the airways (Table 1.1), the branching is asymmetric and not dichotomous, and so the vessels are grouped according to orders and not generations as in Table 1.1. (Modified from Singhal S, Henderson R, Horsfield K, et al. Morphometry of the human pulmonary arterial tree. *Circ Res.* 1973;33:190-197.)

The normal human pulmonary circulation also contains intrapulmonary arteriovenous anastomoses involving pulmonary arterioles of 25 to 50 μm diameter. These pathways are normally closed, and open only when cardiac output increases, for example during exercise (page 185)[19] or in response to hypoxia.[20] Their presence has clinical implications for the lung as a filtration system within the circulation (page 164).

Pulmonary Capillaries

Pulmonary capillaries tend to arise abruptly from much larger vessels, the pulmonary metarterioles. The capillaries form a dense network over the walls of one or more alveoli, and the spaces between the capillaries are similar in size to the capillaries themselves (Fig. 1.7). In the resting state, around 75% of the capillary bed is filled but the percentage is higher in the dependent parts of the lungs. Inflation of the alveoli reduces the cross-sectional area of the capillary bed and increases resistance to blood flow (Chapter 6). One capillary network is not confined to one alveolus, but passes

from one alveolus to another, and blood traverses a number of alveolar septa before reaching a venule. This clearly has a bearing on the efficiency of gas exchange. From the functional standpoint it is often more convenient to consider the pulmonary microcirculation rather than just the capillaries. The microcirculation is defined as the vessels that are devoid of a muscular layer, and it commences with arterioles with a diameter of 75 μm and continues through the capillary bed as far as venules with a diameter of 200 μm. Special roles of the microcirculation are considered in Chapters 11 and 29.

Pulmonary Venules and Veins

Pulmonary capillary blood is collected into venules that are structurally almost identical to the arterioles. In fact, Duke[21] obtained satisfactory gas exchange when an isolated cat lung was perfused in reverse. The pulmonary veins do not run alongside the pulmonary arteries, but lie some distance away, close to the septa which separate the segments of the lung.

Bronchial Circulation[22]

The conducting airways (from trachea to the terminal bronchioles) and the accompanying blood vessels receive their nutrition from the bronchial circulation, which arises from the systemic circulation. The bronchial circulation therefore provides the heat required for warming and humidification of inspired air, and cooling of the respiratory epithelium causes vasodilation and an increase in the bronchial artery blood flow. About one-third of the bronchial circulation returns to the systemic venous system, with the remainder draining into the pulmonary veins, constituting a form of venous admixture (page 100). The bronchial circulation also differs from the pulmonary circulation in its capacity for angiogenesis.[23] Pulmonary vessels have very limited ability to remodel themselves in response to pathological changes, whereas bronchial vessels, like other systemic arteries, can undergo prolific angiogenesis. As a result, the blood supply to most lung cancers (Chapter 30) is derived from the bronchial circulation.

Pulmonary Lymphatics

There are no lymphatics visible in the interalveolar septa, but small lymph vessels commence at the junction between alveolar and extraalveolar spaces. There is a well-developed lymphatic system around the bronchi and pulmonary vessels, capable of containing up to 500 mL of lymph, and draining towards the hilum. Down to airway generation 11 the lymphatics lay in a potential space around the air passages and vessels, separating them from the lung parenchyma. This space becomes distended with lymph in pulmonary oedema and accounts for the characteristic butterfly shadow of the chest radiograph. In the hilum of the lung, the lymphatic drainage passes through several groups of tracheobronchial lymph glands, where they receive tributaries from the superficial subpleural plexus. Most of the lymph from the left lung usually enters the thoracic duct, whereas the right side drains into the right lymphatic duct. However, the pulmonary lymphatics often cross the midline and pass independently into the junction of the internal jugular and subclavian veins on the corresponding sides of the body.

References

1. Patel SR, Frame JM, Larkin EK, et al. Heritability of upper airway dimensions derived using acoustic pharyngometry. *Eur Respir J.* 2008;32:1304-1308.
2. Weibel ER. Why measure lung structure? *Am J Respir Crit Care Med.* 2001;163:314-315.
3. Sauret V, Halson PM, Brown IW, et al. Study of the three-dimensional geometry of the central conducting airways in man using computed tomographic (CT) images. *J Anat.* 2002;200:123-134.
4. Sapoval B, Filoche M, Weibel ER. Smaller is better—but not too small: a physical scale for the design of the mammalian pulmonary acinus. *Proc Natl Acad Sci USA.* 2002;99:10411-10416.
5. Tilley AE, Walters MS, Shaykhiev R, et al. Cilia dysfunction in lung disease. *Annu Rev Physiol.* 2015;77:379-406.
6. Widdicombe JH, Wine JJ. Airway gland structure and function. *Physiol Rev.* 2015;95:1241-1319.
7. Barnes PJ. Club cells, their secretory protein, and COPD. *Chest.* 2015;147:1447-1448.
8. Hajari AJ, Yablonskiy DA, Sukstanskii AL, et al. Morphometric changes in the human pulmonary acinus during inflation. *J Appl Physiol.* 2012;112:937-943.
9. McDonough JE, Knudsen L, Wright AC. Regional differences in alveolar density in the human lung are related to lung height. *J Appl Physiol.* 2015;118:1429-1434.
10. Gil J, Bachofen H, Gehr P, et al. Alveolar volume-surface area relation in air and saline filled lungs fixed by vascular perfusion. *J Appl Physiol.* 1979;47:990-995.
11. Weibel ER. It takes more than cells to make a good lung. *Am J Respir Crit Care Med.* 2013;187:342-346.
12. Toshima M, Ohtani Y, Ohtani O. Three-dimensional architecture of elastin and collagen fiber networks in the human and rat lung. *Arch Histol Cytol.* 2004;67:31-40.
13. Nieman G. Amelia Earhart, alveolar mechanics, and other great mysteries. *J Appl Physiol.* 2012;112:935-936.
14. Maina JN, West JB. Thin and strong! The bioengineering dilemma in the structural and functional design of the blood-gas barrier. *Physiol Rev.* 2005;85:811-844.
*15. **Weibel ER. On the tricks alveolar epithelial cells play to make a good lung. *Am J Respir Crit Care Med.* 2015;191:504-513.**
16. Hogan B. Stemming lung disease? *N Engl J Med.* 2018;378: 2439-2440.
17. Weibel ER. Morphological basis of alveolar-capillary gas exchange. *Physiol Rev.* 1973;53:419-495.
18. Staples KJ. Lung macrophages: old hands required rather than new blood? *Thorax.* 2016;71:973-974.
19. Kennedy JM, Foster GE, Koehle MS, et al. Exercise-induced intrapulmonary arteriovenous shunt in healthy women. *Respir Physiol Neurobiol.* 2012;181:8-13.
20. Duke JW, Davis JT, Ryan BJ, et al. Decreased arterial PO$_2$, not O$_2$ content, increases blood flow through intrapulmonary arteriovenous anastomoses at rest. *J Physiol.* 2016;594:4981-4996.
21. Duke HN. The site of action of anoxia on the pulmonary blood vessels of the cat. *J Physiol.* 1954;125:373.
22. Paredi P, Barnes PJ. The airway vasculature: recent advances and clinical implications. *Thorax.* 2009;64:444-450.
23. Mitzner W, Wagner EM. Vascular remodeling in the circulations of the lung. *J Appl Physiol.* 2004;97:1999-2004.

2

Elastic Forces and Lung Volumes

KEY POINTS

- Inward elastic recoil of the lung opposes outward elastic recoil of the chest wall, and the balance of these forces determines static lung volumes.
- Surface tension within the alveoli contributes significantly to lung recoil and is reduced by the presence of surfactant, although the mechanism by which this occurs is poorly understood.

- Compliance is defined as the change in lung volume per unit change in pressure gradient, and may be measured for the lung, the thoracic cage or both.
- Various static lung volumes may be measured, and the volumes obtained are affected by a variety of physiological and pathological factors.

An isolated lung will tend to contract until eventually all the contained air is expelled. In contrast, when the thoracic cage is opened it tends to expand to a volume about 1 L greater than functional residual capacity (FRC). Thus in a relaxed subject with an open airway and no air flowing, for example, at the end of expiration or inspiration, the inward elastic recoil of the lungs is exactly balanced by the outward recoil of the thoracic cage.

The movements of the lungs are entirely passive and result from forces external to the lungs. With spontaneous breathing, the external forces are the respiratory muscles, whereas artificial ventilation is usually in response to a pressure gradient developed between the airway and the environment. In each case, the pattern of response by the lung is governed by the physical impedance of the respiratory system. This impedance, or hindrance, has numerous origins, the most important of which are the following:

- Elastic resistance of lung tissue and chest wall
- Resistance from surface forces at the alveolar gas–liquid interface
- Frictional resistance to gas flow through the airways
- Frictional resistance from deformation of thoracic tissues (viscoelastic tissue resistance)
- Inertia associated with movement of gas and tissue.

The last three may be grouped together as nonelastic resistance or respiratory system resistance; they are discussed in Chapter 3. They occur while gas is flowing within the airways, and work performed in overcoming this 'frictional' resistance is dissipated as heat and lost.

The first two forms of impedance may be grouped together as 'elastic' resistance. These are measured when gas is not flowing within the lung. Work performed in overcoming elastic resistance is stored as potential energy, and elastic deformation during inspiration is the usual source of

energy for expiration during both spontaneous and artificial breathing.

This chapter is concerned with the elastic resistance afforded by the lungs and chest wall, which will be considered separately and then together. When the respiratory muscles are totally relaxed, these factors govern the resting end-expiratory lung volume or FRC; therefore lung volumes will also be considered in this chapter.

Elastic Recoil of the Lungs[1]

Lung compliance is defined as the change in lung volume per unit change in transmural pressure gradient (i.e., between the alveolus and pleural space). Compliance is usually expressed in litres (or millilitres) per kilopascal (or centimetres of water), with a normal value of 1.5 L.kPa^{-1} (150 mL.cmH$_2$O^{-1}). Stiff lungs have a low compliance.

Compliance may be described as static or dynamic, depending on the method of measurement (page 23). Static compliance is measured after the lungs have been held at a fixed volume for as long as is practicable, whereas dynamic compliance is usually measured in the course of normal rhythmic breathing. Elastance is the reciprocal of compliance and is expressed in kilopascals per litre. Stiff lungs have a high elastance.

The Nature of the Forces Causing Recoil of the Lung

For many years it was thought that the recoil of the lung was caused entirely by stretching of the yellow elastin fibres present in the lung parenchyma. In 1929 von Neergaard (see section on *Lung Mechanics* in Chapter 35) showed that a lung completely filled with and immersed in water had an elastance that was much less than the normal value obtained when the lung was filled with air. He correctly concluded that much of the 'elastic recoil' was caused by surface tension acting throughout the vast air/water interface lining the alveoli.

Surface tension at an air/water interface produces forces that tend to reduce the area of the interface. Thus the gas pressure within a bubble is always higher than the surrounding gas pressure because the surface of the bubble is in a state of tension. Alveoli resemble bubbles in this respect, although the alveolar gas is connected to the exterior by the air passages. The pressure inside a bubble is higher than the surrounding pressure by an amount depending on the surface tension of the liquid and the radius of curvature of the bubble according to the Laplace equation:

$$P = \frac{2T}{R}$$

where P is the pressure within the bubble (dyn.cm^{-2}), T is the surface tension of the liquid (dyn.cm^{-1}) and R is the radius of the bubble (cm). In coherent SI units (see Appendix A), the appropriate units would be pressure in pascals (Pa), surface tension in newtons/metre (N.m^{-1}) and radius in metres (m).

Figure 2.1, A, left, shows a typical alveolus with a radius of 0.1 mm. Assuming that the alveolar lining fluid has a normal surface tension of 20 mN.m^{-1} (20 dyn.cm^{-1}), the pressure within the alveolus will be 0.4 kPa (4 cmH$_2$O), which is rather less than the normal transmural pressure at FRC. If the alveolar lining fluid had the same surface tension as water (72 mN.m^{-1}), the lungs would be very stiff.

The alveolus in Figure 2.1, A, right, has a radius of only 0.05 mm, and the Laplace equation indicates that, if the surface tension of the alveolus is the same, its pressure should be double the pressure in the left-hand alveolus. Thus gas would tend to flow from smaller alveoli into larger alveoli and the lung would be unstable which, of course, is not true. Similarly, the retractive forces of the alveolar lining fluid would increase at low lung volumes and decrease at high lung volumes, which is exactly the reverse of what is observed. These paradoxes were clear to von Neergaard, and he concluded that the surface tension of the alveolar lining

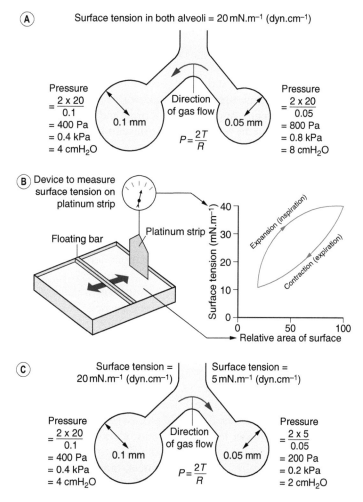

• **Fig. 2.1** Surface tension and alveolar transmural pressure. **(A)** Pressure relations in two alveoli of different size but with the same surface tension of their lining fluids. **(B)** The changes in surface tension in relation to the area of the alveolar lining film. **(C)** Pressure relations of two alveoli of different size when allowance is made for the probable changes in surface tension induced by surfactant.

fluid must be considerably less than would be expected from the properties of simple liquids and, furthermore, that its value must be variable. Observations 30 years later confirmed this when alveolar extracts were shown to have a surface tension much lower than water and which varied in proportion to the area of the interface. Figure 2.1, *B,* shows an experiment in which a floating bar is moved in a trough containing an alveolar extract. As the bar is moved to the right, the surface film is concentrated and the surface tension changes, as shown in the graph on the right of the figure. During expansion, the surface tension increases to 40 mN.m^{-1}, a value which is close to that of plasma but, during contraction, the surface tension falls to 19 mN.m^{-1}, a lower value than any other body fluid. The course of the relationship between pressure and area is different during expansion and contraction, and a loop is described.

The consequences of these changes are important. In contrast to a bubble of soap solution, the pressure within an alveolus tends to decrease as the radius of curvature is decreased. This is illustrated in Figure 2.1, *C,* in which the right-hand alveolus has a smaller diameter and a much lower surface tension than the left-hand alveolus. Gas tends to flow from the larger to the smaller alveolus, and stability is maintained.

The Alveolar Surfactant

The low surface tension of the alveolar lining fluid and its dependence on alveolar radius are because of the presence of a surface-active material known as surfactant. Approximately 90% of surfactant consists of lipids, and the remainder is proteins and small amounts of carbohydrate. Most of the lipid is phospholipid, of which 70% to 80% is dipalmitoyl phosphatidyl choline (DPPC), the main constituent responsible for the effect on surface tension. The fatty acids are hydrophobic and generally straight, lying parallel to each other and projecting into the gas phase. The other end of the molecule is hydrophilic and lies within the alveolar lining fluid. The molecules are thus confined to the surface where, being detergents, they lower surface tension in proportion to the concentration at the interface.

Approximately 2% of surfactant by weight consists of surfactant proteins (SPs), of which there are four types labelled A to D.[2,3] SP-B and SP-C are small proteins vital to the stabilization of the surfactant monolayer (see later); a congenital lack of SP-B results in severe and progressive respiratory failure,[3] and genetic abnormalities of SP-C lead to pulmonary fibrosis in later life.[4] SP-A, and to a lesser extent SP-D, are involved in the control of surfactant release, and possibly the prevention of pulmonary infection (see later).[5]

Synthesis of Surfactant

Surfactant is both formed in and liberated from the alveolar epithelial type II cell (page 11). The lamellar bodies (see Fig. 1.11) contain stored surfactant that is released into the alveolus by exocytosis in response to high volume lung inflation, increased ventilation rate or endocrine stimulation.

After release, surfactant initially forms areas of a lattice structure termed tubular myelin, which is then reorganized into monolayered or multilayered surface films. This conversion into the functionally active form of surfactant is critically dependent on SP-B and SP-C (see later).[3,4] The alveolar half-life of surfactant is 15 to 30 h, with most of its components recycled by type II alveolar cells. SP-A is intimately involved in controlling the surfactant present in the alveolus, with type II alveolar cells having SP-A surface receptors, the stimulation of which exerts negative feedback on surfactant secretion and increases reuptake of surfactant components into the cell.

Action of Surfactant

To maintain the stability of alveoli as shown in Figure 2.1, surfactant must alter the surface tension in the alveoli as their size varies with inspiration and expiration. A simple explanation of how this occurs is that during expiration, as the surface area of the alveolus diminishes, the surfactant molecules are packed more densely, and so exert a greater effect on the surface tension, which then decreases as shown in Figure 2.1, *B.* In reality, the situation is more complex, and at present poorly elucidated.[3] The classical explanation, referred to as the 'squeeze out' hypothesis, is that as a surfactant monolayer is compressed, the less stable phospholipids are squeezed out of the layer, increasing the amount of stable DPPC molecules which have the greatest effect in reducing surface tension.[6] Surfactant phospholipid is also known to exist in vivo in both monolayer and multilayer forms,[2] and it is possible that in some areas of the alveoli the surfactant layer alternates between these two forms as alveolar size changes during the respiratory cycle. This aspect of surfactant function is entirely dependent on the presence of SP-B, a small hydrophobic protein that can be incorporated into a phospholipid monolayer, and SP-C, a larger protein with a hydrophobic central portion allowing it to span a lipid bilayer.[3] When alveolar size reduces and the surface film is compressed, SP-B molecules may be squeezed out of the lipid layer, changing its surface properties, whereas SP-C may serve to stabilize bilayers of lipid to act as a reservoir from which the surface film reforms when alveolar size increases.

Other Effects of Surfactant

Pulmonary transudation is also affected by surface forces. Surface tension causes the pressure within the alveolar lining fluid to be less than the alveolar pressure. Because the pulmonary capillary pressure in most of the lung is greater than the alveolar pressure (page 340), both factors encourage transudation, a tendency checked by the oncotic pressure of the plasma proteins. Thus the surfactant, by reducing surface forces, diminishes one component of the pressure gradient and helps to prevent transudation.

Surfactant also plays an important part in the immunology of the lung.[7] The lipid component of surfactant has antioxidant activity and may attenuate lung damage from a variety of causes, suppressing some groups of lymphocytes, theoretically protecting the lungs from autoimmune damage. In vitro studies have shown that SP-A or SP-D can bind to a wide range of pulmonary pathogens, including viruses, bacteria, fungi, *Pneumocystis jirovecii* and *Mycobacterium tuberculosis*. Polymorphisms of the surfactant genes are associated with the severity of some respiratory diseases; for example, the likelihood of developing severe pulmonary manifestations of an influenza infection is influenced by a single nucleotide polymorphism of the gene encoding SP-B.[8] Acting via specific surface receptors, both SP-A and SP-D activate alveolar neutrophils and macrophages and enhance the phagocytic actions of the latter during lung inflammation.[7]

Alternative Models to Explain Lung Recoil

Treating surfactant-lined alveoli as bubbles that obey Laplace's law has aided the understanding of lung recoil in health and disease for many decades (see section on *Lung Mechanics* in online Chapter 35: The History of Respiratory Physiology). This 'bubble model' of alveolar stability is not universally accepted,[9] and there is evidence that the real situation is more complex. Arguments against the bubble model include the following:

- In theory, differing surface tensions in adjacent alveoli cannot occur if the liquid lining the alveoli is connected by a continuous liquid layer.
- When surfactant layers are compressed at 37°C, multilayered 'rafts' of dry surfactant form, although inclusion of surfactant proteins reduces this physicochemical change.
- Alveoli are not shaped like perfect spheres with a single entrance point; they are variable polyhedrons with convex bulges in their walls where pulmonary capillaries bulge into them (see Fig. 1.7).

Two quite different alternative models have been proposed:
Morphological model. Hills' model proposes that the surfactant lining alveoli results in a 'discontinuous' liquid lining.[10] Based on knowledge of the physical chemistry of surfactants, this model shows that surfactant phospholipids are adsorbed directly onto the epithelial cell surface, forming multilayered rafts of surfactant (Fig. 2.2). These rafts cause patches of the surface to become less wettable, and these areas are interspersed with fluid pools. Surface forces generated by the interaction between the 'dry' areas of surfactant and the areas of liquid are theoretically large enough to maintain alveolar stability. The rafts of surfactant may be many layers thick, and are believed to form and disperse with each breath; their function is almost certainly dependent on both SP-B and SP-C.
Foam model. Scarpelli developed different techniques for preparing lung tissue for microscopy.[11] By maintaining tissue in a more natural state than previous studies, including keeping lung volume close to normal, he suggested that in vivo there are bubble films across alveolar entrances, across alveolar ducts and within respiratory bronchioles. In this model, each acinus may be considered as a series of interconnected, but closed, bubbles forming a stable 'foam'. The bubble films are estimated to be thin enough to offer minimal resistance to gas diffusion, the normal mechanism by which gas movement occurs in a single pulmonary acinus (page 7).

More research is clearly needed to either confirm or refute these models.

Transmural Pressure Gradient and Intrathoracic Pressure

The transmural pressure gradient is the difference between intrathoracic (or 'intrapleural') and alveolar pressure. The

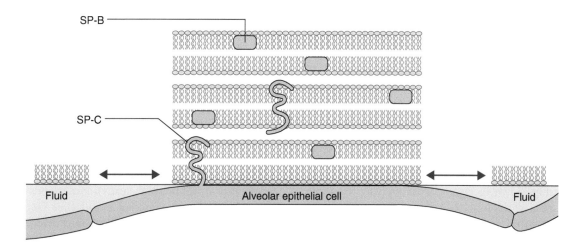

• **Fig. 2.2** Morphological model of alveolar surfactant. Multilayered, less wettable rafts of surfactant are interspersed with fluid pools. Surfactant proteins lie within (SP-B) or across (SP-C) the lipid bilayers, facilitating the formation and dispersion of the rafts with each breath to modify the surface forces within the alveolus. (From Webster NR, Galley HF. *Anaesthesia Science*. Oxford: Blackwell Publishing; 2006. With permission.)

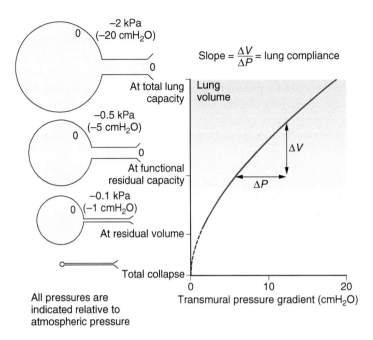

All pressures are indicated relative to atmospheric pressure

• **Fig. 2.3** Relationship between lung volume and the difference in pressure between the alveoli and the intrathoracic space (transmural pressure gradient). The relationship is almost linear over the normal tidal volume range. The calibre of small air passages decreases in parallel with alveolar volume. Airways begin to close at the closing capacity, and there is widespread airway closure at residual volume. Values in the diagram relate to the upright position and to *decreasing* pressure. The opening pressure of a closed alveolus is not shown.

pressure within an alveolus is always greater than the pressure in the surrounding interstitial tissue, except when the volume has been reduced to zero. By increasing lung volume, the transmural pressure gradient steadily increases, as shown for the whole lung in Figure 2.3. If an appreciable pneumothorax is present, the pressure gradient from alveolus to pleural cavity provides a measure of the overall transmural pressure gradient. Otherwise, the oesophageal pressure may be used to indicate the pleural pressure, but there are conceptual and technical difficulties. The technical difficulties are considered at the end of this chapter, whereas some of the conceptual difficulties are indicated in Figure 2.4.

The alveoli in the upper regions of the lung have a larger volume than those in the lower regions, except at total lung capacity. The greater degree of expansion of the alveoli in the upper part results in a greater transmural pressure gradient, which decreases steadily down the lung at approximately 0.1 kPa (or 1 cmH$_2$O) per 3 cm of vertical height; such a difference is indicated in Figure 2.4, *A*. Because the pleural cavity is normally empty, it is not strictly correct to speak of an intrapleural pressure; furthermore, it would not be constant throughout the pleural 'cavity'. One should think rather of the relationship shown in Figure 2.3 as applying to various horizontal strata of the lung, each with its own volume and therefore its own transmural pressure gradient on which its own intrapleural pressure would depend. The transmural pressure gradient has an important influence on many aspects of pulmonary function, so its horizontal stratification confers a regional difference on many features of pulmonary function, including airway closure and ventilation/perfusion

ratios, and therefore gas exchange. These matters are considered in detail in Chapters 3 and 7.

At first sight it might be thought that the subatmospheric intrapleural pressure would result in the accumulation of gas evolved from solution in blood and tissues. In fact the total of the partial pressures of gases dissolved in blood, and therefore tissues, is always less than 1 atm (see Table 25.2), and this factor keeps the pleural cavity free of gas.

Time Dependence of Pulmonary Elastic Behaviour

If an excised lung is rapidly inflated and then held at the new volume, the inflation pressure falls exponentially from its initial value to reach a lower level attained after a few seconds. This also occurs in the intact subject, and is readily observed during an inspiratory pause in a patient receiving artificial ventilation (page 25). It is broadly true to say that the volume change divided by the initial change in transmural pressure gradient corresponds to the dynamic compliance, whereas the volume change divided by the ultimate change in transmural pressure gradient (i.e., measured after it has become steady) corresponds to the static compliance. Static compliance will thus be greater than the dynamic compliance by an amount determined by the degree of time dependence in the elastic behaviour of a particular lung. The respiratory frequency has been shown to influence dynamic lung compliance in the normal subject, but frequency dependence is much more pronounced in the presence of lung disease.

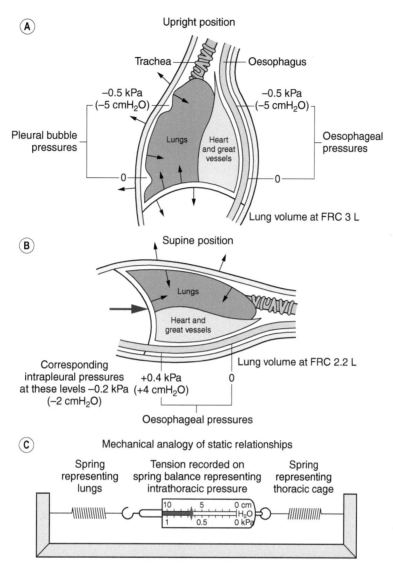

• **Fig. 2.4** Intrathoracic pressures: static relationships in the resting end-expiratory position. The lung volume corresponds to the functional residual capacity *(FRC)*. **(A)** and **(B)** indicate the pressure relative to ambient (atmospheric). Arrows show the direction of elastic forces. The heavy arrow in **(B)** indicates displacement by the abdominal viscera. **(C)** The tension in the two springs is the same and will be indicated on the spring balance. In the supine position: *1*, the FRC is reduced; *2*, the intrathoracic pressure is raised; *3*, the weight of the heart raises the oesophageal pressure above the intrapleural pressure.

Hysteresis

If the lungs are slowly inflated and then slowly deflated, the pressure/volume curve for static points during inflation differs from that obtained during deflation. The two curves form a loop, which becomes progressively broader as the tidal volume is increased (Fig. 2.5). Expressed in words, the loop in Figure 2.5 means that rather more than the expected pressure is required during inflation, and rather less than the expected recoil pressure is available during deflation. This resembles the behaviour of perished rubber or polyvinyl chloride, both of which are reluctant to accept deformation under stress but, once deformed, are again reluctant to assume their original shape. This phenomenon is present to a greater or lesser extent in all elastic bodies, and is known as elastic hysteresis.

Causes of Time Dependence of Pulmonary Elastic Behaviour

There are many possible explanations of the time dependence of pulmonary elastic behaviour, the relative importance of which may vary in different circumstances.

Changes in surfactant activity. It has been explained previously that the surface tension of the alveolar lining fluid is greater at larger lung volume and also during inspiration than at the same lung volume during expiration (Fig. 2.1, *B*). This is probably the most important cause of the observed hysteresis in the intact lung (Fig. 2.5).

Stress relaxation. If a spring is pulled out to a fixed increase in its length, the resultant tension is maximal at first and then declines exponentially to a constant value. This is

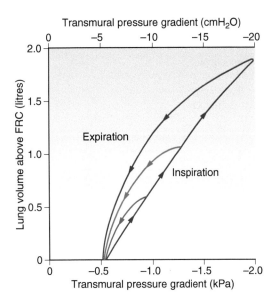

• **Fig. 2.5** Static plot of lung volume against transmural pressure gradient (intraoesophageal pressure relative to atmospheric at zero air flow). Note that inspiratory and expiratory curves form a loop that gets wider the greater the tidal volume. These loops are typical of elastic hysteresis. For a particular lung volume, the elastic recoil of the lung during expiration is always less than the distending transmural pressure gradient required during inspiration at the same lung volume.

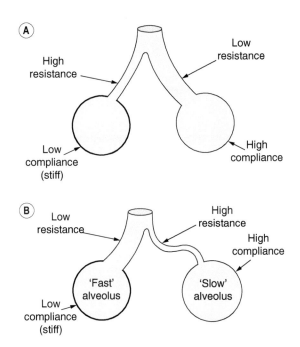

• **Fig. 2.6** Schematic diagrams of alveoli to illustrate conditions under which static and dynamic compliance may differ. **(A)** Represents a theoretically ideal state in which there is a reciprocal relationship between resistance and compliance resulting in gas flow being preferentially delivered to the most compliant regions, regardless of the state of inflation. Static and dynamic compliance are equal. This situation is probably never realized even in the normal subject. **(B)** Illustrates a state that is typical of many patients with respiratory disease. The alveoli can be conveniently be divided into fast and slow groups. The direct relationship between compliance and resistance results in inspired gas being preferentially delivered to the stiff alveoli if the rate of inflation is rapid. An end-inspiratory pause then permits redistribution from the fast alveoli to the slow alveoli.

an inherent property of elastic bodies, known as stress relaxation. Thoracic tissues display stress relaxation, and these 'viscoelastic' properties contribute significantly to the difference between static and dynamic compliance, as well as forming a component of pulmonary resistance (page 29). The crinkled structure of collagen in the lung (see Fig. 1.10) is likely to favour stress relaxation, and excised strips of human lung show stress relaxation when stretched.

Redistribution of gas. In a lung consisting of functional units with identical time constants* of inflation, the distribution of gas should be independent of the rate of inflation, and there should be no redistribution when the lungs are held inflated. However, if different parts of the lungs have different time constants, the distribution of inspired gas will be dependent on the rate of inflation, and redistribution (pendelluft) will occur when inflation is held. This problem is discussed in detail on page 90, but for the time being we can distinguish 'fast' and 'slow' alveoli (the term *alveoli* here refers to functional units rather than the anatomical entity). The fast alveolus has a low airway resistance and/or low compliance (or both), whereas the slow alveolus has a high airway resistance and/or a high compliance (Fig. 2.6, *B*). These properties mean that the fast alveolus has a shorter time constant

and is preferentially filled during a short inflation. This preferential filling of alveoli with low compliance gives an overall higher pulmonary transmural pressure gradient. A slow or sustained inflation permits increased distribution of gas to slow alveoli and tends to distribute gas in accord with the compliance of the different functional units. There should then be a lower overall transmural pressure and no redistribution of gas when inflation is held. The extreme difference between fast and slow alveoli shown in Figure 2.6, *B,* applies to diseased lungs, and no such difference exists in normal lungs. Gas redistribution is therefore unlikely to be a major factor in healthy subjects, but it can be important in patients with airways disease.

Recruitment of alveoli. Below a certain lung volume, some alveoli tend to close and only reopen at a greater lung volume and in response to a higher transmural pressure gradient than that at which they closed. Despite this need for higher pressure to open lung units, recruitment of alveoli is a plausible explanation for the time-dependent phenomena described earlier, and there is now some evidence that this does occur in healthy lungs at FRC.

---

*Time constants are used to describe the exponential filling and emptying of a lung unit. One time constant is the time taken to achieve 63% of maximal inflation or deflation of the lung unit. See Appendix E for details.

Factors Affecting Lung Compliance

Lung volume. It is important to remember that compliance is related to lung volume. This factor may be excluded by relating compliance to FRC to yield the specific compliance (i.e., compliance/FRC), which in humans is almost constant for both sexes and all ages down to neonates. The relationship between compliance and lung volume is true not only within an individual lung, but also between species. Larger animal species have thicker alveolar septa containing increased amounts of collagen and elastin, resulting in larger alveolar diameters, so reducing the pressure needed to expand them. An elephant therefore has larger alveoli and higher compliance than a mouse.

Posture. Lung volume, and therefore compliance, changes with posture (page 22). There are, however, problems in the measurement of intrapleural pressure in the supine position, and when this is considered it seems unlikely that changes of posture have any significant effect on the specific compliance.

Pulmonary blood volume. The pulmonary blood vessels probably make an appreciable contribution to the stiffness of the lung. Pulmonary venous congestion from whatever cause is associated with reduced compliance.

Age. There is a small increase in lung compliance with increasing age, believed to be caused by changes to the structure,[12] or microstructural distribution, of lung collagen and elastin.[13] Both of these changes will affect lung tissue elasticity, but the latter also leads to the enlargement of lung airspaces[13] and so reduces surface forces, mitigating the gradual loss of tissue elasticity.

Bronchial smooth muscle tone. Animal studies[14] have shown that an infusion of methacholine sufficient to result in a doubling of airway resistance decreases dynamic compliance by 50%. The airways might contribute to overall compliance or, alternatively, bronchoconstriction could enhance time dependence and reduce dynamic, but perhaps not static, compliance (Fig. 2.6). This interdependence between small airways and their surrounding alveoli also affects airway resistance (page 29).

Disease. Important changes in lung pressure–volume relationships are found in some lung diseases, and these are described in Part 3, Physiology of pulmonary disease.

Elastic Recoil of the Thoracic Cage

The thoracic cage comprises the ribcage and the diaphragm. Each is a muscular structure and can be considered as an elastic structure only when the muscles are relaxed, which is not easy to achieve except under the conditions of paralysis. Relaxation curves have been prepared relating pressure and volumes in the supposedly relaxed subject, but it is now doubted whether total relaxation was ever achieved. For example, in the supine position the diaphragm is not fully relaxed at the end of expiration but maintains a resting tone to prevent the abdominal contents from pushing the diaphragm cephalad.

Compliance of the thoracic cage is defined as change in lung volume per unit change in the pressure gradient between atmosphere and the intrapleural space. The units are the same as for pulmonary compliance. The measurement is seldom made but the value is of the order of 2 $L.kPa^{-1}$ (200 $mL.cmH_2O^{-1}$).

Factors Influencing Compliance of the Thoracic Cage

Anatomical factors include the ribs and the state of ossification of the costal cartilages, which explains the progressive reduction in chest wall compliance with increasing age. Obesity and even pathological skin conditions may also have an appreciable effect. In particular, scarring of the skin overlying the front of the chest, for example from burns, may impair breathing.

In terms of compliance, a relaxed diaphragm simply transmits pressure from the abdomen that may be increased in obesity (Chapter 15) and abdominal distension. Posture clearly has a major effect, and this is considered below in relation to FRC. Compared with the supine position, thoracic cage compliance is 30% greater in the seated subject, and the total static compliance of the respiratory system is reduced by 60% in the prone position because of the diminished elasticity of the ribcage and diaphragm when prone.

Pressure–Volume Relationships of the Lung Plus Thoracic Cage

Compliance is analogous to electrical capacitance, and in the respiratory system the compliance of lungs and thoracic cage are in series. Therefore the total compliance of the system obeys the same relationship as that for capacitances in series, in which reciprocals are added to obtain the reciprocal of the total value, thus

$$\frac{1}{\text{total compliance}} = \frac{1}{\text{lung compliance}} + \frac{1}{\text{thoracic cage compliance}}$$

typical static values ($L.kPa^{-1}$) for the supine paralysed patient are

$$\frac{1}{0.85} = \frac{1}{1.5} + \frac{1}{2}$$

Instead of compliance, we may consider its reciprocal, elastance. The relationship is then much simpler:

Total elastance =
lung elastance + thoracic cage elastance

The corresponding values ($kPa.L^{-1}$) are then

$$1.17 = 0.67 + 0.5$$

Relationship Between Alveolar, Intrathoracic and Ambient Pressures

At all times the alveolar/ambient pressure gradient is the sum of the alveolar/intrathoracic (or transmural) and intrathoracic/ambient pressure gradients. This relationship is independent of whether the patient is breathing spontaneously or being ventilated by intermittent positive pressure. Actual values depend on compliances, lung volume and posture, and typical values are shown for the upright, conscious relaxed subject in Figure 2.7. The values in the illustration are static and relate to conditions when no gas is flowing.

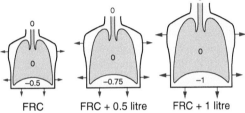

Spontaneous respiration

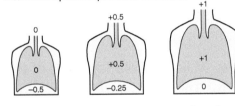

Intermittent positive-pressure ventilation

Figures denote pressure relative to atmosphere (kPa)

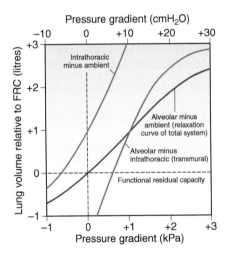

• **Fig. 2.7** Static pressure/volume relations for the intact thorax for the conscious subject in the upright position. The transmural pressure gradient bears the same relationship to lung volume during both intermittent positive pressure ventilation and spontaneous breathing. The intrathoracic-to-ambient pressure difference, however, differs in the two types of ventilation because of muscle action during spontaneous respiration. At all times: alveolar/ambient pressure difference = alveolar/intrathoracic pressure difference + intrathoracic/ambient pressure difference (due attention being paid to the sign of the pressure difference). *FRC*, Functional residual capacity.

Static Lung Volumes

Certain lung volumes, particularly the FRC, are determined by elastic forces. This is therefore a convenient point at which to consider the various static lung volumes and their subdivision (Fig. 2.8).

Total lung capacity (TLC). This is the volume of gas in the lungs at the end of a maximal inspiration. TLC is achieved when the maximal force generated by the inspiratory muscles is balanced by the forces opposing expansion. It is rather surprising that expiratory muscles are also contracting strongly at the end of a maximal inspiration.

Residual volume (RV). This is the volume remaining after a maximal expiration. In the young, RV is governed by the balance between the maximal force generated by expiratory muscles and the elastic forces opposing reduction of lung volume. However, in older subjects closure of small airways may prevent further expiration.

FRC. This is the lung volume at the end of a normal expiration.

Within the framework of TLC, RV and FRC, the other capacities and volumes shown in Figure 2.8 are self-explanatory. A 'capacity' usually refers to a measurement composed of more than one 'volume'.

Factors Affecting Static Lung Volumes

So many factors affect the FRC and other lung volumes that they require a special section of this chapter.

Body size. FRC and other lung volumes are linearly related to subject height.

Sex. For the same body height, females have an FRC about 10% less than males and a smaller forced vital capacity (FVC), the latter resulting from males having less body fat and a more muscular chest.

Age. FVC, FRC and RV all increase with age, but at different rates, with corresponding changes in the other lung volumes as shown in Figure 2.9. On average, FRC increases by around 16 mL per year.

Posture. Moving from the upright (seated) to the supine position leads to a significantly reduced FRC (see Fig. 15.2). The changes are caused by the increased pressure of the abdominal contents on the diaphragm in the supine position, displacing it in a cephalad direction and reducing thoracic volume. This is demonstrated in Figure 2.10 and Table 2.1 showing the influence of different degrees of body tilting and other body positions on FRC. Values of FRC in these figures and Table 2.1 are typical for a subject of 1.70 m height, and reported mean differences between supine and upright positions ranging from 500 to 1000 mL.

Obesity. The effect of obesity on lung volumes is described on page 200.

Ethnic group. Values for lung volumes vary between the different principal ethnic groups in the world, even after age and stature have been taken into account. Causes of these differences include geographic location, diet and levels of activity in childhood, all of which can influence

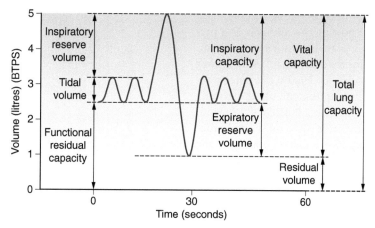

• **Fig. 2.8** Static lung volumes of Dr. Nunn in 1990. The 'spirometer curve' indicates the lung volumes that can be measured by simple spirometry. These are tidal volume, inspiratory reserve volume, inspiratory capacity, expiratory reserve volume and vital capacity. The residual volume, total lung capacity and functional residual capacity cannot be measured by observation of a spirometer without further elaboration of methods. *BTPS,* Body temperature and pressure, saturated.

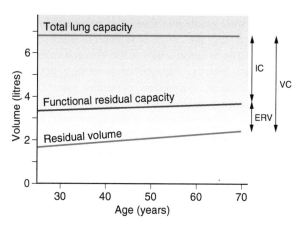

• **Fig. 2.9** Changes in static lung volumes with age. The largest change is in residual volume, the increase in which reduces both expiratory reserve volume and vital capacity whereas inspiratory capacity remains mostly unchanged. (After Janssens JP, Pache JC, Nicod LD. Physiological changes in respiratory function associated with ageing. *Eur Respir J.* 1999;13:197-205)

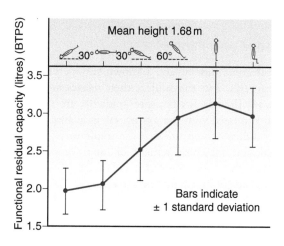

• **Fig. 2.10** Studies by Dr. Nunn and his co-workers of the functional residual capacity in various body positions. *BTPS,* Body temperature and pressure, saturated.

TABLE 2.1	Effect of Posture on Some Aspects of Respiratory Function		
Position	FRC (L) (BTPS)	Ribcage Breathing[a] (%)	Forced Expiratory Volume In 1 s (L) (BTPS)
Sitting	2.91	69.7	3.79
Supine	2.10	32.3	3.70
Supine (arms up)	2.36	33.0	3.27
Prone	2.45	32.6	3.49
Lateral	2.44	36.5	3.67

Data for 13 healthy males aged 24 to 64 years.
[a]Proportion of breathing accounted for by movement of the ribcage.
BTPS, Body temperature and pressure, saturated; *FRC,* functional residual capacity.
(From Lumb AB, Nunn JF. Respiratory function and ribcage contribution to ventilation in body positions commonly used during anesthesia. *Anesth Analg.* 1991;73:422-426.)

lung development. Increasing global migration and interbreeding between ethnic groups is now causing difficulties with interpretation of ethnicity as a component of normal lung volumes.[15]

All of the factors described so far must be taken into account when attempting to ascertain 'normal' values for lung volumes in an individual subject. For example, a predicted normal value for FRC in a Caucasian male aged between 25 to 65 years and in an upright posture may be calculated from:

$$FRC = (5.95 \times height) + (0.019 \times age)$$
$$- (0.086 \times BMI) - 5.3$$

where FRC is in litres, height in meters, age in years and body mass index (BMI) in $kg.m^{-2}$. This type of calculation is routinely performed when measuring lung volumes, and the most common way of reporting the results is as a percentage of predicted, that is, actual measured volume divided by calculated normal for the individual. The diagnosis of many respiratory diseases is dependent on this percentage result (Chapter 28); therefore agreement on the correct formula to use is critical. Extrapolating outside of the population used to develop the predictive equation is a real problem; for example, using an equation based on readings taken from Caucasian subjects aged 25 to 70 years to predict a normal value for a non-Caucasian subject aged 75 will give a misleading result. Furthermore, differences in the predictive equations used can lead to a large variation in the population prevalence of common respiratory diseases which depend on lung volumes for their diagnosis. Other methods of comparing lung volume results with the predicted 'normal' include[16]:

1. Comparison with lower limit of normal (LLN), which is the lower 5th percentile of the reference population, that is, the value below which 5% of that population lies. This is taken to indicate a clinically important abnormal result for diagnosis

2. The z-score is the number of standard deviations (SDs) away from the reference population mean that the individual's result lies. For example, $z = -1.72$ means the result is 1.72 times the SD below the reference population mean. This represents a better measure than percentage predicted of how abnormal the result is relative to the reference population. A z-score of -1.64 is the same as the LLN.

3. Spirometric lung age involves converting the actual results from an unhealthy patient into a hypothetical healthy patient with the same demographics, expressed as the hypothetical patient's age. In any patient with impaired lung volumes, the result is therefore an age greater than their own. 'Lung age' calculations are used mostly to motivate smokers to quit the habit, rather than as a statistically validated way of expressing results.[17]

Functional Residual Capacity in Relation to Closing Capacity

In Chapter 3 it is explained how reduction in lung volume below a certain level results in airway closure with relative or total underventilation in the dependent parts of the lung. The lung volume below which this effect becomes apparent is known as the closing capacity (CC). With increasing age, CC rises until it equals FRC at approximately 70 to 75 years in the upright position but only 44 in the supine position (Fig. 2.11). This is a major factor in the decrease of arterial Po_2 with age (page 148).

Principles of Measurement of Compliance

Compliance is measured as the change in lung volume divided by the corresponding change in the appropriate

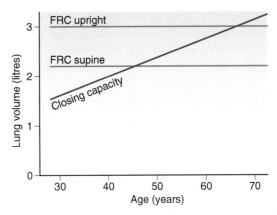

• **Fig. 2.11** Functional residual capacity *(FRC)* and closing capacity as a function of age. (From Leblanc P, Ruff F, Milic-Emili J. Effects of age and body position on 'airway closure' in man. *J Appl Physiol.* 1970; 28:448-453.)

pressure gradient, there being no gas flow when the two measurements are made. For lung compliance, the appropriate pressure gradient is alveolar/intrapleural (or intrathoracic), and for the total compliance, alveolar/ambient. Measurement of compliance of the thoracic cage is seldom undertaken, but the appropriate pressure gradient would then be intrapleural/ambient, measured when the respiratory muscles are totally relaxed.

Volume may be measured with a spirometer, with a body plethysmograph or by integration of a flow rate obtained from a pneumotachogram. Static pressures can be measured with a simple water manometer, but electrical transducers are now more common. Intrathoracic pressure is normally measured as oesophageal pressure which, in the upright subject, is different at different levels. The pressure rises as the balloon descends, and the change is roughly in accord with the specific gravity of the lung (0.3 g.mL^{-1}). It is conventional to measure the pressure 32 to 35 cm beyond the nares, the highest point at which the measurement is free from artefacts because of mouth pressure and tracheal and neck movements. Alveolar pressure equals mouth pressure when no gas is flowing: it cannot be measured directly.

Static Compliance

In the conscious subject, a known volume of air is inhaled from FRC, and the subject then relaxes against a closed airway. The various pressure gradients are then measured and compared with the resting values at FRC. It is, in fact, very difficult to ensure that the respiratory muscles are relaxed, but the measurement of lung compliance is valid because the static alveolar/intrathoracic pressure difference is unaffected by any muscle activity.

In the paralysed subject there are no difficulties with muscular relaxation, and it is very easy to measure static compliance of the whole respiratory system simply using recordings of airway pressure and respiratory volumes. However, because of the uncertainties about interpretation of the oesophageal pressure in the supine position (Fig. 2.4), there is usually some uncertainty about the pulmonary compliance. For static compliance it is therefore easier to measure *lung* compliance in the upright position and total compliance in the anaesthetized paralysed patient, who will usually be in the supine position.

Dynamic Compliance

These measurements are made during rhythmic breathing, but compliance is calculated from pressure and volume measurements made when no gas is flowing, usually at end-inspiratory and end-expiratory 'no-flow' points. The usual method involves creation of a pressure–volume loop by displaying simultaneously as *x*- and *y*-coordinates the required pressure gradient and the respired volume. In the resultant loop, as in Figure 2.12, *A*, the no-flow points are

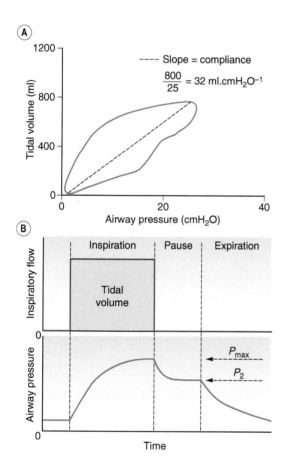

• **Fig. 2.12** Automated measurement of compliance during intermittent positive pressure ventilation. **(A)** Dynamic compliance. Simultaneous measurement of tidal volume and airway pressure creates a pressure–volume loop. End-expiratory and end-inspiratory no-flow points occur when the trace is horizontal. At this point, airway pressure and alveolar pressure are equal, so the pressure gradient is the difference between alveolar and atmospheric pressure. Total respiratory system compliance is therefore the slope of the line between these points. Note that in this patient compliance is markedly reduced. **(B)** Static compliance. Following an end-inspiratory pause, the plateau pressure is recorded (P_2), and along with tidal volume the static compliance easily derived. This manoeuvre also provides an assessment of respiratory system resistance by recording the pressure drop ($P_{max} - P_2$) and the inspiratory flow immediately before the inspiratory pause (see page 39).

where the trace is horizontal and the dynamic compliance is the slope of the line joining these points.

Automated Measurement of Compliance

In a spontaneously breathing awake patient, lung compliance measurement is difficult because of the requirement to place an oesophageal balloon. However, in anaesthetized patients or those patients receiving intermittent positive pressure ventilation (IPPV) in intensive care, the measurement of compliance is considerably easier. Many ventilators and anaesthetic monitoring systems now routinely measure airway pressure and tidal volume. This enables a pressure–volume loop to be displayed (Fig. 2.12, *A*), from which the dynamic compliance of the respiratory system may be calculated on a continuous breath-by-breath basis. When no gas is flowing during IPPV (at the end of inspiration and expiration), the airway pressure equals alveolar pressure. At this point, the airway pressure recorded by the ventilator therefore equals the difference between alveolar and atmospheric pressure, allowing derivation of the total compliance.

Some ventilators will also measure static compliance. The ventilator will inflate the lung with the patient's usual tidal volume and then pause at end-inspiration for between 0.5 and 2 s, until the airway pressure falls to a plateau lasting 300 ms (Fig. 2.12, *B*). Static compliance is then calculated from the volume delivered and pressure recorded during the plateau and may be easily compared with dynamic compliance.

Principles of Measurement of Static Lung Volumes

Vital capacity, tidal volume, inspiratory reserve and expiratory reserve can all be measured with a simple spirometer (Fig. 2.8). Total lung capacity, FRC and RV all contain a fraction (the RV) that cannot be measured by simple spirometry. However, if one of these volumes is measured (most commonly the FRC), the others may easily be derived.

Measurement of Functional Residual Capacity

Three techniques are available. The first uses nitrogen washout by breathing 100% oxygen. The total quantity of nitrogen eliminated is measured as the product of the expired volume collected and the concentration of nitrogen. If, for example, 4 L of nitrogen are collected and the initial alveolar nitrogen concentration was 80%, then the initial lung volume was 5 L.

The second method uses the wash-in of a tracer gas such as helium. If, for example, 50 mL of helium is introduced into the lungs and the helium concentration is then found to be 1%, the lung volume is 5 L. Helium is used for this method because of its low solubility in blood. For the technique to be accurate, the measurement must be made rapidly, or helium dissolving in the tissues and blood will introduce errors.

The third method uses the body plethysmograph. The subject is totally contained within a gas-tight box and attempts to breathe against an occluded airway. Changes in alveolar pressure are recorded at the mouth and compared with the small changes in lung volume, derived from pressure changes within the plethysmograph. Application of Boyle's law then permits calculation of lung volume.

The last method is the only technique for FRC measurement that includes gas trapped within the lung distal to closed airways.

References

1. Faffe DS, Zin WA. Lung parenchymal mechanics in health and disease. *Physiol Rev.* 2009;89:759-775.
*2. **Whitsett JA, Weaver TE. Hydrophobic surfactant proteins in lung function and disease. *N Engl J Med.* 2002;347:2141-2148.**
3. Weaver TE, Conkright JJ. Functions of surfactant proteins B and C. *Annu Rev Physiol.* 2001;63:555-578.
4. van Moorsel CHM, van Oosterhout MFM, Barlo NP, et al. Surfactant protein C mutations are the basis of a significant portion of adult familial pulmonary fibrosis in a Dutch cohort. *Am J Respir Crit Care Med.* 2010;182:1419-1425.
5. Hawgood S, Poulain FR. The pulmonary collectins and surfactant metabolism. *Annu Rev Physiol.* 2001;63:495-519.
*6. **Zuo YY, Possmayer F. How does pulmonary surfactant reduce surface tension to very low values? *J Appl Physiol.* 2007;102:1733-1734.**
7. Janssen WJ, McPhillips KA, Dickinson MG, et al. Surfactant proteins A and D suppress alveolar macrophage phagocytosis via interaction with SIRPa. *Am J Respir Crit Care Med.* 2008; 178:158-167.
8. To KKW, Zhou J, Song Y-Q, et al. Surfactant protein B gene polymorphism is associated with severe influenza. *Chest.* 2014; 145:1237-1243.
*9. **Scarpelli EM, Hills BA. Opposing views on the alveolar surface, alveolar models, and the role of surfactant. *J Appl Physiol.* 2000;89:408-412.**
10. Hills BA. An alternative view of the role(s) of surfactant and the alveolar model. *J Appl Physiol.* 1999;87:1567-1583.
11. Scarpelli EM. The alveolar surface network: a new anatomy and its physiological significance. *Anat Rec.* 1998;251:491-527.
12. Janssens JP, Pache JC, Nicod LD. Physiological changes in respiratory function associated with ageing. *Eur Respir J.* 1999; 13:197-205.
13. Subramaniam K, Kumar H, Tawhai MH. Evidence for age-dependent air-space enlargement contributing to loss of lung tissue elastic recoil pressure and increased shear modulus in older age. *J Appl Physiol.* 2017;123:79-87.
14. Mitzner W, Blosser S, Yager D, et al. Effect of bronchial smooth muscle contraction on lung compliance. *J Appl Physiol.* 1992; 72:158-167.
15. Galanter JM. Bringing lung function prediction equations to diverse populations. *Am J Respir Crit Care Med.* 2017;196: 942-944.
16. Ntima N, Lumb AB. Pulmonary function tests in anaesthetic practice. *Br J Anaesth Educ.* 2019;19:206-211.
17. Khelifa MB, Salem HB, Sfaxi R. "Spirometric" lung age reference equations: A narrative review. *Respir Physiol Neurobiol.* 2018;247:31-42.

3

Respiratory System Resistance

KEY POINTS

- Gas flow in the airway is a mixture of laminar and turbulent flow, becoming more laminar in smaller airways.
- Respiratory system resistance is a combination of resistance to gas flow in the airways and resistance to deformation of tissues of both the lung and chest wall.

- In smaller airways smooth muscle controls airway diameter under the influence of neural, humoral and cellular mechanisms.
- The respiratory system can rapidly compensate for increases in either inspiratory or expiratory resistance.

Elastic resistance, which occurs when no gas is flowing, results from only two of the numerous causes of impedance to inflation of the lung (listed in Chapter 2). This chapter considers the remaining components, which together are referred to as nonelastic resistance or respiratory system resistance. Most nonelastic resistance is provided by frictional resistance to air flow and thoracic tissue deformation (both lung and chest wall), with small contributions from the inertia of gas and tissue and compression of intrathoracic gas. Unlike elastic resistance, work performed against nonelastic resistance is not stored as potential energy (and therefore recoverable), but is lost and dissipated as heat.

Physical Principles of Gas Flow and Resistance

Gas flows from a region of high pressure to one of lower pressure. The rate at which it does so is a function of the pressure difference and the resistance to gas flow, analogous to the flow of an electrical current (Fig. 3.1). The precise relationship between pressure difference and flow rate depends on the nature of the flow, which may be laminar, turbulent or a mixture of the two. It is useful to consider laminar and turbulent flow as two separate entities, but mixed patterns of flow usually occur in the respiratory tract. With a number of important caveats, similar basic considerations apply to the flow of liquids through tubes, which is considered in Chapter 6.

Laminar Flow

With laminar flow, gas flows along a straight unbranched tube as a series of concentric cylinders that slide over one another, with the peripheral cylinder stationary and the

central cylinder moving fastest, the advancing cone forming a parabola (Fig. 3.2, *A*).

The advancing cone front means that some fresh gas will reach the end of a tube, but the volume entering the tube is still less than the volume of the tube. In the context of the respiratory tract, there may be significant alveolar ventilation when the tidal volume is less than the volume of the airways (the anatomical dead space), a fact that is very relevant to high-frequency ventilation (page 384). For the same reason, laminar flow is relatively inefficient for purging the contents of a tube.

In theory, gas adjacent to the tube wall is stationary, so friction between fluid and the tube wall is negligible. The physical characteristics of the airway or vessel wall should therefore not affect resistance to laminar flow. Similarly, the composition of gas sampled from the periphery of a tube during laminar flow may not be representative of the gas advancing down the centre of the tube. To complicate matters further, laminar flow requires a critical length of tubing before the characteristic advancing cone pattern can be established. This is known as the entrance length and is related to the diameter of the tube and the Reynolds number of the fluid (see later).

Quantitative Relationships

With laminar flow, the gas flow rate is directly proportional to the pressure gradient along the tube (Fig. 3.2, *B*); the constant is thus defined as resistance to gas flow:

$$\Delta P = \text{flow rate} \times \text{resistance}$$

where ΔP = pressure gradient.

In a straight unbranched tube, the Hagen–Poiseuille equation allows gas flow to be quantified

$$\text{Flowrate} = \frac{\Delta P \times \pi \times (\text{radius})^4}{8 \times \text{length} \times \text{viscosity}}$$

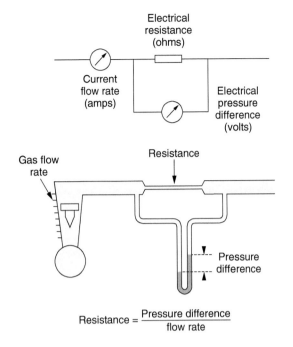

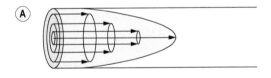

$$\text{Resistance} = \frac{\text{Pressure difference}}{\text{flow rate}}$$

• **Fig. 3.1** Electrical analogy of gas flow. Resistance is pressure difference per unit flow rate. Resistance to gas flow is analogous to electrical resistance (provided that flow is laminar). Gas flow corresponds to electrical current (amps), gas pressure to potential difference (volts), gas flow resistance to electrical resistance (ohms), and Poiseuille's law corresponds to Ohm's law.

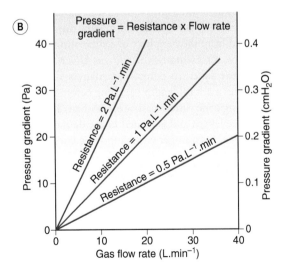

• **Fig. 3.2** Laminar flow. **(A)** In laminar flow gas moves along a straight tube as a series of concentric cylinders of gas with the central cylinder moving fastest and the outside cylinder theoretically stationary. This gives rise to a 'cone front' of gas velocity across the tube. **(B)** The linear relationship between gas flow rate and pressure gradient. The slope of the lines indicates the resistance (1 Pa = 0.01 cmH$_2$O).

by combining these two equations:

$$\text{Resistance} = \frac{8 \times \text{length} \times \text{viscosity}}{\pi \times (\text{radius})^4}$$

In this equation, the fourth power of the radius of the tube explains the critical importance of narrowing of air passages. With constant tube dimensions, viscosity is the only property of a gas relevant under conditions of laminar flow. Helium has a low density but a viscosity close to that of air; therefore it will not improve gas flow if the flow is laminar (page 29).

In the Hagen–Poiseuille equation, the units must be coherent. In CGS units (see Appendix A), dyn.cm^{-2} (pressure), mL.s^{-1} (flow) and cm (length and radius) are compatible with the unit of poise for viscosity (dyn.s.cm^{-2}). In SI units, with pressure in kilopascals, the unit of viscosity is newton.s.m^{-2}. However, in practice it is still customary to express gas pressure in cmH$_2$O and flow in L.s^{-1}. Resistance therefore continues to usually be expressed as cmH$_2$O per litre per second (cmH$_2$O.L^{-1}.s).

Turbulent Flow

High flow rates, particularly through branched or irregular tubes, result in a breakdown of the orderly flow of gas described earlier. An irregular movement is superimposed on the general progression along the tube (Fig. 3.3, *A*), with a square front replacing the cone front of laminar flow. Turbulent flow is almost invariably present when high resistance to gas flow is a problem.

The square front means that no fresh gas can reach the end of a tube until the amount of gas entering the tube is almost equal to the volume of the tube. Turbulent flow is more effective than laminar flow in purging the contents of a tube, and also provides the best conditions for drawing a representative sample of gas from the periphery of a tube. Frictional forces between the tube wall and fluid become more important in turbulent flow.

Quantitative Relationships

The relationship between driving pressure and flow rate differs from the relationship described earlier for laminar flow in three important respects:

1. The driving pressure is proportional to the square of the gas flow rate.
2. The driving pressure is proportional to the density of the gas and is independent of its viscosity.
3. The required driving pressure is, in theory, inversely proportional to the fifth power of the radius of the tube (Fanning equation).

The square law relating driving pressure and flow rate is shown in Figure 3.3, *B*. Resistance, defined as pressure gradient divided by flow rate, is not constant as in laminar flow, but increases in proportion to the flow rate. Units such as cmH$_2$O.L^{-1}.s should therefore be used only when flow is entirely laminar. The following methods of quantification of

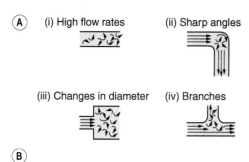

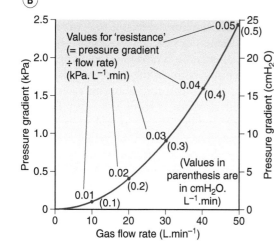

• **Fig. 3.3** Turbulent flow. **(A)** Four circumstances under which gas flow tends to be turbulent. **(B)** The square law relationship between gas flow rate and pressure gradient when flow is turbulent. Note that the value for 'resistance,' calculated as for laminar flow, is quite meaningless during turbulent flow.

'resistance' may be used when flow is totally or partially turbulent.

Two constants. This method considers resistance as comprising two components, one for laminar flow and one for turbulent flow. The simple relationship for laminar flow given previously would then be extended as follows:

$$\text{Pressure gradient} = k_1(\text{flow}) + k_2(\text{flow})^2$$

where k_1 contains the factors of the Hagen–Poiseuille equation and represents the laminar flow component, and k_2 includes factors in the corresponding equation for turbulent flow.

The exponent n. Over a surprisingly wide range of flow rates, the previous equation may be condensed into the following single-term expression with little loss of precision:

$$\text{Pressure gradient} = K(\text{flow})^n$$

where n has a value ranging from 1 with purely laminar flow to 2 with purely turbulent flow; the value of n being a useful indication of the nature of the flow. The constants for the normal human respiratory tract are

$$\text{Pressure gradient (kPa)} = 0.24(\text{flow})^{1.3}$$

TABLE 3.1	**Physical Properties of Clinically Used Gas Mixtures Relating to Gas Flow**		
	Viscosity Relative to Air	Density Relative to Air	Density Viscosity
Oxygen	1.11	1.11	1.00
70% N_2O/30% O_2	0.89	1.41	1.59
80% He/20% O_2	1.08	0.33	0.31

The graphical method. It is often convenient to represent 'resistance' as a graph of pressure difference against gas flow rate, on either linear or logarithmic coordinates. Logarithmic coordinates have the advantage that the plot is usually a straight line whether flow is laminar, turbulent or mixed, and the slope of the line indicates the value of n in the equation above.

Reynolds Number

For long, straight unbranched tubes, the nature of the gas flow may be predicted from the value of the Reynolds number, which is a nondimensional quantity derived from the following expression:

$$\frac{\text{Linear gas velocity} \times \text{tube diameter} \times \text{gas density}}{\text{Gas viscosity}}$$

The property of the gas that affects the Reynolds number is the ratio of density to viscosity. When the Reynolds number is less than 2000, flow is predominantly laminar, whereas at a value greater than 4000, flow is mainly turbulent. Between these values, both types of flow coexist. The Reynolds number also affects the entrance length (i.e., the distance required for laminar flow to become established), which is derived from:

$$\text{Entrance length} = 0.03 \times \text{tube diameter} \times \text{Reynolds number}$$

Thus, for gases with a low Reynolds number, not only will resistance be less during turbulent flow, but laminar flow will become established more quickly after bifurcations, corners and obstructions.

Values for some gas mixtures that a patient may inhale are shown relative to air in Table 3.1. Viscosities of respirable gases do not differ greatly, but there may be very large differences in density.

Respiratory System Resistance

Airway Resistance

This results from frictional resistance in the airways. In the healthy subject, the small airways make only a small contribution to total airway resistance, because their aggregate cross-sectional area increases to very large values after about the eighth generation (see Fig. 1.5). Overall airway resistance is therefore dominated by the resistance of the larger airways.

Gas flow along pulmonary airways is complex compared with the theoretical tubes described earlier and consists of a variable mixture of both laminar and turbulent flow. Both the velocity of gas flow and airway diameter (and therefore Reynolds number) decrease in successive airway generations from a maximum in the trachea to almost zero at the start of the pulmonary acinus (generation 15). In addition, there are frequent divisions with variable lengths of approximately straight airway between. Finally, in large-diameter airways the entrance length is normally greater than the length of the individual airway. As a result of these purely physical factors, laminar flow cannot become established until approximately the 11th airway generation. Predominantly turbulent flow in the conducting airways has two practical implications. First, the physical characteristics of the airway lining will influence frictional resistance more with turbulent than with laminar flow, so changes in airway lining fluid consistency (page 165) will have a significant effect. Second, gas mixtures containing helium (low Reynolds number) are more beneficial in overcoming increased resistance in large airways and of less benefit in small airway disease such as asthma.

Tissue Resistance

In 1955 a component of the work of breathing was attributed to the resistance caused by tissue deformation, and some years later this was measured in anaesthetized and paralysed subjects and termed the viscoelastic or 'tissue' component of respiratory resistance. Figure 3.4 shows the 'spring and dashpot' model, first described by D'Angelo et al.,[1] to illustrate tissue resistance. Dashpots here represent resistance and springs elastance (reciprocal of compliance). Upward movement of the upper bar represents an increase in lung volume, caused by contraction of the inspiratory muscles or the application of inflation pressure as shown in the diagram. There is good evidence that, in humans, the left-hand dashpot represents predominantly airway resistance. The spring in the middle represents the static elastance of the respiratory system. On the right there is a spring and dashpot arranged in series. With a rapid change in lung volume, the spring is extended, while the piston more slowly rises in the dashpot. In due course (2–3 seconds) the spring returns to its original length and so ceases to exert any influence on pressure/volume relationships. This spring therefore represents the time-dependent element of elastance. While it is still under tension at end-inspiration, the combined effect of the two springs results in a high elastance, of which the reciprocal is the dynamic compliance. If inflation is held for a few seconds and movement of the piston through the right-hand dashpot is completed, the right-hand spring ceases to exert any tension, and the total elastance is reduced to that caused by the spring in the middle. The reciprocal of this elastance is the static compliance, which is therefore greater than the dynamic compliance. The system shown in Figure 3.4 is only a simplified scheme to which many further components could be added; nevertheless the model accords well with experimental findings.

The time-dependent change in compliance represented by the spring and dashpot in series could be as a result of many factors. Redistribution of gas makes only a negligible contribution in a healthy human; the major component is because of viscoelastic flow resistance in tissue. In anaesthetized healthy subjects, tissue resistance is of the order of half of the respiratory system resistance, and seems to be largely unaffected by end-expiratory pressure or tidal volume.[1] Tissue resistance originates from both lung and chest wall tissues, with a significant proportion originating in the chest wall.[1,2] The magnitude and importance of this component, particularly in lung disease, is often underestimated, and it is clearly important to distinguish airway resistance from that afforded by the total respiratory system. Separate measurement of tissue resistance is described in the following section.

Inertance as a Component of Respiratory System Resistance

Respired gases, the lungs and the thoracic cage all have appreciable mass, and therefore inertia, which must offer an impedance to change in direction of gas flow, analogous to electrical inductance. This component, termed inertance, is extremely difficult to measure, but inductance and inertance offer an impedance that increases with frequency. Therefore, although inertance is generally believed to be negligible at normal respiratory frequencies, it may become appreciable during high-frequency ventilation (Chapter 32).

Factors Affecting Respiratory Resistance

In normal lungs respiratory resistance is controlled by changes in airway diameter mainly in small airways and bronchioles. This would be expected to alter only the airway component of respiratory resistance, but animal studies

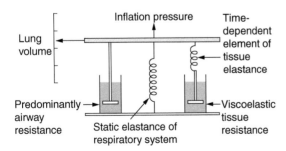

• **Fig. 3.4** The spring and dashpot model of D'Angelo et al.[1] Inflation of the lungs is represented by the bar moving upwards. The springs represent elastance (reciprocal of compliance), and the dashpots represent resistance. The spring and dashpot in series on the right confers time dependence, which is because of viscoelastic tissue resistance.

suggest that contraction of bronchial smooth muscle also causes changes in tissue resistance. Interdependence between the airway and parenchymal components of lung tissue is believed to occur such that airway constriction distorts the surrounding elastic tissue sufficiently to alter its viscoelastic properties.[3] Airway calibre may be reduced by either physical compression (because of a reversal of the normal transluminal pressure leading to airway collapse) or by contraction of the smooth muscle in the airway wall.

Volume-Related Airway Collapse

Effect of Lung Volume on Resistance to Breathing

When lung volume is reduced, there is a proportional reduction in the volume of all air-containing components, including the air passages. Thus if other factors (such as bronchomotor tone) remain constant, airway resistance is an inverse function of lung volume (Fig. 3.5), and there is a direct relationship between lung volume and the maximum expiratory flow rate that can be attained (see later). Quantifying airway diameter is difficult from these curves. It is therefore more convenient to refer to conductance, which is the reciprocal of resistance and is usually expressed as litres per second per cmH2O. Specific airway conductance (sG_{aw}) is the airway conductance relative to lung volume, or the gradient of the line showing conductance as a function of lung volume (Fig. 3.5). Because it takes into account the important effect of lung volume on airway resistance, it is a useful index of bronchomotor tone.

Gas Trapping

At low lung volumes, flow-related airway collapse (see later) occurs more readily, because airway calibre and the transmural pressure are less. Expiratory airway collapse gives rise to a 'valve' effect, and gas becomes trapped distal to the collapsed airway, leading to an increase in residual volume (RV) and functional residual capacity (FRC). Thus in general, increasing lung volume reduces airway resistance and helps to prevent gas trapping. This is most conveniently achieved by the application of continuous positive airway pressure to the spontaneously breathing subject, or positive end-expiratory pressure (PEEP) to the paralysed ventilated patient (Chapter 32). Many patients with obstructive airways disease acquire the habit of increasing their expiratory resistance by exhaling through pursed lips. Alternatively, premature termination of expiration keeps the lung volume above FRC (intrinsic PEEP, page 386). Both manoeuvres have the effect of enhancing airway transmural pressure gradient, thus reducing airway resistance and preventing gas trapping.

Closing Capacity[4,5]

In addition to the overall effect on airway resistance shown in Figure 3.5, there are important regional differences. This is because the airways and alveoli in the dependent parts of the lungs are always smaller than those at the top of the lung, except at total lung capacity or at zero gravity when all are the same size. As the lung volume is reduced towards RV, there is a point at which dependent airways begin to close, and the lung volume at which this occurs is known as the closing capacity (CC). The alternative term, closing volume, equals the CC minus the RV (Fig. 3.6). CC increases linearly with age, and is less than FRC in young adults but increases to become equal to FRC at a mean age of 44 years in the supine position and 75 years in the upright position (see Fig. 2.11).

When the FRC is less than the CC, some of the pulmonary blood flow will be distributed to alveoli with closed airways, usually in the dependent parts of the lungs. This will constitute a shunt (page 100), and must increase the alveolar/arterial Po_2 gradient. This can be seen when volunteers breathe below their FRC, and is particularly marked in older subjects who have a greater CC. Shunting of blood through areas of the lung with closed airways is an

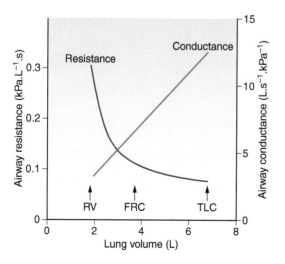

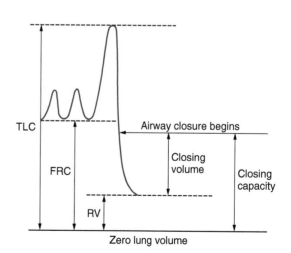

• **Fig. 3.5** Airway resistance and conductance as a function of lung volume (upright posture). The resistance curve is a hyperbola. Specific conductance (sG_{aw}) is the gradient of the conductance line. *FRC*, Functional residual capacity; *RV*, residual volume; *TLC*, total lung capacity.

• **Fig. 3.6** Spirogram to illustrate the relationship between closing volume and closing capacity. This example would be in a young adult with closing capacity less than functional residual capacity (*FRC*). *RV*, Residual volume; *TLC*, total lung capacity.

important cause of decreasing arterial Po_2 with increasing age (page 148) and changes of position (page 250).

Flow-Related Airway Collapse

All the airways can be compressed by reversal of the normal transmural pressure gradient to a sufficiently high level. The cartilaginous airways have considerable structural resistance to collapse, but even the trachea may be compressed with an external pressure in the range of 5 to 7 kPa (50–70 cmH₂O) or when the gas velocity through it becomes suitably high.[6] Airways beyond generation 11 have no structural rigidity (see Table 1.1), and rely instead on the traction on their walls from elastic recoil of the lung tissue in which they are embedded. They can be collapsed by a reversed transmural pressure gradient that is considerably less than that which closes the cartilaginous airways.

Reversal of the transmural pressure gradient may be caused by high levels of air flow during expiration. During all phases of normal breathing, the pressure in the lumen of the air passages should always remain well above the subatmospheric pressure in the thorax, so the airways remain patent. During a maximal forced expiration, the intrathoracic pressure rises to well above atmospheric, resulting in high gas flow rates. Pressure drops as gas flows along the airways, and there will be a point at which airway pressure equals the intrathoracic pressure. At that point (the equal pressure point) the smaller air passages are held open only by the elastic recoil of the lung parenchyma in which they are embedded or, if it occurs in the larger airways, by their structural rigidity. Downstream of the equal pressure point, the transmural pressure gradient is reversed and at some point may overcome the forces holding the airways open, resulting in airway collapse. This effect is also influenced by lung volume (see earlier), and the equal pressure point moves progressively down towards the smaller airways as lung volume is decreased.

Flow-related collapse is best demonstrated on a flow/volume plot. Figure 3.7 shows the normal relationship

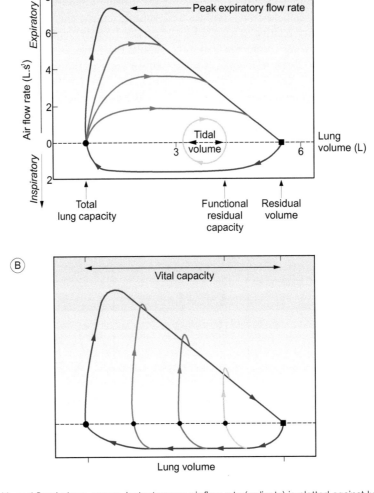

• **Fig. 3.7** Normal flow/volume curves. Instantaneous air flow rate (ordinate) is plotted against lung volume (abscissa). **(A)** The normal tidal excursion is shown as the small loop. In addition, expiration from total lung capacity at four levels of expiratory effort is shown. Within limits, peak expiratory flow rate is dependent on effort but, during the latter part of expiration, all curves converge on an effort-independent section where flow rate is limited by airway collapse. **(B)** The effect of forced expirations from different lung volumes. The pips above the effort-independent section probably represent air expelled from collapsed airways.

between lung volume on the abscissa and instantaneous respiratory flow rate on the ordinate. Time is not directly indicated. In Figure 3.7, *A,* the small loop shows a normal tidal excursion above FRC and with an air flow rate at either side of zero. Arrows show the direction of the trace. At the end of a maximal expiration, the black square indicates RV. The lower part of the large curve then shows the course of a maximal inspiration to total lung capacity (TLC; *black circle*). There follow four expiratory curves, each with different expiratory effort and each attaining a different peak expiratory flow rate. Within limits, the greater the effort, the greater is the resultant peak flow rate. However, all the expiratory curves terminate in a final common pathway, which is independent of effort. In this part of the curves, the flow rate is limited by airway collapse, and the maximal air flow rate is governed by the lung volume (abscissa).

The greater the effort the greater is the degree of airway collapse, and the resultant gas flow rate remains the same. Figure 3.7, *B,* shows the importance of a maximal inspiration before measurement of peak expiratory flow rate. With lung disease, flow-volume loops can help determine where airway obstruction is occurring; some examples are shown in Figure 3.8.

Muscular Control of Airway Diameter

Small airways are the site of most of the important causes of obstruction in a range of pathological conditions described in Chapter 28. Four pathways are involved in controlling muscle tone in small bronchi and bronchioles:
1. Neural pathways
2. Humoral (via blood) control

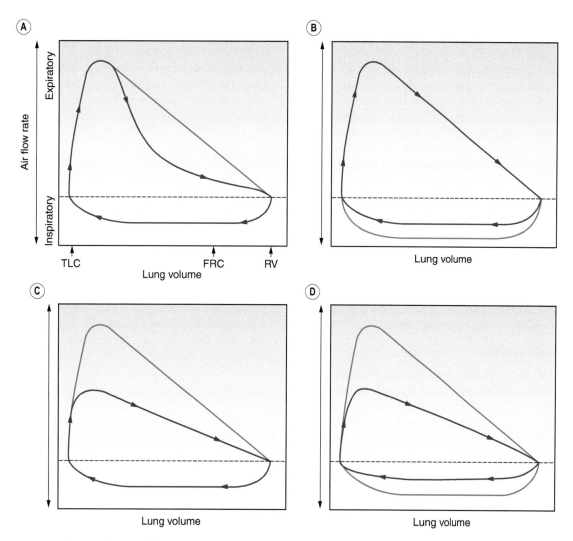

• **Fig. 3.8** Abnormal flow/volume curves. In each case, the normal loop (Fig. 3.7) is shown in blue. **(A)** Small airway obstructive disease such as chronic obstructive pulmonary disease with a concave expiratory phase because of early closure of small airways. **(B)** Variable extrathoracic obstruction with a flattened inspiratory phase and normal expiratory loop. **(C)** Variable intrathoracic obstruction in which the inspiratory phase is normal, but flow limitation occurs early in expiration. **(D)** Fixed large airway obstruction, either intrathoracic or extrathoracic, causes flow limitation in both phases of respiration. *FRC,* Functional residual capacity; *RV,* residual volume; *TLC,* total lung capacity.

3. Direct physical and chemical effects
4. Local cellular mechanisms

These may conveniently be considered as discrete mechanisms, but in practice there is considerable interaction between them, particularly in disease. Neural control is the most important in the normal lung, with direct stimulation and humoral control contributing under some circumstances. Cellular mechanisms, particularly mast cells, have little influence under normal conditions, but are important in airway disease.

Neural Pathways[7]

Parasympathetic System[8]

This system is of major importance in the control of bronchomotor tone and, when activated, the reflex can completely obliterate the lumen of small airways. Both afferent and efferent fibres travel in the vagus nerve with efferent ganglia in the walls of small bronchi. Afferents arise from receptors under the tight junctions of the bronchial epithelium and respond to noxious stimuli acting directly on the receptors (vagal C-fibres), to stimulation of rapidly adapting receptors (page 47) or to cytokines released by cellular mechanisms such as mast cell degranulation. Efferent nerves release acetylcholine (ACh), which acts at M_3 muscarinic receptors to cause contraction of bronchial smooth muscle, while also stimulating M_2 prejunctional muscarinic receptors to exert negative feedback on ACh release. A complex series of second messengers is involved in bringing about smooth muscle contraction in response to ACh (see later). Stimulation of any part of the reflex arc results in bronchoconstriction. Some degree of resting tone is normally present,[7,8] and therefore may permit some degree of bronchodilation when vagal tone is reduced in a similar fashion to vagal control of heart rate. The reflex is not a simple monosynaptic reflex, because there is considerable central nervous system modulation of the response, which offers a potential role for the brain in controlling the degree of airway hyper-responsiveness in lung disease.[9]

Sympathetic System

In contrast to the parasympathetic system, the sympathetic system is poorly represented in the lung and not yet proven to be of major importance in humans. Indeed, it appears unlikely that there is any direct sympathetic innervation of the airway smooth muscle, although there may be an inhibitory effect on cholinergic neurotransmission in some species.

Noncholinergic Parasympathetic Nerves[7]

Airways are provided with a third autonomic control which is neither adrenergic nor cholinergic. This is the only potential bronchodilator nervous pathway in humans, although the exact role of these nerves in humans remains uncertain. The efferent fibres run in the vagus nerve and pass to the smooth muscle of the airway, where they cause slow (several minutes) and prolonged relaxation of bronchi. The neurotransmitter is vasoactive intestinal peptide (VIP), which produces airway smooth muscle relaxation by promoting the production of nitric oxide (NO). How NO brings about smooth muscle relaxation in the airway is not as fully understood as its effect on vascular smooth muscle. It seems likely that NO has its effect without having to cross the cell membrane as a result of some form of cell-surface interaction that produces activation of guanylate cyclase to produce cyclic guanosine monophosphate and muscle relaxation. Resting airway tone does involve bronchodilation by NO, but whether this is from local cellular production of NO or noncholinergic parasympathetic nerves and VIP-mediated release of NO is unknown.

Humoral Control

Despite the minimal significance of sympathetic innervation, bronchial smooth muscle has plentiful β_2-adrenergic receptors, which are highly sensitive to circulating adrenaline, and once again act via complex second messenger systems described later. Basal levels of adrenaline probably do not contribute to bronchial muscle tone, but this mechanism is brought into play during exercise or during the sympathetic 'stress response'. There are a few α-adrenergic receptors which cause bronchoconstriction but are unlikely to be of clinical significance.

Physical and Chemical Effects

Direct stimulation of the respiratory epithelium activates the parasympathetic reflex, as previously described, causing bronchoconstriction. Physical factors known to produce bronchoconstriction include mechanical stimulation of the upper air passages by laryngoscopy and the presence of foreign bodies in the trachea or bronchi. Inhalation of particulate matter, an aerosol of water or just cold air may cause bronchoconstriction, the latter being used as a simple provocation test. Many chemical stimuli result in bronchoconstriction including liquids with low pH such as gastric acid, and gases such as sulphur dioxide, ammonia, ozone and nitrogen dioxide.

Local Cellular Mechanisms

Inflammatory cells in the lung include mast cells, eosinophils, neutrophils, macrophages and lymphocytes, and the role of these cells in lung infection and inflammation is described in Chapters 28, 30 and 31. These inflammatory cells are all stimulated by a variety of pathogens, but some may also be activated by the direct physical factors described in the previous paragraph. Once activated, cytokine production causes amplification of the response, and a variety of mediators are released that can cause bronchoconstriction (Table 3.2). These mediators are produced in normal individuals, but patients with airway disease are usually 'hyper-responsive,' and so develop symptoms of bronchospasm more easily.

TABLE 3.2	Mediators Involved in Alteration of Bronchial Smooth Muscle Tone During Airway Inflammation				
	Bronchoconstriction			Bronchodilatation	
Source	Mediator	Receptor		Mediator	Receptor
Mast cells and other proinflammatory cells	Histamine	H_1		Prostaglandin E_2	EP
	Prostaglandin D_2	TP		Prostacyclin (PGI_2)	EP
	Prostaglandin $F_{2\alpha}$	TP			
	Leukotrienes C_4 D_4 E_4	$CysLT_1$			
	PAF	PAF			
C-fibres	Bradykinin	B_2			
	Substance P	NK_2			
	Neurokinin A	NK_2			
	CGRP	CGRP			
Endothelial and epithelial cells	Endothelin	ET_B			

PAF, Platelet-activating factor; *CGRP*, calcitonin gene-related peptide.

Drug Effects on Airway Smooth Muscle

β₂-Agonists

Nonspecific β-adrenoceptor agonists (e.g., isoprenaline) were the first bronchodilator drugs to be widely used for treating asthma. However, cardiac effects from β₁-receptor stimulation in the heart were believed to be responsible for an increase in mortality during acute asthma, and the development of β₂-specific drugs (e.g., salbutamol) soon followed. Later, long-acting β₂-agonists (e.g., salmeterol) were developed, and are now widely used for treating asthma, with duration of action now allowing once daily dosing.[10] The therapeutic effect of β₂-agonists is more complex than simple relaxation of airway smooth muscle, as they are also known to inhibit the secretion of inflammatory cytokines and most of the bronchoconstrictor mediators shown in Table 3.2,[11] and even to increase surfactant release.[12] Controversy associated with β₂-agonists still continues today—their effect on inflammatory cells and their ability to down-regulate β₂-receptors are both potentially harmful, and concerns exist about the mortality of some groups of patients taking long-acting β₂-agonists.[13]

The β₂-Receptor

The molecular basis of the functional characteristics of the β-adrenoceptor is now clearly elucidated. It contains 413 amino acids and has seven transmembrane helices (Fig. 3.9). The agonist binding site is within this hydrophobic core of the protein, which sits within the lipid bilayer of the cell membrane. This affects the interaction of drugs at the binding site, in that more lipophilic drugs form a depot in the lipid bilayer, from which they can repeatedly interact with the binding site of the receptor, producing a much longer duration of action than hydrophilic drugs. Receptors exist in either activated or inactivated form, the former state occurring when the third intracellular loop is bound to guanosine triphosphate and the α-subunit of the G₅-protein. β₂-receptor agonists probably do not induce a significant conformational change in the protein structure, but simply stabilize the activated form, allowing this to predominate.

Activation of the G-protein by the β₂-receptor in turn activates adenylate cyclase to convert adenosine triphosphate to cyclic adenosine monophosphate (cAMP). cAMP causes relaxation of the muscle cell by inhibiting calcium release from intracellular stores and activating protein kinase A to phosphorylate many of the regulatory proteins involved in the actin–myosin interaction.[11]

Two β₂-receptor genes are present in humans, with a total of 18 polymorphisms described,[14] giving rise to a large number of possible phenotypes. Studies of these phenotypes continue, with some differences observed between individuals in terms of clinical picture or response to therapy, but the contribution that different β₂-receptor phenotypes make to the overall prevalence of asthma appears to be minimal.[14,15]

Phosphodiesterase Inhibitors[16,17]

After its production following β₂-receptor stimulation, cAMP is rapidly hydrolysed by the intracellular enzyme phosphodiesterase (PDE), the inhibition of which will prolong the smooth muscle relaxant effect of β₂-receptor stimulation. Eleven subgroups of PDE have now been identified, with subgroups PDE3, PDE4 and PDE7 found in the lung, but the PDE inhibitors currently used in asthma, such as theophylline, are nonspecific for the different subgroups.

This lack of specificity of currently used PDE inhibitors accounts for their wide-ranging side effects, which continue to limit their therapeutic use. Recent work on PDE inhibitors has found them to have significant antiinflammatory effects in the lung, mediated mostly by PDE4 and occurring at lower blood levels than their bronchodilator effects.[16] This has raised the possibility of a new role for PDE inhibition in treating airway diseases by using PDE4-specific inhibitors (e.g., roflumilast), but clinical results have been disappointing because of frequent side effects.[10,17]

Anticholinergic Drugs

Acetylcholine Receptor

Stimulation of M_3 ACh receptors also activates a G-protein, characterized as G_q. This in turn activates phospholipase C to stimulate the production of inositol triphosphate (IP_3), which then binds to sarcoplasmic reticulum receptors, causing release of calcium from intracellular stores. The elevation of intracellular calcium activates myosin light chain kinase, which phosphorylates part of the myosin chain to activate myosin ATPase and initiate cross-bridging between actin and myosin. IP_3 is converted into the inactive inositol diphosphate by IP_3 kinase. Tachykinin, histamine and leukotriene receptors responsible for bronchoconstriction from other mediators (Table 3.2) act by a very similar mechanism, being linked to G-protein–phospholipase C complexes, which lead to IP_3 formation.

There are now believed to be many molecular interactions between the IP_3 and cAMP signalling pathways. Activation of phospholipase C by the protein G_q also liberates intracellular diacylglycerol, which activates another membrane-bound enzyme, protein kinase C. This enzyme is able to phosphorylate a variety of proteins, including G-proteins and the β_2-receptor itself (Fig. 3.9), causing uncoupling of the receptor from the G-protein and downregulation of the transduction pathway.

Anticholinergic drugs used in the airway are classified into short-acting (e.g., ipratropium) or long-acting (e.g., tiotropium) types. They are more useful in treating chronic obstructive pulmonary disease than asthma (Chapter 28), because only in the former disease is increased parasympathetic activity thought to contribute to symptoms. These drugs have similar binding affinities for both M_2 and M_3 receptors, giving rise to opposing effects on the degree of stimulation of airway smooth muscle. Differences in relative numbers of M_2 and M_3 receptors between individuals and in different disease states will therefore explain the variability in response seen with inhaled anticholinergic drugs.

Leukotriene Antagonists[18]

Even in nonasthmatic individuals, leukotrienes are potent bronchoconstrictors, so the therapeutic potential of leukotriene antagonists has been extensively investigated. Activation of phospholipase A_2 by inflammatory cells initiates the pathway, which ultimately produces three leukotrienes (Table 3.2, Fig. 3.10). In the lung, these all act via a single receptor ($CysLT_1$) on airway smooth muscle cells to cause contraction via the G-protein–IP_3 system described earlier. Leukotrienes have a wide range of activities apart from bronchoconstriction, in particular amplification of the inflammatory response by chemotaxis of eosinophils.

As may be predicted from their actions, antagonists of the $CysLT_1$ receptor (e.g., montelukast, zafirlukast) are not effective in treating acute bronchoconstriction, except that induced by exercise, but are useful in situations when the leukotriene pathway has been activated by stimulation of

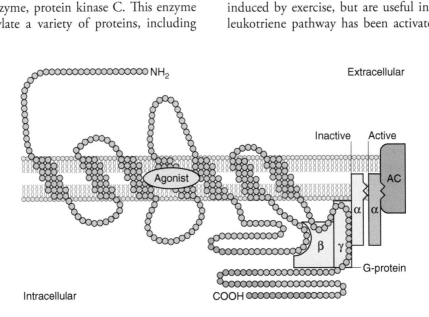

• **Fig. 3.9** Molecular mechanisms of β_2-adrenoceptor stimulation. The receptor exists in activated and inactivated states according to whether or not the α-subunit of the G-protein is bound to adenylate cyclase *(AC)*. The agonist binds to three amino acid residues on the third and fifth transmembrane domains, and by doing so stabilizes the receptor G-protein complex in the activated state. The intracellular C-terminal region of the protein *(green)* is the area susceptible to phosphorylation by intracellular kinases, causing inactivation of the receptor and downregulation.

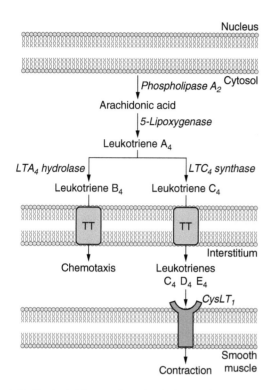

• **Fig. 3.10** The leukotriene pathway in the lung. Inflammatory mediators stimulate phospholipase A_2 to produce arachidonic acid from the phospholipid of the nuclear membrane. Leukotrienes B_4 and C_4 leave the cell via a specific transmembrane transporter (TT) protein. Nonspecific peptidases in the interstitium convert leukotriene C_4 into D_4 and E_4, all of which stimulate the $CysLT_1$ receptor to cause intense bronchoconstriction.

inflammatory cells. They are therefore most likely to be of benefit in the prevention of bronchospasm in chronic asthma, but their place in asthma therapy remains uncertain.[18]

Compensation for Increased Resistance to Breathing

In animals, very little compensation for resistive loading occurs until P_{CO_2} increases, which stimulates ventilation and overcomes the resistance. In humans, the response is more complex.

Inspiratory Resistance

The normal response to increased inspiratory resistance is increased inspiratory muscle effort with little change in the FRC. Accessory muscles may be brought into play according to the degree of resistance.

There are two principal mechanisms of compensation for increased inspiratory resistance. The first operates immediately and even during the first breath in which resistance is applied. It seems probable that the muscle spindles indicate that the inspiratory muscles have failed to shorten by the intended amount, and their afferent discharge then augments the activity in the motoneurone pool of the anterior

horn. This is the typical servo operation of the spindle system with which the intercostal muscles are richly endowed (page 65). This reflex, mediated at the spinal level, is preserved during general anaesthesia (page 260).

In awake humans, the spinal response is accompanied by a further stimulus to ventilation mediated in suprapontine areas of the brain, possibly in the cerebral cortex.[19] This 'behavioural' response defends ventilation even in the face of significant inspiratory loading, preventing any change in P_{CO_2}. If the response does indeed depend on cortical activity, this would explain why resistive loading during physiological sleep can be problematic (Chapter 14).

The fall in intrathoracic pressure associated with increased inspiratory resistance has profound cardiovascular effects, resulting in 'pulsus paradoxus', defined as a greater than 10% fall in systolic blood pressure during inspiration.[20] The degree to which this is observed is an indirect marker of the severity of airway obstruction, for example in acute asthma.

Expiratory Resistance

Expiration against a pressure of up to 1 kPa (10 cmH$_2$O) does not usually result in activation of the expiratory muscles in conscious or anaesthetized subjects. The additional work to overcome this resistance is, in fact, performed by the inspiratory muscles. The subject augments his inspiratory force until he achieves a lung volume (i.e., FRC) at which the additional elastic recoil is sufficient to overcome the expiratory resistance (Fig. 3.11). The mechanism for resetting the FRC at a higher level probably requires accommodation of the intrafusal fibres of the spindles to allow for an altered length of diaphragmatic muscle fibres because of the obstructed expiration. This would reset the developed inspiratory tension in accord with the increased FRC. The conscious subject normally uses his expiratory muscles to overcome expiratory pressures in excess of about 1 kPa (10 cmH$_2$O).

Patients show a remarkable capacity to compensate for acutely increased resistance, such that arterial P_{CO_2} is

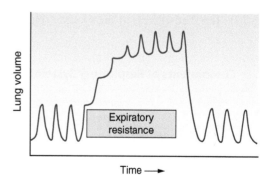

• **Fig. 3.11** Spirogram showing the response of an anaesthetized patient to the sudden imposition of an expiratory resistance. Note that there is an immediate augmentation of the force of contraction of the inspiratory muscles. This continues with successive breaths until the elastic recoil is sufficient to overcome the expiratory resistance. (From Nunn JF, Ezi-Ashi TI. The respiratory effects of resistance to breathing in anaesthetised man. *Anesthesiology.* 1961;22:174-185.)

usually normal. However, the efficiency of these mechanisms in maintaining alveolar ventilation carries severe physiological consequences. In common with other muscles, the respiratory muscles can become fatigued, which is a major factor in the onset of respiratory failure. A raised $P\text{CO}_2$ in a patient with increased respiratory resistance is therefore always serious. Also, intrathoracic pressure will rise during acutely increased expiratory resistance, and so impede venous return and reduce cardiac output (page 390) to the point that syncope may occur.

Principles of Measurement of Respiratory Resistance and Closing Capacity

Respiratory System Resistance

Resistance is determined by the simultaneous measurement of gas flow rate and the driving pressure gradient. In the case of the respiratory tract, the difficulty centres around the measurement of the pressure gradient between mouth and alveolus. Problems also arise because of varying nomenclature and different methods for measuring different components of respiratory system resistance (Table 3.3).[21] In all cases, apparatus resistance must be measured separately and subtracted from the value obtained in the subject.

Normal values for total respiratory system resistance are variable because of the large changes with lung volume and methodological differences, but typical values for a healthy male subject are shown in Table 3.3.

Pressure–Flow Technique

In Chapter 2 it was shown how simultaneous measurement of tidal volume and intrathoracic (oesophageal) pressure yielded the dynamic compliance of the lung (see Fig. 2.12). For this purpose, pressures were selected at the times of zero air flow when pressures were uninfluenced by air flow resistance. The same apparatus may be used for the determination of flow resistance by subtracting the pressure component used in overcoming elastic forces (Fig. 3.12). The shaded areas in the pressure trace indicate the components of the pressure required to overcome flow resistance, and these may be related to the concurrent gas flow rates.

Alternatively, the intrathoracic to mouth pressure gradient and respired volume may be displayed as x- and y-coordinates of a loop. Figure 2.12, A, shows how dynamic compliance could be derived from the no-flow points of such a loop. The area of the loop is a function of the work performed against flow resistance.

The use of an oesophageal balloon makes the method a little invasive, but it does allow continuous measurement of resistance. By measuring intrathoracic pressure, the chest wall component of resistance is excluded, providing a measure of pulmonary resistance, which is airways resistance plus the lung component of tissue resistance.

Oscillating Air Flow

In this technique, a high-frequency oscillating air flow is applied to the airways, with measurement of the resultant pressure and air flow changes. By application of alternating current theory, it is possible to derive a continuous measurement of airway resistance.[22] The technique measures total respiratory resistance and may be used throughout a vital capacity manoeuvre and display resistance as a function of lung volume and derive specific airway conductance.

Body Plethysmograph

During inspiration, alveolar pressure falls below ambient as a function of airway resistance, and the alveolar gas expands in accord with Boyle's law. The increased displacement of the body is then recorded as an increase in pressure in the body plethysmograph. Airway resistance may be derived directly from measurements of air flow and pressure changes, and the method requires the subject to perform either a 'panting' respiratory manoeuvre or to breathe with a small tidal volume. Despite these requirements, plethysmography is generally noninvasive and allows FRC to be measured at the same time,[21] but results for airway resistance may be inconsistent.

TABLE 3.3	**Components of Respiratory System Resistance**[21]

	Mouth and Pharynx	Larynx and Large Airways	Small Airways <3 mm in Diameter	Alveoli and Lung Tissue	Chest Wall	Total
Contribution (kPa.L^{-1}.s)	0.05	0.05	0.02	0.02	0.12	0.26
Airway resistance	Body plethysmograph interrupter technique					0.12
Pulmonary resistance	Pressure flow technique					0.14
Respiratory system resistance	Oscillating air flow technique End-inspiratory interruption					0.26

Blue areas indicate which components contribute to each form of resistance, whereas the text in the blue boxes states the methodology used to measure] each form of resistance.

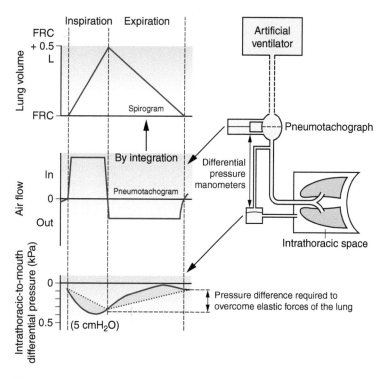

• **Fig. 3.12** The measurement of pulmonary resistance and dynamic compliance by simultaneous measurement of air flow and intrathoracic-to-mouth differential pressure. The spirogram is conveniently obtained by integration of the pneumotachogram. In the pressure trace, the dotted line shows the pressure changes that would be expected in a hypothetical patient with no pulmonary resistance. Compliance is derived as shown. Pulmonary resistance is derived as the difference between the measured pressure differential and that which is required for elastic forces (*green area*) compared with the flow rate shown in the pneumotachograph. Note that the pneumotachogram is a much more sensitive indicator of the no-flow points than the spirogram. *FRC*, Functional residual capacity.

Interrupter Technique

A single manometer may be used to measure both mouth and alveolar pressure if the air passages distal to the manometer are momentarily interrupted with a shutter. This method assumes that, while the airway is interrupted, the mouth pressure comes to equal the alveolar pressure. Resistance is then determined from the relationship between flow rate (measured before interruption) and the pressure difference between mouth (measured before interruption) and alveoli (measured at the end of the interruption). The interruption duration must be short enough to avoid disturbing the subject's breathing pattern but long enough to allow equilibration of pressure along the airway. In practice, interruption is for 50 to 100 milliseconds, occurring repeatedly throughout the respiratory cycle. The technique is adequate for measuring resistance in normal lungs, but it is doubtful if equilibration occurs fully in subjects with diseased airways. The interrupter method measures airway resistance and excludes tissue resistance.

End-Inspiratory Interruption

This method is now widely used for measuring the tissue component of respiratory system resistance.[1,2] It may only be used in anaesthetized paralysed subjects receiving artificial ventilation with accurate control of the respiratory cycle. Following a constant flow inflation of the lung, the airway is occluded for 0.5 to 3 seconds before a passive exhalation occurs. To prevent artefacts during the inspiratory pause, numerous successive breaths may be averaged.[2] Figure 3.13 shows the changes in gas flow, transpulmonary pressure (P_L), oesophageal pressure and lung volume averaged over 33 breaths. Immediately before occlusion, P_L reaches a value of P_{max}, which is governed by both elastic and nonelastic resistance. The fall in pressure following occlusion is biphasic. Immediately after airway occlusion, the P_L falls rapidly to P_1, and $P_{max} - P_1$ is referred to as interrupter resistance and believed to reflect airway resistance as in the interrupter method already described.

In the second phase, a slower decay in pressure occurs from P_1 to P_2, which represents the loss of the time-dependent element of tissue compliance (because of viscoelastic behaviour) and therefore represents tissue resistance:

$$\text{Tissue resistance} = \frac{P_1 - P_2}{\text{Flow rate of inflation}}$$

In practice, the pressure signal may be converted into digital form, and computer analysis calculates the three pressures.[2]

Where these pressures are recorded determines which component of tissue resistance is measured. In Figure 3.13, transpulmonary pressure (tracheal minus oesophageal pressure) is recorded, allowing calculation of the tissue resistance of the

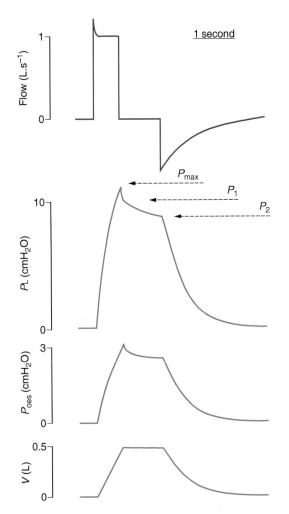

• **Fig. 3.13** End-inspiratory interruption method of measuring resistance. Following a constant flow positive pressure breath, there is an end-inspiratory pause of almost 1 second before passive exhalation. The peak airway pressure (P_{max}) falls initially very quickly to P_1, and thereafter more slowly to a plateau P_2. Tissue resistance, airway resistance and total resistance can then all be calculated (see text for details). In this example, showing the average of 33 consecutive breaths, both transpulmonary (tracheal minus oesophageal) pressure and oesophageal pressure relative to atmosphere have been measured, allowing lung and chest wall components of tissue resistance to be calculated separately. *Flow*, Airway flow rate; *P*L, transpulmonary pressure; P_{oes}, oesophageal pressure; *V*, change in lung volume. (From reference 2.)

lung alone. Oesophageal pressure is also recorded, allowing calculation of the thoracic cage component of tissue resistance.

Finally, measurement of tracheal to atmospheric pressure gradient allows calculation of total respiratory resistance:

Respiratory system resistance

$$= \frac{P_{max} - P_2}{\text{Flow rate of inflation}}$$

This technique is used by the current generation of ventilators to calculate respiratory system resistance. The same static respiratory manoeuvre described in Chapter 2 for the calculation of static compliance (Fig. 2.12, *B*) also allows

measurement of P_{max} and P_2, from which respiratory system resistance is calculated (Fig. 3.13).

Measurement of Closing Capacity[4,21]

CC is the maximal lung volume at which airway closure can be detected in the dependent parts of the lungs (page 31). The measurement is made during expiration and is based on having different concentrations of a tracer gas in the upper and lower parts of the lung. This may be achieved by inspiration of a bolus of tracer gas at the commencement of an inspiration from RV, at which time airways are closed in the dependent part of the lungs (Fig. 3.14). The tracer gas will then be preferentially distributed to the upper parts of the lungs. After a maximal inspiration to TLC, the patient slowly exhales while the concentration of the tracer gas is measured at the mouth. When lung volume reaches the CC and airways begin to close in the dependent parts, the concentration of the tracer gas will rise (phase IV) above the alveolar plateau (phase III). Suitable tracers are ^{133}Xe or 100% oxygen (measured as a fall in nitrogen concentration). This technique can be undertaken in the conscious subject who performs the ventilatory manoeuvres spontaneously or in the paralysed subject in whom ventilation is artificially controlled.

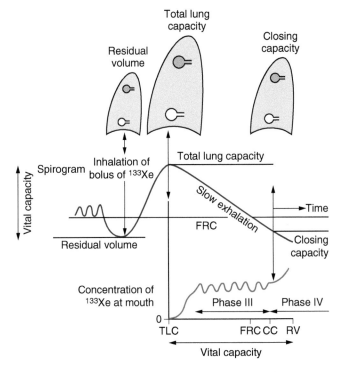

• **Fig. 3.14** Measurement of closing capacity by the use of a tracer gas such as ^{133}Xe. The bolus of tracer gas is inhaled near residual volume and, because of airway closure, is distributed only to those alveoli whose air passages are still open (shown *shaded* in the diagram). During expiration, the concentration of the tracer gas becomes constant after the dead space is washed out. This plateau (phase III) gives way to a rising concentration of tracer gas (phase IV) when there is closure of airways leading to alveoli which did not receive the tracer gas. *CC*, Closing capacity; *FRC*, functional residual capacity; *RV*, residual volume; *TLC*, total lung capacity.

References

1. DAngelo E, Tavola M, Milic-Emili J. Volume and time dependence of respiratory system mechanics in normal anaesthetised paralysed humans. *Eur Respir J.* 2000;16:665-672.

2. D'Angelo E, Prandi E, Tavola M, et al. Chest wall interrupter resistance in anesthetized paralyzed humans. *J Appl Physiol.* 1994;77:883-887.

3. Bossé Y, Riesenfeld EP, Paré PD, et al. It's not all smooth muscle: non-smooth-muscle elements in control of resistance to airflow. *Annu Rev Physiol.* 2010;72:437-462.

4. Milic-Emili J, Torchio R, D'Angelo E. Closing volume: a reappraisal (1967–2007). *Eur J Appl Physiol.* 2007;99:567-583.

5. Drummond GB, Milic-Emili J. Forty years of closing volume. *Br J Anaesth.* 2007;99:772-774.

6. Aljuri N, Venegas JG, Freitag L. Viscoelasticity of the trachea and its effects on flow limitation. *J Appl Physiol.* 2006;100:384-389.

7. Canning BJ. Reflex regulation of airway smooth muscle tone. *J Appl Physiol.* 2006;101:971-985.

*8. **Mazzone SB, Undem BJ. Vagal afferent innervation of the airways in health and disease. *Physiol Rev.* 2016;96:975-1024.**

9. Prabha KC, Martin RJ. Role of central neurotransmission and chemoreception on airway control. *Respir Physiol Neurobiol.* 2010;173:213-222.

10. Gross NJ, Barnes PJ. New therapies for asthma and chronic obstructive pulmonary disease. *Am J Respir Crit Care Med.* 2017;195:159-166.

11. Cazzola M, Page CP, Rogliani P, et al. β2-agonist therapy in lung disease. *Am J Respir Crit Care Med.* 2013;187:690-696.

12. Enhorning G. Surfactant in airway disease. *Chest.* 2008;133:975-980.

13. Dixon AE. Long-acting β-agonists and asthma: the saga continues. *Am J Respir Crit Care Med.* 2011;184:1220-1221.

14. Hall IP, Sayers I. Pharmacogenetics and asthma: false hope or new dawn? *Eur Respir J.* 2007;29:1239-1245.

15. Wjst M. β2-adrenoreceptor polymorphisms and asthma. *Lancet.* 2006;368:710-711.

16. Barnes PJ. Theophylline. *Am J Respir Crit Care Med.* 2013; 188:901-906.

17. Mokry J, Mokra D. Immunological aspects of phosphodiesterase inhibition in the respiratory system. *Respir Physiol Neurobiol.* 2013;187:11-17.

*18. **Scott JP, Peters-Golden M. Antileukotriene agents for the treatment of lung disease. *Am J Respir Crit Care Med.* 2013;188:538-544.**

19. Raux M, Straus C, Redolfi S, et al. Electroencephalographic evidence for pre-motor cortex activation during inspiratory loading in humans. *J Physiol.* 2007;578:569-578.

20. Hamzaoui O, Monnet X, Teboul J-L. Pulsus paradoxus. *Eur Respir J.* 2013;42:1696-1705.

21. Cotes JE, Chinn DJ, Miller MR. *Lung. Physiology, Measurement and Application in Medicine.* Oxford: Blackwell Publishing; 2006.

22. Goldman M, Knudson RJ, Mead J, et al. A simplified measurement of respiratory resistance by forced oscillation. *J Appl Physiol.* 1970;28:113-116.

4

Control of Breathing

KEY POINTS

- The respiratory centre in the medulla generates the respiratory rhythm using an oscillating network of groups of interconnecting neurones.
- Many other diverse areas of the central nervous system influence respiratory control, and these connections are coordinated by the pons.
- Irritant and stretch receptors in the lungs and diaphragm are involved in a series of reflex actions on the respiratory centre to influence respiratory activity.

- Central chemoreceptors respond to changes in pH caused by alterations in carbon dioxide partial pressure, rapidly increasing ventilation in response to elevated arterial P_{CO_2}.
- Peripheral chemoreceptors, principally in the carotid body, increase ventilation in response to reduced arterial P_{O_2}.

Early in pregnancy the foetal brainstem develops a 'respiratory centre', which produces uninterrupted rhythmic breathing activity for many years. Throughout life the subject is mostly unaware of this action, which is closely controlled by a combination of chemical and physical reflexes. In addition, when required, breathing may (within limits) be completely overridden by voluntary control or interrupted by swallowing and involuntary non-rhythmic acts such as sneezing, vomiting, hiccupping or coughing. The control system is complex, with its automatic ability to adapt the action of the respiratory muscles to the changing demands of posture, speech, voluntary movement, exercise and innumerable other circumstances which alter the respiratory requirement or influence the performance of the respiratory muscles.

The Origin of the Respiratory Rhythm[1]

Early attempts to find the site of respiratory control used an anatomical approach involving the removal or stimulation of specific areas of the brainstem in animals (see section on *Control of Ventilation* in Chapter 35). Subsequent development of precise imaging techniques allowed localization of respiratory regions in normal human subjects, confirming much of the historical animal work.

Anatomical Location of the 'Respiratory Centre'

The medulla is the area of brain where the respiratory pattern is generated and where the various voluntary and involuntary demands on respiratory activity are coordinated. There are many neuronal connections both into and out of the medulla, as summarized in Figure 4.1, the functions of which are described later. Respiratory neurones in the medulla are concentrated in two anatomical areas, the ventral and dorsal respiratory groups, which have numerous interconnections (Fig. 4.2). The dorsal respiratory group lies in close relation to the nucleus tractus solitarius, where visceral afferents from cranial nerves IX and X terminate (Fig. 4.2). It is predominantly composed of inspiratory neurones, with upper motor neurones passing to the inspiratory anterior horn cells of the opposite side. The dorsal group is primarily concerned with timing of the respiratory cycle.

The ventral respiratory group comprises a column of respiratory neurones including the following:

- Caudal ventral respiratory group, including the nucleus retroambigualis, which is predominantly expiratory, with upper motor neurones passing to the contralateral expiratory muscles, and the mainly inspiratory nucleus para-ambigualis that controls the force of contraction of the contralateral inspiratory muscles
- Rostral ventral respiratory group, mostly made up of the nucleus ambiguous, which is involved in airway dilator functions of the larynx, pharynx and tongue
- Pre-Bötzinger complex, the anatomical location of the central pattern generator (CPG)
- Bötzinger complex (within the nucleus retrofacialis), which has widespread expiratory functions

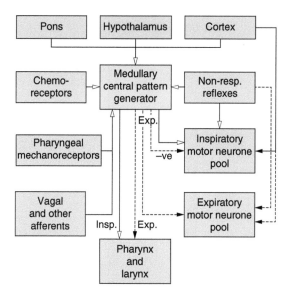

• **Fig. 4.1** Afferent and efferent connections to and from the medullary central pattern generator. The broken lines are 'active' expiratory pathways, which normally remain silent during quiet breathing.

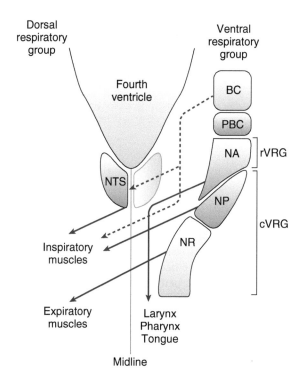

• **Fig. 4.2** Dorsal view of the organization of respiratory neurones in the medulla. For clarity, the dorsal respiratory is shown only on the left, and the ventral respiratory group *(VRG)* is shown only on the right. The VRG consists of the Bötzinger *(BC)* and pre-Bötzinger *(PBC)* complexes, the rostral VRG area *(rVRG)* including the nucleus ambiguous *(NA)* and the caudal VRG area including the nucleus para-ambigualis *(NP)* and nucleus retroambigualis *(NR)*. Areas with predominantly expiratory activity are shaded blue, and those with inspiratory activity shaded brown. Fibres that decussate are shown crossing the midline. The broken lines are expiratory pathways that inhibit inspiratory neurones. *NTS,* Nucleus tractus solitarius.

Central Pattern Generator[1]

Unlike in the heart, there is no single 'pacemaker' neurone responsible for initiating breathing. Instead, a group-pacemaker system exists in which groups of associated neurones generate regular bursts of neuronal activity.[2] For breathing, the group pacemaker involves a complex interaction of at least six groups of neurones with identifiable firing patterns spread throughout the medulla, although concentrated in the region of the pre-Bötzinger complex. Groups of neurones include early inspiratory neurones, inspiratory augmenting (Iaug) neurones, late inspiratory interneurones (putative 'off-switch' neurones), early expiratory decrementing neurones, expiratory augmenting neurones, and late expiratory preinspiratory neurones. Typical firing patterns and the resulting muscle group activity are shown schematically in Figure 4.3. The resultant respiratory cycle may be divided into three phases:

1. *Inspiratory phase.* A sudden onset is followed by ramp increase in Iaug neurones, resulting in motor discharge to the inspiratory muscles, including the pharyngeal dilator muscles. Pharyngeal dilator muscles start to contract shortly before the start of inspiration, possibly by activation of late expiratory (preinspiratory) neurones.

2. *Postinspiratory or expiratory phase I.* This is characterized by declining discharge of the Iaug neurones, and therefore motor discharge to the inspiratory muscles. Early expiratory decrementing neurones also produce declining activity in the laryngeal adductor muscles. This phase therefore represents passive expiration with a gradual let down of inspiratory muscle tone and an initial braking of the expiratory gas flow rate (page 59) by the larynx.

3. *Expiratory phase II.* The inspiratory muscles are now silent and, if required, expiratory augmenting neurones will be activated to produce a gradual increase in expiratory muscle activity.

Alterations in the rate at which spontaneous neuronal activity increases or decreases and the point at which the next group of neurones is activated allow an infinite variation of respiratory patterns. For example, during quiet breathing in the supine position, early expiratory neurones will reduce activity slowly, and expiratory augmenting neurones will be active only briefly, resulting in almost totally passive exhalation. The converse situation will arise following exercise or at a minute volume in excess of approximately 40 L.min^{-1}, when expiration will be immediately and almost totally active.

In practice, many such rhythm-generating networks are represented in parallel, so it is difficult to abolish the respiratory rhythm even with extensive brainstem damage.

Cellular Mechanisms of Central Pattern Generation

Respiratory neurones that exhibit spontaneous activity achieve this by a combination of intrinsic membrane properties and excitatory and inhibitory feedback mechanisms

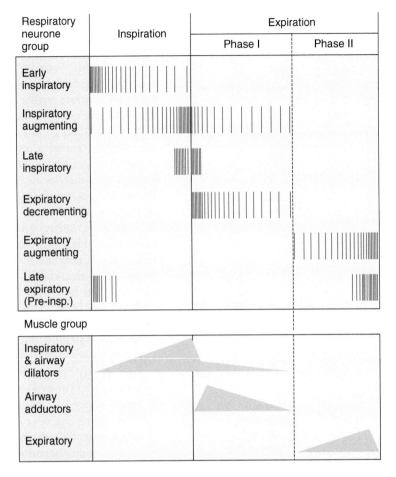

• **Fig. 4.3** Firing patterns of the respiratory neurone groups of the central pattern generator and the corresponding respiratory muscle group activity. Note that expiration is divided into two phases representing passive *(phase I)* and active *(phase II)* expiration. See text for details.

requiring neurotransmitters. In practice, neurotransmitters (both inhibitory and excitatory) have a dual effect: they recruit other cells by direct activation and modulate the spontaneous activity of a single cell by effects on its own membrane ion channels, for example, slowing the rate at which an action potential travels along a dendrite.

Similar to rhythm generation in cardiac tissue, a combination of multiple types of sodium, potassium and calcium ion channels is involved. For instance, in a single Iaug neurone slow membrane depolarization occurs, producing a spontaneous discharge. These cells then 'recruit' other Iaug cells by excitatory postsynaptic potentials, and a crescendo of Iaug activity develops. Calcium-dependent potassium channels then begin to be activated and repolarize the cells, so 'switching off' the Iaug respiratory group. Activation of other cell groups, for instance expiratory augmenting neurones, will result in activation of inhibitory postsynaptic potentials on the Iaug neurones to hyperpolarize the neurone and inhibit the next wave of inspiratory activity. Similar membrane effects occur in all the respiratory neurone groups shown in Figure 4.3.

Neurotransmitters Involved in Central Pattern Generator and Respiratory Control[3]

These neurotransmitters are summarized in Figure 4.4. Central pattern generation requires a combination of excitatory and inhibitory neurotransmitters. Excitatory amino acids (usually glutamate) activate several different receptors. These are divided into two groups: *N*-methyl-D-aspartate (NMDA) receptors, which are fast-acting ion channels, and non-NMDA receptors, which are slower-reacting receptors involving G-protein-mediated effects. Inhibitory neurotransmitters include glycine and γ-aminobutyric acid (GABA), acting via specific glycine receptors and GABA_A receptors, respectively, to hyperpolarize the neurone, thereby inhibiting its activity.

Neuromodulators are substances that can influence the CPG output, but are not involved in rhythm generation. There are numerous neuromodulators of respiration, many of which have several subtypes of receptors. Their exact role in normal human respiration remains unclear, but they are of undoubted relevance in both normal and

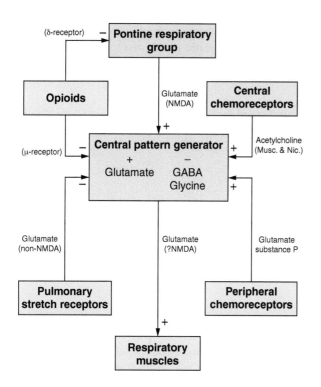

• **Fig. 4.4** Neurotransmitters and neuromodulators in the respiratory centre. Boxes indicate functional neuronal groups, and bold type represents other influences on the respiratory centre. Substances involved in neurotransmission are shown with the most likely receptor subtype, in parentheses, if known. +, indicates excitatory effect increasing respiratory activity; −, indicates inhibitory activity decreasing respiration. Many of the connections shown may not be active during normal resting conditions. NMDA, *N*-methyl-D-aspartate.

Efferent Pathways from the Respiratory Centre

Respiratory motor neurones in the brainstem are pooled into two separate areas, corresponding to inspiratory and expiratory muscle activity (Fig. 4.1). The complex integration of respiratory control seen in the CPG neurones continues to take place at the junction of the upper motor neurone with the anterior horn cell of the lower motor neurone. Three groups of upper motor neurones converge on the anterior horn cells supplying the respiratory muscles. The first group of upper motor neurones is from the dorsal and ventral respiratory groups of the medulla and is concerned with both inspiratory and expiratory output from the CPG. The second group is concerned with voluntary control of breathing (speech, respiratory gymnastics, etc.), and the third group with involuntary nonrhythmic respiratory control (swallowing, cough, hiccup, etc.). Each group of upper motor neurones occupies a specific anatomical location within the spinal cord. Neuronal control of the respiratory muscles is described in Chapter 5.

Central Nervous System Connections to the Respiratory Centre

The Pons

There is no doubt that pontine neurones firing in synchrony with different phases of respiration exist, and these neurones are now referred to as the pontine respiratory group (PRG). Previously known as the pneumotaxic centre, three groups of neurones were identified (inspiratory, expiratory and phase spanning) that were believed to be involved in controlling the timing of the respiratory cycle. The PRG is no longer considered to be essential for the generation of the respiratory rhythm; nevertheless, it does influence the medullary respiratory neurones via a multisynaptic pathway contributing to fine control of the respiratory rhythm as, for example, in setting the lung volume at which inspiration is terminated. There are many central afferent pathways into the PRG, including connections to the hypothalamus, the cortex and the nucleus tractus solitarius. These connections suggest that the pons coordinates the respiratory effects of numerous central nervous system (CNS) activities, including cortical control, peripheral sensory information (odour, temperature) and visceral/cardiovascular inputs.

Cerebral Cortex[4]

Breathing can be voluntarily interrupted, and the pattern of respiratory movements altered, within limits determined mainly by changes in arterial blood gas tensions. This is essential for such acts as speech, singing, sniffing, coughing, making expulsive efforts and performing ventilatory function tests.

Volitional changes in respiration are common, and under some circumstances overcome the usual chemical control of

abnormal breathing. For example, exogenous opioids are known to have a profound depressant effect on respiratory activity in humans (page 55), indicating the presence of opioid receptors in the respiratory centre, but administration of the opioid antagonist naloxone has no effect on respiration in resting normal subjects. Other neuromodulators include acetylcholine, which acts via both muscarinic and nicotinic receptors to mediate the effect of central chemoreceptors on respiration. Serotonin (5-hydroxytryptamine) has many conflicting effects on respiration as a result of the numerous receptor subtypes present. Glutamate acts as a neuromodulator via both NMDA and non-NMDA receptors to mediate the pontine influence on CPG, and is also involved in the influence of pulmonary stretch receptors and peripheral chemoreceptors on the respiratory pattern. Substance P also has an excitatory influence, resulting in an increase in tidal volume in response to peripheral chemoreceptor activity. These diverse neuromodulators probably all ultimately act via a common intracellular signalling pathway within CPG neurones involving protein kinases A and C, which in turn influence the activity of GABA, glycine and glutamate-linked potassium and chloride channels.

respiration. For example, conscious respiratory drive may well maintain breathing in subjects following voluntary hyperventilation when the $P\text{CO}_2$ is below the apnoeic threshold (page 50). The ventilatory response to exercise often occurs before exercise actually starts (page 186), and behavioural responses such as anxiety, pain or panic change the respiratory pattern profoundly.[5,6] There are also minor changes in the respiratory pattern when subjects focus their attention on their breathing, such as when physiological mouth pieces or breathing masks are used.[7]

In addition to volitional changes in the pattern of breathing, there are numerous other suprapontine reflex interferences with respiration, such as sneezing, mastication, swallowing, phonation and coughing.[8,9] Reflex control of respiration during speech is complex.[10] During conversation, respiratory rate and tidal volume must be approximately normal to prevent biochemical disturbance. In addition, for speech to be easily understood, pauses to allow inspiration must occur at appropriate boundaries in the text, for example between sentences. To achieve this, the brain performs complex assessments of the forthcoming speech to select appropriately sized breaths to prevent cumbersome interruptions. This is easier to achieve during reading aloud, when 88% of breaths are taken at appropriate boundaries in the text, compared with a figure of only 63% during spontaneous speech.[10]

Ondine's Curse (Primary Alveolar Hypoventilation Syndrome)

In 1962 Severinghaus and Mitchell[11] described three patients who exhibited long periods of apnoea, even when awake, but who breathed on command. They termed the condition 'Ondine's curse' from its first description in German legend. The water nymph, Ondine, having been jilted by her mortal husband, took from him all automatic functions, requiring him to remember to breathe. When he finally fell asleep, he died. In adults primary alveolar hypoventilation occurs as a feature of many diseases, including chronic poliomyelitis and stroke. Characteristics include a raised $P\text{CO}_2$ in the absence of pulmonary pathology, a flat carbon dioxide/ventilation response curve and periods of apnoea. A similar condition is also produced by overdosage with opioids.

Ondine's curse is also used to describe the rare condition of congenital central hypoventilation syndrome in which babies are born with a permanent defect in automatic respiratory control, leading to apnoea and hypoventilation during sleep.[12] The condition results from a defect in the *PHOX2B* gene which codes for a transcription regulator protein, and affected children have structural defects in the neurones of the retrotrapezoid nucleus where respiratory carbon dioxide sensing occurs (page 48). The children also have abnormal respiratory responses to exercise and, in keeping with the German legend, have abnormalities of cardiac control and thermoregulation. In spite of such severe abnormalities, noninvasive methods of nocturnal ventilation and diaphragmatic pacing have led to almost normal lives for many of these children.

Peripheral Input to the Respiratory Centre and Nonchemical Reflexes

Reflexes Arising from the Upper Respiratory Tract[13]

Nose

Water and stimulants such as ammonia or cigarette smoke may cause apnoea as part of the diving reflex (page 233). Irritants can initiate sneezing which, unlike coughing, cannot be undertaken voluntarily.

Pharynx

Mechanoreceptors that respond to pressure play a major role in activation of the pharyngeal dilator muscles (page 59). There is ample evidence that local anaesthesia of the pharynx impairs their action. Irritants may cause bronchodilatation, hypertension, tachycardia and secretion of mucus in the lower airway.

Larynx

The larynx has a dense sensory innervation with fibres from the subglottic region in the recurrent laryngeal nerve and those from the supraglottic region in the internal branch of the superior laryngeal nerve. Most reflexes arise from the supraglottic area, as a section of the latter nerve abolishes almost all reflex activity. There are three groups of receptors. Mechanoreceptors respond to changes in transmural pressure or laryngeal motion and result in increased pharyngeal dilator muscle activity, particularly during airway obstruction. Cold receptors are found superficially on the vocal folds, and activation generally results in depression of ventilation. The importance of this reflex in adult humans is uncertain, but these receptors may also produce bronchoconstriction in susceptible individuals (Chapter 28). Irritant receptors respond to many substances such as distilled water, cigarette smoke and inhaled anaesthetics, and, in a similar fashion to direct mechanical stimulation of the larynx, cause cough, laryngeal closure and bronchoconstriction.

Cough Reflex[14,15]

This may be elicited by chemical or mechanical stimuli arising in the larynx, trachea, carina or main bronchi. Which of these sites is responsible for the initiation of a cough is difficult to determine. For chemical stimuli the larynx may be of less importance, as superior laryngeal nerve block has little effect on cough stimulated by citric acid inhalation, and in patients following a heart–lung transplant, inhalation of the normally potent stimulant distilled water results in little or no cough (page 409). Coughing can be initiated or partially inhibited voluntarily, but the reflex is complex and comprises three main stages:

1. *Inspiratory phase.* Takes into the lungs a volume of air sufficient for the expiratory activity.
2. *Compressive phase.* Involves a forced expiration against a closed glottis. Transient changes of pressure up to 40 kPa (300 mmHg) may occur in the thorax, arterial blood and the cerebrospinal fluid (CSF) during the act of coughing.
3. *Expulsive phase.* The glottis opens, allowing rapid expiratory flow throughout the respiratory tract.

During this last phase the velocity of gas flow will be greatest in the narrowest section of the airway, usually the large bronchi, trachea and larynx (see Fig. 1.5), an area referred to as the 'choke point'. This high-velocity gas, with its turbulent flow, increases the shear forces between the gas and airway lining fluid, which is dragged from the airway wall and swept up towards the pharynx. The transient high intrathoracic pressure generated during a cough is believed to compress the large airways despite their cartilaginous support, and this narrowing further increases the gas velocity, reaching levels much higher than can be achieved by a voluntary forced expiration. The gas velocity achieved, and so the efficiency of the cough, is highly dependent on the size of breath taken during the inspiratory phase (Fig. 4.5). Finally, a series of smaller expulsive phases after a single inspiration, referred to as a 'peal' of coughs, is commonly seen and may be more effective at removing secretions than a single larger volume cough.[15]

Expiration Reflex[14,16]

Similar to a cough, this reflex originates in the larynx and is believed to exist to prevent material being aspirated into the upper airway. It differs from a cough by the absence of an inspiratory phase, the compressive and expulsive phases occurring immediately and from the lung volume present at the time the larynx is irritated. The distinction between the cough and expiration reflexes is important—a large inspiration as seen at the start of a cough would not be helpful in the presence of solid or liquid at the laryngeal inlet.

Reflexes Arising in the Lung

Pulmonary Stretch Receptors and Their Associated Reflexes[16]

There are many different types of receptors in the lungs sensitive to inflation or deflation, and mechanical or chemical stimulation, afferents from which are mostly conducted by the vagus, although some fibres may be carried in the sympathetic nerves. Slowly adapting stretch receptors (SARs) are found predominantly in the airways rather than in the alveoli, and are closely associated with the tracheobronchial smooth muscle. Lung inflation stimulates the SARs, which are called 'slowly adapting' because of their ability to maintain their firing rate when lung inflation is maintained, thus acting as a form of lung volume sensor. Conversely, rapidly adapting stretch receptors (RARs) are located in the superficial mucosal layer, and are stimulated by changes in tidal volume, respiratory frequency or changes in lung compliance.[16] The RARs also differ from SARs in being nociceptive and chemosensitive, responding to a wide range of chemical irritants, mechanical stimuli and inflammatory mediators.

How these receptors transduce a mechanical change in the tissue into an action potential is unknown. Hypotheses include the release of mediators from nearby associated cells that activate a receptor on the neurone, or ion channels may exist that respond directly to an alteration in their physical shape.[17] Afferent nerves from all these receptors converge on the nucleus tractus solitarius (NTS) of the medulla, where their signals are modulated and coordinated before further polysynaptic pathways communicate with the other regions of the respiratory centre. This processing of the afferent inputs by the NTS is believed to be capable of neuronal plasticity, which means the modulation can be altered by prolonged changes in external environment that influence the afferent inputs.[18]

The reflexes associated with pulmonary stretch receptors have attracted much attention since the associated inflation and deflation reflexes were described by Hering and Breuer in 1868.[19] Breuer was a clinical assistant to Professor Hering, but apparently performed the work at his own instigation. However, Hering, who was a corresponding member of the Vienna Academy of Science, published Breuer's work under his own name, in accord with the custom of the time. Breuer's role was clearly stated in Hering's paper, but he was not a coauthor. Later the same year, Breuer published a much fuller account of his work under his own name.

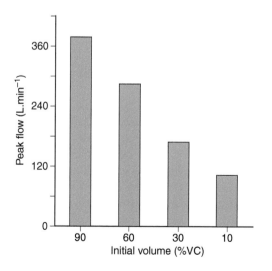

• **Fig. 4.5** Effect of initial lung volume, expressed as a percentage of the subject's vital capacity (%VC), on the peak flow rate achieved during a voluntary cough. Greater gas velocity will improve the efficiency of the cough at removing airway secretions, so coughing from a high lung volume is much more efficient. (Modified from reference 15, The Journal of Physiology © 2012 The Physiological Society. With permission.)

The *inflation reflex* consists of inhibition of inspiration in response to an increased pulmonary transmural pressure gradient (as in sustained inflation of the lung). A similar effect may be obtained by obstructing expiration so that an inspiration is retained in the lungs.

The significance of the Hering–Breuer reflex appears to differ between humans, in whom the reflex is very weak, and laboratory animals, where it is easily demonstrated. Pragmatic evidence that the Hering–Breuer reflex is unimportant in awake humans comes from studies showing normal breathing patterns in volunteers following bilateral vagal nerve block[20] and in patients who have had bilateral lung transplants, when both lungs must be totally denervated (Chapter 33). Conversely, studies in which conscious perception of chest wall position is suppressed by applying imperceptible amounts of assisted ventilation have demonstrated that respiratory pattern is altered within the physiological range, demonstrating the presence of a vagal feedback mechanism.[21] Although the Hering–Breuer inflation reflex appears to exist but has minimal functional significance in adults, it is widely accepted as being present in neonates and infants.[22]

The deflation reflex consists of an augmentation of inspiration in response to deflation of the lung, and can be demonstrated in humans.[23] These results are consistent with the hypothesis that lung deflation has a reflex excitatory effect on breathing, but that the threshold is higher in humans than in other mammalian species.

Head's Paradoxical Reflex

Head, working in Professor Hering's laboratory, described a reversal of the inflation reflex,[24] in which a sudden inflation of the lungs causes a transient inspiratory effort before the onset of apnoea as a result of the inflation reflex. A similar response may also be elicited in newborn infants,[25] but it has not been established whether this 'gasp reflex' is analogous to Head's paradoxical reflex. All anaesthetists have seen that, after administration of respiratory depressants, transient increases in airway pressure often cause an immediate deep, gasping type of inspiration.

Other Pulmonary Afferents

Vagal C-fibre nociceptors are free nerve endings found in close relationship to both bronchi and pulmonary capillaries.[26] They are generally silent during normal breathing, but are stimulated under conditions such as oxidative stress or lung inflammation, or in response to inhaled irritants such as tobacco smoke. Stimulation gives rise to the so-called pulmonary chemoreflex which comprises bradycardia, hypotension, apnoea or shallow breathing, bronchoconstriction and increased mucous secretion.[13] They are believed to be responsible for the sensation of the 'urge-to-cough', and so their inhibition would be beneficial in many respiratory diseases.

High-threshold Aδ-receptors are also present in lungs and are believed to be nociceptors, but their role, particularly in humans, remains unclear.

Reflexes Arising from Outside the Airway and Lungs

Phrenic Nerve Afferents

Approximately one-third of neurones in the phrenic nerve are afferent, mostly arising from muscle spindles and tendon organs forming the spinal reflex arc, which is described on page 65. However, some afferent neurones continue through the ipsilateral spinal cord to the brainstem and somatosensory cortex. Experimental stimulation of phrenic afferent fibres results in a reduction of respiratory efferent activity, but stimulation of some smaller afferent fibres has the opposite effect. Thus the physiological role of phrenic afferents remains obscure, but it is unlikely that they have any influence on normal breathing. The sensory information provided by phrenic afferents is believed to be important in the perception of, and compensation for, increased inspiratory loads, and these afferents are important in the 'breaking point' following a breath hold (page 54).

Baroreceptor Reflexes[27]

The most important groups of arterial baroreceptors are in the carotid sinus and around the aortic arch. These receptors are primarily concerned with regulation of the circulation, but a large decrease in arterial pressure produces hyperventilation, and infusion of vasopressors to increase blood pressure leads to hypoventilation under some circumstances. In humans this barorespiratory coupling is more pronounced in early life, and in adults is related to the state of arousal when studied and the subject's physical fitness.

Afferents from the Musculoskeletal System

These probably do not contribute to normal resting ventilation but have an important role in the hyperventilation of exercise (Chapter 13).

The Influence of Carbon Dioxide on Respiratory Control

For many years it was believed that the respiratory centre itself was sensitive to carbon dioxide. However, it is now known that both central and peripheral chemoreceptors are responsible for the effect of carbon dioxide on breathing, the former accounting for about 80% of the total ventilatory response. Because of their reliance on extracellular pH (see the next section) the central chemoreceptors are regarded as monitors of steady-state arterial $P\text{CO}_2$ and tissue perfusion in the brain, whereas the peripheral chemoreceptors respond more to short-term and rapid changes in arterial $P\text{CO}_2$.[28]

Localization of the Central Chemoreceptors

Studies in animals indicate that central chemosensitive areas are located within 0.2 mm of the ventrolateral surface of the medulla, in a region now referred to as the retrotrapezoid nucleus (RTN). Neurones of the RTN are glutaminergic, and have selective connections to the nearby CPG. Many other areas of the CNS display increased neural activity with carbon dioxide stimulation, including other areas of the medulla, the midline pons, small areas in the cerebellum and the limbic system, although the contribution of these areas to respiratory control is unclear.

Mechanism of Action

An elevation of arterial P_{CO_2} causes an approximately equal rise of extracellular fluid, CSF, cerebral tissue and jugular venous P_{CO_2}, which are all approximately 1.3 kPa (10 mmHg) more than the arterial P_{CO_2}. Over the short term, and without change in CSF bicarbonate, a rise in CSF P_{CO_2} causes a fall in CSF pH. The blood–brain barrier (operative between blood and CSF) is permeable to carbon dioxide but not hydrogen ions, and in this respect resembles the membrane of a P_{CO_2}-sensitive electrode (page 133). In both cases, carbon dioxide crosses the barrier and hydrates to carbonic acid, which then ionizes to give a pH inversely proportional to the log of the P_{CO_2}. A hydrogen ion sensor is thus made to respond to P_{CO_2}.

The mechanism by which a change in pH causes stimulation of chemoreceptor neurones remains disputed. The RTN contains neurons with proton-modulated potassium channels (TASK-2),[29] but recent work suggests complex neuroglial interactions, with astrocytes also being chemosensitive. It is possible that neurons respond to minor changes in P_{CO_2} but as hypercapnia becomes more severe nearby glial cells release adenosine triphosphate (ATP) which acts on P2Y$_1$ purinergic receptors to amplify the response.[30-32]

Compensatory Bicarbonate Shift in the CSF

If the P_{CO_2} of CSF is maintained at an abnormal level, the CSF pH gradually returns towards normal over the course of many hours as a result of changes in the CSF bicarbonate concentration. This is analogous to, and proceeds in parallel with, the partial restoration of blood pH in patients with chronic hyper- or hypocapnia. Compensatory changes in bicarbonate concentrations are similar in both CSF and blood, suggesting a common mechanism. Bicarbonate shift in CSF could therefore result simply from passive ion distribution, although the possibility of active ion transfer cannot be completely excluded. Examples of situations when this normalization of CSF pH may occur include prolonged periods of hypocapnic artificial ventilation and the hypocapnia that occurs in response to hypoxia at altitude (page 207). Once the hypocapnia is reversed, for example when the artificial ventilation is no longer required, hyperventilation may follow for several hours. Compensatory changes in CSF pH are not confined to respiratory alkalosis, but are also found in chronic respiratory acidosis, metabolic acidosis and metabolic alkalosis. If the bicarbonate concentration in CSF is altered by

pathological factors, ventilatory disturbances occur. For example, after intracranial haemorrhage patients may spontaneously hyperventilate, and in these patients the CSF pH and bicarbonate have been shown to be below normal values.

The P_{CO_2}/Ventilation Response Curve

Following a rise in arterial P_{CO_2}, respiratory depth and rate increase until a steady state of hyperventilation is achieved after a few minutes. The response is linear over the range that is usually studied, and may therefore be defined in terms of two parameters: slope and intercept (see Appendix E):

$$\text{ventilation} = S(P_{CO_2} - B)$$

where S is the slope (L.min^{-1}.kPa^{-1} or L.min^{-1}.mmHg^{-1}), and B is the intercept at zero ventilation (kPa or mmHg). The bold red line in Figure 4.6 is a typical normal curve with an intercept (B) of approximately 4.8 kPa (36 mmHg) and a slope (S) of approximately 15 L.min^{-1}.kPa^{-1} (2 L.min^{-1}.mmHg^{-1}). There is in fact a wide variation in both the slope and intercept of individual P_{CO_2}/ventilation response curves. There is a circadian variation within individuals, a reduced intercept with increasing age and a change to the slope in response to hormones, disease or drugs. The dashed curve in Figure 4.6 shows the effect of changing ventilation on arterial P_{CO_2} when the inspired carbon dioxide concentration is negligible, and is a section of a rectangular hyperbola. The normal resting P_{CO_2} and

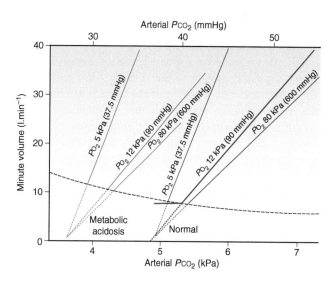

• **Fig. 4.6** Two fans of P_{CO_2}/ventilation response curves at different values of P_{O_2}. The right-hand fan is at normal metabolic acid-base state (zero base excess). The left-hand fan represents metabolic acidosis. The broken line represents the P_{CO_2} produced by the indicated ventilation for zero inspired P_{CO_2}, at basal metabolic rate. The intersection of the broken curve and any response curve indicates the resting P_{CO_2} and ventilation for the relevant metabolic acid-base state and P_{O_2}. The bold red curve is the normal response. See text for details.

ventilation are indicated by the intersection of this curve with the normal P_{CO_2}/ventilation response curve, which is usually obtained by varying the carbon dioxide concentration in the inspired gas.

When subjects hyperventilate voluntarily and reduce their P_{CO_2} below the threshold for carbon dioxide stimulation of respiration, a variety of responses are seen, varying from apnoea to normal respiration or even hyperventilation.[33] Figure 4.6 shows two possible extensions to the normal response curve (*in red*) below the threshold for carbon dioxide stimulation (*dashed line*). The first is an extrapolation of the curve to intersect the *x*-axis (zero ventilation) at a P_{CO_2}, known as the apnoeic threshold (dotted lines in Fig. 4.6). If P_{CO_2} is depressed below this point, apnoea may result, which is seen in some subjects. The second type of extension (shown on the *bold red line*) is horizontal and to the left, like a hockey stick, representing the response of a subject who continues to breathe regardless of the fact that his or her P_{CO_2} has been reduced. The resting arterial point at resting ventilation is normally approximately 0.3 kPa to the left of the extrapolated response curve,[34] supporting the idea of a hockey stick–shaped response curve. When breathing below this threshold for the onset of carbon dioxide–stimulated ventilation (the angle of the hockey stick), hypoxia seems to have no influence.[33] This variable ventilatory response to low P_{CO_2} almost certainly arises from the cortical control of respiration maintaining breathing despite a lack of chemical drive, particularly when awake.

As P_{CO_2} climbs higher, a point of maximal ventilatory stimulation is reached, probably within the range of 13.3 to 26.7 kPa (100–200 mmHg), beyond which respiratory fatigue and carbon dioxide narcosis intervene (Chapter 22). The ventilatory stimulation is reduced until, at very high P_{CO_2}, ventilation is actually depressed below the control value, and finally apnoea results.

The P_{CO_2}/ventilation response curve is the response of the entire respiratory system to the challenge of a raised P_{CO_2}. Apart from reduced sensitivity of the central chemoreceptors, the overall response may be blunted by respiratory muscle weakness or by obstructive or restrictive lung disease. These factors must be considered when drawing conclusions from a reduced response, and diffuse airway obstruction is a most important consideration. Nevertheless the slope of the P_{CO_2}/ventilation response curve remains one of the most valuable parameters in the assessment of the responsiveness of the respiratory system to carbon dioxide and its depression by drugs.

Time Course of P_{CO_2}/Ventilation Response

As described previously, the initial ventilatory response to elevated P_{CO_2} is extremely rapid, occurring within just a few minutes, at which time approximately 75% of the final ventilatory response has occurred. With sustained hypercapnia, the minute ventilation continues to increase for a further hour before reaching a plateau, which is sustained for at least 8 hours in healthy subjects.

The Influence of Oxygen on Respiratory Control

As for carbon dioxide, it was initially thought that hypoxia stimulated respiration by a direct effect on the respiratory centre, until the respiratory role of the peripheral chemoreceptors in the carotid body (CB) was established by Heymans,[35] who received a Nobel prize for his work.

Peripheral Chemoreceptors[36]

The peripheral chemoreceptors are fast-responding monitors of the arterial blood, responding to a fall in arterial P_{O_2}, a rise in arterial P_{CO_2} or H^+ concentration, or a reduction in their perfusion. An increase in ventilation is the result of stimulation. The bilaterally paired CBs, rather than the aortic bodies, are almost exclusively responsible for the respiratory response. Human CBs are approximately 20 mm^3 in volume[37] and are located close to the bifurcation of the common carotid artery. The CBs undergo hyperplasia under conditions of chronic hypoxia, even if intermittent, such as with sleep-disordered breathing (Chapter 14) and are usually lost following carotid endarterectomy (see later).

Histology shows the CBs to contain large sinusoids with a high rate of perfusion, about 10 times the level that would be proportional to their metabolic rate, which is also high. Therefore the arterial/venous P_{O_2} difference is small. This accords with their role as a sensor of arterial blood gas tensions, as well as with their rapid response, which is within the range of 1 to 3 s. At the cellular level, their main feature is the glomus or type I cell, which is in synaptic contact with the carotid sinus nerve endings, derived from axons with their cell bodies in the petrosal ganglion of the glossopharyngeal nerve. Efferent nerves, which are known to modulate receptor afferent discharge, include preganglionic sympathetic fibres from the superior cervical ganglion, amounting to 5% of the nerve endings on the glomus cell. Discharge rate in the afferent nerves from the CB increases in response to the following forms of stimulation.

Hypoxaemic stimulation is by decreased P_{O_2} and not by reduced oxygen content (at least down to about half the normal value). Thus there is little stimulation in anaemia, carboxyhaemoglobinaemia or methaemoglobinaemia. Quantitative aspects of the hypoxic ventilatory response are described in detail next.

Acidaemia of perfusing blood causes stimulation, the magnitude of which is the same whether from respiratory or metabolic acidosis. Quantitatively, the change produced by elevated P_{CO_2} on the peripheral chemoreceptors is only about one-sixth of that caused by the action on the central chemosensitive areas (see later). This response does, however, occur very rapidly,[28] and only develops when a 'threshold' value of arterial P_{CO_2} is exceeded.[33]

Hypoperfusion, for example, from severe systemic hypotension, causes stimulation, possibly by causing a 'stagnant hypoxia' of the chemoreceptor cells (as discussed later).

Blood temperature elevation causes stimulation of breathing via the peripheral chemoreceptors. In addition, the ventilatory responses to both hypoxia and CO_2 are enhanced by a modest (1.4°C) rise in body temperature.

In vitro animal studies have found type I cells to be sensitive to glucose concentration, but the implications for this in vivo remain unclear.[38]

Chemical stimulation by a wide range of substances is known to cause increased ventilation through the medium of the peripheral chemoreceptors. These substances fall into two groups. The first comprises agents such as nicotine and acetylcholine that stimulate sympathetic ganglia. The second group of chemical stimulants comprises substances such as cyanide and carbon monoxide which block the cytochrome system, preventing oxidative metabolism. Drugs which stimulate respiration via the peripheral chemoreceptors are described in following sections.

Mechanism of Action of Peripheral Chemoreceptors[36,39]

There is now agreement that oxygen-sensitive potassium channels are responsible for the hypoxic response of type I cells,[40] and similar channels are found in most cells of the body that respond to hypoxia.[38,39] Many different oxygen-sensitive potassium channels exist, with varying types occurring in different species, in different tissues and under different circumstances within a species. Hypoxia inhibits the activity of the potassium channel, which alters the membrane potential of the cell and stimulates calcium channels to open, allowing an influx of extracellular calcium, which stimulates transmitter release. The molecular mechanism by which potassium channels respond to Po_2 is unknown, including whether or not there is a direct effect on the channel or whether other hypoxia-induced molecules are responsible. Contenders for this role include the following:

- Reactive oxygen species (Chapter 25) produced either from mitochondria or from reduced nicotinamide adenine dinucleotide phosphate oxidase.
- Hydrogen sulphide (H_2S) gas is produced in tissues by the enzyme cystothionine γ-lyase, and studies in knock-out mice without the gene encoding cystothionine γ-lyase found a severely impaired response to hypoxia.[41] Further evidence for a role for H_2S comes from enhancing the response to hypoxia by infusing H_2S donor molecules, although the mechanism of action remains unknown.
- Carbon monoxide produced by haem oxygenase, an antioxidant enzyme constitutively expressed in most cells and closely associated with the potassium channels in type I cells. Carbon monoxide inhibits the sensory activity of the CB, but under hypoxic conditions haem oxygenase is impaired and carbon monoxide production decreases, resulting in increased H_2S production.[42]

These molecular interactions all take place close to the membrane of the type I cells, where the mitochondria, potassium channels and numerous other proteins are co-located.[42]

Various neurotransmitters have been identified within the CB, but acetylcholine and ATP act as the principal excitatory transmitter molecules between the type I cells and the carotid sinus neurones.[39] Many other molecules are present in CBs, but these seem to have an autocrine rather than a neurotransmitter role, in that their release into the CB tissues modulates the response of the cells to the various stimuli. Examples include the following:

- Dopamine, which is abundant in type I cells and released in response to hypoxia, causes inhibition of neurotransmitter release by both presynaptic and postsynaptic mechanisms, in effect 'damping' the response. Low-dose infusion in humans impairs both the hypoxic ventilatory response and the haemodynamic response normally seen with acute hypoxia.[43]
- ATP, as well as acting as a neurotransmitter, has a role in modulating CB stimulation. Accumulation of ATP, and its breakdown product adenosine, within the CB seems to cause the type II cells to release further ATP, enhancing the response. Adenosine may be most important in mild hypoxia, and ATP in severe hypoxia.[44]
- Nitric oxide is released in the CB from neurones containing neuronal nitric oxide synthase (page 80) which form an efferent inhibitory pathway acting on the CB. Once released, NO inhibits CB activity indirectly by affecting vascular tone and directly by inhibiting calcium channels and exerting a negative feedback effect on ATP release.[39] There is evidence that changes in this system of CB modulation are responsible for alterations in oxygen sensitivity in some diseases such as heart failure and sleep-disordered breathing.[45]

Other Effects of Stimulation

Apart from the well-known increase in depth and rate of breathing, peripheral chemoreceptor stimulation causes a number of other effects, including bradycardia, peripheral vasoconstriction, hypertension, increase in bronchiolar tone and adrenal secretion. These interactions between CB activity and sympathetic outflow provide the physiological link for the frequent associations between pulmonary and cardiovascular diseases.[46]

Time Course of the Ventilatory Response to Hypoxia[47]

By controlling the concentration of inhaled oxygen, arterial oxygen saturation can be reduced and then maintained at a constant level of hypoxia, usually with an oxygen saturation (Sa_{O_2}) of about 80%. To separate the effects on ventilation of hypoxia and Pco_2, most studies use isocapnic conditions, where the subject's alveolar Pco_2 is maintained at his or her control (resting ventilation) level by the addition of carbon dioxide to the inspired gas. The interaction of Pco_2 and hypoxia in ventilatory control is discussed later. With a moderate degree of sustained hypoxia, the ventilatory response is triphasic, as shown in Figure 4.7. The three phases are described separately.

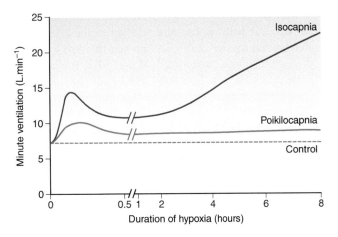

• **Fig. 4.7** Time course of the ventilatory response to hypoxia (Sa_{O_2} 80%). Practical problems prevent the continuous and rapid measurement of minute volume and respiratory gases for 8 hours, so the curves are produced from combining the data from three studies. When arterial Pco_2 is maintained at normal levels (isocapnia), the response is triphasic. When arterial Pco_2 is not controlled (poikilocapnia), the magnitude of the response is damped because the hypoxia-induced hyperventilation reduces Pco_2 and therefore respiratory drive. See Figure 16.3 for respiratory effects of prolonged hypoxia.

Acute Hypoxic Ventilatory Response

This is the first immediate and rapid increase in ventilation. Sudden imposition of hypoxia results in stimulation of ventilation within the lung-to-carotid body circulation time (about 6 s), but in most studies the response appears slower because of the delay between reducing inspired oxygen and the reduction in alveolar and then arterial Po_2. Ventilation continues to increase for between 5 and 10 minutes, rapidly reaching high levels.

Many factors affect the acute hypoxic ventilatory response (AHVR). There are wide variations between individuals, within an individual on different days, between male and female subjects and with the hormonal changes of the menstrual cycle. The response is reduced in older subjects.[48] A small number of otherwise normal subjects lack a measurable AHVR when studied at normal Pco_2. This is of little importance under normal circumstances, because the Pco_2 drive from the central chemoreceptors will normally ensure a safe level of Po_2. However, in certain therapeutic and abnormal environmental circumstances, such as at high altitude, it could be dangerous.

Hypoxic Ventilatory Decline

Shortly after the acute hypoxic response reaches a peak, minute ventilation begins to decline, reaching a plateau level, still above the resting ventilation, after 20 to 30 minutes (Fig. 4.7). The degree of hypoxic ventilatory decline (HVD) in an individual correlates with the acute hypoxic response—the greater the initial increase in ventilation, the greater the subsequent decline. Although not completely elucidated yet, the mechanism of HVD appears to be a centrally mediated change in ventilatory drive rather than a decline in the sensitivity of the CB receptors to hypoxia.[49,50] Animal work suggests that neuroglial interactions are responsible, in a similar way to the involvement of astrocytes in central pH responsiveness and glomus cells in the carotid body. Potential neurotransmitters for these cell-to-cell interactions are D-serine, glutamate and ATP.[51]

Response to Sustained Hypoxia

Once HVD is complete, continued isocapnic hypoxia results in a second slower rise in ventilation over several hours (Fig. 4.7). Ventilation continues to increase for at least 8 hours and reaches a plateau by 24 hours. Species differences in this response again make elucidation of the mechanism in humans difficult, but the most likely explanation is a direct effect of hypoxia on the CBs, possibly mediated by angiotensin II (page 170).

Hypoxia for more than 2 to 3 days only occurs following ascent to altitude, and the effects of this are described in Chapter 16.

Ventilatory Response to Progressive Hypoxia

Instead of maintaining a constant degree of hypoxia, ventilation may be measured during a progressive reduction in Po_2. Once again, by controlling inspired gas concentrations, alveolar Po_2 may be reduced from to 5 kPa (40 mmHg) over 15 minutes, and ventilation increases progressively throughout this period. The response under these circumstances probably equates to the AHVR. If alveolar Po_2 is plotted against minute ventilation, a Po_2/ventilation response curve is produced (Fig. 4.8). A Po_2/ventilation response curve approximates to a rectangular hyperbola (see Appendix E), asymptotic to the ventilation at high arterial Po_2 (zero hypoxic drive) and to the arterial Po_2, at which ventilation theoretically becomes infinite (known as 'C' and approximately 4.3 kPa). Figure 4.8 shows a typical example, but there are very wide individual variations. Note that there is a small but measurable difference in ventilation between normal and very high Po_2.

The initial ventilatory response to Po_2 may be expressed as:

$$\frac{W}{Pa_{O_2} - C}$$

where W is a multiplier (i.e., the gain of the system) and partly dependent on the Pco_2. The ventilatory response here is the difference between the actual ventilation and the ventilation at high Po_2, Pco_2 being unchanged.

The inconvenience of the nonlinear relationship between ventilation and Po_2 may be overcome by plotting ventilation against oxygen saturation. The relationship is then linear with a negative slope, at least down to a saturation of 70%. This approach is the basis of a simple noninvasive method of measurement of the hypoxic ventilatory response (see the following section).

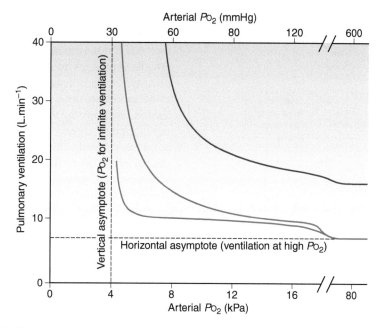

• **Fig. 4.8** Ventilatory response to progressive hypoxia. The green curve represents the normal P_{O_2}/ventilation response under isocapnic conditions, that is with P_{CO_2} maintained at the resting value. It has the form of a rectangular hyperbola asymptotic to the ventilation at high P_{O_2} and the P_{O_2} at which ventilation becomes infinite. The curve is displaced upwards by both hypercapnia and exercise at normal P_{CO_2} (*red line*). Hypocapnia displaces the curve downwards (*blue line*) regardless of whether the hypocapnia results from not controlling P_{CO_2} (poikilocapnia) or by deliberately reducing P_{CO_2}.

Iatrogenic Loss of Peripheral Chemoreceptor Sensitivity[52]

Nerves from the CBs are usually divided during bilateral carotid endarterectomy, and in most patients this abolishes the acute hypoxic response,[53] providing evidence that the CBs are not essential for normal breathing under conditions of rest and mild exercise. Indeed, there is some evidence that the common finding of atheromatous disease at the carotid bifurcation may reduce chemoreceptor function, and that a careful, 'nerve-sparing', carotid endarterectomy can increase the ventilatory response to hypoxia.[54]

Central Hypoxic Depression of Breathing

In addition to its effects on peripheral chemoreceptors, hypoxia also has a direct effect on the respiratory centre. Central respiratory neurone activity is depressed by hypoxia, and apnoea follows severe medullary hypoxia whether because of ischaemia or to hypoxaemia. With denervated peripheral chemoreceptors, phrenic motor activity becomes silent when the medullary P_{O_2} falls to approximately 1.7 kPa (13 mmHg). More intense hypoxia causes a resumption of breathing with an abnormal pattern, possibly driven by a 'gasping' centre. This pattern of central hypoxic depression appears to be particularly marked in neonates and may be the relic of a mechanism to prevent the foetus from attempting to breathe in utero.

Integration of the Chemical Control of Breathing

The two main systems contributing to chemical control of breathing have been described quite separately, but in the intact subject this is not possible. For example, the peripheral chemoreceptors respond (slightly) to changes in P_{CO_2}, and hypoxia affects the respiratory centre directly as well as via the CB receptors. An overall view of the chemical control of breathing is shown schematically in Figure 4.9.

It was originally thought that the various factors interacted according to the algebraic sum of the individual effects caused by changes of P_{CO_2}, P_{O_2}, pH, and so on.[55] Hypoxia and hypercapnia were, for example, thought to be simply additive in their effects, but it is now realized that this was a very simplistic view of a complex system.[56,57]

Effects of P_{CO_2} and pH on the Hypoxic Ventilatory Response

The acute hypoxic response is enhanced at elevated P_{CO_2}, as shown by the upper red curve in Figure 4.8, the mechanism being indicated by broken line B in Figure 4.9. This interaction contributes to the ventilatory response in asphyxia being greater than the sum of the response to be expected from the rise in P_{CO_2} and the fall in P_{O_2} if considered separately.

Responses to both acute and prolonged hypoxia are depressed by hypocapnia, as shown in the lower blue curve in Figure 4.8 and the lower green curve in Figure 4.7. This results

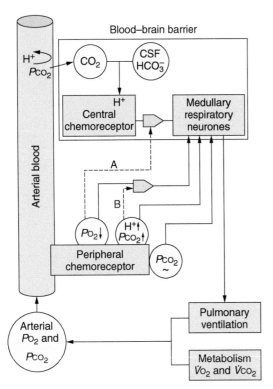

• **Fig. 4.9** Scheme of connections between individual aspects of chemical control of breathing. See text for details. *CSF,* Cerebrospinal fluid.

from opposing effects on the CPG of increased chemoreceptor input because of the hypoxia and decreased central chemoreceptor drive from the hypocapnia. A similar situation exists with poikilocapnia during hypoxic ventilation, when no attempt is made to control Pco_2 and the hypoxia-induced hyperventilation immediately gives rise to hypocapnia. Although rarely studied by physiologists, this situation is important, as poikilocapnia will occur in clinical situations. Poikilocapnic conditions attenuate, but do not abolish, all the phases of the ventilatory response to constant hypoxia (Fig. 4.7). On prolonged exposure to hypoxia at altitude, this effect continues until acclimatization takes place (page 207).

Exercise enhances the response to hypoxia even if the Pco_2 is not raised, possibly because of lactic acidosis, oscillations of arterial Pco_2 (page 187), afferent input from muscle or catecholamine secretion. The upper red curve in Figure 4.8 would also correspond to the response during exercise at an oxygen consumption of approximately 800 mL.min^{-1}. It is important to note that the slope of the curve at normal Po_2 is considerably increased in both these circumstances, so there will then be an appreciable 'hypoxic' drive to ventilation at normal Po_2. Enhanced response to Po_2 during exercise seems to be an important component in the overall ventilatory response to exercise (Chapter 13).

Effects of Po_2 and pH on Central Chemoreceptor Response[33,58]

The broken line (A) in Figure 4.9 shows the influence of the peripheral chemoreceptor drive on the gain of the central

ventilatory response to Pco_2. Typical quantitative relationships are shown in Figure 4.6, with hypoxia at the left of each fan and hyperoxia on the right. The curve marked Po_2 80 kPa represents total abolition of chemoreceptor drive obtained by the inhalation of 100% oxygen.

Metabolic acidosis displaces the whole fan of curves to the left, as shown by the blue lines in Figure 4.6. The intercept (apnoeic threshold) is reduced, but the slope of the curves at each value of Po_2 is virtually unaltered. Display of the fan of Pco_2/ventilation response curves at different Po_2 values is a particularly complete method of representing the state of respiratory control in a patient but is impractical to determine.

Periodic Breathing

This term describes a respiratory pattern in which ventilation waxes and wanes in a regular sequence. It is normal in neonates (page 180), but is seen only during sleep in adults, occurring more frequently in the elderly[59] and in all ages when sleeping at altitude (page 213). The cause of periodic breathing is unknown, but may involve an abnormality of the chemical control of breathing, a poorly responsive control system or an abnormality of the interaction between neurone groups in the CPG.[60] Cheyne–Stokes respiration is an extreme form of periodic breathing in which apnoea occurs during the hypoventilation phase, and is seen most commonly in patients with heart failure. In the case of Cheyne–Stokes respiration, abnormalities of respiratory control and lung function contribute, but the slow circulation time seen in patients with heart failure introduces further periodicity and resonance into the breathing pattern.[61]

Breath Holding

Consciously attempting to stop breathing for as long as possible, usually after taking in a large breath, represents a complex physiological challenge. Although initially quite comfortable, after a variable amount of time the urge to breathe increases, involuntary breathing movements begin, and respiratory discomfort and distress develop before the glottis is opened and the breath hold 'breaks'.[62] Multiple factors affect the duration of a breath hold.

Influence of Pco_2 and Po_2

When the breath is held after air breathing, the arterial and alveolar Pco_2 are remarkably constant at the breaking point, and values are normally close to 6.7 kPa (50 mmHg). This does not mean that Pco_2 is the sole or dominant factor, and concomitant hypoxia is probably more important. Preliminary oxygen breathing delays the onset of hypoxia, and breath-holding times may be greatly prolonged, with consequent elevation of Pco_2 at the breaking point. The relationship between Pco_2 and Po_2 at breaking point, after starting from different levels of oxygenation, is shown in Figure 4.10.

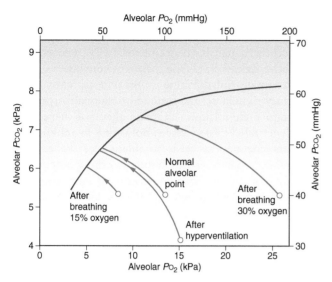

• **Fig. 4.10** The 'breaking point' curve defines the coexisting values of alveolar P_{O_2} and P_{CO_2}, at the breaking point of breath holding, starting from various states. The normal alveolar point is shown, and the curved blue arrows show the changes in alveolar gas partial pressures that occur during breath holding. Starting points are displaced to the right by preliminary breathing of oxygen-enriched gases, and to the left by breathing mixtures containing less than 21% oxygen. Hyperventilation displaces the point representing alveolar gas to the right and downwards. The length of the arrows from the starting point to the breaking point curve gives an approximate indication of the duration of breath hold. This can clearly be prolonged by oxygen breathing or by hyperventilation, with maximal duration occurring after hyperventilation with 100% oxygen.

On the basis of changing blood gas tensions and the great variability of individuals' responses, it might be predicted that subjects with 'flat' ventilatory responses to oxygen and carbon dioxide would be able to hold their breath longer.

Effect of Lung Volume

Breath-holding time is directly proportional to the lung volume at the onset of breath holding, partly because this has a major influence on oxygen stores. There are, however, other effects of lung volume and its change, which are mediated by afferents arising from the chest wall, the diaphragm and the lung itself. Prolongation of breath-holding times is seen after bilateral vagal and glossopharyngeal nerve block, and following complete muscular paralysis of conscious subjects. These observations suggest that much of the distress leading to the termination of breath holding is caused by frustration of the involuntary contractions of the respiratory muscles, which increase progressively during breath holding. Fowler's experiment in 1954 easily demonstrated the importance of frustration of involuntary respiratory movements.[63] After normal air breathing, the breath is held until breaking point. If the expirate is then exhaled into a bag and immediately reinhaled, there is a marked

sense of relief, although it may be shown that the rise of P_{CO_2} and fall of P_{O_2} are uninfluenced.

Extreme durations of breath holding may be attained after hyperventilation and preoxygenation. Times of 14 minutes have been reached, and the limiting factor is then reduction of lung volume to residual volume, as oxygen is removed from the alveolar gas. The physiology of breath-hold diving is described on page 221.

Drug Effects on the Control of Breathing

Considering the therapeutic potential of drugs that could specifically influence respiratory drive, it is surprising that so few drugs affecting respiratory control have been developed. The large number of different receptors involved in normal respiratory control (Fig. 4.4) means that drugs affecting a single receptor may have little effect, or unpredictable effects, on respiration, and so be of little clinical use. In addition, the neurotransmitters and neuromodulators involved are widely distributed throughout the CNS, so agonists or antagonists of their receptors are likely to have diverse effects resulting in unacceptable adverse effects.

Many other factors apart from the drug itself affect respiratory activity, so the effect that a drug exerts on the respiration of an individual patient is complex and unpredictable. For example, in a healthy patient recovering from surgery under general anaesthesia, pain, anxiety, stress and changes in blood chemistry will stimulate breathing, whereas sedation, sleep and residual anaesthetic or analgesic agents will tend to depress respiration.

Respiratory Depressants

Any drug that depresses CNS activity may depress respiration, either individually or in combination with other CNS depressants such as alcohol. Almost all general anaesthetic agents reduce ventilation in a dose-dependent fashion and are described on page 244. Two specific groups of drugs that have well-documented depressant effects on ventilation are opioid analgesics and benzodiazepines.

Opioids[64]

Figure 4.4 shows that both μ- and δ-opioid receptors are present in the respiratory centre. As previously indicated, the role of these receptors in normal respiratory control is unknown. Animal studies suggest that μ-receptors in the pre-Bötzinger complex (Fig. 4.2) may be involved in normal respiratory control.[64] In humans, the evidence is less clear. In healthy subjects, administration of the nonspecific opioid receptor antagonist naloxone has no effect on respiration.

Agonists of μ-opioid receptors, such as morphine, cause dose-dependent depression of respiration normally characterized by a slow respiratory rate, but tidal volume is also commonly reduced. Ventilatory responses to hypoxia and hypercapnia are also severely impaired, removing the physiological safety mechanism for patients, and the cough reflex is suppressed. Partial agonists at the μ-receptor, such as nalbuphine and buprenorphine, have a ceiling effect for their analgesic efficacy that is associated with a lesser effect on ventilation than full agonists. Most of the analgesic effects of clinically used opioids are also mediated by the μ-receptor, so the respiratory depressant effect of opioid drugs is currently inseparable from their therapeutic effect. Equianalgesic doses of different opioids show similar degrees of respiratory depression, but the speed of onset of the drug does affect the clinical pattern of respiratory depression that occurs. With rapidly acting opioids such as fentanyl, apnoea normally follows its intravenous administration, but when an equianalgesic dose of the slower acting morphine is administered, apnoea is unusual, because hypercapnia develops to counteract the respiratory depression. Female subjects show a greater susceptibility to the respiratory depressant effects of opioids.[64,65] A subject's baseline ventilatory response to hypercapnia may, in part, determine his or her likelihood of developing opioid-induced respiratory depression.[66] Neonates have greater numbers of opioid receptors in the their brainstems, possibly indicating a role for endogenous opioids in depressing respiratory activity in utero, but also making them more susceptible to apnoea if given exogenous opioids.[65] Although not directly studied, indirect evidence suggests that this increased susceptibility to opioid-induced respiratory depression continues into childhood. This may have severe consequences, including death,[67] particularly in the postoperative period in children who also have renal failure, altered metabolism of opioids or obstructive sleep apnoea.[68]

Benzodiazepines

Benzodiazepines exert their effect by binding directly to $GABA_A$ receptors and increasing the inhibitory effect of endogenous GABA. Figure 4.4 shows that GABA is involved in respiratory CPG, so it is unsurprising that benzodiazepines affect respiration. Parenterally administered benzodiazepine drugs, such as midazolam or diazepam, cause a dose-dependent reduction in resting ventilation and reduce the ventilatory response to hypoxia and hypercapnia. The degree of respiratory impairment seen correlates well with their effect on consciousness. Reduced resting ventilation with midazolam can be reversed with the benzodiazepine antagonist flumazenil, although the responses to hypoxia and hypercapnia may still be abnormal despite the subjects no longer being sedated.[69] Unlike for opioids, the respiratory depressant effects of benzodiazepines seem to have a ceiling effect, with massive overdoses of these drugs rarely causing life-threatening respiratory depression unless other CNS depressants, commonly alcohol, are ingested simultaneously.

Respiratory Stimulants[70]

Nonspecific CNS stimulant drugs have existed for many years, and, as part of their general stimulant effects, also increase respiratory drive. Early drugs of this type such as nikethamide were used as respiratory stimulants, but at doses effective for stimulating respiration they had an unacceptably high incidence of toxic CNS effects such as headache, agitation, muscle spasms or convulsions.

Doxapram and almitrine are the only currently used respiratory stimulants, and seem to be reasonably specific for respiratory stimulation, although they still have a high incidence of CNS side effects. Both work by inhibiting potassium channels to cause stimulation of the peripheral chemoreceptors to increase respiratory drive; this effect occurs at lower doses than those causing more generalized CNS stimulation. In healthy subjects, infusion of a standard dose of doxapram approximately doubles resting minute volume, and also substantially increases the ventilatory responses to hypoxia and hypercapnia. Despite this impressive action on respiratory control, when used to treat patients with type 2 ventilatory failure (page 316), generalized CNS stimulation undoubtedly contributes to the therapeutic effect by reversing the sedative effects of hypercapnia (page 269) and increasing the patient's perception of his or her breathlessness.[71]

Methods for Assessment of Breathing Control

In assessing the control of breathing under ideal conditions, arterial blood gas tensions would be measured continuously. In practice, this is invasive, and rapid measurements are impossible, so in almost all cases end-tidal gas concentration is measured and converted to partial pressure. In normal healthy subjects with reasonable slow respiratory rates, these measurements will equate well to alveolar and therefore arterial tension, but this may not be the case in patients.

Sensitivity to Carbon Dioxide

A lack of ventilatory response to carbon dioxide may result from impaired function of the respiratory system anywhere between the medullary neurones and the mechanical properties of the lung (see Fig. 27.2). Thus it cannot be assumed that a decreased $P\text{CO}_2$/ventilation response is necessarily because of failure of the central chemoreceptor mechanism.

Steady-State Method

This technique requires the simultaneous measurement of minute volume and $P\text{CO}_2$ after $P\text{CO}_2$ has been raised by increasing the concentration of carbon dioxide in the inspired gas. The ventilation is usually reasonably stable after 5 minutes of inhaling a fixed concentration of carbon dioxide. Severinghaus's pseudo steady-state method[72] measures ventilation after 4 minutes and is a useful compromise giving highly repeatable results.[34] Several points are needed to define the $P\text{CO}_2$/ventilation response curve, and it is a time-consuming process, which may be distressing to some patients.

Rebreathing Method

Introduced by Read in 1967, this technique greatly simplified determination of the slope of the $P\text{CO}_2$/ventilation response curve.[73] The subject rebreathes for up to 4 minutes from a 6-L bag originally containing 7% carbon dioxide and approximately 50% oxygen (the remainder is nitrogen). The carbon dioxide concentration rises steadily during rebreathing, whereas the oxygen concentration should remain above 30%. Thus there will be no appreciable hypoxic drive, and ventilation will be driven solely by the rising arterial $P\text{CO}_2$, which should be very close to the $P\text{CO}_2$ of the gas in the bag. Ventilation is measured by any convenient means and plotted against the $P\text{CO}_2$ of the gas in the bag. The $P\text{CO}_2$/ventilation response curve measured by the rebreathing technique is displaced to the right by approximately 0.7 kPa (5 mmHg) compared with the steady-state method, but the slope agrees closely with the steady-state method,[34,64] and the technique is much easier to perform.

Sensitivity to Hypoxia[74]

There is often some reluctance to test sensitivity to hypoxia because of the reduced $P\text{O}_2$ to which the patient is exposed. Various approaches to the problem have been described, of which three are used (albeit rarely) in practice.

Steady-State Method

This is the classical technique and is best undertaken by preparing $P\text{CO}_2$/ventilation response curves at different levels of $P\text{O}_2$, which are presented as a fan (Fig. 4.6). The spread of the fan is an indication of peripheral chemoreceptor sensitivity, but it is also possible to present the data in the form of the rectangular hyperbola (Fig. 4.8) by plotting the ventilatory response for different values of $P\text{O}_2$ at the same $P\text{CO}_2$.

Rebreathing Method

Read's rebreathing method is described earlier, and has been adapted to measure the response to hypoxia. The oxygen concentration of the rebreathed gas is reduced by the oxygen consumption of the subject, but active steps have to be taken to maintain the $P\text{CO}_2$ at a constant level. Calculation of the response is greatly simplified by measuring the oxygen saturation (usually noninvasively by means of a pulse oximeter) and plotting the response as ventilation against saturation. This normally approximates to a straight line, and the slope is a function of the chemoreceptor sensitivity. However, even if $P\text{CO}_2$ is held constant, the response is directly influenced by the patient's sensitivity to $P\text{CO}_2$.

Intermittent Inhalation of High Oxygen Concentration

This method avoids exposing subjects to hypoxia. Temporary withdrawal of peripheral chemoreceptor drive by inhalation of oxygen should reduce ventilation by approximately 15%. This may be used as an indication of the existence of CB activity, but clearly it is much less sensitive than the steady-state method.

References

1. Richter DW, Smith JC. Respiratory rhythm generation in vivo. *Physiol.* 2014;29:58-71.
2. Del Negro CA, Hayes JA. A 'group pacemaker' mechanism for respiratory rhythm generation. *J Physiol.* 2008;586:2245-2246.
3. Ramirez JM, Telgkamp P, Elsen FP, et al. Respiratory rhythm generation in mammals: synaptic and membrane properties. *Respir Physiol.* 1997;110:71-85.
4. Horn EM, Waldrop TG. Suprapontine control of respiration. *Respir Physiol.* 1998;114:201-211.
5. Kinkead R, Tenorio L, Drolet G, et al. Respiratory manifestations of panic disorder in animals and humans: A unique opportunity to understand how supramedullary structures regulate breathing. *Respir Physiol Neurobiol.* 2014;204:3-13.
6. Tipton MJ, Harper A, Paton JFR, et al. The human ventilatory response to stress: rate or depth? *J Physiol.* 2017;595:5729-5752.
7. Western PJ, Patrick JM. Effects of focusing attention on breathing with and without apparatus on the face. *Respir Physiol.* 1988;72:123-130.
8. Matsuo K, Hiiemae KM, Gonzalez-Fernandez M, et al. Respiration during feeding on solid food: alterations in breathing during mastication, pharyngeal bolus aggregation, and swallowing. *J Appl Physiol.* 2008;104:674-681.
9. Traser L, Özen AC, Burk F, et al. Respiratory dynamics in phonation and breathing—A real-time MRI study. *Respir Physiol Neurobiol.* 2017;236:69-77.
10. Winkworth AL, Davis PJ, Adams RD, et al. Breathing patterns during spontaneous speech. *J Speech Hear Res.* 1995;38:124-144.
11. Severinghaus JW, Mitchell RA. Ondines curse: failure of respiratory centre automaticity while asleep. *Clin Res.* 1962;10:122.
12. Ramanantsoa N, Gallego J. Congenital central hypoventilation syndrome. *Respir Physiol Neurobiol.* 2013;189:272-279.
13. Widdicombe JG. Afferent receptors in the airways and cough. *Respir Physiol.* 1998;114:5-15.
14. Widdicombe J, Fontana G. Cough. Whats in a name? *Eur Respir J.* 2006;28:10-15.
15. Smith JA, Aliverti A, Quaranta M, et al. Chest wall dynamics during voluntary and induced cough in healthy volunteers. *J Physiol.* 2012;590:563-574.
16. Tatar M, Hanacek J, Widdicombe J. The expiration reflex from the trachea and bronchi. *Eur Respir J.* 2008;31:385-390.
17. Taylor-Clark T, Undem BJ. Transduction mechanisms in airway sensory nerves. *J Appl Physiol.* 2006;101:950-959.
18. Bonham AC, Chen C-Y, Sekizawa S, et al. Plasticity in the nucleus tractus solitarius and its influence on lung and airway reflexes. *J Appl Physiol.* 2006;101:322-327.
19. Ullman E. About Hering and Breuer. In: Porter R, ed. *Breathing: Hering-Breuer Centenary Symposium.* Edinburgh and London: Churchill Livingstone; 1970:3.
20. Guz A, Noble MIM, Trenchard D, et al. Studies on the vagus nerves in man: their role in respiratory and circulatory control. *Clin Sci.* 1964;27:293-304.
21. BuSha BF, Stella MH, Manning HL, et al. Termination of inspiration by phase dependent respiratory vagal feedback in awake normal humans. *J Appl Physiol.* 2002;93:903-910.
22. Rabbette PS, Fletcher ME, Dezateux CA, et al. Hering-Breuer reflex and respiratory system compliance in the first year of life: a longitudinal study. *J Appl Physiol.* 1994;76:650-656.
23. Guz A, Noble MIM, Eisle JH, et al. The effect of lung deflation on breathing in man. *Clin Sci.* 1971;40:451-461.
24. Head H. On the regulation of respiration. *J Physiol (Lond).* 1889;10:1-70.
25. Cross KW, Klaus M, Tooley WH, et al. The response of the new-born baby to inflation of the lungs. *J Physiol (Lond).* 1960;151:551-565.

26. Adriaensen D, Timmermans J-P. Breath-taking complexity of vagal C-fibre nociceptors: implications for inflammatory pulmonary disease, dyspnea and cough. *J Physiol.* 2011;589:3-4.

27. McMullan S, Pilowsky PM. The effects of baroreceptor stimulation on central respiratory drive: a review. *Respir Physiol Neurobiol.* 2010;174:37-42.

28. Nattie E. Why do we have both peripheral and central chemoreceptors? *J Appl Physiol.* 2006;100:9-10.

29. Guyenet PG, Bayliss DA, Stornetta RL, et al. Proton detection and breathing regulation by the retrotrapezoid nucleus. *J Physiol.* 2016;594:1529-1551.

30. Rajani V, Zhang Y, Revill AL, et al. The role of P2Y1 receptor signaling in central respiratory control. *Respir Physiol Neurobiol.* 2016;226:3-10.

31. Garg SK, Lioy DT, Knopp SJ, et al. Conditional depletion of methyl-CpG-binding protein 2 in astrocytes depresses the hypercapnic ventilatory response in mice. *J Appl Physiol.* 2015;119:670-676.

32. Sobrinho CR, Wenker IC, Poss EM, et al. Purinergic. Signalling contributes to chemoreception in the retrotrapezoid nucleus but not the nucleus of the solitary tract or medullary raphe. *J Physiol.* 2014;592:1309-1323.

33. Mohan R, Duffin J. The effect of hypoxia on the ventilatory response to carbon dioxide in man. *Respir Physiol.* 1997;108:101-115.

34. Lumb AB, Nunn JF. Ribcage contributions to CO2 response during rebreathing and steady state methods. *Respir Physiol.* 1991;85:97-110.

35. Heymans C, Bouckaert JJ, Dautrebande L. Sinus carotidien et réflexes respiratoire. *Arch Int Pharmacodyn Ther.* 1930;39:400.

36. López-Barneo J, Ortega-Sáenz P, Pardal R, et al. Carotid body oxygen sensing. *Eur Respir J.* 2008;32:1386-1398.

37. Ortega-Sáenz P, Pardal R, Levitsky K, et al. Cellular properties and chemosensory responses of the human carotid body. *J Physiol.* 2013;591:6157-6173.

*38. **Conde SV, Peers C. Carotid body chemotransduction gets the human touch. *J Physiol.* 2013;591:6131-6132.**

39. Nurse CA. Neurotransmitter and neuromodulatory mechanisms at peripheral arterial chemoreceptors. *Exp Physiol.* 2010;95:657-667.

40. López-Barneo J. All for one – O2-sensitive K+ channels that mediate carotid body activation. *J Physiol.* 2018;596:2951-2952.

*41. **Prabhakar NR. Carbon monoxide (CO) and hydrogen sulfide (H2S) in hypoxic sensing by the carotid body. *Respir Physiol Neurobiol.* 2012;184:165-169.**

42. Rakoczy RJ, Wyatt CN. Acute oxygen sensing by the carotid body: a rattlebag of molecular mechanisms. *J Physiol.* 2018;596:2969-2976.

43. Niewinski P, Tubek S, Banasiak W, et al. Consequences of peripheral chemoreflex inhibition with low-dose dopamine in humans. *J Physiol.* 2014;592:1295-1308.

44. Conde SV, Monteiro EC, Rigual R, et al. Hypoxic intensity: a determinant for the contribution of ATP and adenosine to the genesis of carotid body chemosensory activity. *J Appl Physiol.* 2012;112:2002-2010.

45. Porzionatoa A, Macchia V, De Caroa R, et al. Inflammatory and immunomodulatory mechanisms in the carotid body. *Respir Physiol Neurobiol.* 2013;187:31-40.

46. Bock JM. Carotid chemoreceptors: the link between pulmonary and cardiovascular disease? *J Physiol.* 2018;596:2965-2966.

47. Powell FL, Milsom WK, Mitchell GS. Time domains of the hypoxic ventilatory response. *Respir Physiol.* 1998;112:123-134.

48. Hartmann SE, Waltz X, Kissel CK, et al. Cerebrovascular and ventilatory responses to acute isocapnic hypoxia in healthy aging and lung disease: effect of vitamin C. *J Appl Physiol.* 2015;119:363-373.

49. Funk GD. CrossTalk proposal: a central hypoxia sensor contributes to the excitatory hypoxic ventilatory response. *J Physiol.* 2018;596:2935-2938.

50. Teppema LJ. CrossTalk opposing view: the hypoxic ventilatory response does not include a central, excitatory hypoxia sensing component. *J Physiol.* 2018;596:2939-2941.

*51. **Ramirez JM, Severs LJ, Ramirez SC, et al. Advances in cellular and integrative control of oxygen homeostasis within the central nervous system. *J Physiol.* 2018;596:3043-3065.**

52. Timmers HJLM, Wieling W, Karemaker JM, et al. Denervation of carotid and baro-chemoreceptors in humans. *J Physiol.* 2003;553:3-11.

53. Gourine AV, Funk GD. On the existence of a central respiratory oxygen sensor. *J Appl Physiol.* 2017;123:1344-1349.

54. Vanmaele RG, De Backer WA, Willeman MJ, et al. Hypoxic ventilatory response to carotid endarterectomy. *Eur J Vasc Surg.* 1992;6:241-244.

55. Duffin J, Mateika JH. Cross talk opposing view: peripheral and central chemoreflexes have additive effects on ventilation in humans. *J Physiol.* 2013;591:4351-4353.

56. Teppema LJ, Smith CA. Cross talk opposing view: peripheral and central chemoreceptors have hyperadditive effects on respiratory motor control. *J Physiol.* 2013;591:4359-4361.

57. Wilson RJA, Day TA. Cross talk opposing view: peripheral and central chemoreceptors have hypoadditive effects on respiratory motor output. *J Physiol.* 2013;591:4355-4357.

58. Blain GM, Smith CA, Henderson KS, et al. Peripheral chemoreceptors determine the respiratory sensitivity of central chemoreceptors to CO2. *J Physiol.* 2010;588:2455-2471.

59. Wellman A, Malhotra A, Jordan AS, et al. Chemical control stability in the elderly. *J Physiol.* 2007;581:291-298.

60. Lovering AT, Fraigne JJ, Dunin-Barkowski WL, et al. Tonic and phasic drive to medullary respiratory neurons during periodic breathing. *Respir Physiol Neurobiol.* 2012;181:286-301.

61. Sands SA, Mebrate Y, Edwards BA, et al. Resonance as the mechanism of daytime periodic breathing in patients with heart failure. *Am J Respir Crit Care Med.* 2017;195:237-246.

62. Breskovic T, Lojpur M, Maslov PZ, et al. The influence of varying inspired fractions of O2 and CO2 on the development of involuntary breathing movements during maximal apnoea. *Respir Physiol Neurobiol.* 2012;181:228-233.

63. Fowler WS. Breaking point of breath-holding. *J Appl Physiol.* 1954;6:539-545.

64. Pattinson KTS. Opioids and the control of respiration. *Br J Anaesth.* 2008;100:747-758.

65. Lalley PM. Opioidergic and dopaminergic modulation of respiration. *Respir Physiol Neurobiol.* 2008;164:160-167.

66. Potter JVF, Moon RE. Why do some patients stop breathing after taking narcotics? Ventilatory chemosensitivity as a predictor of opioid-induced respiratory depression. *J Appl Physiol.* 2015;119:420-422.

67. Brown KA, Brouillette RT. The elephant in the room: lethal apnea at home after adenotonsillectomy. *Anesth Analg.* 2014;118:1157-1159.

68. Waters KA, McBrien F, Stewart P, et al. Effects of OSA, inhalational anesthesia, and fentanyl on the airway and ventilation of children. *J Appl Physiol.* 1992;92:1987-1994.

69. Gross JB, Blouin RT, Zandsberg S, et al. Effect of flumazenil on ventilatory drive during sedation with midazolam and alfentanil. *Anesthesiology.* 1996;85:713-720.

70. Golder FJ, Hewitt MH, McLeod JF. Respiratory stimulant drugs in the post-operative setting. *Respir Physiol Neurobiol.* 2013;189:395-402.

71. Ebihara S, Ogawa H, Sasaki H, et al. Doxapram and perception of dyspnea. *Chest.* 2002;121:1380-1381.

72. Severinghaus JW. Proposed standard determination of ventilatory responses to hypoxia and hypercapnia in man. *Chest.* 1976;70:129.

73. Read DJC. A clinical method for assessing the ventilatory response to carbon dioxide. *Australas Ann Med.* 1967;16:20-32.

74. Duffin J. Measuring the ventilatory response to hypoxia. *J Physiol.* 2007;584:285-293.

5

Pulmonary Ventilation

KEY POINTS

- Pharyngeal and laryngeal muscles display both tonic and phasic contraction to maintain airway patency and to regulate airflow.
- The diaphragm, the intercostal muscles and some neck muscles bring about inspiration by a complex combination of actions, varying with different postures.
- Expiration is normally passive, except during exercise or at minute volumes several times higher than normal, when

intercostal and abdominal wall muscle contraction causes active expiration.
- The 'work of breathing' describes the power needed to overcome both the elastic recoil of the respiratory system and the nonelastic resistance to gas flow, and is normally generated by the respiratory muscles used for inspiration.

Breathing consists of rhythmic changes in lung volume brought about by the medullary respiratory neurones described in Chapter 4. Several muscle groups are involved in effecting the change in lung volume. First, muscles of the pharynx and larynx control upper airway resistance; second, the diaphragm, rib cage, spine and neck muscles bring about inspiration; and finally, muscles of the abdominal wall, rib cage and spine are used when active expiration is required. Many of these muscle groups have common origins and attachments, such that their activity is complex and dependent both on each other and many nonrespiratory factors including posture, locomotion and voluntary activity.

Upper Airway Muscles

During inspiration through the nose, the pressure in the pharynx must fall below atmospheric by an amount equal to the product of inspiratory gas flow rate and the flow resistance afforded by the nose (see Fig. 3.1). This development of only a few kilopascals of subatmospheric pressure in the pharynx tends to cause the pharynx to collapse.

Pharyngeal obstruction in response to these pressure changes during inspiration is opposed by reflex contraction of pharyngeal dilator muscles during inspiration.[1] The afferent side of the reflex arises from mechanoreceptors in the pharynx and larynx. These pressure receptors respond in a graded manner to subatmospheric pressure and have myelinated afferent fibres to facilitate a rapid response. Based on the observation that the pharyngeal dilator reflex is less active during sleep (page 192), the reflex pathway is believed to involve higher centres of the brain. Nevertheless, the reflex is

extremely rapid, with both genioglossus and tensor palati electromyographic (EMG) activity increasing less than 50 milliseconds after a negative pressure is applied to the pharynx. This compares with a reaction time for voluntary tongue movements of 190 milliseconds. The efferent side of the reflex involves most of the pharyngeal dilator muscles, which display both tonic contraction and phasic inspiratory activity,[2] with the former predominating at rest and the latter developing with increased respiratory drive, for example during exercise.[3] Airway diameters are well maintained down to pressures of 1.5 kPa (15 cmH$_2$O) below atmospheric during active, but not passive, breathing manoeuvres.

There is no significant narrowing of the airway when changing from the erect to the supine posture in the normal subject. Genioglossus EMG activity is increased by 34% in the supine position, presumably to counteract the effect of gravity on the tongue.[4] Anatomical considerations suggest that patency of the nasopharynx in the supine position is maintained by the tensor palati, palatoglossus and palatopharyngeus muscles, and tonic but not phasic respiratory activity has been detected in the levator palate muscle. The soft palate tends to fall back against the posterior pharyngeal wall in the supine position without contraction of these muscles.

Failure of the various mechanisms that preserve pharyngeal airway patency may occur in sleep or anaesthesia; their occurrence and prevention are discussed in Chapters 14 and 21.

Laryngeal Control of Airway Resistance

During quiet breathing, movement of the vocal folds is used as a choke for fine control of airway resistance. On inspiration, phasic activity of the posterior cricoarytenoid muscles, acting by rotating the arytenoid cartilages, abducts the vocal cords to minimize resistance. A greater effect occurs during expiration, when phasic electrical activity in thyroarytenoid muscles indicates adduction of the vocal cords,[5] and therefore an increase in resistance. This may help to prevent collapse of the lower airways (page 32).

Respiratory Muscles of the Trunk

Nomenclature in this area can be confusing, with different authors using different terms. The trunk (referred to as chest wall by some studies) may be divided into the rib cage and abdomen. These two compartments are separated by the diaphragm, and both are therefore greatly influenced by its activity.

Diaphragm

The diaphragm is a membranous muscle separating the abdominal cavity and chest, and in adults has a total surface area[6] of approximately 900 cm². It is the most important

inspiratory muscle, with motor innervation solely from the phrenic nerves (C3–C5). In comparison with other skeletal muscles, the diaphragm is extremely active. Muscle fibres within the diaphragm can reduce their length by up to 40% between residual volume and total lung capacity, and spend 35% of each day contracting, compared with only 14% for the soleus muscle.[7] The diaphragm has considerable reserve of function, and unilateral phrenic block causes little decrement of overall ventilatory capacity. Despite the importance of the diaphragm to respiration, bilateral phrenic interruption is still compatible with good ventilatory function.

Mechanics of Diaphragmatic Function

The origins of the crural part of the diaphragm are the lumbar vertebrae and the arcuate ligaments, whilst the costal parts arise from the lower ribs and xiphisternum. Both parts are inserted into the central tendon. Studies of human subjects using magnetic resonance imaging or fast computed tomography scanning, illustrated in Figure 5.1, have enabled the in vivo actions of the diaphragm to be better defined.[6] Under normal circumstances, a zone of apposition

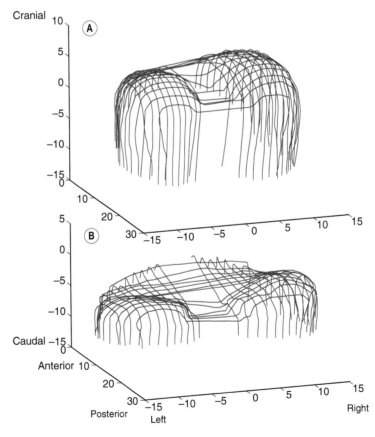

• **Fig. 5.1** Three-dimensional reconstructions of the human diaphragm at functional residual capacity using fast computed tomography scanning (dimensions in centimetres). **(A)** Normal subject showing extensive zone of apposition and normal curvature of the diaphragm domes. **(B)** Patient with hyperinflated chest as a result of chronic obstructive pulmonary disease (page 332). Note the reduced zone of apposition and the flattened diaphragm domes. The subject was supine during the scans. (From Cassart M, Pettiaux N, Gevenois PA, et al. Effect of chronic hyperinflation on diaphragm length and surface area. *Am J Respir Crit Care Med.* 1997;156:504-508 by permission of the authors and the publishers of *American Journal of Respiratory and Critical Care Medicine.*)

exists around the outside of the diaphragm where it is in direct contact with the internal aspect of the rib cage, with no lung in between, with the parietal pleura still allowing free movement of the diaphragm. At upright functional residual capacity (FRC) in humans, approximately 55% of the diaphragm surface area is in the zone of apposition.

There are many ways by which diaphragm contraction may bring about an increase in lung volume,[8] and these are illustrated schematically in Figure 5.2. These may be considered using a 'piston in a cylinder' analogy, with the trunk representing the cylinder and the diaphragm the piston (Fig. 5.2, *A*). Figure 5.2, *B*, illustrates the first possible mechanism, involving downward movement of the diaphragm simply by shortening the zone of apposition around the whole cylinder and leaving the dome shape unchanged. This is a pure 'piston-like' action and has the advantage of very efficient conversion of diaphragm muscle fibre shortening into changes in lung volume. Figure 5.2, *C*, illustrates 'nonpiston-like' behaviour in which the zone of apposition remains unchanged, but an increase in the tension of the diaphragm dome reduces the curvature, thus expanding the lung. This is likely to be less efficient than piston-like behaviour, because much of the muscle tension developed simply opposes the opposite side of the diaphragm rather than moving the diaphragm downwards, such that, in theory, when the diaphragm becomes flat, further contraction will have no effect on lung volume. Finally, Figure 5.2, *D*, incorporates both types of behaviour already described, but also now includes expansion of the lower rib cage (known as 'piston in an expanding cylinder') that occurs with diaphragmatic contraction, particularly in the supine position. This action results from a combination of abdominal pressure pushing the rib cage outwards ('appositional' force) and the diaphragm muscle attachment to the ribs displacing them outwards ('insertional' force).[9]

In the supine position, diaphragm action is a combination of all these above mechanisms, as well as a change in shape involving a tilting and flattening of the diaphragm in the anteroposterior direction.[6]

Rib Cage Muscles[10]

As already described, the rib cage may be regarded as a cylinder whose length is governed primarily by the diaphragm and secondarily by flexion and extension of the spine. The cross-sectional area of the cylinder is governed by movement of the ribs. This movement involves mainly rotation of the neck of the rib about the axis of the costovertebral joints, and their shape is such that elevation of the ribs in this way increases both the lateral and anteroposterior diameter of the rib cage. Elevation of the ribs by the intercostal muscles tends to result in a 'bucket handle' action, whilst elevation of the anterior rib cage by, for example, the sternomastoid muscles elevating the sternum results in a 'pump-handle' type of movement. These two actions tend to occur together and depend also on other requirements such as posture and upper limb movements. Upper ribs are inserted into the sternum and do not necessarily behave in quite the same way as the lower 'floating' ribs, which are inserted into the more flexible costal cartilage.

The intercostal muscles are divided into the external group, fibres of which run in a caudal–ventral direction from their upper rib and are deficient anteriorly, and the less powerful internal group, which have fibres running caudal–dorsal from their upper rib and are deficient posteriorly. Internal intercostal muscles of the upper rib cage become thicker anteriorly, where they are known as the parasternal intercostal muscles. In the 18th century mechanical considerations suggested that the external intercostals were primarily inspiratory, and the internal intercostals primarily expiratory. Although an oversimplification,[10] this has generally been confirmed by EMG. The parasternal portions of the internal intercostals are inspiratory in both humans and animals, and the inspiratory activity of external intercostals, although minimal during quiet breathing, becomes increasingly important during stimulated breathing. Posture plays an important role in intercostal activity in humans. For example, during the rather extreme postural challenge of rotating the trunk, which changes the mechanical properties of the ribs, the respiratory activity of internal and external intercostals is reversed, with internal intercostals becoming expiratory and vice versa.[11]

Scalene muscles are active in inspiration during quiet breathing in humans,[12] particularly when upright. Their role is to elevate the rib cage, and this counteracts the tendency of the diaphragm to cause inward displacement of the upper ribs. Innervation is from C1 to C5.

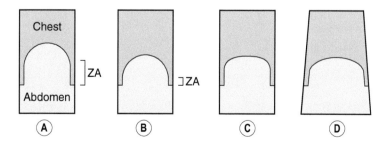

• **Fig. 5.2** Piston in a cylinder analogy of the mechanisms of diaphragm actions on the lung volume. **(A)** Resting end-expiratory position. **(B)** Inspiration with pure piston-like behaviour. **(C)** Inspiration with pure non–piston-like behaviour. **(D)** Combination of piston-like and non–piston-like behaviour in an expanding cylinder, which equates most closely with inspiration in vivo. *ZA*, Zone of apposition.

Accessory Muscles

These are silent during normal breathing in humans, but as ventilation increases the inspiratory muscles contract more vigorously, and accessory muscles are recruited. Considerable hyperventilation (about 50 L.min^{-1}) or severe increases in respiratory loading are usually present before the accessory muscles become active. Accessory muscles include the sternomastoids, the extensors of the vertebral column, the pectoralis minor, the trapezius and the serrati muscles. Many of these muscles, for example the pectorals, reverse their usual origin/insertion and help to expand the chest, provided the arms and shoulder girdle are fixed by grasping a suitable support.

Abdominal Muscles

With the exception of gas within the bowel lumen, the abdomen is an incompressible volume held between the diaphragm and the abdominal muscles. Contraction of either will cause a corresponding passive displacement of the other. Thus abdominal muscles are generally expiratory, and play an important respiratory role during exercise and hypercapnia.[13]

Rectus abdominis, external oblique, internal oblique and transversalis muscles are the most important expiratory muscles, whilst the muscles of the pelvic floor have a supportive role. Contraction of these muscles results in an increase in abdominal pressure, displacing the diaphragm in a cephalad direction. In addition, their insertion into the costal margin results in a caudad movement of the rib cage, assisting expiration by opposing the rib cage muscles. Gastric pressure is a valuable index of their activity because their contraction will always cause an increase in intraabdominal pressure.

In the supine position, the abdominal muscles are normally inactive during quiet breathing and become active only when the minute volume exceeds approximately 40 L.min^{-1}, in the face of substantial expiratory resistance, during phonation or when making expulsive efforts. When upright, their use in breathing is complicated by their role in the maintenance of posture.

Integration of Respiratory Muscle Activity

Breathing

Figure 5.3 shows the radiographic appearance of the rib cage at residual volume, at the normal expiratory level and at maximal inspiration, and illustrates the enormous range of movement within the semirigid rib cage. Expiration normally proceeds passively to the FRC, which may be considered as the equilibrium position governed by the balance of elastic forces, unless modified by residual end-expiratory tone in certain muscle groups. Inspiration is the active phase, entering the inspiratory capacity but normally leaving a substantial volume unused (the inspiratory reserve volume). Similarly, there is a substantial volume (the expiratory reserve volume) between FRC and the residual volume (see Fig. 2.8). By voluntary effort it is possible to affect a satisfactory tidal exchange anywhere within the vital capacity (VC), but the work of breathing is minimal at FRC.

Although we tend to think of the respiratory muscles individually, it is important to remember that they act together in an extraordinarily complex interaction that is influenced by factors including posture, minute volume, respiratory load, disease and anaesthesia. Figure 5.4 illustrates some features of the interaction.[11,14]

Inspiration. In Figure 5.4 it can be seen that the rib cage inspiratory muscles (external intercostals and scalenes) and diaphragm act in parallel to inflate the lungs, with posture affecting which muscle group is dominant (see later). In either position, diaphragm activity alone results in a widening of the lower rib cage and an

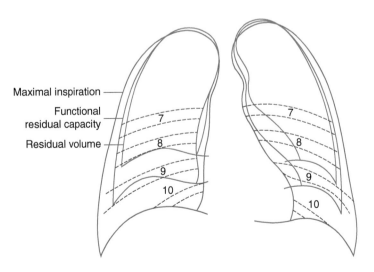

Maximal inspiration

Functional residual capacity

Residual volume

• **Fig. 5.3** Outlines of chest radiographs of a normal subject at various levels of lung inflation. The numbers refer to ribs as seen in the position of maximal inspiration.

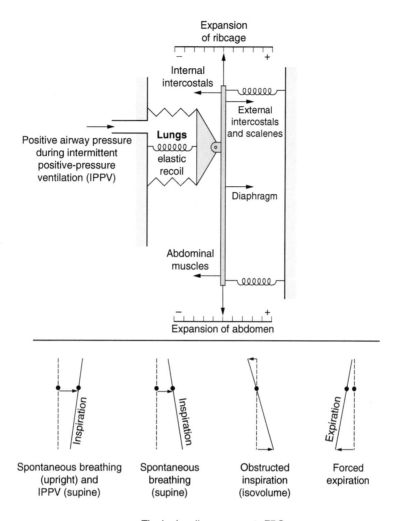

The broken line represents FRC

• **Fig. 5.4** A model of the balance of static and dynamic forces acting on the respiratory system. The central bar, attached to the lungs, is floating freely, held in equilibrium by the elastic forces at the end-expiratory position as shown. It may be displaced by the actions of the various muscles shown, with movement to the right generally indicating inspiration and movement to the left generally indicating expiration. Action of the various inspiratory or expiratory muscles causes changes, not only in the lung volume but also in the inclination of the bar, which represents relative changes in the cross-sectional area of the ribcage and abdomen. See text for details. IPPV, intermittent positive pressure ventilation; FRC, functional residual capacity. (Derived from references 14 and 15.)

indrawing of the upper rib cage, which must be countered by the intercostal and neck muscles contracting simultaneously.

Expiration. Requires no muscular activity during quiet breathing in the supine position, because the elastic recoil of the lungs provides the energy required, aided by the weight of the abdominal contents pushing the diaphragm in a cephalad direction. In the upright posture and during stimulated ventilation, the internal intercostal muscles and the abdominal wall muscles are active in returning the rib cage and diaphragm to the resting position. In extreme hyperventilation, for example following exercise, the expiratory muscles become progressively more important until ventilation assumes a quasi sine wave push-pull pattern.

Separation of Volume Contribution of Rib Cage and Abdomen

Konno and Mead originally proposed that the separate contributions to tidal volume of changes in rib cage (RC) and abdominal (AB) compartments could be measured.[16] Essentially similar results may be obtained by measuring either anteroposterior distance (magnetometers), circumference (strain gauge), cross-sectional area (respiratory inductance plethysmography [RIP]) or multiple points on the trunk (optoelectronic plethysmography[17]). Once initially calibrated to convert measurements of trunk dimensions into volumes, the sum of RC and AB movements correlates well with tidal volume, and provides a noninvasive measure of ventilation. RC/(RC + AB) indicates

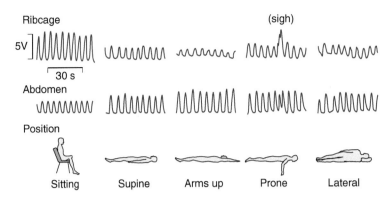

• **Fig. 5.5** Normal respiratory inductance plethysmography traces. The amplitude (in volts) of the signal reflects the cross-sectional area of the rib cage (RC) and abdomen (AB). The sum of the RC and AB signals correlates closely with tidal volume. The figure shows normal breathing in five different positions, demonstrating the predominantly RC contribution when upright and the AB contribution in all horizontal positions. Note the spontaneous sigh occurring in the prone position, resulting entirely from rib cage expansion. (From Lumb AB, Nunn JF. Respiratory function and ribcage contribution to ventilation in body positions commonly used during anaesthesia. *Anesth Analg.* 1991;73:422-426. by permission of the publishers of *Anesthesia and Analgesia.*)

the proportion of tidal volume that can be attributed to expansion of the rib cage (usually expressed as %RC). However, such is the complexity of the muscular system described earlier that changes in %RC cannot be attributed to changes in the force of contraction of any particular muscle. Figure 5.5 shows RIP traces during normal breathing in different positions.

Effect of Posture on Respiratory Muscles

Upright posture, whether standing or sitting, is associated with greater expansion of the rib cage, such that %RC is around two-thirds (Fig. 5.5). To account for this, increased EMG activity has been demonstrated in both the scalene and parasternal intercostal muscles when upright.

Supine Position

When supine, the weight of the abdominal contents pushes the diaphragm upwards, so that in the supine position the diaphragm tends to lie some 4 cm higher, which accords with the reduction in FRC when supine (see Fig. 2.10). With the diaphragm higher in the chest, its fibre length is greater, and it can therefore contract more effectively, counteracting the tendency to airway closure at the reduced FRC. The dimensions of the rib cage are probably little altered, and the increased diaphragm activity therefore results in a reduced %RC of approximately one-third in the supine position. In the prone and lateral position, RC contribution does not differ significantly from that in the supine position (Fig. 5.5).

Lateral Position

In this position (Fig. 5.6), only the lower dome of the diaphragm is pushed higher into the chest by the weight of the abdominal contents, while the upper dome is flattened. It

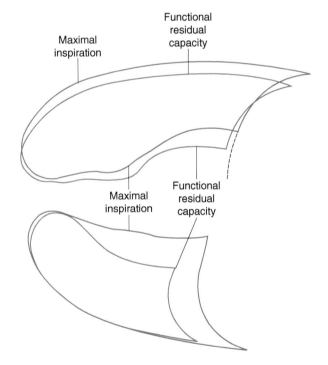

• **Fig. 5.6** Radiographic outlines of the lungs at two levels of lung volume in a conscious subject during spontaneous breathing in the lateral position (right side down). This is the same subject as in Figure 5.3: comparison will show that, in the lateral position at functional residual capacity, the lower lung is close to residual volume, while the upper lung is close to inspiratory capacity. The diaphragm therefore lies much more cephalad in the lower half of the chest. Both these factors contribute to the greater volume changes that occur in the lower lung during inspiration.

follows that the lower dome can contract more effectively than the upper, and the ventilation of the lower lung is about twice that of the upper. This is fortunate because gravity causes a preferential perfusion of the lower lung (page 92).

Chemoreceptor Activation

In animals, clear differences have been demonstrated in the respiratory muscle response to hyperventilation induced either by hypoxia or hypercapnia. For an equivalent minute volume, hypoxia stimulates mostly inspiratory muscles, whereas hypercapnia stimulates both inspiratory and expiratory groups.[13] Similar responses occur in humans, with diaphragm EMG activity increasing in response to both hypercapnia and hypoxia, but more rapidly in the latter, and expiratory muscle activity increasing almost exclusively during hypercapnic hyperventilation.[18]

Neuronal Control of Respiratory Muscles

The respiratory muscles, in common with other skeletal muscles, have their tension controlled by a servo mechanism mediated by muscle spindles. They appear to play a more important role in the intercostal muscles than in the diaphragm, but muscle spindles do exist in both. Their function is largely inferred from knowledge of their well-established role in other skeletal muscles not concerned with respiration.

Two types of cells can be distinguished in the motor neurone pool of the anterior horn cell. The alpha motor neurone has a thick efferent fibre (12–20 μm diameter) and passes in the ventral root directly to the neuromuscular junction of the muscle fibre (Fig. 5.7, *A*). The gamma motor neurone has a thin efferent fibre (2–8 μm), which also passes in the ventral root, but terminates in the intrafusal fibres of the muscle spindle. Contraction of the intrafusal fibres alone (without overall shortening of the muscle) increases the tension in the central part of the spindle (the nuclear bag), causing stimulation of the annulospiral endings. Impulses so generated are then transmitted via fibres that lie in the dorsal root to reach the anterior horn, where

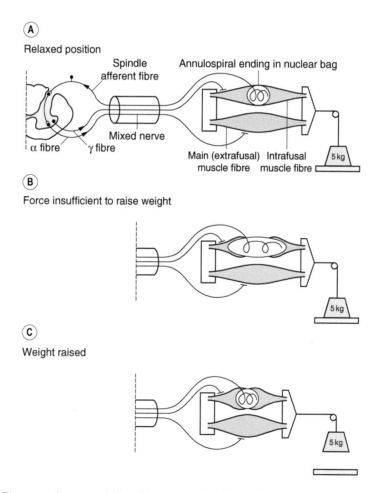

• **Fig. 5.7** Diagrammatic representation of the servo mechanism mediated by the muscle spindles. **(A)** The resting state with muscle and intrafusal fibres of spindle relaxed. **(B)** The muscle is attempting to lift the weight after discharge of both alpha and gamma systems. The force developed by the muscle is insufficient: the weight is not lifted, and the muscle cannot shorten. However, the intrafusal fibres are able to shorten and stretch the annulospiral endings in the nuclear bag of the spindle. Afferent discharge causes increased excitation of the motor neurone pool in the anterior horn. **(C)** Alpha discharge is augmented, and the weight is finally lifted by the more powerful contraction of the muscle. When the weight is lifted, the tension on the nuclear bag is relieved, and the afferent discharge from the spindle ceases. This series of diagrams relates to the lifting of a weight, but it is thought that a similar action of spindles is brought into play when inspiratory muscles contract against increased airways resistance.

they have an excitatory effect on the alpha motor neurones. Using this system, an efferent impulse transmitted by the gamma system causes reflex contraction of the main muscle mass by an arc through the annulospiral afferent and the alpha motor neurone. Thus contraction of the whole muscle may be controlled entirely by efferents travelling in the gamma fibres, and this is believed to occur in relation to breathing.

Alternatively, muscle contraction may in the first instance result from discharge of both the alpha and gamma motor neurones. If shortening of the muscle is unopposed, main (extrafusal) and intrafusal fibres will contract together, and the tension in the nuclear bag of the spindle will be unchanged. If, however, the shortening of the muscle is opposed, the intrafusal fibres will shorten more than the extrafusal fibres, causing the nuclear bag to be stretched (Fig. 5.7, B). The consequent stimulation of the annulospiral endings results in afferent activity that raises the excitatory state of the motor neurones, causing the main muscle fibres to increase their tension until the resistance is overcome, allowing the muscle to shorten and the tension in the nuclear bag of the spindle to be reduced (Fig. 5.7, C).

By this mechanism, fine control of muscle contraction is possible. The message from the upper motor neurone is 'muscles should contract with whatever force may be found necessary to effect the requested shortening', and not simply 'muscles should contract with the requested force'. The former message is typical of input into a servo system, and is far more satisfactory when the load is not known in advance. For respiratory muscles, a servo system is very advantageous. The message conveyed by the efferent tract from the inspiratory neurones of the medulla would be 'inspiratory muscles should contract with whatever force may be necessary to effect a required change in length (corresponding to a certain tidal volume)'. A servo system also provides an excellent mechanism for rapid response to sudden changes in airway resistance. The nature and magnitude of the response of the inspiratory muscles to added resistance to breathing is described in Chapter 3, and the immediate effectiveness of the response is easily explicable in terms of muscle spindles.

Muscle Fibre Subtypes[19]

Respiratory muscles, like all skeletal muscle, contain different types of muscle fibres classified according to which isoform of myosin heavy chain (MHC) is expressed. Table 5.1 shows the three fibre types known to exist in human respiratory muscles and their contractile and biochemical features. Which isoform of MHC is expressed in a muscle fibre determines the velocity of contraction (Table 5.1). Different isoforms of enzymes involved in muscle relaxation also exist in the different fibre types, influencing the rate at which relaxation occurs, and therefore the ability of the cell to maintain a tetanic contraction. Type I fibres contract and relax slowly, but can maintain tension for long periods using aerobic metabolic pathways and are fatigue-resistant. In contrast, type IIb fibres rely mainly on glycolytic metabolic

	Type I	Type IIa	Type IIb
TABLE 5.1 — Properties of Muscle Fibre Types Found in Human Respiratory Muscle, and Their Relative Proportions in Normal and Pathological Situations[19,21,22]			
Contractile Properties			
Velocity of shortening	+	++	++++
Tetanic force	+	+	++
Fatigue resistance	++++	+++	+
Biochemical Properties			
Mitochondrial density	+++	+++	+
ATP consumption rate	+	++	++++
Oxidative enzymes	+++	+++	+
Glycolytic enzymes	+	++	++++
Glycogen content	+	++	+++
Relative Proportions in			
Normal subjects	45%	39%	16%
COPD	↑↑	↓	↓↓
Steroid myopathy	↔	↔	↓↓↓
Artificial ventilation[a]	↓	↑	↔

[a]Animal studies only.
ATP, Adenosine triphosphate; *COPD*, chronic obstructive pulmonary disease (Chapter 28);

pathways for energy supply, their contraction is quicker and stronger in bursts of activity, and they fatigue easily. Type IIa fibres have properties intermediate between these two extreme fibre types. The proportions of different fibre types in a muscle therefore reveal the sort of work normally undertaken by the muscle; for example, in muscles mainly involved in maintaining posture, type I fibres predominate, whilst in those requiring intermittent activity, such as hand muscles, type IIa or IIb fibres predominate.

Relative proportions of the different fibre types in human respiratory muscle are shown in Table 5.1, but it is unclear which types of fibre are responsible for different respiratory muscle activities. In animal respiratory muscles, which tend to have fewer type II fibres than human respiratory muscles, both eupnoeic and stimulated breathing can be achieved solely by using type I fibres, and type II fibres are only required for expulsive efforts such as sneezing and coughing.[7] A high proportion of type I fibres (45% in human diaphragm) indicates that they are probably responsible for both posture and respiration in humans, and that type II fibres are again only required for expulsive efforts and active movements such as running, jumping and so on. Ageing leads to selective atrophy of type II fibres,[20] and respiratory disease, drugs and artificial ventilation all cause changes in the relative proportions of the different fibre types (Table 5.1).

Respiratory Muscle Fatigue and Disuse[19]

The diaphragm, like other striated muscles, is subject to fatigue, which is defined as an inability to sustain tension with repeated activity. For nonrespiratory skeletal muscle, fatigue may be 'central'—that is, the subject is not trying hard enough (either consciously or subconsciously)—but this is unlikely to be significant in respiration because subjects with respiratory failure usually have a high central respiratory drive. Peripheral fatigue occurs when the frequency of motor nerve action potentials becomes chronically increased in an attempt to increase muscle tension. Eventually, when working against an unsustainable load, relaxation of the muscle fibre, the energy-requiring part of contraction, becomes excessively prolonged, and the muscle is unable to respond to the next action potential to generate the required tension. In the diaphragm, resistive loads less than 40% of maximum may be sustained indefinitely, but loads greater than 40% of maximum can only be sustained for a short time.

Blood supply to respiratory muscles may be important in fatigue. Patients with severe congestive cardiac failure, and therefore low cardiac output, have weakened respiratory muscles compared with matched controls, despite having similar muscle strength in the arms. The high rate of activity of respiratory muscles seems to leave them more susceptible to weakness in the face of reduced oxygen supply compared with other muscles, a situation that often causes problems in intensive care when trying to wean patients from artificial ventilation before their cardiovascular function is adequate (page 385).

Effect of Disuse[23]

The diaphragm may be rested by artificial ventilation with or without neuromuscular blockade, and the effect on diaphragmatic performance is clearly important. After only 18 hours of mechanical ventilation there are histological and gene-expression changes indicating muscle fibre atrophy,[24] and within days diaphragm strength is substantially reduced (Table 5.1).[19] Extrapolating these results to all artificially ventilated patients is difficult because there are numerous factors affecting respiratory muscle strength in critically ill patients, particularly the presence of sepsis.[23,25] Even so, it is now clear that complete inactivity of the normally very active respiratory muscles is detrimental to their function. Recent developments in artificial ventilation are now focused on allowing diaphragm activity to continue at a critical level of activity to best preserve its function.[26]

The Work of Breathing

When expiration is passive during quiet breathing, the work of breathing is performed entirely by the inspiratory muscles. Approximately half of this work is dissipated during inspiration as heat in overcoming the frictional forces opposing inspiration. The other half is stored as potential energy in the deformed elastic tissues of lungs and chest wall. This potential energy is thus available as the source of energy for expiration and is then dissipated as heat in overcoming the frictional forces resisting expiration. Energy stored in deformed elastic tissue thus permits the work of expiration to be transferred to the inspiratory muscles. This remains true with moderate increases of either inspiratory or expiratory resistance; lung volume and therefore elastic recoil are increased in the latter condition (page 37).

The actual work performed by the respiratory muscles is very small in the healthy resting subject. Under these circumstances the oxygen consumption of the respiratory muscles is approximately 3 mL.min^{-1}, or less than 2% of the metabolic rate. Furthermore, the efficiency of the respiratory muscles is only about 10%. The efficiency is further reduced in many forms of respiratory disease, certain deformities, pregnancy and when the minute volume is increased (Fig. 5.8). When maximal ventilation is approached, the efficiency falls to such a low level that additional oxygen made available by further increases in ventilation will be entirely consumed by the respiratory muscles.

Units of Measurement of Work

Work is performed when a force moves its point of application, and the work is equal to the product of force and distance moved. Similarly, work is performed when force is applied to the plunger of a syringe, raising the pressure of

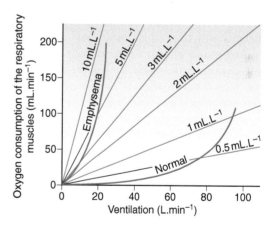

• **Fig. 5.8** Oxygen consumption of the respiratory muscles plotted against minute volume of respiration. The isopleths indicate the oxygen cost of breathing in millilitres of oxygen consumed per litre of minute volume. The curve obtained from the normal subject shows the low oxygen cost of breathing up to a minute volume of 70 L.min^{-1}. Thereafter the oxygen cost rises steeply. In a patient with chronic obstructive pulmonary disease, the oxygen cost of breathing is not only much higher at the resting minute volume, but also rises more steeply as ventilation increases. At a minute volume of 20 L.min^{-1}, the respiratory muscles are consuming 200 mL of oxygen per minute, and a further increase of ventilation would consume more oxygen than it would make available to the rest of the body. (From Campbell EJM, Westlake EK, Cherniak RM. Simple methods of estimating oxygen consumption and the efficiency of the muscles of breathing. *J Appl Physiol.* 1957;11:303-308. By permission of the *Journal of Applied Physiology.*)

gas contained therein. In this case the work is equal to the product of the mean pressure and the change in volume, or alternatively the product of the mean volume and the change in pressure. The units of work are identical whether the product is force $\times$ distance or pressure $\times$ volume. A multiplicity of units have been used for measuring work, and these units are listed in Appendix A.

Power is a measure of the rate at which work is (or can be) performed. The term *work of breathing*, as it is normally used and when expressed in watts, is thus a misnomer because we are referring to the rate at which work is performed, and *power* is the correct term. Work of breathing would be appropriate for a single event such as one breath, and joules would then be the appropriate units.

Dissipation of the Work of Breathing

The work of breathing overcomes two main sources of impedance. The first is the elastic recoil of the lungs and chest wall (Chapter 2), and the second is the nonelastic resistance to gas flow (Chapter 3).

Work Against Elastic Recoil

When an elastic body is deformed, no work is dissipated, as heat and all work are stored as potential energy. Figure 5.9, *A*, shows a section of the alveolar pressure/volume plot for the total respiratory system, showing only the straight part of the curve from near FRC (see Fig. 2.7). As the lungs are inflated, the plot forms the hypotenuse of a triangle, whose area represents the work done against elastic resistance. The area of the triangle (half the base times the height) will thus equal either half the tidal volume times the pressure change or the mean pressure times the volume change. Either product has the units of work or energy (joules) and represents the potential energy available for expiration. In Figure 5.9, *B*, the pressure/volume curve is flatter, indicating stiffer or less compliant lungs. For the same tidal volume, the area of the triangle is increased. This indicates the greater amount of work performed against elastic resistance and the greater potential energy available for expiration.

Work Against Resistance to Gas Flow

Frictional resistance was ignored in Figure 5.9. Additional pressure is required to overcome frictional resistance to gas flow that is reflected in the mouth pressure, which, during inspiration, is greater than the alveolar pressure by the driving pressure required to overcome frictional resistance. When mouth pressure is plotted as in Figure 5.10, the inspiratory curve is bowed to the right, and the darker brown area to the right of the pressure volume curve indicates the additional work performed in overcoming inspiratory frictional resistance. Figure 5.10, *B*, represents a patient with increased airway resistance. The expiratory curve, not shown in Figure 5.10, would be bowed to the left, as the mouth-to-alveolar pressure gradient is reversed during expiration.

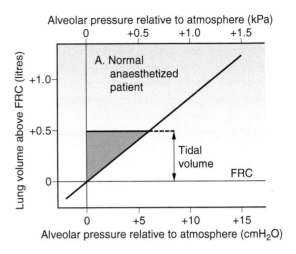

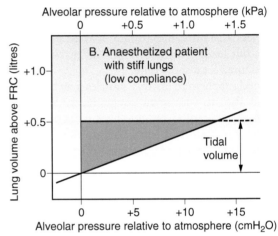

• **Fig. 5.9** Work of breathing against elastic resistance during passive inflation. The lines show pressure/volume plots of the lungs of anaesthetized patients (conscious subjects are shown in Fig. 2.7). The length of the pressure/volume curve covered during inspiration forms the hypotenuse of a right-angled triangle whose area equals the work performed against elastic resistance. Note that, compared with the healthy patient **(A)**, the area is greater when the pressure/volume curve is flatter, as shown in the patient with stiffer or less compliant lungs **(B)**. FRC, functional residual capacity.

The Minimal Work of Breathing

For a constant minute volume, the work performed against elastic resistance is increased when breathing is slow and deep. Conversely, the work performed against airflow resistance is increased when breathing is rapid and shallow. If the two components are summated and the total work is plotted against respiratory frequency, it will be found that there is an optimal frequency at which the total work of breathing is minimal (Fig. 5.11). If there is increased elastic resistance (as in patients with pulmonary fibrosis), the optimal frequency is increased, whereas in the presence of increased airflow resistance the optimal frequency is decreased. Humans and animals tend to select a respiratory frequency close to that which minimizes respiratory work. This applies to different species, different age groups and to pathological conditions.

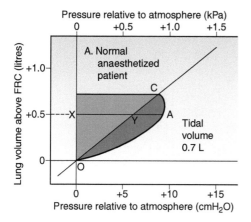

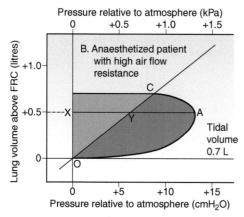

• **Fig. 5.10** Work of breathing against airflow resistance during passive inflation. The sloping line OYC is the alveolar pressure/volume curve. The curve OAC is the mouth pressure/volume curve during inflation of the lungs. The darker brown area indicates the work of inspiration performed against airflow resistance. Compared with the healthy patient (**A**), this work is increased in the patient with high resistance (**B**). At the point when 500 mL of gas has entered the patient, XY represents the pressure distending the lungs, whereas YA represents the pressure overcoming airflow resistance. XA is the inflation pressure at that moment. The lighter brown areas represent the work done against elastic resistance (see Fig. 5.9). FRC, functional residual capacity.

Measurement of Ventilation

Volume may be measured either directly or by the continuous integration of instantaneous gas flow rate (Fig. 5.12).

Direct Measurement of Respired Volumes[27]

Inspiratory and expiratory tidal volumes (and therefore minute volume) may be markedly different, and the difference is important in calculations of gas exchange. The normal respiratory exchange ratio of about 0.8 means that inspiratory minute volume is approximately 50 mL larger than the expiratory minute volume in the resting subject. Much larger differences can arise during exercise and during uptake or wash-out of an inert gas such as nitrogen or, to a greater extent, nitrous oxide.

Water-sealed spirometers provide the reference method for the measurement of ventilation (Fig. 5.12) and may be precisely calibrated by water displacement. They provide negligible resistance to breathing and, by suitable design, may have a satisfactory frequency response up to very high respiratory frequencies.

Dry spirometers are hinged bellows, usually with electronic displays of both volume and instantaneous flow rate. Their accuracy approaches that of a water-filled spirometer, and they are far more convenient in use.

Impellers and Turbines

The best known of these instruments is the respirometer developed by Wright in 1955.[28] The mechanism is entirely mechanical, with indication of volume on a dial, but the output may be converted to an electrical signal to indicate either tidal volume or minute volume. In general the respirometer is accurate and tends to read low at low minute volumes and high at high minute volumes; departure from normality is thus exaggerated, and the instrument is essentially safe.

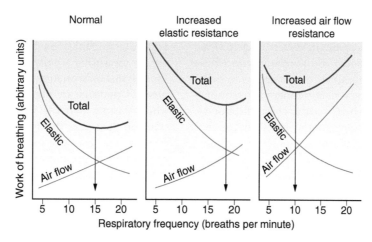

• **Fig. 5.11** Minimal work of breathing. The diagrams show the work done against elastic and airflow resistance separately and summated to indicate the total work of breathing at different respiratory frequencies. The total work of breathing has a minimum value at about 15 breaths per minute under normal circumstances. For the same minute volume, minimum work is performed at higher frequencies with stiff (less compliant) lungs and at lower frequencies when the airflow resistance is increased.

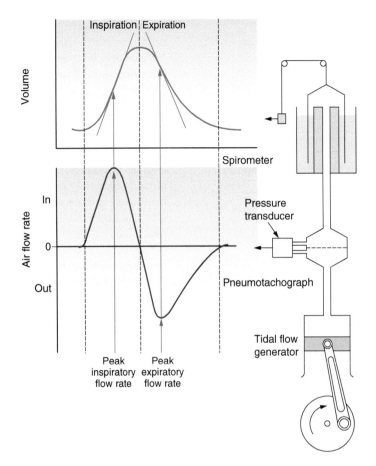

• **Fig. 5.12** Relationship between volume and flow rate. The top graph shows volume plotted against time; this type of tracing is obtained from a spirometer. The bottom graph shows instantaneous airflow rate plotted against time; this type of tracing is obtained from a pneumotachograph. At any instant, the flow-rate trace indicates the slope of the volume trace, while the volume trace indicates the cumulative area under the flow-rate trace. Flow is the differential of volume; volume is the integral of flow rate. Differentiation of the spirometer trace gives a 'pneumotachogram'; integration of the pneumotachogram gives a 'spirometer' trace.

Noninvasive Measurement of Ventilation

A variety of techniques are now available for measuring ventilation from changes in the shape of the chest wall and abdomen, avoiding the use of a mouthpiece, mask or noseclip. Reference has been made previously (page 63) to techniques that allow assessment of the relative contributions of the rib cage and abdominal compartments to each breath. Respiratory inductance plethysmography requires the subject to wear flexible belts on the chest and abdomen, and electrical inductance in the belt reflects the cross-sectional area within it. Optoelectronic plethysmography[17,29] requires the subject to wear a number of reflective markers on the chest and abdominal walls, which reflect infrared light to several cameras placed around the subject, allowing the exact three-dimensional position of the markers to be measured, and so body shape to be calculated. Once initially calibrated against a spirometer, the changes in these measurements can easily be converted to volume. Continuous measurements can be made in varied circumstances, for example in different body positions or during sleep (Fig. 5.5).

Measurement of Ventilatory Volumes by Integration of Instantaneous Gas Flow Rate

Electronics has made measurement of ventilatory volumes by integration of instantaneous flow rate a widespread technique in clinical environments. There are many methods for measuring rapidly changing gas flow rates, of which the original was pneumotachography. This uses measurement of the pressure gradient across a laminar resistance, which ensures that the pressure drop is directly proportional to flow rate. This is illustrated in Figure 5.12, where the resistance is a wire mesh screen. It is necessary to take precautions to prevent errors caused by different gas compositions and temperatures, and to prevent condensation of moisture on the screen. The pressure drop need not exceed a few millimetres of water, and the volume can be very small. Therefore the pneumotachograph should not interfere with respiration.

Most ventilators and anaesthetic machines currently in use can measure respiratory volumes. A pneumotachograph or electronic turbine system is used, normally on the expired limb of the breathing system, and is designed to be of very low resistance to allow measurements during spontaneous respiration. In this way, each expired tidal volume may be measured, from which respiratory rate and minute volume can be derived, and a useful method of detecting apnoea or disconnection is therefore provided.

Measurement of Ventilatory Capacity[27,30]

Measurement of ventilatory capacity is the most commonly performed test of respiratory function. The ratio of ventilatory capacity to actual ventilation is a measure of ventilatory reserve and of the comfort of breathing.

Maximal Voluntary Ventilation

Maximal voluntary ventilation (MVV), also referred to as maximal breathing capacity (MBC), is defined as the maximum minute volume of ventilation that the subject can maintain for 12 to 15 seconds. In the normal subject, MVV is about 15 to 20 times the resting minute volume. The subject simply breathes in and out of a spirometer without the need for removal of carbon dioxide; although simple, the test is exhausting to perform and is now seldom used. The average fit young male adult should have an MBC of about 170 $L.min^{-1}$, but normal values depend on body size, age and sex.

Forced Expiration

A more practical test of ventilatory capacity is the forced expiratory volume in 1 second (FEV_1), which is the maximal volume exhaled in the first second starting from a maximal inspiration. A simple spirometer is all that is required. It is far more convenient to perform than the MVV and less exhausting for the patient. It correlates well with the MVV, which is normally about 35 times the FEV_1. A variety of similar measurements relating to a single forced expiration are described, including forced expiratory volume in 0.5 seconds or 0.75 seconds, which may be useful in children, or forced expiratory volume in 6 seconds, which is a surrogate for forced VC.[30] The effects of age and smoking on FEV_1 are described on page 238.

Peak Expiratory Flow Rate

Most convenient of all the indirect tests of ventilatory capacity is the peak expiratory flow rate. This can be measured with simple and inexpensive hand-held devices and is an easy method for assessing large airway calibre. Interpretation of measurements of maximal expirations may be misleading. It should be remembered that these tests measure active expiration, which plays no part in normal breathing. They are most commonly performed as a measure of airway obstruction and are extensively used in patients with airway diseases (Chapter 28). However, the results also depend on many other factors, including chest restriction, motivation and muscular power. The measurements may also be inhibited by pain. A more specific indication of airway resistance is the ratio of FEV_1 to VC, which should exceed 75% in the normal subject.

Assessment of the Respiratory Muscles

Severe abnormalities of muscle function may be assessed by simple observation of spontaneous breathing. During inspiration, paradoxical movements of the trunk may occur, such as inward displacement of the abdominal wall (diaphragm failure) or inward movement of the upper chest (intercostal failure). Fluoroscopy or ultrasound imaging of the diaphragm provides a more subtle form of observation, and is helpful in detecting phrenic nerve damage, particularly if unilateral, when the body surface changes will be less obvious.

Vital capacity (see Fig. 2.8) is accepted as the best 'bedside' monitor of respiratory muscle function, particularly when performed supine. Performance of a VC manoeuvre requires patient cooperation and coordination, and a single low reading is nonspecific. However, repeated measurement allows the observation of a trend in VC to be followed, and a 25% reduction is unequivocally abnormal. Despite the many causes of a reduced VC, this method of assessing respiratory muscle function is very useful for monitoring the development of progressive muscle weakness in conditions such as myasthenia gravis and Guillain–Barré syndrome (page 318).

Pressure measurements, when breathing against an imposed resistance, are used to assess both inspiratory and expiratory muscle strength. All require some patient compliance and involve a degree of respiratory discomfort, so these tests, although more specific than VC for respiratory muscle function, are not widely used. Mouth pressure may be measured while a slow inspiration or expiration is performed against a moderate respiratory resistance, or mouth pressure may be measured during a rapid 'sniff' procedure in which the nasal airway acts as the resistance.

References

1. Cheng S, Butler JE, Gandevia SC, et al. Movement of the tongue during normal breathing in awake healthy humans. *J Physiol.* 2008;586:4283-4294.
2. Bailey EF. Activities of human genioglossus motor units. *Respir Physiol Neurobiol.* 2011;179:14-22.
3. Walls CE, Laine CM, Kidder IJ, et al. Human hypoglossal motor unit activities in exercise. *J Physiol.* 2013;591:3579-3590.
4. Douglas NJ, Jan MA, Yildirim N, et al. Effect of posture and breathing route on genioglossal EMG activity in normal subjects and in patients with the sleep apnea/hypopnea syndrome. *Am Rev Respir Dis.* 1993;148:1341-1345.
5. Kuna ST, Insalaco G, Woodson GE. Thyroarytenoid muscle activity during wakefulness and sleep in normal adults. *J Appl Physiol.* 1988;65:1332-1339.
6. Gauthier AP, Verbanck S, Estenne M, et al. Three-dimensional reconstruction of the in vivo human diaphragm shape at different lung volumes. *J Appl Physiol.* 1994;76:495-506.

7. Mantilla CB, Sieck GC. Phrenic motor unit recruitment during ventilatory and non-ventilatory behaviors. *Respir Physiol Neurobiol.* 2011;179:57-63.

8. Petroll WM, Knight H, Rochester DF. A model approach to assess diaphragmatic volume displacement. *J Appl Physiol.* 1990;69:2175-2182.

9. De Troyer A, Wilson TA. Action of the diaphragm on the rib cage. *J Appl Physiol.* 2016;121:391–400.

10. De Troyer A, Kirkwood PA, Wilson TA. Respiratory action of the intercostal muscles. *Physiol Rev.* 2005;85:717-756.

11. Rimmer KP, Ford GT, Whitelaw WA. Interaction between postural and respiratory control of human intercostal muscles. *J Appl Physiol.* 1995;79:1556-1561.

12. Hudson AL, Gandevia SC, Butler JE. The effect of lung volume on the co-ordinated recruitment of scalene and sternomastoid muscles in humans. *J Physiol.* 2007;584:261-270.

13. Drummond G. Like breathing out and breathing in…. *J Physiol.* 2010;588:3345.

14. Hillman DR, Finucane KE. A model of the respiratory pump. *J Appl Physiol.* 1987;63:951-961.

15. Drummond GB. Chest wall movements in anaesthesia. *Eur J Anaesthiol.* 1989;6:161-196.

16. Konno K, Mead J. Measurement of the separate volume changes of ribcage and abdomen during breathing. *J Appl Physiol.* 1967;22:407-422.

17. Romei M, Lo Mauro A, D'Angeloa MG, et al. Effects of gender and posture on thoraco-abdominal kinematics during quiet breathing in healthy adults. *Respir Physiol Neurobiol.* 2010;172:184-191.

18. Xie S, Takasaki Y, Popkin J, et al. Chemical and postural influence on scalene and diaphragmatic activation in humans. *J Appl Physiol.* 1991;70:658-664.

19. Laghi F, Tobin MJ. Disorders of the respiratory muscles. *Am J Respir Crit Care Med.* 2003;168:10-48.

20. Elliott JE, Greising SM, Mantilla CB. Functional impact of sarcopenia in respiratory muscles. *Respir Physiol Neurobiol.* 2016;226:137-146.

21. Gayan-Ramirez G, Decramer M. Effects of mechanical ventilation on diaphragm function and biology. *Eur Respir J.* 2002;20:1579-1586.

22. Levine S, Kaiser L, Leferovich J, et al. Cellular adaptations in the diaphragm in chronic obstructive pulmonary disease. *N Engl J Med.* 1997;337:1799-1806.

23. Petrof BJ. Diaphragm weakness in the critically ill. Basic mechanisms reveal therapeutic opportunities. *Chest.* 2018;154:1395-1403.

24. Levine S, Nguyen T, Taylor N, et al. Rapid disuse atrophy of diaphragm fibers in mechanically ventilated humans. *N Engl J Med.* 2008;358:1327-1335.

*25. **Supinski GS, Morris PE, Dhar S. Diaphragm dysfunction in critical illness. Chest. 2018;153:1040-1051.**

26. Heunks L, Ottenheijm C. Diaphragm-protective mechanical ventilation to improve outcomes in ICU Patients? *Am J Respir Crit Care Med.* 2018;197:150-152.

27. Miller MR, Hankinson J, Brusasco V, et al. Standardisation of spirometry. *Eur Respir J.* 2005;26:319-338.

28. Wright BM. A respiratory anemometer. *J Physiol.* 1955;127:25P.

29. Nozoea M, Maseb K, Takashimab S, et al. Measurements of chest wall volume variation during tidal breathing in the supine and lateral positions in healthy subjects. *Respir Physiol Neurobiol.* 2014;193:38-42.

30. Cotes JE, Chinn DJ, Miller MR. *Lung Function. Physiology, Measurement and Application in Medicine.* Oxford, UK: Blackwell Publishing; 2006.

6

The Pulmonary Circulation

KEY POINTS

- Pulmonary blood flow approximates to cardiac output and can increase several-fold with little change in pulmonary arterial pressure.
- Passive distension and recruitment of closed pulmonary capillaries, particularly in the upper zones of the lung, allow pulmonary vascular resistance to fall as blood flow increases.

- Active control of pulmonary vascular resistance has only a minor role in controlling pulmonary vascular resistance and involves intrinsic responses in vascular smooth muscle, modulated by numerous neural and humoral factors.
- Hypoxic pulmonary vasoconstriction of pulmonary arterioles is a fundamental difference from the systemic circulation, although the mechanism of this response to hypoxia remains uncertain.

The evolution of warm-blooded animals led to a 10-fold increase in oxygen requirements, which may only be achieved through having a pulmonary circulation almost completely separate from the systemic circulation (page 302).

Pulmonary Blood Flow

The flow of blood through the pulmonary circulation is approximately equal to the flow through the whole of the systemic circulation. It therefore varies from approximately 6 L.min^{-1} under resting conditions to as much as 25 L.min^{-1} during strenuous exercise. It is remarkable that such an increase can normally be achieved with minimal increase in pressure. Pulmonary vascular pressures and vascular resistance are much less than those of the systemic circulation. Consequently the pulmonary circulation has only limited ability to control the regional distribution of blood flow within the lungs, and is affected by gravity, which results in overperfusion of dependent regions of the lungs. Maldistribution of the pulmonary blood flow has important consequences for gaseous exchange, and these are considered in Chapter 7.

In fact, the relationship between the inflow and outflow of the pulmonary circulation is much more complicated (Fig. 6.1). The lungs receive a significant quantity of blood from the bronchial arteries, which usually arise from the arch of the aorta. Blood from the bronchial circulation returns to the heart in two ways. From a plexus around the hilum, blood from the pleurohilar part of the bronchial circulation returns to the superior vena cava via the azygos veins, and this fraction (about one-third) may thus be regarded as normal systemic flow, neither arising from nor returning to the pulmonary circulation. However, another fraction of the bronchial circulation, distributed more peripherally in the lung, passes

through postcapillary anastomoses to join the pulmonary veins, constituting an admixture of venous blood with the oxygenated blood from the alveolar capillary networks.

The situation may be further complicated by blood flow through precapillary anastomoses from the bronchial arteries to the pulmonary arteries. These communications (so-called *Sperr arteries*) have muscular walls, and are thought to act as sluice gates, opening when increased pulmonary blood flow is required. Their functional significance in normal subjects is unknown, but in diseased lungs flow through these anastomoses may be crucial. For example, in situations involving pulmonary oligaemia (e.g., pulmonary artery stenosis, pulmonary embolism) blood from the bronchial arteries will flow through the anastomoses to supplement pulmonary arterial flow.[1] It should be noted that a Blalock–Taussig shunt operation achieves the same purpose for palliation of patients with cyanotic congenital heart disease.

Pulmonary Blood Volume

As a first approximation the right heart pumps blood into the pulmonary circulation, and the left heart pumps away the blood that returns from the lungs. Therefore provided that the output of the two sides is the same, the pulmonary blood volume will remain constant. However, very small differences in the outputs of the two sides must result in large changes in pulmonary blood volume if they are maintained for more than a few beats.

Factors Influencing Pulmonary Blood Volume
Posture

Change from the supine to the erect position decreases the pulmonary blood volume by almost one-third, which is

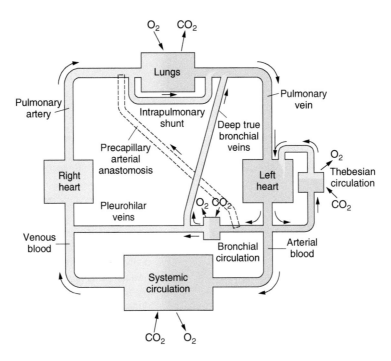

• **Fig. 6.1** Schema of bronchopulmonary anastomoses and other forms of venous admixture in a normal subject. Part of the bronchial circulation returns venous blood to the systemic venous system, while another part returns venous blood to the pulmonary veins constituting venous admixture. Other forms of venous admixture are the Thebesian circulation of the left heart and flow through atelectatic parts of the lungs. It is clear from this diagram why the output of the left heart must be slightly greater than that of the right heart.

about the same as the corresponding change in cardiac output. Both changes result from pooling of blood in dependent parts of the systemic circulation.

Systemic Vascular Tone

Because the systemic circulation has much greater vasomotor activity than the pulmonary circulation, an overall increase in vascular tone will tend to squeeze blood from the systemic into the pulmonary circulation. This may result from the release of endogenous catecholamines, administration of vasoconstrictor drugs or passive compression of the body in a G-suit. The magnitude of the resulting volume shift will depend on many factors such as position, overall blood volume and activity of the numerous humoral and nervous mechanisms controlling pulmonary vascular tone at the time (see later). Conversely, it seems likely that pulmonary blood volume would be diminished when systemic tone is diminished, for example during sepsis or with regional anaesthesia when systemic vascular resistance is decreased.

Pulmonary Vascular Pressures

Pulmonary arterial pressure is only about one-sixth of systemic arterial pressure, although the capillary and venous pressures are not greatly different for the two circulations (Fig. 6.2). Thus there is only a small pressure drop along the pulmonary arterioles, and therefore a reduced potential for active regulation of the distribution of the pulmonary blood flow. This also explains why there is little damping of the arterial pressure wave, and the pulmonary capillary blood flow is markedly pulsatile.

Consideration of pulmonary vascular pressures carries a special difficulty in the selection of the reference pressure. Systemic pressures are customarily measured with reference to ambient atmospheric pressure, but this is not always appropriate when considering the pulmonary arterial pressure, which is relatively small in comparison with the intrathoracic and pulmonary venous pressures. This may be important in two circumstances. First, the extravascular (intrathoracic) pressure may have a major influence on the intravascular pressure and should be considered. Second, the driving pressure through the pulmonary circulation may be markedly influenced by the pulmonary venous pressure, which must be considered when measuring pulmonary vascular resistance. We must therefore distinguish between pressures within the pulmonary circulation expressed in the three different forms listed in the following paragraphs. Measurement techniques may be adapted to indicate these pressures directly (Fig. 6.3).

Intravascular pressure is the pressure at any point in the circulation relative to atmosphere. This is the customary way of expressing pressures in the systemic circulation, and is also the commonest method of indicating pulmonary vascular pressures.

Transmural pressure is the difference in pressure between the inside of a vessel and the tissue surrounding the vessel. In

Systemic circulation			Pulmonary circulation	
mmHg	cmH$_2$O		mmHg	cmH$_2$O
90	120	Arteries	17	22
		Arterioles		
30	40		13	17
		Capillaries		
10	13		9	12
		Veins		
2	3	Atria	6	8

• **Fig. 6.2** Comparison of typical mean pressure gradients along the systemic and pulmonary circulations (mean pressures relative to atmosphere).

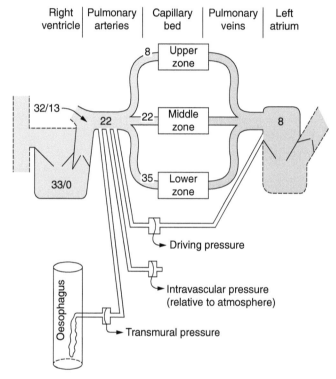

• **Fig. 6.3** Normal values for pressures in the pulmonary circulation relative to atmospheric pressure (cmH$_2$O). Systolic and diastolic pressures are shown for the right ventricle and pulmonary trunk, and mean pressures elsewhere. Note the effect of gravity on pressures at different levels in the lung fields. Three different connected manometers are shown to indicate driving pressure, intravascular pressure and transmural pressure.

the case of the larger pulmonary vessels, the outside pressure is the intrathoracic pressure (commonly measured as the oesophageal pressure, as shown in Fig. 6.3). This method should be used to exclude the physical effect of major changes in intrathoracic pressure.

Driving pressure is the difference in pressure between one point in the circulation and another point downstream. The driving pressure of the pulmonary circulation as a whole is the pressure difference between pulmonary artery and left atrium. This is the pressure that overcomes the flow resistance and should be used for determination of vascular resistance.

These differences are far from solely academic. For example, an increase in intrathoracic pressure because of positive pressure ventilation will increase the pulmonary arterial intravascular pressure, but will also similarly increase pulmonary venous intravascular pressure; therefore driving pressure (and therefore flow) remains unchanged. Similarly, if the primary problem is a raised left atrial pressure, blood will 'back up' through the pulmonary circulation, and pulmonary arterial intravascular pressure will also be raised, but the driving pressure will again not be increased. Therefore for assessing pulmonary blood flow (and so resistance) driving pressure is the correct measurement, but this requires pulmonary venous (left atrial) pressure to be recorded, which is difficult to achieve (page 85). Pulmonary arterial intravascular pressure is usually measured, and the value must therefore be interpreted with caution.

Typical normal values for pressures within the pulmonary circulation are shown in Figure 6.3.

Effect of Intraalveolar Pressure

Alteration of intraalveolar pressure causes changes in intrathoracic pressure according to the following relationship:

Intrathoracic pressure =
alveolar pressure − alveolar transmural pressure.

Alveolar transmural pressure is a function of lung volume (see Fig. 2.7), and when the lungs are passively inflated, the intrathoracic pressure will normally increase by rather less than half the inflation pressure. The increase will be even less if the lungs are stiff, and thus a low compliance protects the circulation from inflation pressure (page 391). Intravascular pressures are normally increased directly and instantaneously by the effects of changes in intrathoracic pressure, and this explains the initial rise in systemic arterial pressure during a Valsalva manoeuvre (page 389). It also explains the cyclical changes in pulmonary arterial pressure during spontaneous respiration, with pressures greater during expiration than during inspiration. Such changes would not be seen if transmural pressure was measured (Fig. 6.3).

In addition to the immediate physical effect of an increase in intrathoracic pressure on intravascular pressures, there is a secondary physiological effect because of interference with venous return. This accounts for the secondary decline in systemic pressure seen in the Valsalva manoeuvre.

Pulmonary Vascular Resistance

Vascular resistance is an expression of the relationship between driving pressure and flow, as in the case of resistance to gas flow. It may be expressed in similar terms as follows:

Pulmonary vascular resistance
$$= \frac{\text{pulmonary driving pressure}}{\text{cardiac output}}.$$

There are, however, important caveats, and the concept of pulmonary vascular resistance is not a simple parallel to Ohm's law, appropriate to laminar flow (page 28). First, the tubes through which the blood flows are not rigid, but tend to expand as flow is increased, particularly in the pulmonary circulation with its low vasomotor tone. Consequently the resistance tends to fall as flow increases, and the plot of pressure against flow rate is neither linear (see Fig. 3.2) nor curved with the concavity upwards (see Fig. 3.3), but curved with the concavity downwards. The second complication is that blood is a non-Newtonian fluid (because of the presence of the red blood cells), and its viscosity varies with the shear rate, which is a function of its linear velocity. For accurate measurement of pulmonary vascular resistance, corrections should be made for haematocrit at the time of measurement.[2]

Vascular Resistance in the Lung

Although the relationship between flow and pressure in blood vessels is far removed from simple linearity, there is a widespread convention that pulmonary vascular resistance should be expressed in a form of the previous equation. This is directly analogous to electrical resistance, as though there were laminar flow of a Newtonian fluid through rigid pipes. It would, of course, be quite impractical in the clinical situation to measure pulmonary driving pressure at different values of cardiac output to determine the true nature of their relationship.

Vascular resistance is expressed in units derived from those used for expression of pressure and flow rate. Using conventional units, vascular resistance is usually expressed in units of mmHg per litre per minute. In absolute centimetre per gram per second units, vascular resistance is usually expressed in units of dynes per square centimetre per cubic centimetre per second (i.e., $dyn.s.cm^{-5}$). The appropriate SI units will probably be $kPa.L^{-1}.min$. Normal values for the pulmonary circulation in the various units are shown in Table 6.1.

Localization of the Pulmonary Vascular Resistance

In the systemic circulation the greatest part of resistance is in the arterioles, along which the pressure falls from a mean

TABLE 6.1	Normal Values for the Pulmonary Circulation		
	Driving Pressure	Pulmonary Blood Flow	Pulmonary Vascular Resistance
SI units	1.2 kPa	5 L.min^{-1}	0.24 kPa.L^{-1}.min
Conventional units	9 mmHg	5 L.min^{-1}	1.8 mm Hg.L^{-1}.min
Absolute CGS units	12,000 dyn.cm^{-2}	83 cm^3.s^{-1}	144 dyn. s.cm^{-5}

See Appendix A for explanation of units

value of approximately 12 kPa (90 mmHg) down to approximately 4 kPa (30 mmHg; Fig. 6.2). This pressure drop largely obliterates the pulse pressure wave, and the systemic capillary flow is not pulsatile to any great extent. In the pulmonary circulation, the pressure drop along the arterioles is very much smaller than in the systemic circulation and, as an approximation, the pulmonary vascular resistance is equally divided between arteries, capillaries and veins. Pulmonary arteries and arterioles, with muscular vessel walls, are mostly extraalveolar and involved in active control of pulmonary vascular resistance by mechanisms such as nervous, humoral or gaseous control. In contrast, pulmonary capillaries are intimately associated with the alveolus (see Fig. 1.8), so resistance of these vessels is therefore greatly influenced by alveolar pressure and volume. Thus in the pulmonary circulation, vessels without the power of active vasoconstriction play a major role in governing total vascular resistance and the distribution of the pulmonary blood flow.

Passive Changes in Pulmonary Vascular Resistance

Effect of Pulmonary Blood Flow (Cardiac Output)

The pulmonary circulation can adapt to large changes in cardiac output with only small increases in pulmonary arterial pressure. Thus pulmonary vascular resistance must decrease as flow increases. Reduced resistance implies an increase in the total cross-sectional area of the pulmonary vascular bed, and particularly the capillaries. These adaptations to increased flow occur partly by passive distension of vessels and partly by recruitment of collapsed vessels, and the former is the more important factor.

Recruitment of previously unperfused pulmonary vessels occurs in response to increased pulmonary flow. This is particularly true of the capillary bed, which is devoid of any vasomotor control, so allowing the opening of new passages in the network of capillaries lying in the alveolar septa, and is most likely to occur in the upper part of the lung where capillary pressure is lowest (zone 1, see later). Capillary recruitment was first described in histological studies involving sections cut in lungs rapidly frozen while perfused with blood, which showed that the number of open capillaries increased with rising pulmonary arterial pressure. Recruitment of capillaries in the intact lung remains poorly understood. Animal studies using colloidal particles in the blood demonstrate that there is perfusion in all pulmonary capillaries, including in zone 1, during normal ventilation, but when airway pressure is increased there is no flow in almost two-thirds of capillaries in zone 1. It therefore seems that, with increased alveolar pressure unperfused capillaries are available for recruitment, but that under normal circumstances, with low airway pressures, there is flow in all capillaries. However, these studies using colloidal particles cannot discriminate between plasma or blood flow, and have led to speculation that some, *almost* collapsed, capillaries may contain only plasma ('plasma skimming') or even blood flow from the bronchial circulation.[3]

Distension in the entire pulmonary vasculature occurs in response to increased transmural pressure gradient and is again most likely to occur in capillaries devoid of muscular control. In one animal study, capillary diameter increased from 5 to 10 μm as the transmural pressure increased from 0.5 to 2.5 kPa (5–25 cmH$_2$O).[4] As described in the previous section, it now seems likely that capillaries never collapse completely, and therefore passive distension is clearly the more important adaptation to increased flow.

A striking example of the ability of the pulmonary vasculature to adapt to changing flow occurs after pneumonectomy (page 401), when the remaining lung will normally take the entire resting pulmonary blood flow without a rise in pulmonary arterial pressure. There is, inevitably, a limit to the flow that can be accommodated without an increase in pressure, and this will be less if the pulmonary vascular bed is affected by disease. The most important pathological cause of increased pulmonary blood flow is left-to-right shunting through a patent ductus arteriosus or through atrial or ventricular septal defects. Under these circumstances the pulmonary blood flow may be several-fold greater than the systemic flow before pulmonary hypertension develops. Despite this, remodelling of the pulmonary vessels commonly results in an increase in vascular resistance, causing an earlier and more severe rise in pulmonary arterial pressure.

Effect of Lung Inflation

Reference has been made earlier to the effect of alveolar pressure on pulmonary vascular pressures. The effect on pulmonary vascular resistance is complex. Confusion has arisen in the past because of failure to appreciate that pulmonary vascular resistance must be derived from driving pressure and not from pulmonary arterial or transmural pressure (Fig. 6.3). This is important because inflation of the lungs normally influences the pressure in the oesophagus, pulmonary artery and left atrium, and so can easily conceal the true effect on vascular resistance.

When pulmonary vascular resistance is correctly calculated from the driving pressure, there is reasonable agreement that the pulmonary vascular resistance is minimal at functional residual capacity, and that changes in lung volume in either direction cause a small increase in resistance, particularly at high lung volumes (Fig. 6.4). These observations may be explained by considering pulmonary capillaries as belonging to three distinct groups:

Alveolar capillaries are sandwiched between two adjacent alveolar walls, usually bulging into one alveolus (see Fig. 1.8), and supported from collapse only by the pressure in the capillary and flimsy septal fibrous tissue. Expansion of the alveolus will therefore compress these capillaries and increase their contribution to pulmonary vascular resistance. If the lung consisted entirely of alveolar capillaries,

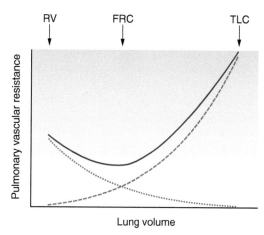

• **Fig. 6.4** Relationship between pulmonary vascular resistance (PVR) and lung volume. The solid red line represents total PVR and is minimal at the functional residual capacity *(FRC)*. Compression of alveolar capillaries *(dashed blue line)* is responsible for the increased PVR as lung volume approaches total lung capacity *(TLC)*. Increasing PVR as lung volume approaches residual volume *(RV)* may result from compression of corner capillaries *(dotted yellow line)* or extraalveolar vessels, or from hypoxia-induced vasoconstriction in collapsed lung units. It should be noted that this graph is derived from studies mainly involving isolated animal lungs, and may not be applicable to the intact animal or human subject.

then pulmonary vascular resistance would be directly related to lung volume.

Corner capillaries lie within the junction between three or more alveoli, and are not therefore sandwiched between alveolar walls. In this area, the alveolar wall is believed to form 'pleats' during lung deflation (see Fig. 1.10), which are then stretched out longitudinally (rather than expanded outwards) during inspiration, and so have little effect on the blood vessels nearby. Indeed, blood vessels in this area are generally uninfluenced by alveolar pressure, but may expand at high lung volume and constrict at very small lung volumes, possibly secondary to local hypoxia surrounding the collapsed alveoli.

Extraalveolar vessels provide an additional explanation for the increased pulmonary vascular resistance at small lung volumes. Compression of larger pulmonary vessels at low lung volumes may result in reduced flow in dependent parts of the lung (page 92), and this is likely to contribute to the overall change in pulmonary vascular resistance.

The anatomical difference between these capillaries is undoubted, whilst the effect of the anatomical features on physiology is unproven. Much of the work has involved mathematical modelling based on animal studies in the open-chested or isolated preparation, and the relevance of these to the intact human remains uncertain.

Effect of Gravity on Alveolar and Vascular Pressures

Vascular Weir

The interplay of alveolar pressure, flow rate and vascular resistance is best considered by dividing the lung field into

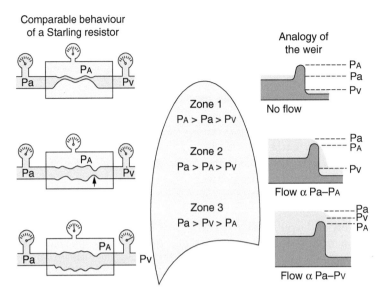

Comparable behaviour
of a Starling resistor

Analogy of
the weir

Zone 1
$P_A > P_a > P_v$

Zone 2
$P_a > P_A > P_v$

Zone 3
$P_a > P_v > P_A$

No flow

Flow α $P_a – P_A$

Flow α $P_a – P_v$

• **Fig. 6.5** The effect of gravity on pulmonary vascular resistance is shown by comparison with a Starling resistor (left) and with a weir (right). P_a, Pulmonary artery pressure; P_A, alveolar pressure; P_v, pulmonary venous pressure (all pressures relative to atmosphere). See text for full discussion.

three zones, a concept first described by West in 1965.[5] Figure 6.5 shows behaviour as a Starling resistor and also the analogy of a weir. A Starling, or threshold, resistor can be visualized as a length of compressible tubing within a rigid chamber, such that flow occurs only when the upstream pressure (left gauges in Fig. 6.5) exceeds the pressure within the chamber (middle gauges), and a reduction in the downstream pressure (right gauges) cannot initiate flow. In zone 1 of Figure 6.5, the pressure within the arterial end of the collapsible vessels is less than the alveolar pressure, and therefore insufficient to open the vessels that remain collapsed as in a Starling resistor. The upstream water is below the top of the weir, so there can be no flow. The downstream (venous) pressure is irrelevant. Zone 1 corresponds to conditions that may apply in the uppermost parts of the lungs.

In the midzone of the lungs (zone 2 of Fig. 6.5), the pressure at the arterial end of the collapsible vessels exceeds the alveolar pressure and, under these conditions, a collapsible vessel, behaving like a Starling resistor, permits flow in such a way that the flow rate depends on the arterial/alveolar pressure difference. Resistance in the Starling resistor is concentrated at the point marked with the arrow in Figure 6.5. The greater the difference between arterial and alveolar pressure, the more widely the collapsible vessels will open and the greater will be the flow. Note that the venous pressure is still not a factor that affects flow or vascular resistance. This condition is still analogous to a weir, the upstream depth (head of pressure) corresponding to the arterial pressure, and the height of the weir corresponding to alveolar pressure. Flow depends solely on the difference in height between the upstream water level and the top of the weir. The depth of water below the weir (analogous to venous pressure) cannot influence the flow of water over the weir unless it rises above the height of the weir.

In the lower zone of the lungs (zone 3 of Fig. 6.5), the pressure in the venous end of the capillaries is above the alveolar pressure, and under these conditions a collapsible vessel behaving like a Starling resistor will be held wide open, and the flow rate will, as a first approximation, be governed by the arterial/venous pressure difference (the driving pressure) in the normal manner for the systemic circulation. However, as the intravascular pressure increases in relation to the alveolar pressure, the collapsible vessels will be further distended, and their resistance will be correspondingly reduced. Returning to the analogy of the weir, the situation is now one in which the downstream water level has risen until the weir is completely submerged and offers little resistance to the flow of water, which is largely governed by the difference in the water level above and below the weir. However, as the levels rise further, the weir is progressively more and more submerged, and what little resistance it offers to water flow is diminished still further.

Active Control of Pulmonary Vascular Resistance

In addition to the passive mechanisms described, pulmonary blood vessels are also able to control vascular resistance by active vasoconstriction and vasodilatation, and there is some evidence that the pulmonary vasculature is normally kept in a state of active vasodilatation.

Cellular Mechanisms Controlling Pulmonary Vascular Tone[6]

There are many mechanisms by which pulmonary vascular tone may be controlled (Table 6.2), but the role of many of these in the human lung is uncertain. Some of the

TABLE 6.2   Receptors and Agonists Involved in Active Control of Pulmonary Vascular Tone

Receptor Group	Subtypes	Principal Agonists	Responses	Endothelium-Dependent?
Adrenergic	α_1	Noradrenaline	Constriction	No
	α_2	Noradrenaline	Dilatation	Yes
	β_2	Adrenaline	Dilatation	Yes
Cholinergic	M_3	Acetylcholine	Dilatation	Yes
Amines	H_1	Histamine	Variable	Yes
	H_2	Histamine	Dilatation	No
	$5\text{-}HT_1$	5-HT	Variable	Variable
Purines	P_{2x}	ATP	Constriction	No
	P_{2y}	ATP	Dilatation	Yes
	A_1	Adenosine	Constriction	No
	A_2	Adenosine	Dilatation	No
Eicosanoids	TP	Thromboxane A_2	Constriction	No
	IP	Prostacyclin	Dilatation	?
Peptides	NK_1	Substance P	Dilatation	Yes
	NK_2	Neurokinin A	Constriction	No
	?	VIP	Relaxation	Variable
	AT	Angiotensin	Constriction	No
	ANP	ANP	Dilatation	No
	B_2	Bradykinin	Dilatation	Yes
	ET_A	Endothelin	Constriction	No
	ET_B	Endothelin	Dilatation	Yes
	?	Adrenomedullin	Dilatation	?
	V_1	Vasopressin	Dilatation	Yes

The existence of many of the substances listed is at present only established in animals, and their physiological or pathological relevance in humans therefore remains uncertain.

5-HT, 5-hydroxytryptamine; *ATP*, adenosine triphosphate; *ANP*, Atrial natriuretic peptide; *VIP*, vasoactive intestinal peptide.

receptor–agonist systems in Table 6.2 have only been demonstrated in vitro using animal tissue but may eventually emerge as important in humans either for normal maintenance of pulmonary vascular tone or during hypoxia or lung injury (Chapter 31). Activity of some, although not all, of the mechanisms listed in Table 6.2 is dependent on the endothelial lining of the pulmonary blood vessels. It seems likely that many basic control mechanisms occur within the smooth muscle cell, whilst the endothelium acts as a modulator of the response. Some control mechanisms, such as the autonomic nervous system and hypoxic pulmonary vasoconstriction, have been extensively investigated in humans, and are described separately in later sections.

Receptors

Endothelial and smooth muscle cells of the pulmonary vasculature each have numerous receptor types, and the agonists for these receptors may originate from nerve endings (e.g., acetylcholine (ACh), noradrenaline), be produced locally (e.g., eicosanoids, endothelin) or arrive via the blood (e.g., peptides). In addition, many similar or identical compounds produce opposing effects by their actions on differing subgroups of receptors, for example α_1 (vasoconstrictor) and β_2 (vasodilator) adrenergic receptors. There remain therefore a large number of poorly understood systems acting together to bring about control of pulmonary vascular smooth muscle.

Second Messengers

Pulmonary vasodilators that act directly on the smooth muscle, such as prostaglandins, vasoactive intestinal peptide and, under some circumstances, β_2-agonists, mostly activate adenyl cyclase to produce cyclic adenosine $3',5'$ monophosphate (cAMP) as a second messenger. In turn, cAMP causes a host of intracellular activity via activation of protein kinase enzymes that reduce both the phosphorylation of myosin and intracellular calcium levels to bring about relaxation of the muscle cell.

Receptors that cause contraction of pulmonary vascular smooth muscle are usually G-protein-coupled. Activation produces a second messenger, inositol 1,4,5-triphosphate (IP_3), which releases calcium from intracellular stores and activates myosin phosphorylation to produce contraction.

Role of the Endothelium and Nitric Oxide

In 1980 Furchgott and Zawadzki were the first to demonstrate that endothelial cells were required for ACh-induced relaxation in isolated aortic tissue. The messenger passing between the endothelium and smooth muscle cells was termed endothelium-derived relaxing factor,[7] the major part of which was subsequently shown to be nitric oxide (NO). Many pulmonary vasodilator mechanisms have been shown to be endothelium-dependent (Table 6.2), and it is likely that NO is a common pathway for producing relaxation of vascular smooth muscle from a variety of stimuli.

Nitric oxide synthase (NOS) produces NO by the conversion of L-arginine to L-citrulline, via a highly reactive hydroxy-arginine intermediate. NOS is involved in both stages, and requires many cofactors including calmodulin and nicotinamide adenine dinucleotide phosphate (NADPH), and probably other flavine-derived factors such as flavine adenine dinucleotide. Control of NOS activity depends on the availability of the substrate, arginine, and the concentrations of the various cofactors. The biological disposal of NO is described on page 148.

NOS exists in multiple forms; the major ones are constitutive, inducible and neuronal. Inducible NOS (iNOS) is produced in many cells, but only in response to activation by inflammatory mediators and other cytokines, and once activated can produce large amounts of NO for long periods. Constitutive NOS (cNOS) is permanently present in some cells, including pulmonary endothelium, and produces short bursts of low levels of NO in response to changes in calcium and calmodulin levels. In systemic vessels, sheer stress of the blood vessel wall may directly activate calcium-dependent potassium channels to activate cNOS, but in the pulmonary circulation receptor stimulation is the usual source of altered calcium levels and cNOS activation. Neuronal NOS is responsible for the production of the NO released from neurones as a neurotransmitter or neuromodulator, such as in the carotid body (page 51).

The mechanism by which receptor activation leads to muscle relaxation is illustrated in Figure 6.6. NO diffuses from the site of production to the smooth muscle cell, where it activates guanylate cyclase to produce cyclic guanosine 3′,5′ monophosphate (cGMP), which in turn activates a protein kinase enzyme. This system is similar to the cAMP pathway previously described, and causes relaxation by a combination of effects on cytosolic calcium levels and the activity of enzymes controlling myosin activity.

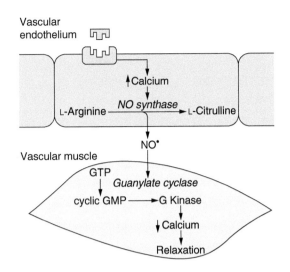

• **Fig. 6.6** Schematic pathway for the activation of constitutive NOS and the action of NO in the pulmonary vasculature. There are many different receptors thought to act via this mechanism to bring about vasodilatation. See text for details. GTP, guanosine triphosphate; GMP, guanosine monophosphate.

There is good evidence that basal production of NO occurs in normal human lungs and contributes to the maintenance of low pulmonary vascular resistance.

Hypoxic Pulmonary Vasoconstriction[6,8,9]

When vasoconstriction occurs in response to hypoxia, pulmonary blood vessels are displaying their fundamental difference from systemic vessels. Hypoxic pulmonary vasoconstriction (HPV) is mediated both by mixed venous (pulmonary arterial) Po_2 and alveolar Po_2 (Fig. 6.7), and the greater influence is from the alveolus. The overall response to Po_2 is nonlinear. This may be deduced from Figure 6.7 by noting the pressure response for different values of the isobaric Po_2 (the broken green line), and it will be seen that the general shape of the response curve resembles an oxyhaemoglobin dissociation curve with a P_{50} of approximately 4 kPa (30 mmHg). The combined effect of hypoxia in alveolar gas and mixed venous blood may be considered as acting at a single point,[10] which exerts a 'stimulus' Po_2 as follows:

$$P(\text{stimulus})O_2 \times P\bar{v}_{O_2}{}^{0.375} \times PA_{O_2}{}^{0.626}$$

Regional hypoxic pulmonary vasoconstriction is beneficial as a way of diverting the pulmonary blood flow away from regions in which the oxygen partial pressure is low, and is an important factor in the optimization of ventilation/perfusion relationships (see Chapter 7), even in healthy normoxic lung.[11] It is also important in the fetus to minimize perfusion of the unventilated lung. However, long-term continuous or intermittent HPV leads to remodelling of the pulmonary vasculature and pulmonary hypertension, and this response is disadvantageous in a range of clinical conditions (see Chapter 29).

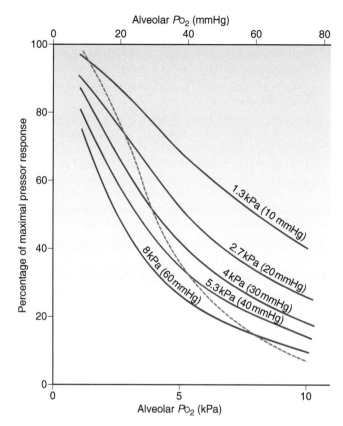

• **Fig. 6.7** Influence of mixed venous P_{O_2} on hypoxic pulmonary vasoconstriction. The intensity of pulmonary vasoconstriction (ordinate) is shown as a function of alveolar P_{O_2} (abscissa) for different values of mixed venous P_{O_2} (indicated for each curve). The broken line shows the response when the alveolar and mixed venous P_{O_2} are identical. (From Marshall BE, Marshall C. Anesthesia and the pulmonary circulation. In: Covino BG, Fozzard HA, Rehder K, et al., eds. *Effects of Anesthesia.* Bethesda, MD: American Physiological Society; 1983.)

The pressor response to hypoxia results from constriction of small arterioles of 30 to 200 μm in diameter and begins within a few seconds of the P_{O_2} decreasing. In humans, hypoxia in a single lobe of the lung results in a rapid decline in perfusion of the lobe, such that after a few minutes regional blood flow is half that during normoxia. With prolonged hypoxia, HPV is biphasic, and the initial rapid response reaches a plateau after about 5 minutes, with the second phase occurring approximately 40 minutes later[12] (Fig. 6.8) and reaching a maximal response 2 to 4 hours after the onset of hypoxia.[13]

In healthy subjects, HPV within the lung is heterogeneous,[14] with intense vasoconstriction in some areas and relative overperfusion elsewhere (Fig. 6.9), the degree to which this occurs varying between individuals, which has important implications when travelling to high altitude (page 213).

Mechanism of Hypoxic Pulmonary Vasoconstriction[6,9,15,16]

Neural connections to the lung are not required because HPV occurs in isolated lung preparations and in humans

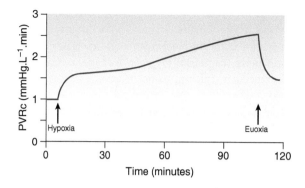

• **Fig. 6.8** Time course of the hypoxic pulmonary vasoconstriction response to prolonged isocapnic hypoxia in humans (end-tidal P_{O_2} 6.7 kPa, 50 mmHg). Phase 1 of the response is complete within a few minutes, and the phase 2 response occurs approximately 40 minutes later. *PVRc,* Pulmonary vascular resistance corrected for cardiac output. Note that after prolonged hypoxia PVRc does not return to baseline immediately. (From reference 12.)

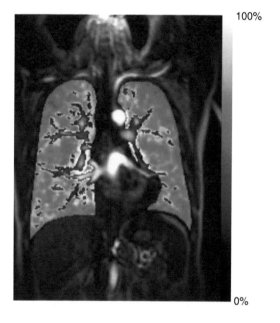

• **Fig. 6.9** Contrast-enhanced magnetic resonance (MR) imaging in a healthy subject who is supine and breathing 12% oxygen (oxygen saturation 73%–77%) showing the heterogeneous nature of hypoxic pulmonary vasoconstriction. The colours indicate percentage of 'peak signal intensity' after intravenous injection of MR contrast, and represent perfusion of parenchymal lung tissue from zero (*black*) to maximal (*white*). (From reference 14. With permission.)

after lung transplantation. Attempts to elucidate the mechanism of HPV have been hampered by species differences, the multitude of systems affecting pulmonary vascular tone and a lack of appreciation of the biphasic nature of the response. Uncertainties remain on the cellular mechanism of HPV, but there is now agreement that contraction of pulmonary artery smooth muscle cells (PASMCs) in response to hypoxia is an inherent property of these cells, and that pulmonary endothelial cells only act to modulate the PASMC response.[17]

Oxygen Sensing in Pulmonary Artery Smooth Muscle Cells

This is similar to the mechanisms already described in the carotid body (page 51). Hypoxia leads to a small increase in intracellular calcium concentration, and also a Rho kinase–mediated increase in the calcium sensitivity of the contractile proteins of the cell. These changes in calcium activity result from opening of voltage-dependent L-type calcium channels, stimulated in turn by hypoxia-induced inhibition of voltage-gated potassium (Kv) channels. As in the carotid body, the molecular oxygen sensor that affects the Kv channel remains controversial. This may be an inherent property of the Kv channel itself, although other mechanisms undoubtedly contribute, including:

- *Redox state in the cytoplasm.* This includes ratios of the redox couples of glutathione and nicotinamide adenine dinucleotide. It is suggested that, when normoxic, the redox state of the cell maintains the Kv channels in the open position, creating the normal resting membrane potential, and that during hypoxia the channels close, altering membrane potential and activating the calcium channels.
- *Mitochondrial reactive oxygen species (ROS).* ROS production is described in Chapter 25. It is likely that hypoxia is directly sensed by the mitochondrial complexes of the electron transport chain (page 152), leading to an increase in ROS production at complex III of the chain,[15,18] which acts as an important signalling mechanism for HPV.[19]
- *Cellular energy state.* In hypoxic cells, when glucose remains available, levels of high-energy molecules such as adenosine triphosphate (ATP) are maintained mostly by glycolysis (page 151). An alternative pathway for maintaining ATP levels involves adenylate kinase converting any available adenosine diphosphate molecules into ATP, which increases adenosine monophosphate (AMP) levels. High levels of AMP activate an oxygen-sensitive enzyme AMP-activated kinase which initiates a range of intracellular changes to reduce ATP consumption, and may also lead to release of Ca^{2+} from sarcoplasmic reticulum.
- *Hypoxia-inducible factor (HIF).*[20] This is a ubiquitous enzyme which, under hypoxic conditions, initiates transcription of many different genes to help the cell survive hypoxia (page 276). HIF comprises two subunits, an α-subunit which is oxygen sensitive and a constitutive β-subunit. In normoxic cells the α-subunit of active HIF has a half-life of only 5 min because of its rapid inactivation by hydroxylation; this reaction is dependent on prolyl hydroxylase-domain (PHD) enzymes. PHD activity is dependent on Po_2 across a wide range of values, and the effects of HIF on transcription is also oxygen-dependent,[6] so both its existence and activity are oxygen-sensitive.
- *Cyclooxygenase and lipoxygenase (page 170).* These use molecular oxygen as a substrate, so are inherently oxygen-sensitive. Activity of these enzymes generates many vasoactive metabolites, so modification of their activity by hypoxia can have multiple effects on the pulmonary vasculature. Evidence suggests that cyclooxygenase and lipoxygenase activity are not primarily responsible for oxygen sensing in HPV, but may be involved in modulating the response.

Despite extensive research there is still no consensus on how oxygen sensing in pulmonary blood vessels occurs.[6] Many of these molecular mechanisms are interconnected, and in vivo it is inevitable that multiple different systems are involved.

Modulation by the Endothelial Cell of the Pulmonary Artery Smooth Muscle Cells[17]

Endothelial cell activity may either enhance or inhibit HPV. Inhibitors of HPV include prostacyclin (PGI_2) and NO, both of which may exist to maintain some perfusion of hypoxic lung regions, although their role in normal lung is uncertain. For example, PGI_2 is a potent pulmonary vasodilator, but cyclooxygenase, which is required for its production, is inhibited by hypoxia, which may therefore diminish the vasodilator effects.

Similarly, basal NO secretion by endothelial cells may act to moderate HPV, but hypoxia also inhibits endothelial NO production enhancing HPV. Molecules that enhance HPV include thromboxane A_2 (see later) and endothelin. Endothelin is a 21 amino acid peptide released by endothelial cells in response to hypoxia.[21] It is a potent vasoconstrictor peptide which has a prolonged effect on pulmonary vascular tone, such that this mechanism is probably involved in the second slow phase of HPV (Fig. 6.8). Endothelin is believed to be involved in producing the pulmonary hypertension associated with altitude hypoxia (see Chapter 16), although attempts to enhance HPV with endothelin infusions have not been successful.[13] Two groups of endothelin receptors are described, ET_A and ET_B, and the ratio of these two receptors varies between the central and peripheral vasculature of the lung. Apart from its vasoconstrictor effects, endothelin can also stimulate cellular proliferation of either vascular endothelial cells or pulmonary fibroblasts, and has an important role in the pulmonary vascular remodelling that accompanies long-term hypoxia.

Iron and Hypoxic Pulmonary Vasoconstriction[20,22]

Increased iron availability (achieved by intravenous infusion) attenuates HPV, whereas reducing iron availability by administration of desferrioxamine enhances the response. Administration of intravenous iron results in a prolonged attenuation of HPV for at least 43 days.[22] The mechanism of this effect is that PHD activity (see previous section) is critically dependent on iron concentration within the cytoplasm. These observations may be highly significant for patients, given that normal subjects have widely varying iron levels, depending on such factors as sex, diet and chronic illness, providing the potential to use iron to modify pulmonary hypertension in disease states.[23,24]

Effects of P_{CO_2} and pH on Pulmonary Vascular Resistance

Elevated P_{CO_2} has a slight pressor effect in the pulmonary circulation, and both respiratory and metabolic acidosis augment HPV. Alkalosis, whether respiratory (hypocapnia) or metabolic in origin, causes pulmonary vasodilatation and attenuates HPV.[25]

Neural Control

There are three systems involved in autonomic control of the pulmonary circulation, which are similar to those controlling airway tone (page 33).

Adrenergic sympathetic nerves originate from the first five thoracic nerves and travel to the pulmonary vessels via the cervical ganglia and a plexus of nerves around the trachea and smaller airways. They act mainly on the smooth muscle of arteries and arterioles down to a diameter of less than 60 μm. There are both α_1-receptors, which mediate vasoconstriction, usually in response to noradrenaline release, and β_2-receptors, which produce vasodilatation, mainly in response to circulating adrenaline. Overall, α_1 effects predominate, causing sympathetic stimulation that increases pulmonary vascular resistance. The influence of the sympathetic system is not as strong as in the systemic circulation and seems to have little influence under resting conditions. There is no obvious disadvantage in this respect in patients with lung transplant (see Chapter 33).

Cholinergic nerves of the parasympathetic system travel in the vagus nerve and cause pulmonary vasodilatation by release of ACh and stimulation of M_3 muscarinic receptors. ACh-mediated vasodilatation is accepted as endothelium- and NO-dependent, and in the absence of endothelium, ACh is a vasoconstrictor. The significance of cholinergic nerves in humans is less clear than that of adrenergic systems.

Noncholinergic parasympathetic (NCP) nerves are closely related anatomically to the other autonomic mechanisms, but with different neurotransmitters, and are similar to the NCP nerves controlling airway smooth muscle (page 34). In the lung, most NCP nerves are inhibitory, causing vasodilatation via release of NO, possibly in conjunction with peptides (Table 6.2). The functional significance of this system is unknown.

Humoral Control

Pulmonary vascular endothelium is involved in the metabolism of many circulating substances (see Chapter 11), some of which cause changes in vascular tone (Table 6.2). Which of these are involved in the control of normal pulmonary vascular resistance is unclear, and it is quite possible that very few are, but some are undoubtedly involved in pulmonary vascular disease (see Chapter 29).

Catecholamines. Circulating adrenaline following sympathetic stimulation acts on both α- and β-receptors and results in a predominantly vasoconstrictor response. Exogenous adrenaline and related inotropes such as dopamine have a similar effect.

Eicosanoids. Arachidonic acid metabolism via the cyclo-oxygenase pathway (to prostaglandins (PG) and thromboxane) and lipoxygenase pathway (to leukotrienes (LT)) has been demonstrated in pulmonary vessels in animals. The products of arachidonic acid metabolism have diverse biological effects in many physiological systems, and the pulmonary vasculature is no exception. Arachidonic acid, thromboxane A_2, $PGF_{2\alpha}$, PGD_2, PGE_2 and LTB_4 are all vasoconstrictors, whereas PGI_2 is usually a vasodilator. These pathways are believed to be involved in pathological pulmonary hypertension resulting from sepsis, reperfusion injury or congenital heart disease.

Amines. Histamine relaxes pulmonary vascular smooth muscle during adrenaline-induced constriction, but constricts resting smooth muscle. Constriction is in response to H_1 stimulation on smooth muscle cells, whilst relaxation occurs either via H_1 receptors on endothelium (NO dependent) or H_2 receptors on smooth muscle cells. 5-hydroxytryptamine (5-HT; serotonin) is liberated from activated platelets and is a potent vasoconstrictor. It may be involved in pulmonary hypertension secondary to emboli (page 345).

Peptides. Numerous peptides that are vasoactive in the pulmonary circulation are shown in Table 6.2. Responses are again diverse, with many systems producing vasodilatation via endothelium receptors and vasoconstriction via direct effects on smooth muscle (e.g., substance P and neurokinin A).

Purine nucleosides such as adenosine and ATP are highly vasoactive, again with variable responses according to the amount of tone in the pulmonary blood vessel. Adenosine is a pulmonary vasodilator in normal subjects.

Drug Effects on the Pulmonary Circulation

A higher than normal pulmonary arterial pressure occurs rarely as a primary disease, but commonly develops as a secondary consequence of chronic hypoxia from a variety of lung diseases (see Chapter 29). Considering the wide range of receptor–agonist systems present in the pulmonary vasculature (Table 6.2), it is surprising that there are only a few effective drugs available. One reason for this is the nonspecific nature of many of the receptors found in the pulmonary vasculature, such that drugs acting on these receptors have widespread effects elsewhere in the body that make them therapeutically unacceptable. Another problem with pulmonary vasodilators in respiratory disease is that abolishing HPV removes the body's main mechanisms for compensating for poor ventilation perfusion matching. For example, nifedipine administered sublingually in patients with severe airways disease causes a significant reduction in pulmonary hypertension, but this is associated with a worsening of arterial hypoxaemia. As a way of avoiding both these problems, delivering drugs by inhalation has had some success, particularly if the drug is inactivated before reaching the systemic circulation.

Inhaled Drugs

Nitric Oxide

Inhaled NO (iNO) in patients with severe lung disease is a selective pulmonary vasodilator, with the systemic circulation unaffected because of its rapid inactivation by haemoglobin (page 148). NO therefore increases blood flow to well-ventilated areas of the lung, diverting blood flow away from poorly ventilated areas, decreasing ventilation–perfusion mismatch and improving arterial oxygenation.

iNO in the presence of oxygen is rapidly oxidized to NO_2; the rate of oxidation is directly related to oxygen concentration and the square of NO concentration. NO_2 can react with water to form highly injurious nitric and nitrous acids that can cause severe lung damage. Hence, to minimize the production of NO_2, both the concentration of oxygen and NO, and the contact time between the two, should be minimized. Some of the beneficial effects of iNO may be short-lived, whilst rapid discontinuation of iNO leads to a rebound phenomenon, probably as a result of inhibition of endogenous NO, with decreased oxygenation and increased pulmonary artery pressures. Hence, iNO should be withdrawn in a slow, stepwise fashion. Despite these numerous drawbacks, therapeutic iNO in some groups of patients with acute lung injury can be beneficial for oxygenation, but unfortunately this does not result in improved survival.[26]

Prostacyclin (PGI2)[27]

Intravenous PGI_2 has been used for some time for treatment of pulmonary hypertension and to reduce PA pressure in critically ill patients, but its lack of selectivity for the pulmonary vasculature causes significant adverse effects. When delivered by inhalation, metabolism of PGI_2 by the lung is negligible, so systemic absorption occurs. However, the dose required by inhalation is very small, and despite its systemic absorption, clinically significant adverse effects are minimal.

Systemic Drugs[28]

PGI_2 or its analogues may be administered continuously by the intravenous or subcutaneous routes. PGI_2 has a half-life of less than 5 min, so a variety of longer-acting synthetic analogues have been developed, such as iloprost (half-life ~30 min) and treprostinil (half-life ~4.5 hours). An oral PGI_2 receptor agonist, selexipag, is now available.

Angiotensin-converting enzyme inhibitors reduce pulmonary vascular resistance in patients with pulmonary hypertension secondary to lung disease, but only with long-term treatment. These drugs are also believed to reduce pulmonary vascular remodelling (page 347). Losartan, an angiotensin II receptor antagonist, reduces pulmonary artery pressure within hours of administration.

Phosphodiesterase (PDE) inhibitors can inhibit the breakdown of both cAMP and cGMP, and so enhance the activity of these cellular messengers that bring about PASMC relaxation from a variety of pathways (see earlier discussion), including all those mediated by NO. These drugs have been used to reduce pulmonary hypertension by both the intravenous and inhaled routes. Of particular interest for the pulmonary circulation are selective inhibitors of type 5 PDE, which is specific for pulmonary cGMP breakdown. Sildenafil, more well known for its use as a treatment for impotence, is an oral inhibitor of PDE5 with few side effects that acts as a pulmonary vasodilator by enhancing the effects of endogenous NO.[29]

Calcium antagonists such as nifedipine reduce secondary pulmonary hypertension in a dose-dependent fashion by inhibition of the L-type calcium channels on PASMCs (described earlier). However, as already described, in some patient groups hypoxaemia may worsen, and at the large doses often needed to reduce pulmonary hypertension, the negative inotropic effects of calcium antagonists become significant, and right heart failure caused by the pulmonary hypertension can deteriorate.

Endothelin receptor antagonists[21,28] competitively antagonize both ET_A and ET_B receptors, although in the clinical situation ET_B effects seem to predominate and reduce PA pressure. Endothelin has been implicated in vascular remodelling of pulmonary vessels with chronic hypoxia, so these drugs may also slow this harmful process. Bosentan and ambrisentan are currently used to treat patients with pulmonary hypertension, and more long-acting drugs such as macitentan are now available.[28]

Pulmonary vasoconstrictors[30] include the sympathomimetics with α-receptor activity, such as noradrenaline, phenylephrine and metaraminol, which affect pulmonary and systemic vessels with similar potency. The systemic vasoconstrictor vasopressin has no effect on pulmonary vessels.

Principles of Measurement of the Pulmonary Circulation

Detailed consideration of haemodynamic measurement techniques lies outside the scope of this book. The following section presents only the broad principles of measurement such as may be required in relation to respiratory physiology.

Pulmonary Vascular Pressures

Pressure measurements within the pulmonary circulation are almost always made with electronic pressure transducers, which measure instantaneous pressure against time (Fig. 6.10). Systolic and diastolic pressures are measured from the peaks and troughs of this trace, and the mean pressure is derived electronically.

Figure 6.3 shows the sites at which pressure must be measured to obtain the various forms of pulmonary vascular pressure (page 75). Driving pressure, the most useful of

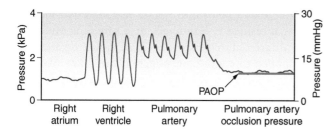

• **Fig. 6.10** Pressure traces obtained when inserting a balloon flotation catheter in a patient receiving intermittent positive pressure ventilation. With the balloon inflated, the catheter tip follows blood flow through the right atrium, right ventricle and pulmonary artery until it occludes a branch of the pulmonary artery. The pulmonary artery occlusion pressure *(PAOP)* is the pressure measured distal to the balloon, and equates to pulmonary venous and left atrial pressures. Note the respiratory swings in the trace caused by positive pressure ventilation. PAOP is measured as the mean pressure at end expiration.

these, requires measurement of pulmonary arterial and pulmonary venous (left atrial) pressures.

Pulmonary arterial pressure may be measured using a balloon flotation catheter. Following insertion into the right atrium via a central vein, a balloon of less than 1 mL volume is inflated to encourage the catheter tip to follow the flow of blood through the right ventricle and pulmonary valve into the pulmonary artery (Fig. 6.10). The most commonly used catheter is the Swan–Ganz, named after the two cardiologists who devised the catheter after Dr Swan watched sailboats being propelled by the wind in 1967.[31]

Left atrial pressure represents pulmonary venous pressure, and is measured in humans by one of three possible techniques, of which only the first is used commonly in clinical practice.

• Pulmonary artery occlusion pressure (PAOP) is obtained by advancing the Swan–Ganz catheter into a branch of the pulmonary artery, with the balloon inflated, until the arterial pulsation disappears (Fig. 6.10). There should then be no flow in the column of blood between the tip of the catheter and the left atrium, and the manometer will indicate left atrial pressure.

• A left atrial catheter may be sited during cardiac surgery and passed through the chest wall for use postoperatively.

• A catheter may be passed retrogradely from a peripheral systemic artery.

Clinical assessment of pulmonary vascular pressures only rarely involves invasive techniques such as these.[32] Echocardiography enhanced with Doppler flow measurements is a much less invasive technique suitable for screening patients for pulmonary hypertension. The technique relies on there being some degree of tricuspid regurgitation, which is present in most patients, and the size and velocity of blood flowing back into the atrium allows right ventricular systolic pressure to be estimated. In the absence of significant pulmonary stenosis, which is easily assessed during the echocardiography, the right ventricular systolic pressure equates to that in the pulmonary artery.

Pulmonary Blood Flow

The method used for measurement of pulmonary blood flow will affect whether or not the result includes venous admixture such as the bronchial circulation and intrapulmonary shunts shown in Figure 6.1. Although of minimal relevance in normal subjects, in patients with lung disease venous admixture may be highly significant. In general, methods involving uptake of an inert gas from the alveoli will exclude venous admixture, and all other methods include it.

The Fick principle states that the amount of oxygen extracted from the respired gases equals the amount added to the blood which flows through the lungs. Thus the oxygen uptake of the subject must equal the product of pulmonary blood flow and arteriovenous oxygen content difference:

$$\dot{V}O_2 = \dot{Q}\left(Ca_{O_2} - C\bar{v}_{O_2}\right),$$

therefore

$$\dot{Q} = \frac{\dot{V}O_2}{\left(Ca_{O_2} - C\bar{v}_{O_2}\right)}$$

All the quantities on the right-hand side can be measured, although determination of the oxygen content of the mixed venous blood requires catheterization of the right ventricle or, preferably, the pulmonary artery, as described earlier. Interpretation of the result is less easy. The calculated value includes the intrapulmonary arteriovenous shunt, but the situation is complicated beyond the possibility of an easy solution if there is appreciable extrapulmonary admixture of venous blood (Fig. 6.1). The second major problem is that spirometry measures the total oxygen consumption, including that of the lung. The Fick equation excludes the lung (see page 161), but the difference is negligible with healthy lungs. There is evidence that the oxygen consumption of infected lungs may be very large (page 161), and therefore the Fick method of measurement of cardiac output would appear to be invalid under such circumstances.

Methods based on uptake of inert tracer gases include the modified Fick method. This measurement of cardiac output may be used with any fairly soluble inert gas. The tracer gas is inhaled either continually or for a single breath, and the end-tidal partial pressure of tracer gas then measured. Analysis of volume and composition of expired tracer gas permits measurement of gas uptake. Because the duration of the procedure is short and does not permit recirculation, it may be assumed that the mixed venous concentration of the tracer gas is zero. The Fick equation then simplifies to the following:

Cardiac output = tracer gas uptake/
arterial tracer gas concentration.

The arterial tracer gas concentration equals the product of the arterial gas tension (assumed equal to the alveolar [end-tidal] gas tension) and the solubility coefficient of the tracer gas in blood. Thus, arterial blood sampling may be avoided, so the method is relatively noninvasive.

All the methods based on the uptake of inert tracer gases have the following characteristics:

- They measure pulmonary capillary blood flow, excluding any flow through shunts. This is in contrast to the Fick and dye methods.
- The assumption that the partial pressure of the tracer gas is the same in end-expiratory gas and arterial blood is invalid in the presence of either alveolar dead space or shunt (see Chapter 7).
- Some of the tracer gas dissolves in the tissues lining the respiratory tract and is carried away by blood perfusing these tissues. The indicated blood flow is therefore greater than the actual pulmonary capillary blood flow.

The tracer gas used most recently is freon. In this case argon (highly insoluble gas) is added to the gas mixture to ensure complete mixing of the freon with alveolar gas, and to detect subjects with a large respiratory dead space (see Chapter 7) in whom the method is invalid.[33]

Dye or Thermal Dilution

The most popular technique for measurement of cardiac output is by dye dilution. An indicator substance is introduced as a bolus into a large vein, and its concentration is measured continuously at a sampling site in the systemic arterial tree. Figure 6.11, A, shows the method as it is applied to continuous noncirculating flow like fluids through a pipeline. The downstream concentration of dye is displayed on the y-axis of the graph against time on the x-axis. The dye is injected at time t_1 and is first detected at the sampling point at time t_2. The uppermost curve shows the form of a typical curve. There is a rapid rise to maximum concentration followed by a decay that is an exponential washout in form (see Appendix E), reaching insignificant levels at time t_3. The second graph shows the concentration (y-axis) on a logarithmic scale when the exponential part of the decay curve becomes a straight line (see Fig. E.5). Between times t_2 and t_3, the mean concentration of dye equals the amount of dye injected, divided by the volume of fluid flowing past the sampling point during the interval $t_2 - t_3$, which is the product of the fluid flow rate and the time interval $t_2 - t_3$. The equation may now be rearranged to indicate the flow rate of the fluid as seen in the following expression:

$$\frac{\text{amount of dye injected}}{\text{mean concentration of dye} \times \text{time interval } t_2 - t_3}$$

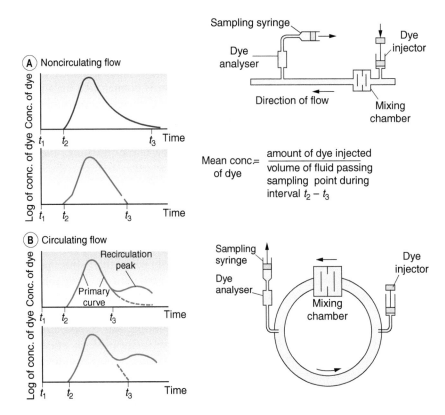

$$\text{Mean conc. of dye} = \frac{\text{amount of dye injected}}{\text{volume of fluid passing sampling point during interval } t_2 - t_3}$$

• **Fig. 6.11** Measurement of flow by dye dilution. **(A)** The measurement of continuous noncirculating flow rate of fluid in a pipeline. The bolus of dye is injected upstream, and its concentration is continuously monitored downstream. The relationship of the relevant quantities is shown in the equation. Mean concentration of dye is determined from the area under the curve. **(B)** The more complicated situation when recirculation occurs and the front of the circulating dye laps its own tail, giving a recirculation peak. Reconstruction of the primary curve is based on extrapolation of the primary curve before recirculation occurs. This is facilitated by the fact that the down curve is exponential, and therefore a straight line on a logarithmic plot.

The amount of dye injected is known, and the denominator is the area under the curve.

Figure 6.11, *B*, shows the more complicated situation when fluid is flowing round a circuit. Under these conditions, the front of the dye-laden fluid may lap its own tail, so that a recirculation peak appears on the graph before the primary peak has decayed to insignificant levels. This commonly occurs when cardiac output is determined in humans, and steps must be taken to reconstruct the tail of the primary curve as it would have been had recirculation not taken place. This is done by extrapolating the exponential washout which is usually established before the recirculation peak appears. This is shown as the broken lines in the graphs in Figure 6.11, *B*. The calculation of cardiac output then proceeds as previously described for nonrecirculating flow. This previously laborious procedure is now performed electronically as an integral part of the apparatus for measuring cardiac output.

Many different indicators have been used for the dye dilution technique, but currently the most satisfactory appears to be 'coolth'. A bolus of cold saline is injected, and the dip in temperature is recorded downstream, with the temperature record corresponding to the dye curve. No blood sampling is required, and temperature is measured directly with a thermometer mounted on the catheter. The coolth is dispersed in the systemic circulation, so there is no recirculation peak to complicate the calculation. The thermal method is particularly suitable for repeated measurements.

References

1. Hasegawa I, Kobayashi K, Kohda E, et al. Bronchopulmonary arterial anastomosis at the precapillary level in human lung. *Acta Radiol*. 1999;39:578-584.
2. Vanderpool RR, Naeije R. Hematocrit-corrected pulmonary vascular resistance. *Am J Respir Crit Care Med*. 2018;198:305-309.
3. Johnson RL, Hsai CCW. Functional recruitment of pulmonary capillaries. *J Appl Physiol*. 1994;76:1405-1407.
4. Sobin SS, Fung YC, Tremer HM, et al. Elasticity of the pulmonary alveolar microvascular sheet in the cat. *Circ Res*. 1972;30:440-450.
5. West JB, Dollery CT. Distribution of blood flow and the pressure-flow relations of the whole lung. *J Appl Physiol*. 1965;20:175-183.
*6. Sylvester JT, Shimoda LA, Aaronson PI, et al. Hypoxic pulmonary vasoconstriction. *Physiol Rev*. 2012;92:367-520.
7. Cherry PD, Furchgott RF, Zawadzki JV, et al. Role of endothelial cells in relaxation of isolated arteries by bradykinin. *Proc Natl Acad Sci U S A*. 1982;79:2106-2110.
8. Lumb AB, Slinger P. Hypoxic pulmonary vasoconstriction: physiology and anesthetic implications. *Anesthesiology*. 2015;122:932-946.
9. Dunham-Snary KJ, Wu D, Sykes EA, et al. Hypoxic pulmonary vasoconstriction: from molecular mechanisms to medicine. *Chest*. 2017;151:181-192.
10. Marshall BE, Marshall C, Frasch HF. Control of the pulmonary circulation. In: Stanley TH, Sperry RJ, eds. *Anesthesia and the Lung*. Dordrecht: Kluwer; 1992:9-18.
11. Asadi AK, Sá RC, Kim NH, et al. Inhaled nitric oxide alters the distribution of blood flow in the healthy human lung, suggesting active hypoxic pulmonary vasoconstriction in normoxia. *J Appl Physiol*. 2015;118:331-343.
12. Talbot NP, Balanos GM, Dorrington KL, et al. Two temporal components within the human pulmonary vascular response to approximately 2 h of isocapnic hypoxia. *J Appl Physiol*. 2005;98:1125-1139.
13. Talbot NP, Balanos GM, Robbins PA, et al. Can intravenous endothelin-1 be used to enhance hypoxic pulmonary vasoconstriction in healthy humans? *Br J Anaesth*. 2008;101:466-472.
14. Dehnert C, Risse F, Ley S, et al. Magnetic resonance imaging of uneven pulmonary perfusion in hypoxia in humans. *Am J Respir Crit Care Med*. 2006;174:1132-1138.
*15. Strielkov I, Pak O, Sommer N, et al. Recent advances in oxygen sensing and signal transduction in hypoxic pulmonary vasoconstriction. *J Appl Physiol*. 2017;123:1647-1656.
16. Sommer N, Dietrich A, Schermuly RT, et al. Regulation of hypoxic pulmonary vasoconstriction: basic mechanisms. *Eur Respir J*. 2008;32:1639-1651.
17. Grimmer B, Kuebler WM. The endothelium in hypoxic pulmonary vasoconstriction. *J Appl Physiol*. 2017;123:1635-1646.
*18. Smith KA, Schumacker PT. Sensors and signals: the role of reactive oxygen species in hypoxic pulmonary vasoconstriction. *J Physiol*. 2019;597(4):1033-1043.
19. Gillespie MN, Al-Mehdi AB, McMurtry IF. Mitochondria in hypoxic pulmonary vasoconstriction. Potential importance of compartmentalized reactive oxygen species signaling. *Am J Respir Crit Care Med*. 2013;187:338-340.
20. Frise MC, Robbins PA. Iron, oxygen, and the pulmonary circulation. *J Appl Physiol*. 2015;119:1421-1431.
21. Dupuis J, Hoeper MM. Endothelin receptor antagonists in pulmonary arterial hypertension. *Eur Respir J*. 2008;31:407-415.
22. Bart NK, Curtis MK, Cheng HY, et al. Elevation of iron storage in humans attenuates the pulmonary vascular response to hypoxia. *J Appl Physiol*. 2016;121:537-544.
23. Smith TG, Talbot NP, Privat C, et al. Effects of iron supplementation and depletion on hypoxic pulmonary hypertension. Two randomized controlled trials. *JAMA*. 2009;302:1444-1450.
24. Smith TG, Talbot NP, Dorrington KL, et al. Intravenous iron and pulmonary hypertension in intensive care. *Intensive Care Med*. 2011;37:1720.
25. Loeppky JA, Scotto P, Riedel CE, et al. Effects of acid-base status on acute hypoxic pulmonary vasoconstriction and gas exchange. *J Appl Physiol*. 1992;72:1787-1797.
26. Afshari A, Brok J, Møller AM, et al. Inhaled nitric oxide for acute respiratory distress syndrome and acute lung injury in adults and children: a systematic review with meta-analysis and trial sequential analysis. *Anesth Analg*. 2011;112:1411-1421.
27. Gomberg-Maitland M, Olschewski H. Prostacyclin therapies for the treatment of pulmonary arterial hypertension. *Eur Respir J*. 2008;31:891-901.
*28. Hensley MK, Levine A, Gladwin MT, et al. Emerging therapeutics in pulmonary hypertension. *Am J Physiol Lung Cell Mol Physiol*. 2018;314:L769-L781.
29. Galiè N, Ghofrani HA, Torbicki A, et al. Sildenafil citrate therapy for pulmonary arterial hypertension. *N Engl J Med*. 2005;353:2148-2157.
30. Currigan DA, Hughes RJ, Wright CE, et al. Vasoconstrictor responses to vasopressor agents in human pulmonary and radial arteries. An in vitro study. *Anesthesiology*. 2014;121:930-936.
31. Swan HJC, Ganz W. Hemodynamic monitoring: a personal and historical perspective. *Can Med Assoc J*. 1979;121:868-871.
32. De Backer D, Bakker J, Cecconi M, et al. Alternatives to the Swan–Ganz catheter. *Intensive Care Med*. 2018;44:730-741.
33. Winter SM. Clinical non-invasive measurement of effective pulmonary blood flow. *Int J Clin Monit Comput*. 1995;12:121-140.

7

Distribution of Pulmonary Ventilation and Perfusion

KEY POINTS

- Both ventilation and perfusion are distributed preferentially to dependent regions of the lung as a result of gravity and lung structure, and vary with posture and lung volume.
- In healthy lungs ventilation and perfusion are closely matched, with little variation of the ventilation to perfusion $(\dot{V}/\dot{Q})$ ratio in different lung regions.

- Regions of lung with a $\dot{V}/\dot{Q}$ ratio of 0 represent intrapulmonary shunting of mixed venous blood, whilst regions with a $\dot{V}/\dot{Q}$ ratio of infinity contribute to the alveolar dead space.
- Physiological dead space describes the part of each tidal volume that does not take part in gas exchange, and is made up of alveolar and anatomical dead space components.

The lung may be considered as a simple exchanger with a gas inflow and outflow, and a blood inflow and outflow (Fig. 7.1). There is near-equilibrium of oxygen and carbon dioxide tensions between the two outflow streams from the exchanger itself. This theoretical model assumes that gas flow in and out of the alveolus and blood flow through the pulmonary capillary are both continuous. This assumption may be true within some human alveoli where, at normal tidal volumes, gas movement is by diffusion (page 6), but pulmonary capillary blood flow is pulsatile (page 74). This model has been deliberately drawn without countercurrent flow, which would be far more efficient. Such a system operates in the gills of fishes and the lungs of birds (page 301), and brings the P_{O_2} of arterial blood close to the P_{O_2} of their environment.

Gas exchange will clearly be optimal if ventilation and perfusion are distributed in the same proportion to one another throughout the lung. Conversely, to take an extreme example, if ventilation was distributed entirely to one lung and perfusion to the other, there could be no gas exchange, although total ventilation and perfusion might each be normal. This chapter begins with consideration of the spatial and temporal distribution of ventilation, followed by similar treatment for the pulmonary circulation. Distributions of ventilation and perfusion are then considered in relation to one another. Finally, the concepts of dead space and shunt are presented.

Distribution of Ventilation

Spatial and Anatomical Distribution of Inspired Gas

Distribution between the two lungs in the normal subject is influenced by posture and by the manner of ventilation. By

virtue of its larger size, the right lung normally enjoys a ventilation slightly greater than the left lung in both the upright and the supine positions (Table 7.1). In a conscious patient in the lateral positions, the lower lung is always better ventilated, regardless of the side on which the subject is lying, although there still remains a bias in favour of the right side.[1] Fortunately, the preferential ventilation of the lower lung accords with increased perfusion of the same lung, so the ventilation/perfusion ratios of the two lungs are not greatly altered on assuming the lateral position. However, the upper lung tends to be better ventilated in the anaesthetized patient in the lateral position, regardless of the mode of ventilation and particularly with an open chest (Table 7.1).

In addition to causing postural differences between ventilation of the left and right lungs, gravity also influences the distribution of ventilation within each lung. Lung tissue may be considered as a semifluid or gel-like substance confined within the chest cavity, and the weight of the tissue above compresses the tissue below such that the density of the lung increases as vertical height reduces (Fig. 7.5).[5] Thus in dependent areas lung tissue is less expanded than in nondependent areas, and so is more compliant and receives more ventilation.

Distribution of ventilation to horizontal slices of lung has been studied for many years by inhalation of radioactive isotopes, and more recently by advanced computerized tomography techniques.[6] In the upright position, with slow vital capacity inspirations, uppermost slices of the lung have a ventilation of around one-third that of slices at the bases. A slow inspiration from functional residual capacity (FRC), as occurs during normal resting ventilation, results in a smaller vertical gradient down the lung, with the ratio of basal to apical ventilation being approximately 1.5:1.

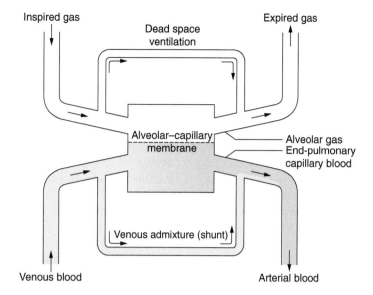

• **Fig. 7.1** In this functional representation of gas exchange in the lungs, the flow of gas and blood is considered as a continuous process with movement from left to right. Under most circumstances equilibrium is obtained between alveolar gas and end-pulmonary capillary blood, and the gas tensions in the two phases are almost identical. However, alveolar gas is mixed with dead space gas to give expired gas, and end-pulmonary capillary blood is mixed with shunted venous blood to give arterial blood. Thus both expired gas and arterial blood have gas partial pressures that differ from those in alveolar gas and end-pulmonary capillary blood.

TABLE 7.1 Distribution of Resting Lung Volume (Functional Residual Capacity) and Ventilation Between the Two Lungs in Humans

	Supine		Right Lateral (Left Side Up)		Left Lateral (Right Side Up)	
	Right Lung	Left Lung	Right Lung	Left Lung	Right Lung	Left Lung
Conscious[1]	1.69	1.39	1.68	2.07	2.19	1.38
	53%	47%	61%	39%	47%	53%
Anaesthetized spontaneous breathing[2]	1.18	0.91	1.03	1.32	1.71	0.79
	52%	48%	45%	55%	56%	44%
Anaesthetized artificial ventilation[3]	1.36	1.16	1.33	2.21	2.29	1.12
	52%	48%	44%	56%	60%	40%
Anaesthetized thoracotomy[4]					—	—
					83%	17%

The first figure is the unilateral functional residual capacity (litres), and the second the percentage partition of ventilation. Each study refers to separate subjects or patients.

In any horizontal position the vertical height of the lung is reduced by about 30%, and therefore the gravitational force generating maldistribution is much less. A variety of scanning techniques have been described that quantify regional ventilation in the supine position (page 105), and have confirmed earlier findings that normal tidal breathing results in a small degree of preferential ventilation of the posterior slices of the lungs compared with the anterior slices.

Gravity is not the only factor influencing regional ventilation; lung structure also contributes. A study of normal human lungs, rapidly frozen at a constant transpulmonary pressure and assessed using microcomputed tomographic imaging, found that the density of alveoli present in the parenchyma varies with lung height and volume. At total lung capacity (TLC) in the upright position was found to be 32 alveoli per mm^3 at the lung apex and 21 at the lung base.[7] This difference in alveolar density will tend to mitigate the effect of the different transpulmonary pressure between apex and base, with a smaller number of alveoli at the lung base each receiving more ventilation. This may explain why there is such a small difference in regional ventilation at FRC. However, when these anatomical results were scaled down to lung volume at FRC, the authors estimated similar alveolar density at apex and base (approximately 47 alveoli per mm³), which contradicts many other earlier studies described below suggesting a greater alveolar density in dependent regions. Scanning techniques with the ability to measure ventilation in areas of lung only a few cubic millimetres in size have also demonstrated increased ventilation in central, compared with peripheral, lung regions.[5] This is likely to result from unequal branching patterns of the airways in a similar fashion to that seen in pulmonary blood vessels (see later).

Distribution of Inspired Gas in Relation to the Rate of Alveolar Filling

Starting from FRC, preferential ventilation of the dependent parts of the lung is only present at inspiratory flow rates below 1.5 L.s⁻¹. At higher flow rates, distribution becomes approximately uniform. Fast inspirations from FRC reverse the distribution of ventilation, with preferential ventilation of the upper parts of the lungs, which is contrary to the distribution of pulmonary blood flow (see later). Normal inspiratory flow rate is, however, much less than 1.5 L.s⁻¹ (~0.5 L.s⁻¹), so there will be a small vertical gradient of ventilation during normal breathing.

The rate of inflation of the lung as a whole is a function of inflation pressure, compliance and airway resistance. It is convenient to think in terms of the time constant (explained in Appendix E), which is the product of the compliance and resistance and is (1) the time required for inflation to 63% of the final volume attained if inflation is prolonged indefinitely or (2) the time that would be required for inflation of the lungs if the initial gas flow rate were maintained throughout inflation (see Appendix E, Fig. E.6).

These considerations apply equally to large and small areas of the lungs; Figure 2.6 shows fast and slow alveoli, the former with a short time constant and the latter with a long time constant. Figure 7.2 shows some of the consequences of different functional units of the lung having different time constants. For simplicity, Figure 7.2 describes the response to passive inflation of the lungs by development of a constant mouth pressure, but the considerations are fundamentally similar for both spontaneous respiration and artificial ventilation.

Figure 7.2, *A*, shows two functional units of identical compliance and resistance. If the mouth pressure is increased to a constant level, there will be an increase in volume of each unit equal to the mouth pressure multiplied by the compliance of the unit. The time course of inflation will follow the wash-in type of exponential function (Appendix E), and the time constants will be equal to the product of compliance and resistance of each unit, and

therefore identical. If the inspiratory phase is terminated at any instant, the pressure and volume of each unit will be identical, and no redistribution of gas will occur between the two units.

Figure 7.2, *B*, shows two functional units, one of which has half the compliance but twice the resistance of the other. The time constants of the two will thus be equal. If a constant inflation pressure is maintained, the one with the lower compliance will increase in volume by half the volume change of the other. Nevertheless, the pressure build-up within each unit will be identical. Thus, as in the previous example, the relative distribution of gas between the two functional units will be independent of the rate or duration of inflation. If the inspiratory phase is terminated at any point, the pressure in each unit will be identical, and no redistribution will occur between the different units.

In Figure 7.2, *C*, the compliances of the two units are identical, but the resistance of one is twice that of the other. Therefore its time constant is double that of its fellow, and it will fill more slowly, although the volume increase in both units will be the same if inflation is prolonged indefinitely. Relative distribution between the units is thus dependent on the rate and duration of inflation. If inspiration is checked by closure of the upper airway after 2 seconds (for example), the pressure will be higher in the unit with the lower resistance. Gas will then be redistributed from one unit to the other, as shown by the arrow in the diagram.

Figure 7.2, *D*, shows a pair of units with identical resistances, but the compliance of one is half that of the other. Its time constant is thus half that of its fellow, and it has a faster time course of inflation. However, because its compliance is half that of the other, the ultimate volume increase will only be half that of the other unit when inflation is prolonged indefinitely. The relative distribution of gas between the two units is dependent on the rate and duration of inflation. Pressure rises more rapidly in the unit with the lower compliance, and if inspiration is checked by closure of the upper airway at 2 seconds (for example), gas will be redistributed from one unit to the other, as shown by the arrow.

An interesting and complex situation occurs when one unit has an increased resistance and the other a reduced compliance (Fig. 7.2, *E*). This combination also features in the presentation of the concept of fast and slow alveoli in Figure 2.7. In the present example the time constant of one unit is four times that of the other, whereas the ultimate volume changes are determined by the compliance as in Figure 7.2, *D*. When the inflation pressure is sustained, the unit with the lower resistance (the 'fast alveolus') shows the greater volume change at first, but rapidly approaches its equilibrium volume. Thereafter the other unit (the 'slow alveolus') undergoes the major volume changes, the inflation of the two units being out of phase with one another. Throughout inspiration, the pressure build-up in the unit with the shorter time constant is always greater and, if inspiration is checked by closure of the upper airway, gas will be

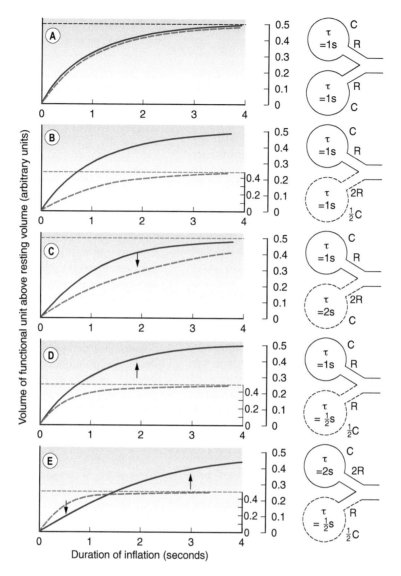

• **Fig. 7.2** The effect of mechanical characteristics on the time course of inflation of different functional units of the lung when exposed to a sustained constant inflation pressure. The *y*-coordinate is volume change, but a scale showing intraalveolar pressure is shown on the right. Separate pressure scales are necessary when the compliances are different. In each case two functional units are shown; the continuous red curve relates to the upper unit, and the broken blue curve to the lower unit. Arrows show the direction of gas redistribution if inflow is checked by closure of the upper airway at the times indicated. See text for explanation of the changes. τ = time constant. R = resistance, C = compliance.

redistributed from one unit to the other, as shown by the arrows in Figure 7.2, *E*.

These complex relationships may be summarized as follows. If the inflation pressure is sustained indefinitely, the volume change in different units of the lungs will depend solely upon their regional compliances. If their time constants are equal, the build-up of pressure in the different units will be identical at all times during inflation, and therefore:

• Distribution of inspired gas will be independent of the rate, duration or frequency of inspiration.
• Dynamic compliance (so far as it is influenced by considerations discussed in relation to Fig. 2.6) will not be

affected by changes in frequency and should not differ greatly from static compliance.
• If inspiration is checked by closure of the upper airway, there will be no redistribution of gas within the lungs.

If, however, the time constants of different units are different, it follows that:

• Distribution of inspired gas will be dependent on the rate, duration and frequency of inspiration.
• Dynamic compliance will be decreased as respiratory frequency is increased and should differ significantly from static compliance.
• If inspiration is checked by closure of the upper airway, gas will be redistributed within the lungs.

Effect of Maldistribution on the Alveolar 'Plateau'

If different functional units of the lung empty synchronously during expiration, the composition of the expired air will be approximately constant after the gas in the airways (anatomical dead space) has been flushed out. However, this will not occur when there is maldistribution with fast and slow units, as shown in Figure 2.6. The slow units are slow both to fill and to empty, and thus are hypoventilated for their volume; therefore they tend to have a high P_{CO_2} and low P_{O_2}, and are slow to respond to a change in the inspired gas composition. This forms the basis of the single-breath test of maldistribution, in which a single breath of 100% oxygen is used to increase alveolar P_{O_2} and decrease alveolar P_{N_2}. The greatest increase of P_{O_2} will clearly occur in the functional units with the best ventilation per unit volume, which will usually have the shortest time constants. The slow units will make the predominant contribution to the latter part of exhalation, when the mixed exhaled P_{O_2} will decline, and the P_{N_2} will increase. Thus the expired alveolar plateau of nitrogen will be sloping upwards in patients with maldistribution. It should, however, be stressed that this test will only be positive if maldistribution is accompanied by sequential emptying of units because of differing time constants. For example, Figure 7.2, B, shows definite maldistribution because of the different regional compliances that directly influence the regional ventilation. However, because time constants are equal, there will be a constant mix of gas from both units during the course of expiration (i.e., no sequential emptying), and therefore the alveolar plateau would remain flat in spite of P_{O_2} and P_{N_2} being different for the two units. However, maldistribution because of the commoner forms of lung disease is usually associated with different time constants and sequential emptying. Routine continuous monitoring of expired carbon dioxide concentration during anaesthesia allows some assessment of maldistribution of ventilation. As for the single-breath nitrogen test, an upward sloping expiratory plateau of carbon dioxide indicates sequential emptying of alveoli with different time constants (page 135), but a level plateau does not indicate normal distribution of ventilation, just equal time constants of lung units.

Distribution of Perfusion

Because the pulmonary circulation operates at low pressure, it is rarely distributed evenly to all parts of the lung, and the degree of nonuniformity is usually greater than for gas.

Distribution Between the Two Lungs

Measuring unilateral pulmonary blood flow in humans is difficult, but indirect methods show that unilateral pulmonary blood flow is similar to the distribution of ventilation observed in the supine position (Table 7.1). In the lateral position, the diameter of the thorax is of the order of 30 cm, and so the column of blood in the pulmonary circulation exerts a hydrostatic pressure that is high in relation to the mean pulmonary arterial pressure. A fairly gross maldistribution therefore occurs, with much of the upper lung comprising zone 2 and much of the lower lung comprising zone 3 (see Fig. 6.5).

Gravitational Effects on Regional Pulmonary Blood Flow

In the previous chapter, it was shown how the pulmonary vascular resistance is mainly in the capillary bed and is governed by the relationship between alveolar, pulmonary arterial and pulmonary venous pressures. Early studies with radioactive tracers in the blood took place at TLC and showed flow increasing progressively down the lung in the upright position. However, Hughes et al. later found that there was also a significant reduction of flow in the most dependent parts of the lung, which became known as zone 4,[8] an effect that became progressively more important as lung volume was reduced from TLC towards the residual volume (RV). Figure 7.3 is derived from the work of Hughes' group, and shows that pulmonary perfusion per alveolus is, in fact, reasonably uniform at the lung volumes relevant to normal tidal exchange. However, the dependent parts of the lung contain slightly larger numbers of smaller alveoli than the apices at FRC, and the perfusion per unit lung volume is therefore increased at the bases. The mechanism of reduced blood flow in zone 4 remains uncertain, possibilities including compression of extraalveolar vessels (page 77), hypoxic pulmonary vasoconstriction (page 80) or the local branching structure of pulmonary blood vessels.[9]

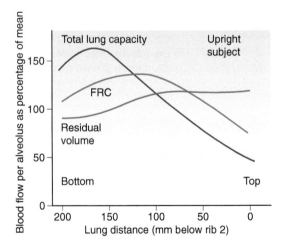

• **Fig. 7.3** Pulmonary perfusion per alveolus as a percentage of that expected if all alveoli were equally perfused (in the upright position). At total lung capacity, perfusion increases down to 150 mm, below which perfusion is slightly decreased (zone 4). At functional residual capacity *(FRC)*, zone 4 conditions apply below 100 mm, and at residual volume the perfusion gradient is actually reversed. It should be noted that perfusion has been calculated per alveolus. If shown as perfusion per unit lung volume, the nonuniformity at total lung capacity would be the same, because alveoli are all the same size at total lung capacity. At FRC there are more but smaller alveoli at the bases, and the nonuniformity would be greater. (From reference 8.)

In the supine position the differences in blood flow between apices and bases are replaced by differences between anterior and posterior regions. Supine subjects can be studied using the same variety of scanning techniques as used for assessing ventilation (page 106), revealing the same height-dependent gradients in alveolar size and perfusion as seen in earlier observations in upright subjects. Blood flow per unit lung volume increases by 11% per centimetre of descent through the lung,[10] whereas ventilation increases but less dramatically (Fig. 7.4),[11] resulting in a smaller

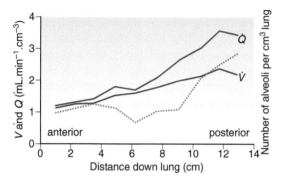

• **Fig. 7.4** Vertical gradients in ventilation and perfusion in the supine position. Data are mean results from positron emission tomography scans of eight subjects during normal breathing, and for each vertical level represent the average value for a horizontal slice of lung. The solid lines relate to the left ordinate and are ventilation ($\dot{V}$) and perfusion ($\dot{Q}$) per cubic centimetre of lung tissue. Ventilation and perfusion both increase on descending through the lung. The dotted line relates to the right ordinate and represents the number of alveoli per unit lung volume, which increases in dependent areas such that the blood flow per alveolus remains fairly constant. (From references 10 and 11.)

ventilation to perfusion $\dot{V}/\dot{Q}$) ratio in dependent areas.[10] These studies also showed that the number of alveoli per cubic centimetre of lung was approximately 30% greater in the posterior compared with anterior lung (Fig. 7.4).[11] Thus the increased perfusion in dependent areas of lung is again mainly caused by an increase in the number of (relatively small) alveoli.

Lung volume also affects regional blood flow distribution. Differences in the density of lung between nondependent and dependent regions are maximal at RV and almost absent at TLC, and when this is taken into account to calculate regional blood flow, the gravitational variation is small and unaffected by lung volume (Fig. 7.5).[9] A similar study using magnetic resonance imaging in healthy subjects demonstrated the variation in lung perfusion with lung height at FRC, FRC+ 500 mL and FRC + 1000 mL to replicate tidal ventilation. Changes in transmural and hydrostatic pressures at different lung volumes appeared to be more important factors in the redistribution of pulmonary perfusion than changes in pulmonary vascular resistance within different lung regions.[12]

Gravity-Independent Regional Blood Flow[5]

It is now accepted that gravity is not the only cause of the variability of regional pulmonary blood flow, although its relative contribution remains controversial. Physiological studies in space some years ago showed that, at microgravity, regional blood flow becomes more uniform than on Earth, but residual nonuniformity still persists (page 229). Also, many studies have measured pulmonary blood flow in the prone position, and found that although blood flow

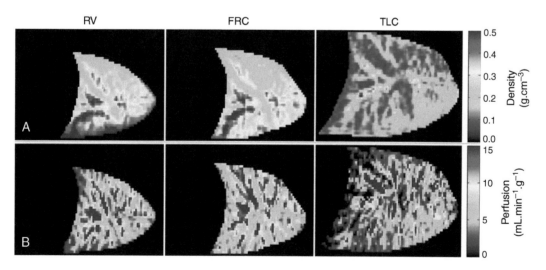

• **Fig. 7.5** Magnetic resonance images showing regional variation in lung density and perfusion in a healthy supine subject at different lung volumes. Figures show a single sagittal slice through the right lung. **(A)** Lung density is increased in dependent regions because of gravity, the variation being maximal at residual volume, intermediate at functional residual capacity, and lung density becomes almost uniform at total lung capacity. **(B)** Regional lung perfusion per gram of lung tissue is mostly unaffected by gravity at all lung volumes, being more influenced by distance from the hilum. *FRC,* Functional residual capacity; *TLC,* total lung capacity; *RV,* residual volume. (From reference 9 with permission of the author and publishers of *Journal of Physiology.*)

becomes more uniform, the flow distribution when prone is not simply a reversal of the supine position, as may be expected if gravity was the only influence.[13] A tilt table has also been used to assess gravitational effects on lung blood flow at FRC by moving subjects from upright to the extreme position of 80 degrees head down.[14] Gravity-dependent variation in blood flow was clearly demonstrated between the two positions, but lung structure remained a more important determinant of regional blood flow distribution.

Some groups estimate that gravity is responsible for only 25% of the regional blood flow variability seen.[5] Pulmonary blood flow may vary in a radial fashion, with greater flow to central compared with peripheral lung regions in each horizontal slice of lung (Fig. 7.5). Regional flow is believed to be influenced by vascular architecture, with the branching pattern of the pulmonary vasculature responsible for the observed gravity-independent variation (the fractal hypothesis).[15] Two aspects of vascular structure contribute to the variations in flow. First, bifurcations of pulmonary arteries into two slightly different size vessels will have a large effect on the flow rates in each.[5] Second, pulmonary arteries are more numerous than pulmonary airways, as a result of small extra branches, often given off at right angles, throughout the pulmonary arterial tree. Mathematical modelling indicates that these 'supernumerary' branches contribute significantly to the heterogeneity of regional perfusion.

Ventilation in Relation to Perfusion

It is convenient to consider the relationship between ventilation and perfusion in terms of the $\dot{V}/\dot{Q}$ ratio. Each quantity is measured in litres per minute, and, taking the lungs as a whole, typical resting values might be 4 $L.min^{-1}$ for alveolar ventilation and 5 $L.min^{-1}$ for pulmonary blood flow. Thus the overall ventilation/perfusion ratio would be 0.8. If ventilation and perfusion of all alveoli were uniform, then each alveolus would have an individual $\dot{V}/\dot{Q}$ ratio of 0.8. In fact, ventilation and perfusion are not uniformly distributed, but may range all the way from unventilated alveoli to unperfused alveoli, with every gradation in between. Unventilated alveoli will have a $\dot{V}/\dot{Q}$ ratio of 0, and the unperfused alveoli a $\dot{V}/\dot{Q}$ ratio of infinity.

Alveoli with no ventilation $\dot{V}/\dot{Q}$ ratio of 0) will have P_{O_2} and P_{CO_2} values that are the same as those of mixed venous blood, because the trapped air in the unventilated alveoli will equilibrate with mixed venous blood. Alveoli with no perfusion ($\dot{V}/\dot{Q}$ ratio of infinity) will have P_{O_2} and P_{CO_2} values that are the same as those of the inspired gas, because there is no gas exchange to alter the composition of the inspired gas that is drawn into these alveoli. Alveoli with intermediate $\dot{V}/\dot{Q}$ ratio values will thus have P_{O_2} and P_{CO_2} values that are intermediate between those of mixed venous blood and inspired gas. Figure 7.6 is a P_{O_2}/P_{CO_2} plot, with the red line joining the mixed venous point to the inspired gas point. This line covers all possible combinations of

alveolar P_{O_2} and P_{CO_2}, with an indication of the $\dot{V}/\dot{Q}$ ratio that determines them.

The inhalation of higher than normal partial pressures of oxygen moves the inspired point of the curve to the right. The mixed venous point also moves to the right, but only by a small amount, for reasons that are explained on page 285. A new curve must be prepared for each combination of values for mixed venous blood and inspired gas. The curve can then be used to demonstrate the gas tensions in the horizontal strata of the lung according to their different $\dot{V}/\dot{Q}$ ratios (Fig. 7.6).

Computational models of ventilation and perfusion based on computed tomography (CT) imaging have shown that the effects of gravity are the most important in ensuring passive $\dot{V}/\dot{Q}$ matching in the supine adult human lung.[16] Such gravitational effects include tissue deformation, regional compliance distribution and the effect of the hydrostatic pressure gradient on vessel size. The geometric matching of the arterial tree and the airways has a more minor role in $\dot{V}/\dot{Q}$ matching during supine normal breathing.

Body Position and Ventilation and Perfusion Ratios

As already described, both ventilation and perfusion increase in more dependent regions of the lung, with perfusion increasing slightly more than ventilation. In upright positions in healthy, young subjects breathing at FRC, the $\dot{V}/\dot{Q}$ ratio is approximately 2 at the lung apex and 0.8 at the lung bases (Fig. 7.7).[17] In horizontal positions, there is no major difference in $\dot{V}/\dot{Q}$ ratio between cranial and caudal (Fig. 7.7) or dependent and nondependent lung regions.

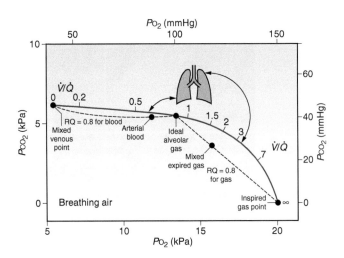

• **Fig. 7.6** The heavy line indicates all possible values for P_{O_2} and P_{CO_2} of alveoli with ventilation/perfusion ratios ranging from zero to infinity (subject breathing air). Values for normal alveoli are distributed as shown in accord with their vertical distance up the lung field. Mixed expired gas may be considered as a mixture of ideal alveolar and inspired gas (dead space). Arterial blood may be considered as a mixture of blood with the same gas partial pressures as ideal alveolar gas and mixed venous blood (shunt).

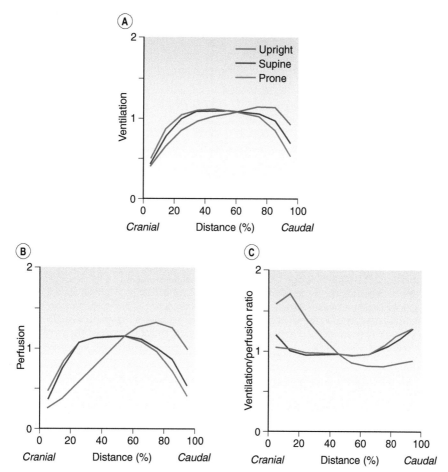

• **Fig. 7.7** Measurement of ventilation/perfusion relationships in healthy volunteers breathing at normal lung volume using single-photon emission computed tomography (page 106). **(A)** Ventilation (V̇), **(B)** perfusion (Q̇) and **(C)** V̇/Q̇ ratios. In each case, the lung has been divided into 10 sections in the cranial to caudal direction. Ventilation and perfusion refer to the ventilation in the region under consideration relative to the ventilation of the whole lung. Note the excellent matching of ventilation and perfusion in the supine (*red*) and prone (*blue*) positions, with less good matching when upright (*yellow*), with perfusion increasing more than ventilation in the dependent lung regions. (From reference 17).

Multiple Inert Gas Elimination Technique[18]

Techniques either employing radioactive tracers or using scanning modalities (page 105) measure regional ventilation and perfusion in three dimensions. The older approaches in particular could only discriminate between functionally fairly large regions of lung tissue. A different approach is the multiple inert gas elimination technique (MIGET), the methodology of which is outlined on page 107, which plots the distribution of pulmonary ventilation and perfusion, not in relation to anatomical location, but in a large number of compartments defined by their V̇/Q̇ ratios, expressed on a logarithmic scale.

Figure 7.8 shows typical plots for healthy subjects.[19] For the young adult (Fig. 7.8, *A*), both ventilation and perfusion are mainly confined to alveoli with V̇/Q̇ ratios in the range 0.5 to 2.0. There is no measurable distribution to areas of infinite V̇/Q̇ (i.e., alveolar dead space) or zero V̇/Q̇ ratio (i.e., intrapulmonary shunt), but the method does not detect extrapulmonary shunt, which must be present to a small extent (page 100). For the older subject (Fig. 7.8, *B*),

there is a widening of the distribution of V̇/Q̇ ratios, with the main part of the curve now in the range of V̇/Q̇ ratios 0.3 to 5.0. In addition, there is the appearance of a 'shelf' of distribution of blood flow to areas of low V̇/Q̇ ratio in the range 0.01 to 0.3. This probably represents underventilation of dependent areas of the lung because of airway closure when the closing capacity exceeds the functional residual capacity (see Fig. 2.11). The effect of increased spread of V̇/Q̇ ratios on gas exchange is considered in the next section (page 104).

The pattern of distribution of V̇/Q̇ ratios shows characteristic changes in a number of pathological conditions such as pulmonary oedema and pulmonary embolus. Some examples are shown in Figure 7.9.

Quantification of Spread of V̇/Q̇ Ratios Using Three-Compartment Model

The MIGET method of analysis illustrated in Figures 7.8 and 7.9 is technically complex. A less precise but highly practical approach was described in the 1940s by groups

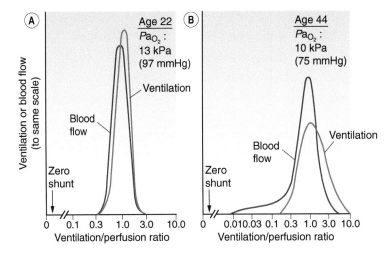

• **Fig. 7.8** The distribution of ventilation and blood flow in relation to ventilation/perfusion *(V̇/Q̇)* ratios in two normal subjects. **(A)** A male aged 22 years with typical narrow spread and no measurable intrapulmonary shunt or alveolar dead space. **(B)** The wider spread of *V̇/Q̇* ratios in a male aged 44 years. There is still no measurable intrapulmonary shunt or alveolar dead space, but the appreciable distribution of blood flow to underperfused alveoli is sufficient to reduce the arterial P_{O_2} to 10 kPa (75 mmHg) while breathing air. (From reference 19 with permission of the authors and copyright permission of the American Society for Clinical Investigation.)

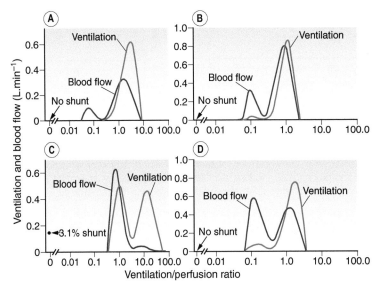

• **Fig. 7.9** Examples of abnormal patterns of maldistribution of ventilation and perfusion, to be compared with the normal curves in Figure 7.8. **(A)** Chronic obstructive pulmonary disease, the blood flow to units of very low ventilation/perfusion ratio would cause arterial hypoxaemia and simulate a shunt. **(B)** Asthma, with a more pronounced bimodal distribution of blood flow than the patient shown in **(A)**. **(C)** Bimodal distribution of ventilation seen in a 60-year-old patient with chronic obstructive pulmonary disease, predominantly emphysema. A similar pattern is seen after pulmonary embolism. **(D)** Pronounced bimodal distribution of perfusion after a bronchodilator was administered to the patient shown in **(B)**. (From West JB. *Ventilation: Blood Flow and Gas Exchange.* Oxford: Blackwell Scientific; 1990.With permission of the author and publishers.)

including those led by Riley and Cournard.[20] The essence of what has generally become known as the Riley approach is to consider the lung as if it were a three-compartment model (Fig. 7.10) comprising (1) ventilated but unperfused alveoli (alveolar dead space), (2) perfused but unventilated alveoli (intrapulmonary shunt) and (3) ideally perfused and ventilated alveoli.

Gas exchange can only occur in the 'ideal' alveolus. There is no suggestion that this is an accurate description of the actual state of affairs, which is better depicted by the type of plot shown in Figure 7.8, where the analysis would comprise about 50 compartments in contrast to the three compartments of the Riley model. However, the parameters of the three-compartment model may be easily determined,

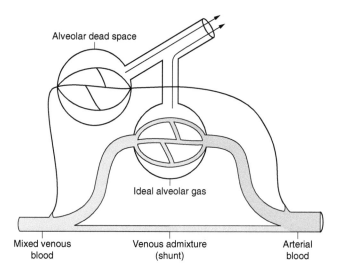

• Fig. 7.10 Three-compartment (Riley) model of gas exchange. The lung is imagined to consist of three functional units comprising alveolar dead space, ideal alveoli and venous admixture (shunt). Gas exchange occurs only in the ideal alveoli. The measured alveolar dead space consists of true alveolar dead space together with a component caused by ventilation/perfusion ($\dot{V}/\dot{Q}$) scatter. The measured venous admixture consists of true venous admixture (shunt) together with a component caused by $\dot{V}/\dot{Q}$ scatter. Note that ideal alveolar gas is exhaled contaminated with alveolar dead space gas, so it is not possible to sample ideal alveolar gas.

and the values obtained are of direct relevance to therapy. Thus an increased dead space can usually be offset by an increased minute volume, and arterial P_{O_2} can be restored to normal with shunts up to about 30% by an appropriate increase in the inspired oxygen concentration (Fig. 7.13).

Methods for calculating dead space and shunt for the three-compartment model are described at the end of the chapter, but no analytical techniques are required beyond measurement of blood and gas P_{CO_2} and P_{O_2}. It is then possible to determine what fraction of the inspired tidal volume does not participate in gas exchange and what fraction of the cardiac output constitutes a shunt. However, it is most important to remember that the measured value for 'dead space' will include a fraction representing ventilation of *relatively* underperfused alveoli ($\dot{V}/\dot{Q} >1$ and $\dot{V}/\dot{Q} <\infty$), and the measured value for 'shunt' will include a fraction representing perfusion of relatively underventilated alveoli ($\dot{V}/\dot{Q} >0$ and $\dot{V}/\dot{Q} <1$). Furthermore, although perfusion of relatively underventilated alveoli will reduce arterial P_{O_2}, the pattern of change, in relation to the inspired oxygen concentration, is quite different from that of a true shunt (Fig. 7.14).

The concept of ideal alveolar gas is considered on page 107, but it will be clear from Figure 7.10 that ideal alveolar gas cannot be sampled for analysis. There is a convention that ideal alveolar P_{CO_2} is assumed to be equal to the arterial P_{CO_2}, and that the respiratory exchange ratio of ideal alveolar gas is the same as that of expired air.

Dead Space

It was realized in the 19th century that an appreciable part of each inspiration did not penetrate to those regions of the lungs in which gas exchange occurred, and was therefore exhaled unchanged. This fraction of the tidal volume has long been known as dead space, whereas the effective part of the minute volume of respiration is known as the alveolar ventilation. The relationship is as follows:

alveolar ventilation = respiratory frequency
$$\times \left(\text{tidal volume} - \text{dead space}\right)$$
$$\dot{V}_A = f\left(V_T - V_D\right).$$

It is often useful to think of two ratios. The first is the dead space/tidal volume ratio (often abbreviated to V_D/V_T and expressed as a percentage). The second useful ratio is the alveolar ventilation/minute volume ratio. The first ratio indicates the wasted part of the breath, and the second gives the used portion of the minute volume. The sum of the two ratios is unity, and so one may easily be calculated from the other.

Components of Dead Space

The preceding section considers dead space as though it were a single homogeneous component of expired air. The situation is actually more complicated, and Figure 7.11 shows in diagrammatic form the various components of a single expired breath.

The first part to be exhaled will be the apparatus dead space if the subject is using any form of external breathing apparatus. The next component will be from the anatomical dead space, which is the volume of the conducting air passages with the qualifications considered next. Thereafter gas is exhaled from the alveolar level, and the diagram shows two representative alveoli corresponding to the two ventilated compartments of the three-compartment lung model shown in Figure 7.10. One alveolus is perfused, and, from this, ideal alveolar gas is exhaled. The other alveolus is unperfused and so without gas exchange, and, from this alveolus, the composition of the exhaled gas therefore approximates that of inspired gas. This component of the expirate is known as *alveolar dead space* gas, which is important in many pathological conditions. The physiological dead space is the sum of the anatomical and alveolar dead spaces and is defined as the sum of all parts of the tidal volume that do not participate in gas exchange.

In Figure 7.11, the final part of the expirate is called an end-tidal or, preferably, an end-expiratory sample, and consists of a mixture of ideal alveolar gas and alveolar dead space gas. The proportion of alveolar dead space gas in an end-expiratory sample is variable. In a healthy resting subject the composition of such a sample will be close to that of ideal alveolar gas. However, in many pathological states (and during anaesthesia) an end-expiratory sample may contain a substantial proportion of alveolar dead space gas, and thus be unrepresentative of the alveolar (and therefore arterial) gas partial pressures. For symbols, the small capital A relates

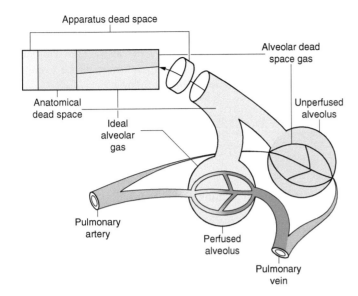

• **Fig. 7.11** Components of a single breath of expired gas. The rectangle is an idealized representation of a single expired breath. The physiological dead space equals the sum of the anatomical and alveolar dead spaces. The alveolar dead space does not equal the volume of unperfused spaces at alveolar level, but only the part of their contents that is exhaled. This varies with tidal volume.

to ideal alveolar gas, as in $P_{A_{CO_2}}$, end-expiratory gas is distinguished by a small capital E suffixed with a prime ($P_{E'_{CO_2}}$), and mixed expired gas is indicated by a small capital E with a bar ($P_{\bar{E}_{CO_2}}$). The term 'alveolar/arterial P_{O_2} difference' always refers to ideal alveolar gas. Unqualified, the term 'alveolar' may mean either end-expiratory or ideal alveolar, depending on the context. This is a perennial source of confusion, and it is better to specify either ideal alveolar gas or end-expiratory gas.

It must again be stressed that Figure 7.11 is only a model to simplify quantification, and there may be an infinite gradation of $\dot{V}/\dot{Q}$ ratios between zero and infinity. However, it is often helpful from the quantitative standpoint, particularly in the clinical field, to consider alveoli as if they fell into the three categories shown in Figure 7.10.

Anatomical Dead Space

The anatomical dead space is now generally defined as the volume of gas exhaled before the carbon dioxide concentration rises to its alveolar plateau, according to the technique of Fowler[21] outlined at the end of this chapter (Fig. 7.18).

The volume of the anatomical dead space, in spite of its name, is not constant, and is influenced by many factors, some of which are of considerable clinical importance. Most of these factors influence the anatomical dead space by changing the volume of the conducting airways, except for changes in tidal volume and respiratory rate, which affect the flow pattern of gas passing along the airways.

Factors Influencing the Anatomical Dead Space

Size of the subject must clearly influence the dimensions of the conducting air passages, and anatomical dead space increases with body size.

Age is another factor. In early infancy, anatomical dead space is approximately 3.3 mL.kg^{-1}, and by the age of 6 years this has decreased to the adult value of approximately 2 mL.kg^{-1}. Throughout this period of development, intrathoracic anatomical dead space remains constant at 1 mL.kg^{-1}, whereas the volumes of the nose, mouth and pharynx change relative to body weight.[22] From early adulthood, anatomical dead space increases by approximately 1 mL per year.

Posture influences many lung volumes, including the anatomical dead space, with typical values for healthy subjects when supine being a third less than when sitting.

Position of the neck and jaw has a pronounced effect on the anatomical dead space, with mean values in conscious subjects of 143 mL with the neck extended and jaw protruded, 119 mL in the normal position and 73 mL with the neck flexed and chin depressed.[23] It is noteworthy that the first position is the one used by resuscitators and anaesthetists to procure the least possible airway resistance. Unfortunately, it also results in the maximum dead space.

Lung volume at the end of inspiration affects the anatomical dead space, because the volume of the air passages changes in proportion to the lung volume. The increase is of the order of 20 mL additional anatomical dead space for each litre increase in lung volume.

Tracheal intubation, tracheostomy or laryngeal mask airway use will bypass much of the extrathoracic anatomical dead space, which is normally approximately 70 mL. These methods of airway maintenance bypass about half of the total anatomical dead space.[23] Any advantage gained is usually lost by the addition of further apparatus dead space to the breathing system, for example by the use of a breathing system filter or a heat- and moisture-exchanging humidifier.

Drugs acting on the bronchiolar musculature will affect the anatomical dead space, with any bronchodilator drug (page 35) causing a small increase in anatomical dead space.

Tidal volume and respiratory rate. A reduction in tidal volume results in a marked reduction of the anatomical dead space as measured by Fowler's method, and this limits the fall of alveolar ventilation resulting from small tidal volumes. This is important in spontaneously breathing comatose or anaesthetized patients who will often have tidal volumes smaller than the normal anatomical dead space of 150 mL.

Reduced anatomical dead space with small tidal volumes is unlikely to result from changes in the physical dimensions of the airways and results mostly from changes in the flow patterns and mixing of gases within the airways.

First, at low flow rates there is a greater tendency towards laminar flow of gas through the air passages (page 30). Inspired gas advances with a cone front, and the tip of the cone penetrates the alveoli before all the gas in the conducting passages has been washed out. Second, with a slow respiratory rate and/or a prolonged inspiratory time, there is more time for mixing of gases between the alveoli and the smaller airways. Mixing will occur by simple diffusion, possibly aided by a mixing effect of the heartbeat, which tends to mix all gas lying below the carina. This effect is negligible at normal rates of ventilation, but becomes marked during hypoventilation.

Alveolar Dead Space

Alveolar dead space may be defined as the part of the inspired gas that passes through the anatomical dead space to mix with gas at the alveolar level but does not take part in gas exchange. The cause of the failure of gas exchange is lack of adequate perfusion of the spaces to which the gas is distributed at the alveolar level. Measured alveolar dead space must sometimes contain a component because of the ventilation of relatively underperfused alveoli, which have a very high (but not infinite) $\dot{V}/\dot{Q}$ ratio (Fig. 7.9). The alveolar dead space is too small to be measured with confidence in healthy supine humans, but becomes appreciable under some circumstances:

Low cardiac output, regardless of the cause, results in pulmonary hypotension and failure of perfusion of the uppermost parts of the lungs (zone 1, see page 78). During anaesthesia with controlled ventilation, sudden changes in end-expiratory carbon dioxide therefore usually indicate changing alveolar dead space secondary to abrupt variations in cardiac output (page 132).

Pulmonary embolism is considered separately in Chapter 29. Apart from its effect on cardiac output, pulmonary embolism is a direct cause of alveolar dead space that may reach massive proportions.

Posture changes have a significant effect on the distribution of pulmonary blood flow (page 92). Fortunately, during normal breathing there are similar changes in the distribution of ventilation, so that $\dot{V}/\dot{Q}$ mismatch is uncommon and there are no significant changes in alveolar dead space. However, if a patient is ventilated artificially in the lateral position, ventilation is distributed in favour of the upper lung (Table 7.1), particularly in the presence of an open chest (page 405),[4] and under these conditions, part of the ventilation of the upper lung will constitute alveolar dead space.

Physiological Dead Space

Physiological dead space is the sum of all parts of the tidal volume that do not participate in gaseous exchange. Today it is universally defined by the Bohr mixing equation with substitution of arterial $P\text{CO}_2$ for alveolar $P\text{CO}_2$, as described later.

Physiological dead space remains a fairly constant fraction of the tidal volume over a wide range of tidal volumes. It is therefore generally more useful to use the V_D/V_T ratio: the alveolar ventilation will then be $(1 - V_D/V_T) \times$ the respiratory minute volume. Thus, if the physiological dead space is 30% of the tidal volume (i.e., $V_D/V_T = 0.3$), then the alveolar ventilation will be 70% of the minute volume. This approach is radically different from the assumption of a constant dead space which is subtracted from the tidal volume, with the difference then being multiplied by the respiratory frequency to indicate the alveolar ventilation.

The Bohr Equation

Bohr introduced his equation in 1891[24] when the dead space was considered simply as gas exhaled from the conducting airways (i.e., anatomical dead space only). It may be simply derived as follows. During expiration, all the carbon dioxide eliminated is contained in the alveolar gas.

Therefore

$$\text{Volume of CO}_2 \text{ eliminated in the alveolar gas} = \text{volume of CO}_2 \text{ eliminated in the mixed expired gas,}$$

that is to say

$$\text{Alveolar CO}_2 \text{ concentration} \times \text{alveolar ventilation} = \text{mixed-expired CO}_2 \text{ concentration} \times \text{minute volume,}$$

or, for a single breath

$$\text{Alveolar CO}_2 \text{ concentration} \times (\text{tidal volume} - \text{dead space}) = \text{mixed-expired CO}_2 \text{ concentration} \times \text{tidal volume.}$$

There are four terms in this equation. There is no serious difficulty in measuring two of them, the tidal volume and the mixed-expired carbon dioxide concentration. This leaves the alveolar carbon dioxide concentration and the dead space. Therefore the alveolar carbon dioxide concentration may be derived if the dead space is known, or, alternatively, the dead space may be derived if the alveolar carbon dioxide concentration is known. Bohr originally described his equation to calculate alveolar carbon dioxide fraction using known values for anatomical dead space derived from cadaver studies.

The use of this equation has been expanded to measure various components of the dead space by varying the interpretation of the term *alveolar*. In the previous equations, the word *alveolar* may be taken to mean end-expiratory gas, and therefore this use of the Bohr equation indicates the anatomical dead space. If the ideal alveolar carbon dioxide concentration were used, then the equation would indicate the physiological dead space comprising the sum of the anatomical and alveolar dead spaces (Fig. 7.11). Ideal alveolar gas cannot be sampled, but in 1938, once blood gas measurements were possible, Enghoff[25] proposed that arterial P_{CO_2} may be substituted for alveolar P_{CO_2} in the Bohr equation, and the value so derived is now widely accepted as the definition of the physiological dead space:

$$\frac{V_D}{V_T} = \frac{\left(Pa_{CO_2} - P_{\bar{E}_{CO_2}}\right)}{Pa_{CO_2}}.$$

The Enghoff modification made measurement of physiological dead space feasible, but caution should be exercised when using this formula in situations where a large shunt exists, as the assumption that ideal alveolar and arterial P_{CO_2} are equal may no longer be true.[26]

In the healthy, conscious, resting subject, there is no significant difference between the P_{CO_2} of end-expiratory gas and arterial blood. The former may therefore be used as a substitute for the latter, because the anatomical and physiological dead spaces should be the same (the normal alveolar dead space is too small to measure). However, the use of the end-expiratory P_{CO_2} in the Bohr equation may cause difficulties in certain situations. In exercise, in acute hyperventilation or if there is maldistribution of inspired gas with sequential emptying, the alveolar P_{CO_2} rises, often steeply, during expiration of the alveolar gas, and the end-tidal P_{CO_2} will depend on the duration of expiration. The dead space so derived will not necessarily correspond to any of the compartments of the dead space shown in Figure 7.9.

Factors Influencing Physiological Dead Space

This section summarizes factors that affect physiological dead space in normal subjects, but reasons for the changes have been considered earlier in the sections on the anatomical and alveolar dead space.

Age and sex. There is a tendency for V_D and also the V_D/V_T ratio to increase with age, as a result of changes in the anatomical component. The volume of V_D in men is around 50 mL greater than in women, but the former group has larger tidal volumes, and there is therefore little difference between sexes in the V_D/V_T ratios.

Body size. As described previously, it is evident that anatomical dead space and therefore V_D, in common with other pulmonary volumes, will be larger in larger people.

Posture. The V_D/V_T ratio decreases from a mean value of 34% in the upright position to 30% in the supine position.[27] This is largely explained by the change in anatomical dead space described earlier.

Pathology. Changes in dead space are important features of many causes of lung dysfunction such as pulmonary embolism, smoking, anaesthesia, artificial ventilation and heart failure.[28] These topics are discussed in Part 3 of this book.

Effects of an Increased Physiological Dead Space

Regardless of whether an increase in physiological dead space is in the anatomical or the alveolar component, alveolar ventilation is reduced unless there is a compensatory increase in respiratory minute volume. Reduction of alveolar ventilation because of an increase in physiological dead space produces changes in the ideal alveolar gas tensions that are identical to those produced when alveolar ventilation is decreased by reduction in respiratory minute volume (see Fig. 9.9).

It is usually possible to counteract the effects of an increase in physiological dead space with a corresponding increase in the respiratory minute volume. If, for example, the minute volume is 10 L.min^{-1} and the V_D/V_T ratio 30%, the alveolar ventilation will be 7 L.min^{-1}. If the patient then experienced a pulmonary embolism resulting in an increase of the V_D/V_T ratio to 50%, the minute volume would need to be increased to 14 L.min^{-1} to maintain an alveolar ventilation of 7 L.min^{-1}. However, should the V_D/V_T increase to 80%, the minute volume would need to be increased to 35 L.min^{-1}. Ventilatory capacity may be a limiting factor with massive increases in dead space, and this is a rare cause of ventilatory failure (see Chapter 27).

Venous Admixture or Shunt

Admixture of arterial blood with poorly oxygenated or mixed venous blood is an important cause of arterial hypoxaemia.

Nomenclature of Venous Admixture

Venous admixture is the degree of admixture of mixed venous blood with pulmonary end-capillary blood that would be required to produce the observed difference between the arterial and the pulmonary end-capillary P_{O_2} (usually taken to equal ideal alveolar P_{O_2}); the principles of the calculation are shown in Figure 7.12. Note that the venous admixture is not the *actual* amount of venous blood that mingles with the arterial blood, but the *calculated* amount that would be required to produce the observed value for the arterial P_{O_2}. Calculated venous admixture and the actual volume of blood mixing differ because of two factors. First, the Thebesian and bronchial venous drainage does not necessarily have the same P_{O_2} as mixed venous blood. Second, venous admixture includes the contribution to the arterial blood from alveoli having a $\dot{V}/\dot{Q}$ ratio greater than 0 but less than 1 (Fig. 7.8), when, again, P_{O_2} will differ from that of mixed venous blood. Venous admixture is thus a convenient index but defines neither the precise volume nor the anatomical pathway of the shunt. Nevertheless, it is often loosely termed *shunt*.

Anatomical (extrapulmonary) shunt refers to the amount of venous blood that mixes with the pulmonary end-capillary

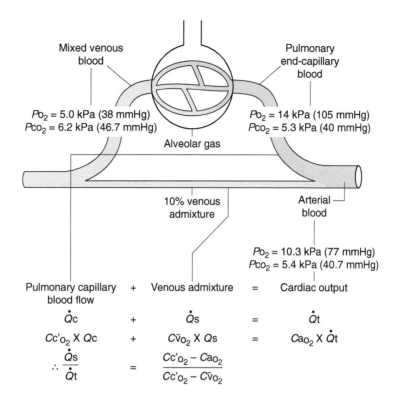

• **Fig. 7.12** A schematic representation of venous admixture. It makes the assumption that all the arterial blood has come either from alveoli with normal ventilation/perfusion ($\dot{V}/\dot{Q}$) ratios or from a shunt carrying only mixed venous blood. This is never true, but it forms a convenient method of quantifying venous admixture from whatever cause. The shunt equation is similar to the Bohr equation and is based on the axiomatic relationship that the total amount of oxygen in 1 minute's flow of arterial blood equals the sum of the amount of oxygen in 1 minute's flow through both the pulmonary capillaries and the shunt. The amount of oxygen in 1 minute's flow of blood equals the product of blood flow rate and the oxygen content of the blood. $\dot{Q}t$, total cardiac output; $\dot{Q}c$, pulmonary capillary blood flow; $\dot{Q}s$, blood flow through shunt; Ca_{O_2}, oxygen content of arterial blood; Cc'_{O_2}, oxygen content of pulmonary end-capillary blood; $C\bar{v}_{O_2}$ oxygen content of mixed venous blood.

blood on the arterial side of the circulation. The term embraces bronchial and Thebesian venous blood flow, and also admixture of mixed venous blood caused by atelectasis, bronchial obstruction, congenital heart disease with right-to-left shunting, and so on. Clearly different components may have different oxygen contents, which will not necessarily equal the mixed venous oxygen content. Anatomical shunt excludes blood draining any alveoli with a $\dot{V}/\dot{Q}$ ratio greater than 0.

Virtual shunt refers to shunt values derived from calculations in which the arterial to mixed-venous oxygen difference is assumed rather than actually measured (see later).

Pathological shunt is sometimes used to describe the forms of anatomical shunt that do not occur in the normal subject.

The term *physiological shunt* is, unfortunately, used in two senses. In the first sense, it is used to describe the degree of venous admixture that occurs in a normal healthy subject. Differences between the actual measured venous admixture and the normal value for the 'physiological shunt' thus indicate the amount of venous admixture

that results from the disease process. In its alternative sense, physiological shunt is synonymous with venous admixture as derived from the mixing equation (Fig. 7.12). This term is probably best avoided.

Forms of Venous Admixture

The contribution of $\dot{V}/\dot{Q}$ mismatch to venous admixture is discussed in detail in the next section. Other important sources of venous admixture, both normal and pathological, include the following:

Venae cordis minimae (Thebesian veins). Some small veins of the left heart drain directly into the chambers of the left heart, and so their contents mix with the pulmonary venous blood. The oxygen content of this blood is probably very low, and therefore the flow (believed to be about 0.3% of cardiac output[29]) causes an appreciable fall in the arterial P_{O_2}.

Bronchial veins. Figure 7.1 shows that part of the venous drainage of the bronchial circulation passes by way of the deep true bronchial veins to reach the pulmonary veins. It is uncertain how large this component is in the healthy subject, but it is probably less than 1% of cardiac output. In bronchial disease and coarctation of the aorta, the flow through this channel may be greatly increased, and in bronchiectasis and emphysema may be as large as 10% of cardiac output. In these circumstances it becomes a major cause of arterial desaturation.

Congenital heart disease. Right-to-left shunting in congenital heart disease is the cause of the worst examples of venous admixture. When there are abnormal communications between right and left heart, shunting will usually be from left to right unless the pressures in the right heart are raised above those of the left heart. This occurs in conditions involving obstruction to the right ventricular outflow tract (e.g., tetralogy of Fallot) or in prolonged left-to-right shunt when the increased pulmonary blood flow causes pulmonary hypertension and eventually a reversal of the shunt (Eisenmenger syndrome).

Pulmonary pathology often results in increased venous admixture, thus causing hypoxaemia. Venous drainage from lung tumours constitutes a pathological shunt, but more commonly venous admixture results from pulmonary blood flow past nonventilated alveoli in conditions such as lobar or bronchopneumonia, pulmonary collapse and acute lung injury. The amount of venous admixture that occurs with lung disease is variable, depending on the balance between hypoxic pulmonary vasoconstriction (page 80) and pathological vasodilation of the pulmonary vessels by inflammatory mediators.

Effect of Venous Admixture on Arterial $P\text{CO}_2$ and $P\text{O}_2$

Qualitatively, it will be clear that venous admixture reduces the overall efficiency of gas exchange and results in arterial blood gas tensions that are closer to those of mixed venous blood than would otherwise be the case. Quantitatively, the effect is simple, provided that we consider the contents of gases in blood. In the case of the anatomical shunt in Figure 7.12, conservation of mass (oxygen) is the basis of the equations, which simply state that the amount of oxygen flowing in the arterial system equals the sum of the amount of oxygen leaving the pulmonary capillaries and the amount of oxygen flowing through the shunt. For each term in this equation the amount of oxygen flowing may be expressed as the product of the blood flow rate and the oxygen content of blood flowing in the vessel (the symbols are explained in Fig. 7.12 and Appendix D). Figure 7.12 shows how the equation may be cleared and solved for the ratio of the venous admixture to the cardiac output. The final equation has a form that is rather similar to that of the Bohr equation for the physiological dead space.

In terms of content, the shunt equation is very simple to solve for the effect of venous admixture on arterial oxygen content. If, for example, pulmonary end-capillary oxygen content is 20 mL.dL^{-1} and mixed venous blood oxygen content is 10 mL.dL^{-1}, then a 50% venous admixture

TABLE 7.2	Effect of 5% Venous Admixture on the Difference Between Arterial and Pulmonary End-Capillary Blood Levels of Carbon Dioxide and Oxygen	
	Pulmonary End-Capillary Blood	Arterial Blood
CO_2 content (mL.dL^{-1})	49.7	50.0
$P\text{CO}_2$ (kPa)	5.29	5.33
$P\text{CO}_2$ (mmHg)	39.7	40.0
O_2 content (mL.dL^{-1})	19.9	19.6
O_2 saturation (%)	97.8	96.8
$P\text{O}_2$ (kPa)	14.0	12.0
$P\text{O}_2$ (mmHg)	105	90

It has been assumed that the arterial/venous oxygen content difference is 4.5 mL.dL^{-1} and that the haemoglobin concentration is 149 g.L^{-1}.

will result in an arterial oxygen content of 15 mL.dL^{-1}, a 25% venous admixture will result in an arterial oxygen content of 17.5 mL.dL^{-1}, and so on. It is then necessary to convert arterial oxygen content to $P\text{O}_2$ by reference to the haemoglobin dissociation curve (see page 145). Because arterial $P\text{O}_2$ is usually on the flat part of the haemoglobin dissociation curve, small changes in content tend to have a very large effect on $P\text{O}_2$, although this effect diminishes at lower arterial $P\text{O}_2$ when the dissociation curve becomes steeper.

The effect of venous admixture on arterial carbon dioxide content is roughly similar in magnitude to that of oxygen content. However, because of the steepness of the carbon dioxide dissociation curve near the arterial point (see Fig. 9.2), the effect on arterial $P\text{CO}_2$ is very small and far less than the change in arterial $P\text{O}_2$ (Table 7.2).

Two conclusions may be drawn:
- Arterial $P\text{O}_2$ is the most useful blood gas measurement for the detection of venous admixture.
- Venous admixture reduces the arterial $P\text{O}_2$ markedly but has relatively little effect on arterial $P\text{CO}_2$ or on the content of either carbon dioxide or oxygen unless the venous admixture is large.

Elevations of arterial $P\text{CO}_2$ are seldom caused by venous admixture, and it is customary to ignore the effect of moderate shunts on $P\text{CO}_2$. In the clinical situation, it is more usual for venous admixture to lower the $P\text{CO}_2$ indirectly, because the decreased $P\text{O}_2$ commonly causes hyperventilation, which more than compensates for the very slight elevation of $P\text{CO}_2$ that would otherwise result from the venous admixture (see Fig. 26.1).

Effect of Cardiac Output on Shunt

Cardiac output influences venous admixture, and its consequences, in two opposing ways. First, a reduction of cardiac output leads to a decrease in mixed venous oxygen content, with the result that a given shunt causes a greater reduction in arterial Po_2 provided the shunt fraction is unaltered, a relationship that is illustrated in Figure 10.5. Second, it has been observed that, in a range of pathological and physiological circumstances, a reduction in cardiac output causes an approximately proportional reduction in the shunt fraction. One possible explanation for the reduced shunt fraction is activation of hypoxic pulmonary vasoconstriction as a result of the reduction in Po_2 of the mixed venous blood flowing through the shunt (page 80). It is remarkable that these two effects tend to have approximately equal and opposite effects on arterial Po_2. Thus with a decreased cardiac output, there is usually a reduced shunt of a more desaturated mixed venous blood, with the result that the arterial Po_2 is scarcely changed.

The Iso-Shunt Diagram

If we assume normal values for arterial Pco_2, haemoglobin and arterial/mixed venous oxygen content difference, the arterial Po_2 is determined mainly by the inspired oxygen concentration and venous admixture considered in the context of the three-compartment model (Fig. 7.10). The relationship between inspired oxygen concentration and arterial Po_2 is a matter for constant attention in clinical situations,

and it is useful to appreciate this relationship at different levels of venous admixture (Fig. 7.13). The arterial/mixed venous oxygen content difference is often unknown in the clinical situation, and therefore the diagram has been prepared for an assumed content difference of 5 mL oxygen per 100 mL of blood. Iso-shunt bands have then been drawn on a plot of arterial Po_2 against inspired oxygen concentration. Because calculation of the venous admixture requires knowledge of the actual arterial/mixed venous oxygen content difference, the iso-shunt lines in Figure 7.13 refer to the virtual shunt, which was defined earlier.

In practice, the iso-shunt diagram is useful for adjusting the inspired oxygen concentration to obtain a required level of arterial Po_2. Under stable pathological conditions, changing the inspired oxygen concentration results in changes in arterial Po_2 that are reasonably well predicted by the iso-shunt diagram. In critical care environments, the iso-shunt graph may therefore be used to determine the optimal inspired oxygen concentration to prevent hypoxaemia while avoiding the administration of an unnecessarily high concentration of oxygen.[30] For example, if a patient is found to have an arterial Po_2 of 30 kPa (225 mmHg) while breathing 90% oxygen, he has a virtual shunt of 20%, and if it is required to attain an arterial Po_2 of 10 kPa (75 mmHg), this should be achieved by reducing the inspired oxygen concentration to 45%.

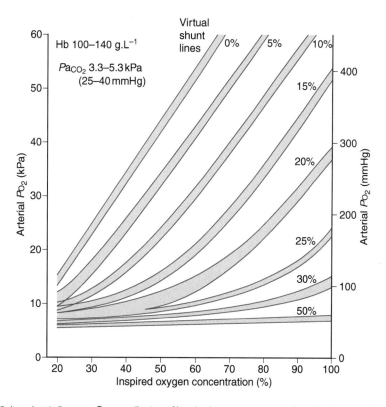

• **Fig. 7.13** Iso-shunt diagram. On coordinates of inspired oxygen concentration (abscissa) and arterial Po_2 (ordinate), iso-shunt bands have been drawn to include all values of haemoglobin (Hb) and arterial Pco_2 shown earlier. Arterial to mixed-venous oxygen content difference is assumed to be 5 mL.dL^{-1}, and normal barometric pressure is assumed. (From reference 30 with permission of the Editor of the *British Journal of Anaesthesia* and Oxford University Press.)

With inspired oxygen concentrations in excess of 40%, perfusion of alveoli with low (but not zero) $\dot{V}/\dot{Q}$ ratios has relatively little effect on arterial P_{O_2}. However, with inspired oxygen concentrations in the range of 21% to 35%, increased scatter of $\dot{V}/\dot{Q}$ ratios has an appreciable effect on arterial P_{O_2} for reasons that are explained in the next section. Therefore in these circumstances the standard iso-shunt diagram is not applicable, because arterial P_{O_2} is less than predicted as the inspired oxygen concentration is reduced towards 21%, and a modified iso-shunt diagram is required, as described later.

The Effect of Scatter of $\dot{V}/\dot{Q}$ Ratios on Arterial P_{O_2}

It is usually extremely difficult to say whether reduction of arterial P_{O_2} is from true shunt (areas of zero $\dot{V}/\dot{Q}$ ratio) or from increased scatter of $\dot{V}/\dot{Q}$ ratios with an appreciable contribution to arterial blood from alveoli with very low (but not zero) $\dot{V}/\dot{Q}$ ratios. In the clinical field, it is quite usual to ignore scatter of $\dot{V}/\dot{Q}$ ratios (which are difficult to quantify) and treat blood-gas results *as if* the alveolar/arterial

P_{O_2} difference was caused entirely by true shunt. In the example shown in Figure 7.14, it is quite impossible to distinguish between scatter of $\dot{V}/\dot{Q}$ ratios and a shunt based on a single measurement of arterial P_{O_2}. However, the two conditions are quite different in the effect of increased inspired oxygen concentrations on the alveolar/arterial P_{O_2} difference, and therefore the apparent shunt.

Figure 7.13 shows that, for a true shunt, with increasing inspired oxygen concentration, the effect on arterial P_{O_2} increases to reach a plateau value of 2 to 3 kPa (15–22 mmHg) for each 1% of shunt. This is more precisely shown in terms of alveolar/arterial P_{O_2} difference, plotted as a function of alveolar P_{O_2} in Figure 10.4.

It is not intuitively obvious why an increased spread of $\dot{V}/\dot{Q}$ ratios should increase the alveolar/arterial P_{O_2} difference. There are essentially two reasons. First, there tends to be more blood from the alveoli with low $\dot{V}/\dot{Q}$ ratio. For example, in Figure 7.14, 57% of the arterial blood comes from the alveoli with low $\dot{V}/\dot{Q}$ ratio and low P_{O_2}, whereas only 10% is contributed by the alveoli with high $\dot{V}/\dot{Q}$ ratio and high P_{O_2}. Therefore the latter cannot compensate for the former, when arterial oxygen levels are determined with due

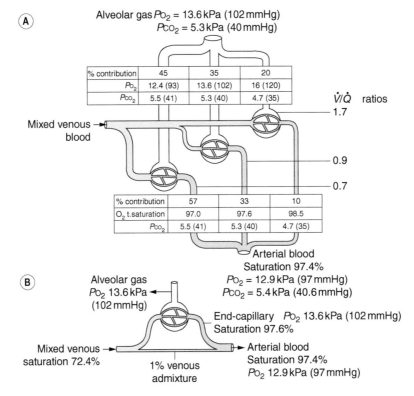

• **Fig. 7.14** Alveolar to arterial P_{O_2} difference caused by scatter of ventilation/perfusion $(\dot{V}/\dot{Q})$ ratios and its representation by an equivalent degree of venous admixture. **(A)** Scatter of $\dot{V}/\dot{Q}$ ratios corresponding roughly to the three zones of the lung in the normal upright subject. Mixed alveolar gas P_{O_2} is calculated with allowance for the volume contribution of gas from the three zones. Arterial saturation is similarly determined, and the P_{O_2} derived. There is an alveolar/arterial P_{O_2} difference of 0.7 kPa (5 mmHg). **(B)** A theoretical situation that would account for the same alveolar to arterial P_{O_2} difference, caused solely by venous admixture. This is a useful method of quantifying the functional effect of scattered $\dot{V}/\dot{Q}$ ratios, but should be carefully distinguished from the actual situation.

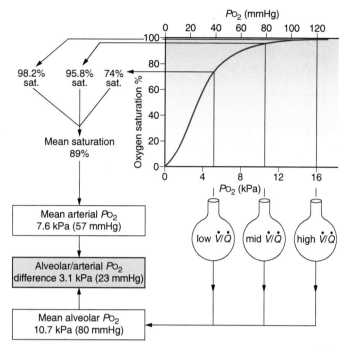

• **Fig. 7.15** Alveolar/arterial Po_2 difference caused by scatter of ventilation/perfusion ($\dot{V}/\dot{Q}$) ratios resulting in oxygen partial pressures along the upper inflexion of the oxygen dissociation curve. The diagram shows the effect of three groups of alveoli with Po_2 values of 5.3, 10.7 and 16.0 kPa (40, 80 and 120 mmHg). Ignoring the effect of the different volumes of gas and blood contributed by the three groups, the mean alveolar Po_2 is 10.7 kPa. However, because of the shape of the dissociation curve, the saturations (sat.) of the blood leaving the three groups are not proportional to their Po_2. The mean arterial saturation is, in fact, 89%, and the Po_2 therefore is 7.6 kPa. The alveolar/arterial Po_2 difference is thus 3.1 kPa. The actual difference would be somewhat greater because gas with a high Po_2 would make a relatively greater contribution to the alveolar gas, and blood with a low Po_2 would make a relatively greater contribution to the arterial blood. In this example, a calculated venous admixture of 27% would be required to account for the scatter of $\dot{V}/\dot{Q}$ ratios in terms of the measured alveolar/arterial Po_2 difference, at an alveolar Po_2 of 10.7 kPa.

allowance for volume contribution. The second reason is illustrated in Figure 7.15. Alveoli with high $\dot{V}/\dot{Q}$ ratios are on a flatter part of the haemoglobin dissociation curve than are alveoli with low $\dot{V}/\dot{Q}$ ratios. Therefore the adverse effect on oxygen content is greater for alveoli with a low $\dot{V}/\dot{Q}$, and therefore low Po_2, than is the beneficial effect of alveoli with a high $\dot{V}/\dot{Q}$, and therefore high Po_2. This shows that, the greater the spread of $\dot{V}/\dot{Q}$ ratios, the larger the alveolar/arterial Po_2 difference.

Modification of the Iso-Shunt Diagram to Include $\dot{V}/\dot{Q}$ Scatter

The iso-shunt diagram previously described does not take into account $\dot{V}/\dot{Q}$ scatter, so it has bands which are too wide for practical use below an inspired oxygen concentration of approximately 40% (Fig. 7.13). This problem was overcome by a two-compartment model including both true shunt and $\dot{V}/\dot{Q}$ scatter components,[31] which for the latter factor assumes a bimodal distribution of $\dot{V}/\dot{Q}$ scatter and uses five grades of $\dot{V}/\dot{Q}$ mismatch 'severity'. Figure 7.16 shows the effect of $\dot{V}/\dot{Q}$ mismatch on the 0% iso-shunt line (*red lines*), clearly displaying the variation in arterial Po_2

with $\dot{V}/\dot{Q}$ scatter at lower inspired oxygen concentrations. Further examples are shown in Figure 7.16 of the effect of $\dot{V}/\dot{Q}$ scatter on the inspired to arterial oxygen gradients. This model is clearly an oversimplification of the situation in lung disease (Fig. 7.9). Nevertheless, the second grade of $\dot{V}/\dot{Q}$ mismatch, when combined with a range of shunt values, was found to provide a close simulation of the relationship between arterial Po_2 and inspired oxygen concentration for a wide variety of patients with moderate respiratory dysfunction.

Principles of Assessment of Distribution of Ventilation and Pulmonary Blood Flow

Regional Distribution of Ventilation and Perfusion
Radioactive Tracers

Regional distribution of ventilation and perfusion may both be conveniently studied with a gamma camera. Ventilation is assessed following inhalation of a suitable radioactive gas that is not too soluble in blood. Both ^{133}Xe and

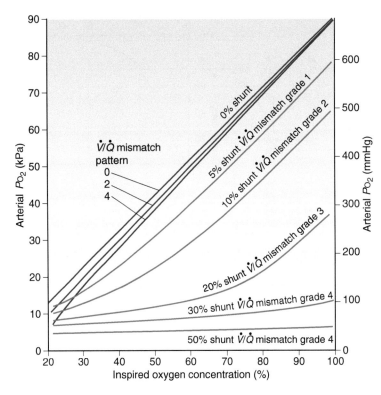

• **Fig. 7.16** Iso-shunt lines modified to incorporate the effect on arterial Po_2 of increasing degrees of ventilation/perfusion $(\dot{V}/\dot{Q})$ mismatch.[41] Blue lines show the effects of differing degrees of $\dot{V}/\dot{Q}$ mismatch in the absence of a true shunt. At lower inspired oxygen the arterial Po_2 is progressively decreased below normal for the reasons shown in Figures 7.14 and 7.15. The other iso-shunt lines shown are examples of progressively more severe degrees of combined shunt and $\dot{V}/\dot{Q}$ mismatch.

[81]Kr are suitable for this purpose, the latter usually used because its short half-life (13 seconds) reduces uptake by the pulmonary circulation. For assessment of regional perfusion, a relatively insoluble gas such as ^{133}Xe or ^{99}Tc may be dissolved in saline and administered intravenously, and its distribution within the lung again recorded with a gamma camera. The technique defines both ventilation and perfusion in zones of the lung that can be related to anatomical subdivisions by comparing anteroposterior and lateral scans.

Scanning Techniques

A variety of scanning techniques are now used, mostly for research purposes, to assess regional ventilation or perfusion including:[32]

• *Magnetic resonance imaging (MRI).* Low proton density in lung tissue because of the presence of air makes MRI scanning of the lungs challenging. However, technological advances in MRI scanning have led to more functionally relevant scans. By using tracer gases, such as [3]He or [129]Xe that have been magnetically 'hyperpolarized', oxygen or fluoride-containing gases, MRI scans can be greatly enhanced in a similar way to the use of contrast for traditional x-rays. All of these tracers are non-radioactive and can be inhaled in gaseous form, providing

high-resolution images of regional ventilation that correlate well with more traditional methods.[33] Intravenous contrast using gadolinium compounds is routinely used in MRI scanning and can provide high-resolution images of lung perfusion (see Figs 6.9 and 7.5).

• *Positron emission tomography (PET).* For this technique radioactive isotopes, for example N_2,[13] are inhaled or injected intravenously, and the radioisotopic concentration in a three-dimensional field is measured during normal breathing. Resolutions of less than 1 cm[3] of lung tissue are now possible, but the radiation exposure limits its use.

• *Single-photon emission computed tomography (SPECT).* This technique also uses inhaled or intravenous radioactive tracers. Although of low resolution compared with the other scans, it does have the advantage of being able to image more than one process simultaneously, for example lung ventilation and perfusion.

• *Four-dimensional computerized tomography and multidetector row computerized tomography (4D CT and MDCT).* Both MRI and SPECT have relatively long acquisition times and low resolution. MDCT shortens acquisition time and can reconstruct lung volumes from specific points in the respiratory cycle when used in combination with 4D CT imaging.[6]

Noninvasive Techniques

Electrical impedance tomography (EIT) involves placing 16 electrodes around the circumference of the chest, through which a high-frequency alternating 5 mA current is applied. Impedance between the multiple pairs of electrodes is affected by both air and fluid volumes, so the technique can produce a two-dimensional image reflecting either pulmonary ventilation or perfusion. Although only a single slice is obtained, and the resolution lower than MRI, the non-invasive nature of the technique means it is now finding clinical applications in the lung function laboratory,[34] during anaesthesia (see Fig. 32.7) and in intensive care. Another novel approach is molecular flow sensing, which employs laser absorption spectroscopy to measure the concentration of oxygen, carbon dioxide and water vapour every 10 milliseconds within the airway.[35] Data derived using this technique have been used to build a mathematical model to enable characterization of inhomogeneity in lung tissue with respect to ventilation, blood flow and dead space. This approach may prove clinically useful, as it does not involve ionizing radiation and is noninvasive.

Measurement of Ventilation and Perfusion as a Function of $\dot{V}/\dot{Q}$ Ratios

The information of the type displayed in Figures 7.8 and 7.9 is obtained by the MIGET,[18] which uses six tracer gases with different blood solubility ranging from very soluble (acetone) to very insoluble (sulphur hexafluoride). Saline is equilibrated with these gases and infused intravenously at a constant rate. Once steady state is achieved, levels of the tracer gases in the arterial blood are then measured by gas chromatography, and levels in the mixed venous blood are derived by use of the Fick principle. It is then possible to calculate the retention of each tracer in the blood passing through the lung and the elimination of each in the expired gas. Retention and elimination are related to the solubility coefficient of each tracer in blood, and therefore it is possible to compute a distribution curve for pulmonary blood flow and alveolar ventilation, respectively, in relation to the spectrum of $\dot{V}/\dot{Q}$ ratios (Fig. 7.8). The technique is technically demanding and laborious and has not become widely used outside of physiology research laboratories.

Direct imaging of regional $\dot{V}/\dot{Q}$ ratios, or even localized Po_2, is now possible with some of the scanning techniques described in the previous section.[36] Proton MRI has recently been used to evaluate $\dot{V}/\dot{Q}$ ratios, and has been compared with MIGET, indicating reliable correlation in results between the two techniques.[37] SPECT scanning has some significant advantages in this respect, in that two radioactive tracers with different energies can be administered together, one intravenously and one by inhalation, to produce images of both ventilation and perfusion simultaneously. Furthermore, some of these tracers have half-lives of several minutes, during which time they remain fixed in lung tissue. Because of this they can be administered outside of the scanner, for example in the sitting or prone positions, and then the subject scanned supine with the images forming a record of ventilation and perfusion in the position adopted when administering the tracers (Fig. 7.7).[17]

Measurement of Venous Admixture

Venous admixture, according to the Riley three-compartment model (Fig. 7.10), is calculated by solution of the equation shown in Figure 7.12. When the alveolar Po_2 is less than approximately 30 kPa (225 mmHg), scatter of $\dot{V}/\dot{Q}$ ratios contributes appreciably to the total calculated venous admixture (Fig. 7.16). When the subject breathes 100% oxygen, the component attributed to scatter of $\dot{V}/\dot{Q}$ ratios is minimal. Nevertheless, the calculated quantity still does not indicate the precise value of shunted blood because some of the shunt consists of blood of which the oxygen content is unknown (e.g., from bronchial veins and venae cordis minimae). The calculated venous admixture is thus at best an index rather than a precise measurement of mixing of arterial blood with venous blood.

To solve the equation shown in Figure 7.12, there are three quantities required:
1. *Arterial oxygen content.* Arterial Po_2 or oxygen saturation may be measured on blood drawn from any convenient systemic artery. If arterial Po_2 is measured, this must first be converted to oxygen saturation (page 145 *et seq.*) before the oxygen content can be calculated (page 154).
2. *Mixed venous oxygen content.* Mixed venous blood must be sampled from the right ventricle or pulmonary artery. Blood from the inferior and superior venae cavae and the coronary sinus, each with quite different oxygen contents, remains separate in the right atrium. Oxygen content may then be calculated from measured Po_2 as for the arterial sample. An assumed value for arterial/mixed venous blood oxygen content difference is often made if it is not feasible to sample mixed venous blood.
3. *Pulmonary end-capillary oxygen content.* This cannot be measured directly, and is assumed equal to the alveolar Po_2 (page 114). If Figure 7.10 is studied in conjunction with Figure 7.12, it will be seen that the alveolar Po_2 required is the ideal alveolar Po_2 and not the end-expiratory Po_2, which may be contaminated with alveolar dead space gas. The ideal alveolar Po_2 is derived by solution of one of the alveolar air equations (see next), and again converted to oxygen content.

Alveolar Air Equation

The difference between inspired and alveolar gas concentrations is equal to the ratio of the output (or uptake) of the gas to the alveolar ventilation according to the universal alveolar air equation:

$$\begin{array}{l} \text{Alveolar} \\ \text{concentration} \\ \text{of gas } X \end{array} = \begin{array}{l} \text{inspired concentration of gas } X \\ \pm \dfrac{\text{output (or uptake) of gas } X}{\text{alveolar ventilation}}. \end{array}$$

This equation uses fractional concentrations and does not correct for any difference between inspired and expired minute volumes (see later). The sign on the right-hand side is plus for output of a gas (e.g., carbon dioxide) and minus for uptake (e.g., oxygen).

For the derivation of Po_2 in ideal alveolar gas, the universal air equation was first modified with some precision by Riley et al. in 1946.[38] The equation exists in several forms that appear very different but give the same result.

Derivation of the ideal alveolar Po_2 is based on the following assumptions.

- Quite large degrees of venous admixture or $\dot{V}/\dot{Q}$ scatter cause relatively little difference between the Pco_2 of ideal alveolar gas (or pulmonary end-capillary blood) and arterial blood (Table 7.2). Therefore ideal alveolar Pco_2 is approximately equal to arterial Pco_2.
- The respiratory exchange ratio of ideal alveolar gas (in relation to inspired gas) equals the respiratory exchange ratio of mixed expired gas (again in relation to inspired gas).

From these assumptions it is possible to derive an equation that indicates the ideal alveolar Po_2 in terms of arterial Pco_2 and inspired gas Po_2. As a very rough approximation, the oxygen and carbon dioxide in the alveolar gas replace the oxygen in the inspired gas. Therefore approximately

$$\text{Alveolar } Po_2 \approx \text{inspired } Po_2 - \text{arterial } Pco_2.$$

This equation is not sufficiently accurate for use, except in the special case when 100% oxygen is breathed. In other situations, three corrections are required to overcome errors because of the following factors:

1. Usually, less carbon dioxide is produced than oxygen is consumed (effect of the respiratory exchange ratio, RQ).
2. The respiratory exchange ratio produces a secondary effect because the expired volume does not equal the inspired volume.
3. The inspired and expired gas volumes may also differ because of inert gas exchange.

The simplest practicable form of the equation corrects the principal effect of the respiratory exchange ratio (1), but not the small supplementary error because of the difference between the inspired and expired gas volumes (2):

$$\text{Alveolar } Po_2 \approx \text{inspired } Po_2 - \text{arterial } Pco_2/\text{RQ}.$$

This form is suitable for rapid bedside calculations of alveolar Po_2, when great accuracy is not required.

One stage more complicated is an equation that allows for differences in the volume of inspired and expired gas because of the respiratory exchange ratio, but still does not allow for differences because of the exchange of inert gases. This equation exists in various forms, all algebraically identical:[38]

$$\text{Alveolar } Po_2 = P_{I_{O_2}} - \frac{Pa_{CO_2}}{\text{RQ}}\left(1 - F_{I_{O_2}}(1 - \text{RQ})\right).$$

This equation is suitable for use whenever the subject has been breathing the inspired gas mixture long enough for the inert gas to be in equilibrium. It is unsuitable for use when the inspired oxygen concentration has recently been changed, when the ambient pressure has recently been changed (e.g., during hyperbaric oxygen therapy) or when the inert gas concentration has recently been changed (e.g., soon after the start or finish of a period of inhaling nitrous oxide).

Perhaps the most satisfactory form of the alveolar air equation is that which was advanced by Filley et al. in 1954.[39] This equation makes no assumption that inert gases are in equilibrium and allows for the difference between inspired and expired gas regardless of the cause. It also proves to be very simple in use and does not require the calculation of the respiratory exchange ratio, although it does require sampling of mixed-expired gas:

$$\text{Alveolar } Po_2 = P_{I_{O_2}} - Pa_{CO_2}\left(\frac{P_{I_{O_2}} - P\overline{E}_{CO_2}}{P\overline{E}_{CO_2}}\right).$$

If the alveolar Po_2 is calculated separately according to the last two equations, the difference (if any) will be that attributed to inert gas exchange.

When using these equations in practice it is important to consider water vapour, as alveolar gas will be saturated with water at body temperature, such that:

$$P_{I_{O_2}} = F_{I_{O_2}} \times \left(P_B - P_{H_2O}\right),$$

where $F_{I_{O_2}}$ is the fractional inspired oxygen concentration, P_B is barometric pressure, and P_{H_2O} is saturated vapour pressure of water at 37° C (6.3 kPa, 47 mmHg).

Distinction Between Shunt and the Effect of $\dot{V}/\dot{Q}$ Scatter

Shunt and scatter of $\dot{V}/\dot{Q}$ ratios will each produce an alveolar/arterial Po_2 difference from which a value for venous admixture may be calculated. It is usually impossible to say to what extent the calculated venous admixture is as a result of a true shunt or to perfusion of alveoli with a low $\dot{V}/\dot{Q}$ ratio. Three methods are available for distinction between the two conditions.

If the inspired oxygen concentration is altered, the effect on the arterial Po_2 will depend on the nature of the disorder. If oxygenation is impaired by a shunt, the arterial Po_2 will increase, as shown in the iso-shunt diagram (Fig. 7.13). If, however, the disorder is attributed to scatter of $\dot{V}/\dot{Q}$ ratios, the arterial Po_2 will approach the normal value for the inspired oxygen concentration as the inspired oxygen concentration is increased (Fig. 7.16). $\dot{V}/\dot{Q}$ scatter has virtually no effect when the subject breathes 100% oxygen. This difference between shunt and $\dot{V}/\dot{Q}$ scatter forms the basis of a noninvasive method for investigating the mechanism of impaired gas exchange in the clinical setting.[40] Oxygen saturation

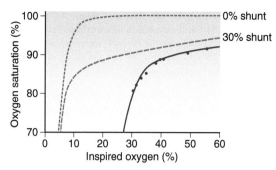

• **Fig. 7.17** Noninvasive evaluation of impaired gas exchange during one-lung anaesthesia and thoracotomy. Oxygen saturation has been measured at nine different inspired oxygen concentrations (*circles*), and a curve fitted to the points (*solid line*). Mathematical modelling (*broken lines*) shows that shunt displaces the curve downwards (0% and 30% shunt shown), and ventilation/perfusion ($\dot{V}/\dot{Q}$) mismatch displaces the curve to the right. A computer algorithm, using an assumed value for arteriovenous oxygen difference, can compute the virtual shunt and the shift because of $\dot{V}/\dot{Q}$ mismatch from the actual curve obtained from the patient, in this case 30% shunt and marked $\dot{V}/\dot{Q}$ mismatch in the patient during one-lung ventilation (page 403). (From reference 40 with permission of the authors and the editor of *Anaesthesia*.)

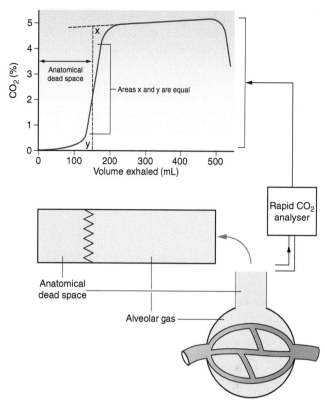

• **Fig. 7.18** Measurement of anatomical dead space using carbon dioxide (CO_2) as the tracer gas. If the gas passing the patient's lips is continuously analysed for CO_2 concentration, there is a sudden rise to the alveolar plateau level, after the expiration of gas from the anatomical dead space. If the instantaneous CO_2 concentration is plotted against the volume exhaled (allowing for delay in the CO_2 analyser), a graph similar to that shown is obtained. A vertical line is constructed so that the two areas *x* and *y* are equal. This line will indicate the volume of the anatomical dead space. Note that the abscissa records *volume* rather than *time* as seen with capnography performed in clinical situations.

is measured at several different inspired oxygen concentrations, and an oxygen saturation versus inspired oxygen curve drawn. Mathematical modelling, again using an assumed value for arteriovenous oxygen difference, and studies during one-lung anaesthesia have shown that the shunt depresses the curve downwards, whereas increasing $\dot{V}/\dot{Q}$ mismatch moves the curve to the right (Fig. 7.17).[40]

The MIGET for analysis of distribution of blood flow in relation to $\dot{V}/\dot{Q}$ ratio is the best method for distinction between shunt and areas of low $\dot{V}/\dot{Q}$ ratio (see earlier section).

Measurement of Dead Space

Anatomical dead space is most conveniently measured by the technique illustrated in Figure 7.18, originally developed for use with a nitrogen analyser by Fowler.[21] The carbon dioxide concentration at the lips is measured continuously with a rapid gas analyser, and then displayed against the volume actually expired. The 'alveolar plateau' of carbon dioxide concentration is not flat, but slopes gently. Anatomical dead space is easily derived from the graph, as shown in Figure 7.18, or by a variety of mathematical methods.[41]

Physiological dead space. Mixed expired air is collected over a period of 2 or 3 minutes, during which time an arterial blood sample is collected, and the $P\text{CO}_2$ of blood and gas are then determined. Provided that the inspired gas is free from carbon dioxide, physiological dead space is indicated by the following form of the Bohr equation:

$$\begin{array}{l}\text{Physiological} \\ \text{dead space}\end{array} = \text{tidal volume}\left(\frac{Pa_{\text{CO}_2} - P\bar{\text{E}}_{\text{CO}_2}}{Pa_{\text{CO}_2}}\right) \\ - \text{apparatus dead space.}$$

Alveolar dead space is measured as the difference between the physiological and anatomical dead space, determined separately but at the same time. When only the physiological dead space is measured, it is often possible to attribute a large increase in physiological dead space to an increase in the alveolar component, because there are few circumstances in which the anatomical dead space is greatly enlarged.

For *clinical measurement of dead space*, methods are now available for the estimation of anatomical, physiological and therefore alveolar dead spaces from a single breath recording of expired carbon dioxide, and a single arterial $P\text{CO}_2$ measurement. The requirement for an arterial blood sample still makes this an invasive measurement, but the bedside assessment of alveolar dead space is now possible in critical care situations.

The arterial/end-expiratory $P\text{CO}_2$ difference is a convenient and relatively simple method of assessing the magnitude of the alveolar dead space. In Figure 7.11, end-expiratory gas is shown to consist of a mixture of ideal alveolar gas and alveolar dead space gas. If the patient has an appreciable alveolar dead space, the end-expiratory P_{CO_2} will be less than the arterial P_{CO_2}, which is assumed equal to the ideal alveolar P_{CO_2}.

If, for example, ideal alveolar gas has a P_{CO_2} of 5.3 kPa (40 mmHg) and the end-expiratory P_{CO_2} is found to be 2.65 kPa (20 mmHg), it follows that the end-expiratory gas consists of equal parts of ideal alveolar gas and alveolar dead space gas. Thus if the tidal volume is 500 mL, and the anatomical dead space 100 mL, then alveolar dead space and ideal alveolar gas components would be 200 mL each.

References

1. Svanberg L. Influence of posture on lung volumes, ventilation and circulation in normals. *Scand J Clin Lab Invest*. 1957;9(suppl 25):1-195.
2. Rehder K, Sessler AD. Function of each lung in spontaneously breathing man anesthetized with thiopental-meperidine. *Anesthesiology*. 1973;38:320-327.
3. Rehder K, Hatch DJ, Sessler AD, et al. The function of each lung of anesthetized and paralyzed man during mechanical ventilation. *Anesthesiology*. 1972;37:16-26.
4. Nunn JF. The distribution of inspired gas during thoracic surgery. *Ann R Coll Surg Engl*. 1961;28:223-237.
5. Galvin I, Drummond GB, Nirmalan M. Distribution of blood flow and ventilation in the lung: gravity is not the only factor. *Br J Anaesth*. 2007;98:420-428.
6. Jahani N, Sanghun C, Choi J, et al. Assessment of regional ventilation and deformation using 4D-CT imaging for healthy human lungs during tidal breathing. *J Appl Physiol*. 2015;119:1064-1074.
7. McDonough J, Knudsen L, Wright A, et al. Regional differences in alveolar density in the human lung are related to lung height. *J Appl Physiol*. 2015;118:1429-1434.
8. Hughes JM, Glazier JB, Maloney JE, et al. Effect of lung volume on the distribution of pulmonary blood flow in man. *Respir Physiol*. 1968;4:58-72.
9. Hopkins SR, Arai TJ, Henderson AC, et al. Lung volume does not alter the distribution of pulmonary perfusion in dependent lung in supine humans. *J Physiol*. 2010;588(23):4759-4768.
10. Brudin LH, Rhodes CG, Valind SO, et al. Interrelationship between regional blood flow, blood volume, and ventilation in supine humans. *J Appl Physiol*. 1994;76:1205-1210.
11. Brudin LH, Rhodes CG, Valind SO, et al. Relationship between regional ventilation and vascular and extravascular volume in supine humans. *J Appl Physiol*. 1994;76:1195-1204.
12. Arai T, Theilmann R, Sá R, et al. The effect of lung deformation on the spatial distribution of pulmonary blood flow. *J Physiol*. 2016;594:6333-6347.
13. Prisk GK, Yamada K, Henderson AC, et al. Pulmonary perfusion in the prone and supine postures in the normal human lung. *J Appl Physiol*. 2007;103:883-894.
14. Ax M, Sanchez-Crespo A, Lindahl S, et al. The influence of gravity on regional lung blood flow in humans: SPECT in the upright and head-down posture. *J Appl Physiol*. 2017;122:1445-1451.
15. Hlastala MP, Glenny RW. Vascular structure determines pulmonary blood flow distribution. *News Physiol Sci*. 1999;14:182-186.
16. Kang W, Clark AR, Tawhai MH. Gravity outweighs the contribution of structure to passive ventilation-perfusion matching in the supine adult human lung. *J Appl Physiol*. 2018;124:23-33.

*17. Petersson J, Rohdin M, Sánchez-Crespo A, et al. Regional lung blood flow and ventilation in upright humans studied with quantitative SPECT. *Respir Physiol Neurobiol*. 2009;166:54-60.
18. Roca J, Wagner PD. Principles and information content of the multiple inert gas elimination technique. *Thorax*. 1993;49:815-824.
19. Wagner PD, Laravuso RB, Uhl RR, et al. Continuous distributions of ventilation perfusion ratios in normal subjects breathing air and 100% O_2. *J Clin Invest*. 1974;54:54-68.
20. Riley RL, Cournand A. 'Ideal' alveolar air and the analysis of ventilation perfusion relationships in the lung. *J Appl Physiol*. 1949;1:825-849.
21. Fowler WS. Lung function studies. II. The respiratory dead space. *Am J Physiol*. 1948;154:405-416.
22. Numa AH, Newth CJL. Anatomic dead space in infants and children. *J Appl Physiol*. 1996;80:1485-1489.
23. Nunn JF, Campbell EJM, Peckett BW. Anatomical subdivisions of the volume of respiratory dead space and effect of position of the jaw. *J Appl Physiol*. 1959;14:174-176.
24. Bohr C. Über die Lungenathmung. *Skand Arch Physiol*. 1891;2:236.
25. Enghoff H. Volumen inefficax. Bemerkungen zur Frage des schädlichen Raumes. *Uppsala Läkareforen Forhandl*. 1938;44:191-218.
*26. Suarez-Sipmann F, Santos A, Böhm SH, et al. Corrections of Enghoff's dead space formula for shunt effects still overestimate Bohr's dead space. *Respir Physiol Neurobiol*. 2013;189:99-105.
27. Craig DB, Wahba WM, Don HF, et al. 'Closing volume' and its relationship to gas exchange in seated and supine positions. *J Appl Physiol*. 1971;31:717-721.
28. Robertson HT. Dead space: the physiology of wasted ventilation. *Eur Respir J*. 2015;45:1704-1716.
29. Ravin MG, Epstein RM, Malm JR. Contribution of thebesian veins to the physiologic shunt in anesthetized man. *J Appl Physiol*. 1965;20:1148-1152.
30. Benator SR, Hewlett AM, Nunn JF. The use of iso-shunt lines for control of oxygen therapy. *Br J Anaesth*. 1973;45:711-718.
31. Petros AJ, Doré CJ, Nunn JF. Modification of the iso-shunt lines for low inspired oxygen concentrations. *Br J Anaesth*. 1994;72:515-522.
32. Simon BA, Kaczka DW, Bankier AA, et al. What can computed tomography and magnetic resonance imaging tell us about ventilation? *J Appl Physiol*. 2012;113:647-657.
33. Sá RC, Asadi AK, Theilmann RJ, et al. Validating the distribution of specific ventilation in healthy humans measured using proton MR imaging. *J Appl Physiol*. 2014;116:1048-1056.
34. Vogt B, Pulletz S, Elke G, et al. Spatial and temporal heterogeneity of regional lung ventilation determined by electrical impedance tomography during pulmonary function testing. *J Appl Physiol*. 2012;113:1154-1161.
35. Mountain J, Santer P, O'Neill D. Potential for noninvasive assessment of lung inhomogeneity using highly precise, highly time-resolved measurements of gas exchange. *J Appl Physiol*. 2017;124:615-631.
36. Petersson J, Glenny RW. Imaging regional PAO_2 and gas exchange. *J Appl Physiol*. 2012;113:340-352.
37. Sá R, Henderson A, Simonson T, et al. Measurement of the distribution of ventilation-perfusion ratios in the human lung with proton MRI: comparison with the multiple inert gas elimination technique. J Appl Physiol. 2017:123:136-146.
38. Riley RL, Lilienthal JL, Proemmel DD, et al. On the determination of the physiologically effective pressures of oxygen and carbon dioxide in alveolar air. *Am J Physiol*. 1946;147:191-198.
39. Filley GF, Macintosh DJ, Wright GW. Carbon monoxide uptake and pulmonary diffusing capacity in normal subject at rest and during exercise. *J Clin Invest*. 1954;33:530-539.
40. de Gray L, Rush EM, Jones JG. A noninvasive method for evaluating the effect of thoracotomy on shunt and ventilation perfusion inequality. *Anaesthesia*. 1997;52:630-635.
41. Tang Y, Turner MJ, Baker AB. Systematic errors and susceptibility to noise of four methods for calculating anatomical dead space from the CO_2 expirogram. *Br J Anaesth*. 2007;98:828-834.

8

Diffusion of Respiratory Gases

KEY POINTS

- For gas to transfer between the alveolus and haemoglobin in the red blood cell it must diffuse across the alveolar and capillary walls, through the plasma and across the red cell membrane.
- The reaction rate for oxygen with haemoglobin also affects the rate at which red blood cells become saturated with oxygen on passing through the pulmonary capillary.

- Transfer of oxygen and carbon dioxide is very rapid, and impairment of this transfer is rarely a cause of impaired gas exchange.
- Carbon monoxide, because of its high affinity for haemoglobin, is used to assess the diffusing capacity of the lungs.

The previous chapters have described in detail how alveolar gases and pulmonary capillary blood are delivered to their respective sides of the alveolar wall. This chapter deals with the final step of lung function by discussing the transfer of respiratory gases between the alveolus and blood.

Nomenclature in this field is confusing. In Europe, measurement of the passage of gases between the alveoli and pulmonary capillaries is referred to as lung 'transfer factor' (e.g., $T_{L_{CO}}$, which represents the lung transfer factor for carbon monoxide). However, the older term 'diffusing capacity' (e.g., $D_{L_{CO}}$, for the lung diffusing capacity for carbon monoxide), which has been used for many years in the United States, is now the recommended term,[1] despite the fact that some of the barrier to oxygen transfer is unrelated to diffusion (see later).

Fundamentals of the Diffusion Process

Diffusion of a gas is a process by which a net transfer of molecules takes place from a zone in which the gas exerts a high partial pressure to a zone in which it exerts a lower partial pressure. The mechanism of transfer is the random movement of molecules, and the term excludes active biological transport, transfer by mass movement of gas in response to a *total* pressure difference (e.g., gas flow as occurs during tidal ventilation) and 'facilitated' mass movement (e.g., transfer of oxygen around the circulation bound to haemoglobin). The partial pressure of a gas in a gas mixture is the pressure it would exert if it occupied the space alone (equal to total pressure multiplied by fractional concentration). Gas molecules pass in each direction but at a rate proportional to the partial pressure of the gas in the zone

from which they are leaving. The net transfer of the gas is the difference in the number of molecules passing in each direction, and is thus proportional to the difference in partial pressure between the two zones. Typical examples of diffusion are shown in Figure 8.1.

In each of the examples shown in Figure 8.1, there is a finite resistance to the transfer of the gas molecules. In Figure 8.1, *A*, the resistance is concentrated at the restriction in the neck of the bottle. Clearly, the narrower the neck, the slower will be the process of equilibration with the outside air. In Figure 8.1, *B*, the site of the resistance to diffusion is less circumscribed, but includes gas diffusion within the alveolus, the alveolar/capillary membrane, the diffusion path through the plasma and the delay in combination of oxygen with the reduced haemoglobin in the red blood cell (RBC). In Figure 8.1, *C*, the resistance commences with the delay in the release of oxygen by haemoglobin and includes all the interfaces between the RBC membrane and the site of oxygen consumption in the mitochondria. There may then be an additional component in the rate at which oxygen enters into chemical reactions.

In the living body oxygen is constantly being consumed while carbon dioxide is being produced, so equilibrium cannot be attained as in the case of the open bottle of oxygen in Figure 8.1, *A*. Instead, a dynamic equilibrium is attained with diffusion down a gradient between the alveolus and the mitochondria for oxygen and the reverse for carbon dioxide. The maintenance of these partial pressure gradients is, in fact, a characteristic of life.

In the case of gases that are not metabolized to any great extent, such as nitrogen, there is always a tendency towards a static equilibrium at which all tissue partial pressures become equal to the partial pressure of the particular gas in the inspired air.

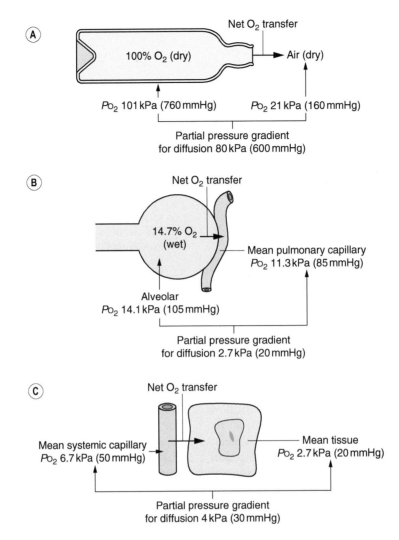

Ⓐ

Net O$_2$ transfer

100% O$_2$ (dry) → Air (dry)

P_{O_2} 101 kPa (760 mmHg) P_{O_2} 21 kPa (160 mmHg)

Partial pressure gradient
for diffusion 80 kPa (600 mmHg)

Ⓑ

Net O$_2$ transfer

14.7% O$_2$
(wet)

Mean pulmonary capillary
P_{O_2} 11.3 kPa (85 mmHg)

Alveolar
P_{O_2} 14.1 kPa (105 mmHg)

Partial pressure gradient
for diffusion 2.7 kPa (20 mmHg)

Ⓒ

Net O$_2$ transfer

Mean systemic capillary
P_{O_2} 6.7 kPa (50 mmHg)

Mean tissue
P_{O_2} 2.7 kPa (20 mmHg)

Partial pressure gradient
for diffusion 4 kPa (30 mmHg)

• **Fig. 8.1** Three examples of diffusion of oxygen. In each case there is a net transfer of oxygen from left to right in accord with the partial pressure gradient. **(A)** Oxygen passes from one gaseous phase to another. **(B)** Oxygen passes from a gaseous phase to a liquid phase. **(C)** Oxygen passes from one liquid to another.

Quantification of Resistance to Diffusion

The propensity of a gas to diffuse as a result of a given pressure gradient is known as its diffusing capacity according to the equation:

$$\text{Diffusing capacity} = \frac{\text{Net rate of gas transfer}}{\text{Partial pressure gradient}}.$$

The usual biological unit of diffusing capacity is mL. min^{-1}.mmHg^{-1} or, in the International System of Units (SI), mL.min^{-1}.kPa^{-1}.

Small molecules diffuse more easily than large molecules. Graham's law states that the rate of diffusion of a gas is inversely proportional to the square root of its density. In addition, gases diffuse more readily at higher temperatures. Apart from these factors, which are inherent in the gas, the resistance to diffusion is related directly to the length of the diffusion path and inversely to the area of interface that is available for diffusion.

Diffusion of Gases in Solution

The partial pressure of a gas in solution in a liquid is defined as equal to the partial pressure of the same gas in a gas mixture that is in equilibrium with the liquid. When a gas is diffusing into or through an aqueous phase, the solubility of the gas in water becomes an important factor, and the diffusing capacity under these circumstances is considered to be directly proportional to the solubility. Nitrous oxide would thus be expected to have about 20 times the diffusing capacity of oxygen in crossing a gas–water interface. High solubility does not confer an increased 'agility' of the gas in its negotiation of an aqueous barrier, but simply means that, for a given partial pressure, more molecules of the gas are present in the liquid.

Partial Pressure Versus Concentration Gradients

Nongaseous substances in solution diffuse in response to concentration gradients. This is also true for gas mixtures at the same total pressure, when the partial pressure of any component gas is directly proportional to its concentration. This is not the case when a gas in solution in one liquid diffuses into a different liquid in which it has a different solubility coefficient. When gases are in solution, the partial pressure they exert is directly proportional to their concentration in the solvent, but inversely to the solubility of the gas in the solvent. Thus, if water and oil have the same concentration of nitrous oxide dissolved in each, the partial pressure of nitrous oxide in the oil will be only one-third of the partial pressure in the water, because the oil/water solubility ratio is about 3:1. If the two liquids are shaken up together, there will be a net transfer of nitrous oxide from the water to the oil until the partial pressure in each phase is the same. At that time the concentration of nitrous oxide in the oil will be about three times the concentration in the water. There is thus a net transfer of nitrous oxide against the concentration gradient, but always with the partial pressure gradient. It is therefore useful to consider partial pressure rather than concentrations in relation to movement of gases and vapours from one compartment of the body to another. The same units of pressure may be used in gas, aqueous and lipid phases.

Diffusion of Oxygen in the Lungs

It is now widely accepted that oxygen passes from the alveoli into the pulmonary capillary blood by a passive process of diffusion according to physical laws, though for a while it was believed that oxygen was actively secreted into the blood (see the 'Oxygen secretion controversy' section in Online Chapter 35(e)). It is believed that diffusion equilibrium is very nearly achieved for oxygen during the normal pulmonary capillary transit time in the resting subject. Therefore, in these circumstances, the uptake of oxygen is limited by pulmonary blood flow and not by diffusing capacity. However, when exercising while breathing gas mixtures deficient in oxygen or at reduced barometric pressure, the diffusing capacity becomes important and may limit oxygen uptake.

Components of the Alveolar/Capillary Diffusion Pathway

Gas Space Within the Alveolus

At functional residual capacity, the diameter of the average human alveolus is of the order of 200 μm (page 8), and it is likely that mixing of normal alveolar gas is almost instantaneous over the small distance from the centre to the periphery. Precise calculations are impossible on account of the complex geometry of the alveolus, but the overall efficiency of gas exchange within the lungs suggests that mixing must be complete within less than 10 milliseconds. Therefore, in practice it is usual to consider alveolar gas of normal composition as uniformly mixed.

This generalization does not hold when subjects inhale gases of widely different molecular weights. This was first demonstrated in normal subjects inhaling mixtures of sulphur hexafluoride (SF_6) and helium, when the SF_6 concentration was found to be higher (relative to helium) earlier in the breath. According to Graham's law, SF_6 (molecular weight 146) would diffuse six times less readily than helium (molecular weight 4), and would therefore tend to remain concentrated at the core of the alveolus. A similar problem is seen with inhaled anaesthetic agents; for example, a large proportion of the end-expiratory/arterial partial pressure gradient for the anaesthetic isoflurane (molecular weight 184.5) cannot be explained by alveolar dead space or shunt, and may be due to failure to achieve uniformity within the alveolus.[2] Nevertheless, it seems unlikely that non-uniformity within a single alveolus is an important factor limiting diffusing capacity under normal conditions with gases such as oxygen, nitrogen and carbon dioxide, which have similar molecular weights.

Alveolar Lining Fluid

Alveoli contain a thin layer of surfactant-rich fluid through which respiratory gases must diffuse.[3] The depth of this fluid layer, and therefore its impediment to diffusion, is quite variable. There are 'pools' of fluid in alveolar corners (see Fig. 1.9) and in the depressions between where the capillaries bulge into the alveolus, with only a very thin layer on the surface of the capillary bulges, thus providing the minimal diffusion barrier in the most vital area.

Tissue Barrier

Electron microscopy reveals details of the actual path between alveolar gas and pulmonary capillary blood, shown in Figure 1.8. Each alveolus is lined with epithelium which, with its basement membrane, is about 0.2 μm thick, except where epithelial cell nuclei bulge into the alveolar lumen. Beyond the basement membrane is the interstitial space, which is very thin where it overlies the capillaries, particularly on the active side; elsewhere it is thicker and contains collagen and elastin fibres. The pulmonary capillaries are lined with endothelium, which has its own basement membrane, and is approximately the same thickness as the alveolar epithelium, except where it is expanded to enclose the endothelial cell nuclei. The total thickness of the active part of the tissue barrier is thus about 0.5 μm, containing two pairs of lipid bilayers separated by the interstitial space.

Plasma Layer

Human pulmonary capillaries are estimated to have a mean diameter of 7 μm, similar to the diameter of an RBC, part of which is therefore forced into contact with the endothelial cell surface (see Fig. 1.8). The diffusion path through plasma may therefore be very short indeed, but only a small proportion of the RBC surface will be in such close proximity with the endothelium, with much of the RBC passing through the middle of the capillary, up to 3.5 μm from the endothelial cell. Furthermore, because the diameter of the capillary is about 14 times the thickness of the tissue barrier, it is clear that the diffusion path within the capillary is likely to be much longer than the path through the alveolar/capillary membrane. A complex pattern of diffusion gradients is therefore established within the plasma depending on the oxygen tension in the alveolus and the number of RBCs present.[4] This is discussed in more detail later with respect to carbon monoxide.

Diffusion into and Within the Red Blood Cell[5]

Confining haemoglobin within the RBC reduces the oxygen-diffusing capacity by 40% in comparison with free haemoglobin solution. There are three possible explanations for this observation. First, there is evidence that the rapid uptake of O_2 and CO by RBCs causes depletion of gas in the plasma layer immediately surrounding the RBC. Referred to as the *unstirred layer*, this phenomenon is most likely to occur at low packed cell volume when adjacent RBCs in the pulmonary capillary have more plasma between them.[6] Second, oxygen must diffuse across the RBC membrane, though this is not normally believed to be a significant diffusion barrier. Third, once in the cell, oxygen must diffuse through a varying amount of intracellular fluid before combining with haemoglobin, a process aided by mass movement of the haemoglobin molecules caused by the deformation of the RBC as it passes through the capillary bed, in effect 'mixing' the oxygen with the haemoglobin.

RBCs change shape as they pass through capillaries, and this plays an important role in the uptake and release of oxygen.[5] The dependence of diffusing capacity on RBC shape changes may result from reducing the unstirred layer by mixing the plasma around the RBC, from changes in the cell membrane surface area to RBC volume ratio or from assisting the mass movement of haemoglobin within the cell. This has led to further studies in which the deformability of RBCs is reduced (using chlorpromazine) or increased (using sodium salicylate), which have demonstrated that diffusing capacity is increased with greater RBC deformability.[6] Of more clinical significance is the effect of plasma cholesterol on RBC function.[7] Elevated cholesterol concentration in the plasma causes increased cholesterol in the RBC membrane, a change that is known to make the membrane thicker and less deformable, both of which lead to reduced efficiency of diffusion across the membrane. Oxygen uptake by RBCs in the lung and its release in the tissues are both believed to be significantly impaired by hypercholesterolaemia, particularly in tissues with high oxygen extraction ratios such as the heart.

Uptake of Oxygen by Haemoglobin

The greater part of the oxygen that is taken up in the lungs enters into chemical combination with haemoglobin. This chemical reaction takes a finite time and forms an appreciable part of the total resistance to the transfer of oxygen.

This important discovery resulted in an extensive reappraisal of the whole concept of diffusing capacity. In particular, it became clear that measurements of diffusing capacity did not necessarily give an indication of the degree of permeability of the alveolar/capillary membrane.

Quantification of the Diffusing Capacity for Oxygen

The diffusing capacity of oxygen is simply the oxygen uptake divided by the partial pressure gradient from alveolar gas to pulmonary capillary blood, where the relevant value is the mean pulmonary capillary Po_2:

Oxygen diffusing capacity

$$= \frac{\text{Oxygen uptake}}{\text{Alveolar } Po_2 - \text{mean pulmonary capillary} Po_2}.$$

The alveolar Po_2 can be derived with some degree of accuracy (page 107), but there are very serious problems in estimating the mean pulmonary capillary Po_2. It is clearly impossible to make a direct measurement of the mean Po_2 of the pulmonary capillary blood, and therefore attempts have been made to derive this quantity indirectly from the presumed changes of Po_2 that occur as blood passes through the pulmonary capillaries.

The earliest analysis of the problem was made by Bohr in 1909.[8] He made the assumption that, at any point along the pulmonary capillary, the rate of diffusion of oxygen was proportional to the Po_2 difference between the alveolar gas and the pulmonary capillary blood at that point. Using this approach, and assuming a value for the alveolar/pulmonary end-capillary Po_2 gradient, it seemed possible to construct a graph of capillary Po_2 plotted against the time the blood had been in the pulmonary capillary. A typical curve drawn on this basis is shown as the broken blue line in Figure 8.2, *A*. Once the curve has been drawn, it is relatively easy to derive the mean pulmonary capillary Po_2, which then permits calculation of the oxygen-diffusing capacity. The validity of the assumption of the alveolar/pulmonary end-capillary Po_2 gradient is considered later.

Unfortunately, this approach, known as the Bohr integration procedure, was shown to be invalid when it was found that the fundamental assumption was untrue. The rate of transfer of oxygen is not proportional to the alveolar/capillary Po_2 gradient at any point along the capillary. It would no doubt be true if the transfer of oxygen were a purely physical process, but the rate of transfer is actually limited by the chemical combination of oxygen with haemoglobin, which is sufficiently slow to comprise a major part of the total resistance to transfer of oxygen.

Studies in vitro of the rate of combination of oxygen with haemoglobin have shown that this is not directly proportional to the Po_2 gradient, for two distinct reasons:
1. The combination of the fourth molecule of oxygen with the haemoglobin molecule ($Hb_4 (O_2)_3 + O_2 \rightleftharpoons Hb_4 (O_2)_4$)

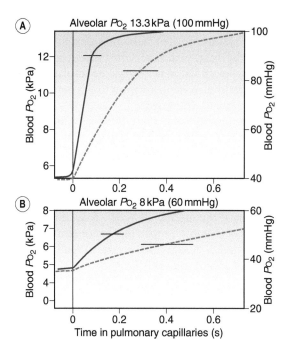

• **Fig. 8.2** Each graph shows the rise in blood P_{O_2} as blood passes along the pulmonary capillaries. The horizontal line at the top of the graph indicates the alveolar P_{O_2} that the blood P_{O_2} is approaching. In **(A)** the subject is breathing air, whereas in **(B)** the subject is breathing about 14% oxygen. The broken blue curve shows the rise in P_{O_2} calculated according to the Bohr procedure on an assumed value for the alveolar/end-capillary P_{O_2} gradient. The continuous red curve shows the values obtained by forward integration. Horizontal bars indicate mean pulmonary capillary P_{O_2} calculated from each curve.

$[(O_2)_4)]$ has a much higher velocity constant than that of the combination of the other three molecules (page 144).
2. As the capillary oxygen saturation rises, the number of molecules of reduced haemoglobin diminishes, and the velocity of the forward reaction must therefore diminish by the law of mass action. This depends on the haemoglobin dissociation curve, and is therefore not a simple exponential function of the actual P_{O_2} of the blood.

When these two factors are combined it is found that the resistance to diffusion because of chemical combination of oxygen within the RBC is fairly constant up to a saturation of about 80% (P_{O_2} = 6 kPa or 45 mmHg). Thereafter it falls very rapidly to become zero at full saturation. In view of these findings the Bohr integration procedure was elaborated to allow for changes in the rate of combination of haemoglobin with oxygen.[9] Assuming traditional values for the alveolar/end-capillary P_{O_2} difference, the resulting curve lies well to the left of the original Bohr curve, as shown by the continuous red curve in Figure 8.2, A. This indicated a mean pulmonary capillary P_{O_2} greater than had previously been believed, and therefore an oxygen-diffusing capacity that was substantially greater than the accepted value. The situation is actually more complicated still, as quick-frozen sections of lung show that the colour of haemoglobin begins to alter to the red colour of oxyhaemoglobin within the pulmonary arterioles before the blood has even entered the pulmonary

capillaries. Furthermore, pulmonary capillaries do not cross only a single alveolus, but may pass over three or more.

Both the classic and the modified Bohr integration procedures for calculation of mean capillary P_{O_2} depended critically on the precise value of the pulmonary end-capillary P_{O_2}. The constructed curve (Fig. 8.2, *A*), and therefore the derived mean capillary P_{O_2}, were considerably influenced by very small variations in the assumed value. The ideal alveolar/arterial P_{O_2} difference could be measured, but the problem was to separate this into its two components, the ideal alveolar/pulmonary end-capillary P_{O_2} difference (attributed to diffusion block) and the pulmonary end-capillary/arterial P_{O_2} difference (attributed to venous admixture). Figure 7.10 will make this clear.

Forward Integration[10]

This involved a new and entirely opposite approach based on the new understanding of the kinetics of the combination of oxygen with haemoglobin and the pattern of blood flow through the pulmonary capillaries. Starting at the arterial end of the pulmonary capillaries, the P_{O_2} of the capillary blood is calculated progressively along the capillary until an estimate is obtained of the remaining alveolar/capillary P_{O_2} gradient at the end of the capillary. This procedure of forward integration was thus the reverse of the classic approach which, starting from the alveolar/end-capillary P_{O_2} gradient, worked backwards to see what was happening along the capillary.

Forward integrations gave important results suggesting that alveolar/end-capillary P_{O_2} gradients were much smaller than had previously been thought. For example, when breathing air the gradient was always less than 0.0001 kPa, and only when exercising and breathing low inspired oxygen concentrations did the gradient become significant.

Capillary Transit Time

Capillary transit time is a most important factor determining both the pulmonary end-capillary P_{O_2} and the diffusing capacity. It is seen from Figure 8.2, *A*, that, if the capillary transit time is reduced to below 0.25 seconds there will be an appreciable gradient between the alveolar and end-capillary P_{O_2}. Because the diffusion gradient from alveolar gas to mean pulmonary capillary blood will be increased, the oxygen-diffusing capacity must be decreased.

The mean pulmonary capillary transit time equals the pulmonary capillary blood volume divided by the pulmonary blood flow (approximately equal to cardiac output). This gives a normal time of the order of 0.8 seconds with a subject at rest, though estimates vary from 0.1 to 3 seconds. It is therefore likely that, in a similar fashion to ventilation and perfusion, there is a wide range of normal capillary transit times affected by many factors such as posture, lung volume, cardiac output, and so on. Blood from capillaries with the shortest time will yield desaturated blood, and this will not be compensated by blood from capillaries with longer than average transit times, for the reason shown in Figure 7.15.

Diffusion of Carbon Dioxide in the Lungs

Carbon dioxide has a much higher water solubility than oxygen, and, although its density is greater, it may be calculated to penetrate an aqueous membrane about 20 times as rapidly as oxygen (Table 8.1). Therefore it was formerly believed that diffusion problems could not exist for carbon dioxide because the patient would have succumbed from hypoxia before hypercapnia could attain measurable proportions. All of this ignored the fact that chemical reactions of the respiratory gases were sufficiently slow to affect the measured diffusing capacity, and in fact were generally the limiting factor in gas transfer. The carriage of carbon dioxide in the blood is discussed in Chapter 9, but for the moment it is sufficient to note the essential reactions in the release of chemically combined carbon dioxide including (1) release of some carbon dioxide from carbamino carriage and (2) conversion of bicarbonate ions to carbonic acid followed by dehydration to release molecular carbon dioxide.

The latter reaction involves the movement of bicarbonate ions across the RBC membrane, but its rate is probably limited by the dehydration of carbonic acid. This reaction would be very slow indeed if it were not catalysed by carbonic anhydrase, which is present in abundance in the RBC and also on the endothelium. The important limiting role of the rate of this reaction was elegantly shown in a study of the effect of inhibition of carbonic anhydrase on carbon dioxide transport. This resulted in a large increase in the arterial/alveolar P_{CO_2} gradient, corresponding to a gross decrease in the apparent diffusing capacity of carbon dioxide.

Equilibrium of carbon dioxide is probably very nearly complete within the normal pulmonary capillary transit time. However, even if it were not so, it would be of little significance because the mixed venous/alveolar P_{CO_2} difference is itself quite small (approximately 0.8 kPa or 6 mmHg). Therefore an end-capillary gradient as large as 20% of the initial difference would still be too small to be of any importance.

TABLE 8.1	The Influence of Physical Properties on the Diffusion of Gases Through a Gas–Liquid Interface		
Gas	Density Relative to Oxygen	Water Solubility Relative to Oxygen	Diffusing Capacity Relative to Oxygen
Oxygen	1.00	1.00	1.00
Carbon dioxide	1.37	24.0	20.5
Nitrogen	0.88	0.515	0.55
Carbon monoxide	0.88	0.75	0.80
Nitrous oxide	1.37	16.3	14.0
Helium	0.125	0.37	1.05
Nitric oxide	0.94	1.70	1.71

Hypercapnia is, in fact, never caused by decreased diffusing capacity, except when carbonic anhydrase is completely inhibited by drugs such as acetazolamide (page 124). Pathological hypercapnia may always be explained by other causes, usually alveolar ventilation that is inadequate for the metabolic rate of the patient.

The assumption that there is no measurable difference between the P_{CO_2} of the alveolar gas and the pulmonary end-capillary blood is used when the alveolar P_{CO_2} is assumed equal to the arterial P_{CO_2} for the purpose of derivation of the ideal alveolar P_{O_2} (page 108). The assumption is also made that there is no measurable difference between end-capillary and arterial P_{CO_2}. We have seen in the previous chapter (Table 7.2) that this is not strictly true, and a large shunt of 50% will cause an arterial/end-capillary P_{CO_2} gradient of approximately 0.4 kPa.

Diffusion of Carbon Monoxide in the Lungs

Diffusing capacity is usually measured for carbon monoxide, for the very practical reason that affinity of carbon monoxide for haemoglobin is so high that the partial pressure of the gas in the pulmonary capillary blood remains effectively zero. The formula for calculation of this quantity then simplifies to

$$\text{Diffusing capacity for carbon monoxide} = \frac{\text{Carbon monoxide uptake}}{\text{Alveolar } P_{CO}}$$

(compare with corresponding equation for oxygen, page 114).

There are no insuperable difficulties in the measurement of either of the remaining quantities on the right-hand side of the equation, and the methods are outlined at the end of the chapter. Traditional units for CO diffusing capacity are $mL.min^{-1}.mmHg^{-1}$, although in SI units the volume of CO is usually described in molar terms, that is, $mmol. min^{-1}.kPa^{-1}$.

Measurement of the carbon monoxide diffusing capacity is firmly established as a valuable routine pulmonary function test, which may show changes in a range of conditions in which other pulmonary function tests yield normal values. It provides an index that shows that something is wrong, and changes in the index provide a useful indication of progress of the disease. However, it is much more difficult to explain a reduced diffusing capacity for carbon monoxide in terms of the underlying pathophysiology (see later).

Diffusion Path for Carbon Monoxide

Diffusion of carbon monoxide within the alveolus, through the alveolar/capillary membrane and through the plasma into the RBC, is governed by the same factors that apply to oxygen, and these were outlined earlier. The quantitative difference is due to the different density and water solubility of the two gases (Table 8.1). These factors indicate that the rate of diffusion of oxygen up to the point of entry into the RBC is 1.25 times the corresponding rate for carbon monoxide.

Diffusion of CO in Plasma

The frequent use of carbon monoxide for measurement of lung diffusing capacity has focused attention on the diffusion pathway for CO, which, in spite of the slight differences in the physical properties of CO and oxygen, is likely to be very similar in vivo. Clearly, direct measurement of diffusion gradients in a pulmonary capillary is not possible, so attempts to elucidate the diffusion pattern of gases in capillary plasma are based on mathematical models. The most helpful analysis assumed that there is a gradient of CO concentration within the capillary, with minimal CO in the centre, and used a 'finite element analysis' to show that diffusion paths for CO are likely to be nonlinear.[4] Figure 8.3 shows a theoretical drawing of the CO flux in the capillary at both high and low haematocrit, showing clearly that, except in severe anaemia, CO uptake is achieved long before diffusion to the centre of the capillary is able to take place. In spite of these detailed models, agreement with observed CO diffusion remains poor under most situations.[4]

Uptake of CO by Haemoglobin

The affinity of haemoglobin for carbon monoxide is about 250 times as great as it is for oxygen. Nevertheless, it does not follow that the rate of combination of carbon monoxide with haemoglobin is faster than the rate of combination of oxygen with haemoglobin: it is, in fact, slower. The reaction is slower still when oxygen must first be displaced from haemoglobin, according to the equation

$$CO + HbO_2 \rightarrow O_2 + HbCO.$$

Therefore the reaction rate of carbon monoxide with haemoglobin is reduced when the oxygen saturation of the haemoglobin is high. The inhalation of different concentrations of oxygen thus causes changes in the reaction rate of carbon monoxide with the haemoglobin of a patient, an observation that has been used to study different components of the resistance to diffusion of carbon monoxide in humans.

Quantification of the Components of the Resistance to Diffusion of CO

When two resistances are arranged in series, the total resistance of the pair is equal to the sum of the two individual resistances.

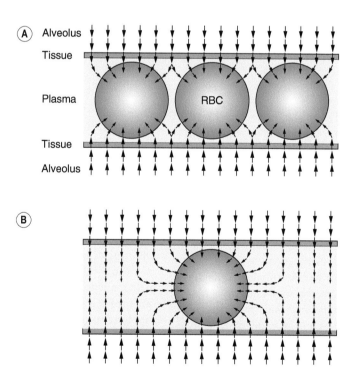

• **Fig. 8.3** Mathematical model of diffusion paths for carbon monoxide (CO) between the alveolus and the red blood cell (RBC). The size and direction of the arrows indicate the magnitude and direction of the CO flux, respectively. The RBC is assumed to be an infinite 'sink' for CO. **(A)** Normal. Packed cell volume 66%, under which conditions CO is absorbed by the RBC mainly at the periphery of the capillary. **(B)** Severe anaemia. Packed cell volume 12%. Diffusion occurs into the centre of the plasma and follows a nonlinear path into the RBC. The thickness of the tissue barrier relative to capillary diameter is drawn to scale, showing the relatively small contribution that the alveolar capillary membrane makes to the diffusion barrier in total. (From reference 4.)

Diffusing capacity is analogous to conductance, which is the reciprocal of resistance. Therefore the reciprocal of the diffusing capacity of the total system equals the sum of the reciprocals of the diffusing capacities of the two components

In theory, the diffusing capacity of CO in the blood includes diffusion across the plasma membrane, diffusion across the RBC membrane, diffusion within the RBC and the chemical combination of CO with haemoglobin. However, in vivo, as in the case of oxygen, the reaction rate of CO with haemoglobin is a significant factor. This diffusing capacity for blood is equal to the product of the pulmonary capillary blood volume (Vc) and the rate of reaction of carbon monoxide with haemoglobin (θco), a parameter which varies with the oxygen saturation of the haemoglobin. The equation may now be rewritten as

$$\frac{1}{\text{total diffusing capacity for CO}} = \frac{1}{\substack{\text{diffusing capacity of CO} \\ \text{for the alveolar/capillary} \\ \text{membrane}}} + \frac{1}{\substack{\text{pulmonary capillary blood} \\ \text{volume reaction rate} \\ \text{of CO with blood}}}.$$

The usual symbols for representation of this equation are as follows:

$$\frac{1}{DL_{CO}} = \frac{1}{DM_{CO}} + \frac{1}{Vc \times \theta_{CO}}.$$

The term Dm is often described simply as membrane diffusing capacity. $Dm_{CO} = 0.8 Dm_{O_2}$ under similar conditions (see Table 8.1).

The total diffusing capacity for carbon monoxide is a routine clinical measurement, and is described at the end of this chapter: θco may be determined, at different values of oxygen saturation, by studies in vitro. This leaves two unknowns—the diffusing capacity through the alveolar/capillary membrane and the pulmonary capillary blood volume. By repeating the measurement of total diffusing capacity at different arterial oxygen saturations (obtained by inhaling different concentrations of oxygen), it is possible to obtain two simultaneous equations with two unknowns which may then be solved to obtain values for Dm_{CO} and pulmonary capillary blood volume. Measurement of pulmonary capillary blood volume by this technique yields normal values between 60 and 110 mL (depending on subject height), which agrees well with a morphometric estimate of about 100 mL.

Factors Affecting Diffusing Capacity

The basic principles of pulmonary diffusion described so far indicate that there are three major mechanisms by which

diffusing capacity may alter: changes in the effective surface area of the gas exchange membrane, a change in the physical properties of the membrane or changes related to the uptake of gases by the RBC. Each of these mechanisms will be discussed individually, and then other factors that affect diffusion capacity by either multiple or unknown mechanisms will be described.

Most of the factors outlined in this section will apply equally to oxygen and CO diffusion, though the majority have been studied using CO for the reasons described in the previous section.

Factors Affecting the Membrane Surface Area

Total lung volume, and therefore the number of alveoli available for gas exchange, will clearly affect diffusing capacity. However, only those alveoli that are adequately ventilated and perfused will contribute to gas exchange, and the scatter of ventilation/perfusion therefore has an important influence on the diffusing capacity.

Body Size

Stature influences diffusing capacity directly due to the relationship between height and lung volume. Normal values for total diffusing capacity may be calculated from the formulae:
Males:

$$DL_{CO} = 10.9 \times \text{height(m)} - 0.067 \\ \times \text{age(years)} - 5.89.$$

Females:

$$DL_{CO} = 7.1 \times \text{height(m)} - 0.054 \\ \times \text{age(years)} - 0.89.$$

A healthy 30-year-old male 1.78 m tall would therefore have a CO-diffusing capacity of 11.5 mmol.min^{-1}.kPa^{-1} (34.4 mL.min.$^{-1}$mmHg^{-1}).

Lung Volume

Diffusing capacity is directly related to lung volume, and so maximal at total lung capacity.[11] Different techniques for the measurement of diffusing capacity use different lung volumes, so it is now standard practice to simultaneously measure lung volume at which diffusing capacity was measured (referred to as *alveolar volume*) by inert gas dilution, usually with helium or methane. Diffusing capacity can then be measured as diffusing capacity per litre alveolar volume, referred to as the diffusion constant (Kco), with units of mmol.min^{-1}.kPa^{-1}.L^{-1} (mL.min.$^{-1}$mmHg^{-1}.L^{-1}).

Ventilation/Perfusion Mismatch

This results in a physiological dysfunction that presents many of the features of a reduction in diffusing capacity. If, for example, most of the ventilation is distributed to the left lung and most of the pulmonary blood flow to the right lung, then the effective interface must be reduced. Minor degrees of maldistribution greatly complicate the interpretation of a reduced diffusing capacity. Both maldistribution and impaired diffusing capacity have a similar effect on the alveolar/arterial Po_2 gradient in relation to inspired oxygen concentration (see Fig. 7.16), and a distinction cannot be made by simple means.

Posture

Diffusing capacity is substantially increased when the subject is supine rather than standing or sitting, in spite of the fact that lung volume is reduced. This change is probably explained by the increase in pulmonary blood volume, and the more uniform distribution of perfusion of the lungs in the supine position.

Pathology

The total area of the alveolar/capillary membrane may be reduced by any disease process or surgery that removes a substantial number of alveoli. For example, emphysema reduces the diffusing capacity mainly by destruction of alveolar septa, such that $D_{L_{CO}}$ correlates with the anatomical degree of emphysematous changes in the lung.

Factors Affecting the Membrane Diffusion Barrier

It will be clear that the oxygen diffusing capacity may be influenced by many factors that have really nothing at all to do with diffusion per se. In fact, there is considerable doubt as to whether a true defect of alveolar/capillary membrane diffusion is ever the limiting factor in transfer of oxygen from the inspired gas to the arterial blood.

Chronic heart failure and pulmonary oedema remain the only likely causes of a membrane diffusion barrier. This may occur either via pulmonary capillary congestion increasing the length of the diffusion pathway for oxygen through plasma, by interstitial oedema increasing the thickness of the membrane or by raised capillary pressure damaging the endothelial and epithelial cells leading to proliferation of type II alveolar cells and thickening of the membrane. The membrane component of diffusing capacity (Dm) is reduced in heart failure, and the reduction correlates with symptom severity, whereas capillary volume increases only in severe heart failure.[12] It is therefore possible that, with heart failure of a suitable severity over a prolonged period, a form of alveolar/capillary block can occur.

Factors Affecting Uptake of Gases by Haemoglobin

Haemoglobin concentration affects diffusing capacity by influencing the rate and amount of oxygen or CO uptake by blood flowing through the pulmonary capillary. Measurements of diffusing capacity are therefore usually mathematically corrected to account for abnormalities in the patient's haemoglobin concentration.

In the previous section, it has been explained how a reduction in capillary transit time may reduce the diffusing capacity. The mean transit time is reduced when cardiac output is raised, and this may increase diffusing capacity substantially, for example during exercise (see next).

Other Determinants of Diffusing Capacity

Age. Even when corrected for changes in lung volume, $D_{L_{CO}}$ declines in a linear fashion with increasing age (see earlier discussion).

Sex. Women have a reduced total pulmonary diffusing capacity in comparison with men. This difference is almost totally explained by differences in stature and haemoglobin concentration. $D_{L_{CO}}$ in women varies throughout the menstrual cycle, reaching a peak before menstruation, and seems to result from changes in θ, the reaction rate of CO with blood. The finding may, however, represent a technical problem with measuring $D_{L_{CO}}$ in that the low value during menstruation could result from a high endogenous production of carboxyhaemoglobin during the catabolism of haem compounds.

Exercise. During exercise diffusing capacity may be double the value obtained at rest, as a result of increased cardiac output causing a reduction in capillary transit time and pulmonary capillary recruitment in nondependent lung zones (page 76). Because of this large effect of cardiac output on the measurement of diffusing capacity, some groups advocate using simultaneous noninvasive measures of cardiac output to aid interpretation of the diffusing capacity result.

Smoking history. This affects diffusing capacity even when most of the other determinants listed in this section are taken into account. $D_{L_{CO}}$ is reduced in proportion to the number of cigarettes per day currently smoked, and the total lifetime number of cigarettes ever smoked. The causes of this decline in lung function with smoking are discussed in Chapter 20.

Diffusion of Oxygen in the Tissues[13,14]

Oxygen leaves the systemic capillaries by the reverse of the process by which it entered the pulmonary capillaries. Chemical release from haemoglobin is followed by diffusion through the capillary wall and thence through the tissues to its site of utilization in the mitochondria.

Krogh, in 1919, was the first to describe the factors that influence the diffusion of oxygen through tissues, and his ideas developed into the first mathematical model to quantify the transfer of oxygen from the capillaries into the tissues (Fig. 8.4).[15] In Krogh's model, an individual capillary is assumed to be surrounded by a cylindrical area of tissue that derives its oxygen from the single capillary under consideration. There is a nonlinear gradient in Po_2 along the length of the capillary, referred to as the axial or longitudinal gradient, from a maximum at the arteriolar end of the capillary to a minimum at the venule. This curve is an inverted form

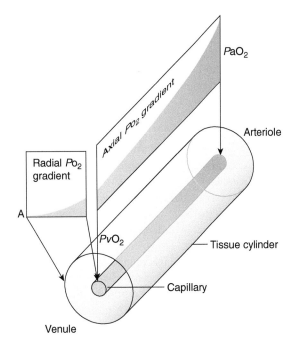

• **Fig. 8.4** Schematic representation of the Krogh model of tissue oxygenation. See text for details. Point A is the lethal corner, or the tissue region where Po_2 will always be the lowest, that is, at the point furthest away from the venular end of the capillary.

of the oxyhaemoglobin dissociation curve (see Fig. 10.9) between oxygen saturation values of 100% and 75%. At each point along the capillary, there is a further nonlinear radial Po_2 gradient where the oxygen diffuses across the capillary wall and surrounding tissues to its site of use in the mitochondria of the cells in the tissue cylinder. Using this model, a theoretical value for the Po_2 at any point in the tissue cylinder can be calculated using the Krogh–Erlang equation.[15] Although Krogh's model did not include axial diffusion within the tissues, this is also believed to occur. With axial gradients along the capillary and in the tissue, and radial gradients throughout, Po_2 is always minimal at the outer edge of the tissue cylinder at the venous end of the capillary, a region referred to as the 'lethal corner'. The concept of the Krogh cylinder makes no pretence to histological accuracy, but it does illustrate the difficulty of talking about the mean tissue Po_2, which is not an entity like the arterial or mixed venous Po_2.

The Krogh model has numerous unrealistic assumptions, for example that capillaries are all straight, parallel and of constant length and radius, with no connections between them. Values obtained for tissue Po_2 from the Krogh–Erlang equation are therefore only theoretical, and measurement of tissue Po_2 on a small enough scale to confirm Krogh's cylinder model remains impossible. Even so, studies of tissue Po_2 have provided some support for Krogh's model. Heterogeneity of tissue Po_2 has been shown to be considerable, and measurements of Po_2 along the length of individual pial capillaries have demonstrated a nonlinear decline in Po_2 along the capillary that closely matches the Krogh model.[16]

Diffusion paths are much longer in tissues than in the lung. In well-vascularized tissue, such as brain, each capillary serves a zone of radius of approximately 20 μm, but the corresponding distance is approximately 200 μm in skeletal muscle and greater still in fat and cartilage. In muscle tissue the effects of this long diffusion distance are mitigated by the presence of myoglobin which facilitates oxygen transport within the cell. No such mechanism exists in fat tissue, and there is ample evidence of cellular hypoxia in white adipocytes, which activates inflammatory pathways, potentially explaining the link between obesity and many systemic diseases.[17]

It is also impracticable to talk about mean tissue Po_2 because this varies from one organ to another and must also depend on perfusion in relation to metabolic activity. Furthermore, within a tissue there must be some cells occupying more favourable sites towards the arterial ends of capillaries, and others must accept oxygen from the venous ends of the capillaries, where the Po_2 is always lower. This is well demonstrated in the liver where the centrilobular cells must exist at a lower Po_2 than those at the periphery of the lobule. Even within a single cell, there can be no uniformity of Po_2. Not only are there 'low spots' around the mitochondria, but those mitochondria in regions of the cell nearest to the capillary presumably enjoy a higher Po_2 than those lying further away.

Principles of Measurement of Diffusing Capacity[18]

All the methods are based on the general equation (for carbon monoxide):

$$D_{CO} = \frac{\dot{V}_{CO}}{P_{A_{CO}} - P\bar{C}_{CO}}.$$

In each case it is usual to assume that the mean partial pressure of carbon monoxide in the pulmonary capillary blood, $P\bar{C}_{CO}$, is effectively zero. It is, therefore, only necessary to measure the carbon monoxide uptake ($\dot{V}_{CO}$) and the alveolar carbon monoxide tension ($P_{A_{CO}}$). The diffusing capacity so measured (D_{CO}) is the total diffusing capacity including that of the alveolar capillary membrane, plasma and the component due to the reaction time of carbon monoxide with haemoglobin.

Nitric oxide may also be used for the measurement of diffusing capacity, and because this gas also combines rapidly with haemoglobin (about 280 times faster than carbon monoxide), the reaction also is independent of the Po_2.[18] This rapid reaction between nitric oxide and blood means that θ_{NO} may be regarded as infinite, and therefore diffusing capacity measured using nitric oxide ($D_{L_{NO}}$) may be a more accurate assessment of Dm, although this is disputed.[19] Carbon monoxide is currently still the usual gas used for diffusing capacity measurements, despite calls for more widespread use of nitric oxide due to its potentially better diagnostic utility.[20]

Steady-State Method

The subject breathes a gas mixture containing approximately 0.3% carbon monoxide for about a minute. After this time, expired gas is collected when the alveolar P_{CO} is steady but the mixed venous P_{CO} has not yet reached a level high enough to require consideration in the calculation.

Carbon monoxide uptake is measured in exactly the same way as oxygen consumption by the open method (page 161): the amount of carbon monoxide expired (expired minute volume × mixed expired CO concentration) is subtracted from the amount of carbon monoxide inspired (inspired minute volume × inspired CO concentration). The alveolar P_{CO} is calculated from the Filley version of the alveolar air equation (page 108) using carbon monoxide in place of oxygen.

The steady-state method requires no special respiratory manoeuvre and is therefore particularly suitable for use in children.

Single-Breath Method[1]

This method is the most frequently used in clinical practice and has a long history of progressive refinement. There are many variations on the exact method used, which yield broadly similar results, but the multitude of techniques and factors affecting the results have led to attempts to standardize the method between centres.

The patient is first required to exhale maximally. He then draws in a vital-capacity breath of a gas mixture containing approximately 0.3% carbon monoxide and approximately 10% helium. The breath is held for 10 seconds, and a gas sample is then taken after the exhalation of the first 0.75 L, which is sufficient to wash out the patient's dead space. The breath-holding time is sufficient to overcome maldistribution of the inspired gas.

It is assumed that no significant amount of helium has passed into the blood. Therefore, the ratio of the concentration of helium in the inspired gas to the concentration in the end-expiratory gas, multiplied by the volume of gas drawn into the alveoli during the maximal inspiration, will indicate the total alveolar volume during the period of breath holding. The alveolar P_{CO} at the commencement of breath holding is equal to the same ratio multiplied by the P_{CO} of the inspired gas mixture. The end-expiratory P_{CO} is measured directly.

From these data, together with the time of breath holding, it is possible to calculate the carbon monoxide uptake and the mean alveolar P_{CO}. Lung diffusing capacity for carbon monoxide can then be calculated and normalized for lung volume using the alveolar volume measured at the same time with helium.

Rebreathing Method

Somewhat similar to the single-breath method is the rebreathing method by which a gas mixture containing approximately 0.3% carbon monoxide and 10% helium is rebreathed rapidly from a bag. The bag and the patient's lungs are considered as a single system, with gas exchange occurring in very much the same way as during breath holding. The calculation proceeds in a similar way to that for the single-breath method.

References

1. Graham BL, Brusasco V, Burgos F, et al. 2017 ERS/ATS standards for single-breath carbon monoxide uptake in the lung. *Eur Respir J.* 2017;49:1600016.
2. Landon MJ, Matson AM, Royston BD, et al. Components of the inspiratory-arterial isoflurane partial pressure difference. *Br J Anaesth.* 1993;70:605-611.
3. Weibel ER, Federspiel WJ, Fryder-Doffey F, et al. Morphometric model for pulmonary diffusing capacity I. Membrane diffusing capacity. *Respir Physiol.* 1993;93:125-149.
4. Hsia CC, Chuong CJ, Johnson RL. Critique of conceptual basis of diffusing capacity estimates: a finite element analysis. *J Appl Physiol.* 1995;79:1039-1047.
5. Sarelius I. Invited editorial on 'Effect of RBC shape and deformability on pulmonary O_2 diffusing capacity and resistance to flow in rabbit lungs'. *J Appl Physiol.* 1995;78:763-764.
6. Betticher DC, Reinhart WH, Geiser J. Effect of RBC shape and deformability on pulmonary O_2 diffusing capacity and resistance to flow in rabbit lungs. *J Appl Physiol.* 1995;78:778-783.
7. Buchwald H, O'Dea TJ, Menchaca HJ, et al. Effect of plasma cholesterol on red blood cell oxygen transport. *Clin Exp Pharmacol Physiol.* 2000;27:951-955.
8. Bohr C. Über die spezifische Tätigkeit der Lungen bei der respiratorischen Gasaufnahme. *Skand Arch Physiol.* 1909;22:221.
9. Staub NC, Bishop JM, Forster RE. Importance of diffusion and chemical reaction rates in O_2 uptake in the lung. *J Appl Physiol.* 1962;17:21-27.
10. Staub NC. Alveolar-arterial oxygen tension gradient due to diffusion. *J Appl Physiol.* 1963;18:673-680.
11. Stam H, Hrachovina V, Stijnen T, et al. Diffusing capacity dependent on lung volume and age in normal subjects. *J Appl Physiol.* 1994;76:2356-2363.
12. Puri S, Baker BL, Dutka DP, et al. Reduced alveolar-capillary membrane diffusing capacity in chronic heart failure. *Circulation.* 1995;91:2769-2774.
13. Tsai AG, Johnson PC, Intaglietta M. Oxygen gradients in the microcirculation. *Physiol Rev.* 2003;83:933-963.
*14. **Goldman D. Theoretical models of microvascular oxygen transport to tissue. *Microcirculation.* 2008;15:795-811.**
15. Kreuzer F. Oxygen supply to the tissues: the Krogh model and its assumptions. *Experientia.* 1982;38:1415-1426.
16. Ivanov KP, Sokolova IB, Vovenko EP. Oxygen transport in the rat brain cortex at normobaric hyperoxia. *Eur J Appl Physiol.* 1999;80:582-587.
17. Trayhurn P. Hypoxia and adipose tissue function and dysfunction in obesity. *Physiol Rev.* 2013;93:1-21.
18. Hughes JM, Pride NB. Examination of the carbon monoxide diffusing capacity (DL_{CO}) in relation to its KCO and VA components. *Am J Respir Crit Care Med.* 2012;186:132-139.
19. Zavorsky GS. No red cell resistance to NO? I think not! *J Appl Physiol.* 2010;108:1027-1029.
20. Zavorsky GS. Nitric oxide uptake in the lung: It is about time that clinicians use this test routinely. *Respir Physiol Neurobiol.* 2017;241:1-2.

9

Carbon Dioxide

KEY POINTS

- Most of the carbon dioxide carried in blood is in the form of bicarbonate, production and breakdown of which is catalysed by the enzyme carbonic anhydrase.
- Formation of bicarbonate is enhanced by the buffering of hydrogen ions by haemoglobin, and by active removal of bicarbonate ions from the red blood cell by band 3 protein.

- Smaller amounts of carbon dioxide are carried in solution in plasma, as carbonic acid or as carbamino compounds formed with plasma proteins and haemoglobin.
- There is normally a small gradient between arterial and alveolar $P\text{CO}_2$ caused by scatter of ventilation/perfusion ratios.

Carbon dioxide is the end product of aerobic metabolism and is produced almost entirely in the mitochondria where the $P\text{CO}_2$ is highest. From its point of origin, there are a series of partial pressure gradients as carbon dioxide passes through the cytoplasm and the extracellular fluid into the blood. In the lungs, the $P\text{CO}_2$ of the blood entering the pulmonary capillaries is normally higher than the alveolar $P\text{CO}_2$; therefore carbon dioxide diffuses from the blood into the alveolar gas, and a dynamic equilibrium is established. The equilibrium concentration equals the ratio between carbon dioxide output and alveolar ventilation (page 107). Blood leaving the alveoli has, for practical purposes, the same $P\text{CO}_2$ as alveolar gas, and arterial blood $P\text{CO}_2$ is usually very close to 'ideal' alveolar $P\text{CO}_2$.

Abnormal levels of arterial $P\text{CO}_2$ occur in a number of pathological states and have many important physiological effects throughout the body, some as a result of changes in pH, and these are discussed in Chapter 22. Fundamental to all problems relating to $P\text{CO}_2$ is the mechanism by which carbon dioxide is carried in the blood.

Carriage of Carbon Dioxide in Blood

In Physical Solution

Carbon dioxide is moderately soluble in water. According to Henry's law of solubility:

$$P\text{CO}_2 \times \text{solubility coefficient} = \text{CO}_2 \text{ concentration in solution.} \quad \text{[Eq. 9.1]}$$

The solubility coefficient of carbon dioxide (α) is expressed in units of $\text{mmol.L}^{-1}\,\text{kPa}^{-1}$ (or $\text{mmol.L}^{-1}.\text{mmHg}^{-1}$). The

value depends on temperature, and examples are listed in Table 9.1. The contribution of dissolved carbon dioxide to the total carriage of the gas in blood is shown in Table 9.2

As Carbonic Acid

In solution, carbon dioxide hydrates to form carbonic acid:

$$\text{CO}_2 + \text{H}_2\text{O} \rightleftharpoons \text{H}_2\text{CO}_3. \quad \text{[Eq. 9.2]}$$

The equilibrium of this reaction is far to the left under physiological conditions, with less than 1% of the molecules of carbon dioxide in the form of carbonic acid. There is a very misleading medical convention by which both forms of carbon dioxide in Equation 9.2 are sometimes shown as carbonic acid. Thus the term H_2CO_3 may, in some situations, mean the total concentrations of dissolved carbon dioxide and H_2CO_3; to avoid confusion it is preferable to use $\alpha P\text{CO}_2$ as in Equation 9.7. This does not apply to Equations 9.4 and 9.5, where H_2CO_3 has its correct meaning.

Carbonic Anhydrase[1]

The reaction of carbon dioxide with water (Eq. 9.2) is non-ionic and slow, requiring a period of minutes for equilibrium to be attained. This would be far too slow for the time available for gas exchange in pulmonary and systemic capillaries if the reaction were not catalysed in both directions by the enzyme carbonic anhydrase (CA). In addition to its role in the respiratory transport of carbon dioxide, CA plays a fundamental role in many body tissues, for example, the generation of hydrogen and bicarbonate ions in secretory organs including the stomach and kidney and the intracellular transfer of carbon dioxide within both skeletal and

TABLE 9.1   Values for Solubility of Carbon Dioxide in Plasma and pK' at Different Temperatures

| Temperature (°C) | Solubility of Carbon Dioxide in Plasma | | pK' | | |
	mmol.L^{-1}.kPa^{-1}	mmol.L^{-1} mmHg^{-1}	at pH 7.6	at pH 7.4	at pH 7.2
40	0.216	0.0288	6.07	6.08	6.09
39	0.221	0.0294	6.07	6.08	6.09
38	0.226	0.0301	6.08	6.09	6.10
37	0.231	0.0308	6.08	6.09	6.10
36	0.236	0.0315	6.09	6.10	6.11
35	0.242	0.0322	6.10	6.11	6.12
25	0.310	0.0413	6.15	6.16	6.17
15	0.416	0.0554	6.20	6.21	6.23

TABLE 9.2   Normal Values for Carbon Dioxide Carriage in Blood

	Arterial Blood (Hb sat. 95%)	Mixed Venous Blood (Hb sat. 75%)	Arterial/Venous Difference
Whole Blood			
pH	7.40	7.37	−0.033
P_{CO_2} (kPa)	5.3	6.1	+0.8
(mmHg)	40.0	46.0	+6.0
Total CO_2 (mmol.L^{-1})	21.5	23.3	+1.8
(mL.dL^{-1})	48.0	52.0	+4.0
Plasma (mmol.L^{-1})			
Dissolved CO_2	1.2	1.4	+0.2
Carbonic acid	0.0017	0.0020	+0.0003
Bicarbonate ion	24.4	26.2	+1.8
Carbamino CO_2	Negligible	Negligible	Negligible
Total	25.6	27.6	+2.0
Red Blood Cell Fraction of 1 L of Blood			
Dissolved CO_2	0.44	0.51	+0.07
Bicarbonate ion	5.88	5.92	+0.04
Carbamino CO_2	1.10	1.70	+0.60
Plasma Fraction of 1 L of Blood			
Dissolved CO_2	0.66	0.76	+0.10
Bicarbonate ion	13.42	14.41	+0.99
Total in 1 L of blood (mmol.L^{-1})	21.50	23.30	+1.80

Hb sat., Haemoglobin saturation.

cardiac muscle. In mammals there are now 16 isozymes of CA identified, of which two are involved in blood carbon dioxide transport.

Red blood cells (RBCs) contain large amounts of CA II, one of the fastest enzymes known, whereas CA IV is a membrane-bound isozyme present in pulmonary capillaries. There is no CA activity in plasma. CA is a zinc-containing enzyme of low molecular weight, and there is now extensive knowledge of the molecular mechanisms of CA. First, the zinc atom hydrolyses water to a reactive $Zn–OH^-$ species, whilst a nearby histidine residue acts as a 'proton shuttle', removing the H^+ from the metal-ion centre and transferring it to any buffer molecules near the enzyme. Carbon dioxide then combines with the $Zn–OH^-$ species, and the HCO_3^- formed rapidly dissociates from the zinc atom. The maximal rate of catalysis is determined by the buffering power in the vicinity of the enzyme, as the speed of the enzyme reactions is so fast that its kinetics are determined mostly by the ability of the surrounding buffers to provide/remove H^+ ions to/from the enzyme.

CA is inhibited by a large number of compounds, including some drugs such as thiazide diuretics and various heterocyclic sulphonamides, of which acetazolamide is the most important. Acetazolamide is nonspecific for the different CA isozymes, and so inhibits CA in all organs at a dose of 5 to 20 $mg.kg^{-1}$, and also has other pharmacological actions which may contribute to its diverse therapeutic uses.[2] Acetazolamide has been used extensively in studies of CA, which have revealed the surprising fact that CA is not essential to life. The quantity and efficiency of RBC CA are such that more than 98% of activity must be blocked before there is any discernible change in carbon dioxide transport, although when total inhibition is achieved, Pco_2 gradients between tissues and alveolar gas are increased, pulmonary ventilation is increased and alveolar Pco_2 is decreased.

As Bicarbonate Ion

The largest fraction of carbon dioxide in the blood is in the form of bicarbonate ion, which is formed by ionization of carbonic acid thus:

$$H_2CO_3 + H^+ + HCO_3^- \rightleftharpoons 2H^+ + CO_3^{2-}.$$ [Eq. 9.3]

The second dissociation occurs only at high pH (>9), and is not a factor in the carriage of carbon dioxide by the blood. The first dissociation is, however, of the greatest importance within the physiological range. The pK_1' is about 6.1, and carbonic acid is about 96% dissociated under physiological conditions.

According to the law of mass action:

$$\frac{[H^+] \times [HCO_3^-]}{[H_2CO_3]} = K_1',$$ [Eq. 9.4]

where K_1' is the equilibrium constant of the first dissociation. The subscript 1 indicates that it is the first dissociation, and the prime indicates that we are dealing with concentrations rather than the more correct thermodynamic activities.

Rearrangement of Equation 9.4 gives the following:

$$[H^+] = K_1' \frac{[H_2CO_3]}{[HCO_3^-]}.$$ [Eq. 9.5]

The left-hand side is the hydrogen ion concentration, and this equation is the nonlogarithmic form of the Henderson–Hasselbalch equation. The concentration of carbonic acid cannot be measured, and the equation may be modified by replacing this term with the total concentration of dissolved carbon dioxide and H_2CO_3, most conveniently quantified as αPco_2, as previously described. The equation now takes the form:

$$[H^+] = K_1' \frac{\alpha Pco_2}{[HCO_3^-]}.$$ [Eq. 9.6]

The new constant K' is the *apparent* first dissociation constant of carbonic acid and includes a factor that allows for the substitution of total dissolved carbon dioxide concentration for carbonic acid.

The equation is now in a useful form and permits the direct relation of plasma hydrogen ion concentration, Pco_2 and bicarbonate concentration, all quantities that can be measured. The value of K' cannot be derived theoretically and is determined experimentally by simultaneous measurements of the three variables. Under normal physiological conditions, if $[H^+]$ is in $nmol.L^{-1}$, Pco_2 in kPa and HCO_3^-, in $mmol.L^{-1}$, the value of the combined parameter $(\alpha K')$ is about 180. If Pco_2 is in mmHg, the value of the parameter is 24.

Most people prefer to use the pH scale and follow the approach described by Hasselbalch in 1916 and take logarithms of the reciprocal of each term in Equation 9.6, with the following familiar result:[3]

$$\begin{aligned} pH &= pK' + \log \frac{[HCO_3^-]}{\alpha Pco_2} \\ &= pK' + \log \frac{[CO_2] - \alpha Pco_2}{\alpha Pco_2} \end{aligned}$$ [Eq. 9.7]

where pK' has an experimentally derived value of the order of 6.1, but varies with temperature and pH (see Table 9.1). $[CO_2]$ refers to the total concentration of carbon dioxide in all forms (dissolved CO_2, H_2CO_3 and bicarbonate) in plasma, and not in whole blood.

As Carbamino Compounds

Amino groups in the uncharged $R–NH_2$ form have the ability to combine directly with carbon dioxide to form a carbamic acid. At body pH, the carbamic acid then dissociates almost completely to carbamate:

$$R-N-H + CO_2 \rightleftharpoons R-N-C-OH \rightleftharpoons R-N-C-O^- + H^+$$

[Eq. 9.8]

In a protein, the amino groups involved in the peptide linkages between amino acid residues cannot combine with carbon dioxide. The potential for carbamino carriage is therefore restricted to the one terminal amino group in each protein chain and to the side chain amino groups that are found in lysine and arginine. Because both hydrogen ions and carbon dioxide compete to react with uncharged amino groups, the ability to combine with carbon dioxide is markedly pH-dependent. The terminal α-amino groups are the most effective at physiological pH, and one binding site per protein monomer is more than sufficient to account for the quantity of carbon dioxide carried as carbamino compounds.

Carbamino Carriage and Haemoglobin

Only very small quantities of carbon dioxide are carried in carbamino compounds with plasma proteins. Almost all carbamino carriage is by binding to haemoglobin, and reduced haemoglobin is about 3.5 times as effective as oxyhaemoglobin (Fig. 9.1), this being a major component

of the Haldane effect (see later). Carbon dioxide binds to α-amino groups at the ends of both the α- and β-chains of haemoglobin. Earlier studies of carbon dioxide haemoglobin reactions using free haemoglobin solution overestimated the magnitude of carbamino binding with haemoglobin, as later work showed that 2,3-diphosphoglycerate (2,3-DPG) present in vivo antagonizes the binding of carbon dioxide with haemoglobin. This antagonism results from direct competition between carbon dioxide and 2,3-DPG for the end-terminal valine of the β-chain of haemoglobin, an effect that is not observed on the α-chains.

Haldane Effect[4]

This is the difference in the quantity of carbon dioxide carried, at constant $P\text{CO}_2$, in oxygenated and deoxygenated blood (Fig. 9.2). Although the amount of carbon dioxide carried in the blood by carbamino carriage is small, the difference between the amount carried in venous and arterial

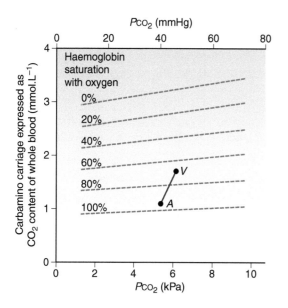

• **Fig. 9.1** The broken blue lines on the graph indicate the carbamino carriage of carbon dioxide at different levels of oxygen saturation of haemoglobin. Note that oxygen saturation has a far greater influence on carbamino carriage than the actual $P\text{CO}_2$ (x-axis). Points A and V represent the saturation and $P\text{CO}_2$ of arterial and venous blood, respectively. Note that the arterial/venous difference in carbamino carriage is large in relation to the actual amounts of carbamino carriage.

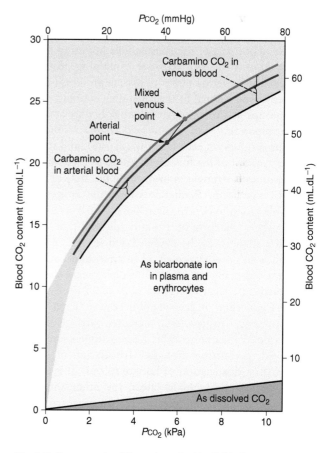

• **Fig. 9.2** Components of the carbon dioxide (CO₂) dissociation curve for whole blood. Dissolved CO₂ and bicarbonate ion vary with $P\text{CO}_2$, but are little affected by the state of oxygenation of the haemoglobin. (Increased basic properties of reduced haemoglobin cause a slight increase in formation of bicarbonate ion.) Carbamino carriage of CO₂ is strongly influenced by the state of oxygenation of haemoglobin, but hardly at all by $P\text{CO}_2$.

blood is about a third of the total arterial/venous difference (Table 9.2). Therefore this accounts for the major part of the Haldane effect, and the remainder is because of the increased buffering capacity of reduced haemoglobin, which is discussed in the next section. When the Haldane effect was described by Christiansen et al. in 1914, they believed that the whole effect was because of altered buffering capacity:[5] Carbamino carriage was not demonstrated until some years later.

Formation of carbamino compounds does not require the dissolved carbon dioxide to be hydrated, and so is independent of CA. The reaction is very rapid and would be of particular importance in a subject who had received a CA inhibitor.

Effect of Buffering Power of Proteins on Carbon Dioxide Carriage

Amino and carboxyl groups concerned in peptide linkages have no buffering power. Neither have most side chain groups (e.g., in lysine and glutamic acid) because their pK values are far removed from the physiological range of pH. In contrast is the imidazole group of the amino acid histidine, which is nearly the only amino acid to be an effective buffer in the normal range of pH. Imidazole groups constitute the major part of the considerable buffering power of haemoglobin, with each tetramer containing 38 histidine residues. The buffering power of plasma proteins is less and is directly proportional to their histidine content. The four haem groups of a molecule of haemoglobin are attached to the corresponding four amino acid chains at one of the histidine residues on each chain (page 143), and the dissociation constant of the imidazole groups of these four histidine residues is strongly influenced by the state of oxygenation of the haem. Reduction causes the corresponding imidazole group to become more basic. The converse is also true: in the acidic form of the imidazole group of the histidine, the strength of the oxygen bond is weakened. Each reaction is of great physiological interest, and both effects were noticed many decades before their mechanisms were elucidated.

1. The reduction of haemoglobin causes it to become more basic. This results in increased carriage of carbon dioxide as bicarbonate, because hydrogen ions are removed, permitting increased dissociation of carbonic acid (first dissociation of Equation 9.3). This accounts for part of the Haldane effect; the other and greater part is because of increased carbamino carriage (see earlier discussion).

2. Conversion to the basic form of histidine causes increased affinity of the corresponding haem group for oxygen. This is, in part, the cause of the Bohr effect (page 146).

Total deoxygenation of the haemoglobin in blood would raise the pH by about 0.03 if the $P\text{CO}_2$ were held constant at 5.3 kPa (40 mmHg), and this would correspond roughly to the addition of 3 mmol of base to 1 L of blood. The normal degree of desaturation in the course of the change from

arterial to venous blood is approximately 25%, corresponding to a pH increase of about 0.007 if $P\text{CO}_2$ remains constant. In fact, $P\text{CO}_2$ rises by approximately 0.8 kPa (6 mmHg), which would cause a decrease of pH of 0.040 if the oxygen saturation were to remain the same. The combination of an increase of $P\text{CO}_2$ of 0.8 kPa and a decrease of saturation of 25% thus results in a fall of pH of 0.033 (Table 9.2).

Distribution of Carbon Dioxide Within the Blood

Table 9.2 shows the forms in which carbon dioxide is carried in normal arterial and mixed venous blood. Although the amount carried in solution is small, most of the carbon dioxide enters and leaves the blood as carbon dioxide itself (Fig. 9.3). Within the plasma there is little chemical combination of carbon dioxide, for three reasons. First, there is no CA in plasma; therefore it is formed only very slowly. Second, there is little buffering power in plasma to promote the dissociation of carbonic acid. Third, the formation of

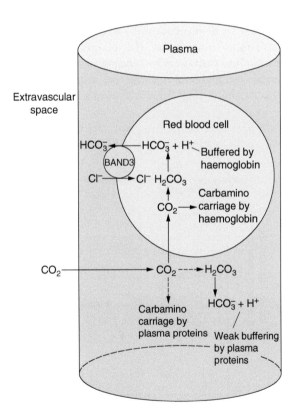

• **Fig. 9.3** How carbon dioxide enters the blood in molecular form. Within the plasma, there is only negligible carbamino carriage by plasma proteins, and a slow rate of hydration to carbonic acid because of the absence of carbonic anhydrase. The greater part of carbon dioxide (CO_2) diffuses into the red blood cell, where conditions for carbamino carriage (by haemoglobin) are more favourable. In addition, more rapid formation of carbonic acid is facilitated by carbonic anhydrase, the removal of hydrogen ions by haemoglobin buffering and the transfer of bicarbonate out of the red blood cell in exchange for chloride by the band 3 ion-exchange protein (Hamburger shift).

carbamino compounds by plasma proteins is not great and must be almost identical for arterial and venous blood.

Carbon dioxide can, however, diffuse freely into the RBC, where two courses are open. First, increasing intracellular $P\text{CO}_2$ will increase carbamino carriage of carbon dioxide by haemoglobin, an effect greatly enhanced by the fall in oxygen saturation, which is likely to be occurring at the same time (Fig. 9.1). The second course is hydration and dissociation of carbon dioxide to produce hydrogen and bicarbonate ions, facilitated by the presence of CA in the RBC. However, accumulation of intracellular hydrogen and bicarbonate ions will quickly tip the equilibrium of the reaction against further dissociation of carbonic acid, a situation that is avoided in the RBC by two mechanisms:

Haemoglobin Buffering

Hydrogen ions produced by CA are quickly buffered by the imidazole groups on the histidine residues of the haemoglobin, as described previously. Once again, the concomitant fall in haemoglobin saturation enhances this effect by increasing the buffering capacity of the haemoglobin.

Hamburger Shift

Hydration of carbon dioxide and buffering of the hydrogen ions results in the formation of considerable quantities of bicarbonate ion within the RBC. These excess bicarbonate ions are actively transported out of the cell into the plasma in exchange for chloride ions to maintain electrical neutrality across the RBC membrane. This ionic exchange was first suggested by Hamburger in 1918,[6] and believed to be a passive process. It is now known to be facilitated by a membrane-bound protein that has been extensively studied and named band 3 after its position on a gel electrophoresis plate. Band 3 exchanges bicarbonate and chloride ions by a 'ping-pong' mechanism in which one ion first moves out of the RBC before the other ion moves inwards, in contrast to most other ion pumps, which simultaneously exchange the two ions. Band 3 protein is also intimately related to other proteins in the RBC (Fig. 9.4):[7,8]

- *RBC cytoskeleton.* The cytoplasmic domain of band 3 acts as an anchoring site for many of the proteins involved in the maintenance of cell shape and membrane stability, such as ankyrin and spectrin. A genetically engineered deficiency of band 3 in animals results in small, fragile spherical RBCs, and in humans an inherited defect of band 3 is responsible for hereditary spherocytosis in which RBCs become spheroidal in shape and fragile.[9] RBC shape and deformability are now known to be important in oxygen transport in the capillaries (page 114), and it is possible that band 3 is involved in bringing about these shape changes.
- *CA.* Band 3 is also closely associated with CA, and the protein complex formed is believed to act as a metabolon, a term describing the channelling of a substrate directly between proteins that catalyse sequential reactions in a metabolic pathway.[7] In this case the substrate is bicarbonate, which after its formation by CA is transferred directly to band 3, which exports it from the cell.
- *Haemoglobin.* Band 3 is also associated with haemoglobin, with which it is believed to form another metabolon system exporting nitric oxide–derived nitrosothiols, possibly to regulate capillary blood flow and oxygen release from haemoglobin (page 148).
- *Glycolytic enzymes.* Some of the enzymes involved in glycolysis (page 151), including glyceraldehyde-3-phosphate dehydrogenase, phosphofructokinase and aldolase, are bound to band 3; the functional significance of this is unknown.

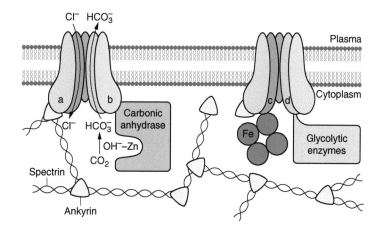

• **Fig. 9.4** Proteins associated with band 3 in the red blood cell membrane. Band 3 has 12 transmembrane domains forming the bicarbonate/chloride exchange ion channel, and four globular cytoplasmic domains (a–d), each of which is associated with different groups of intracellular proteins. *(a)* Ankyrin and spectrin, to maintain and possibly alter red cell shape; *(b)* carbonic anhydrase, with which band 3 acts as a metabolon to directly export bicarbonate ions from the red cell; *(c)* haemoglobin, with which band 3 may act as a metabolon to export nitric oxide; *(d)* glycolytic enzymes (the functional significance of this association is unknown).

In the pulmonary capillary, where $P\text{co}_2$ is low, the series of events previously described goes into reverse, and the carbon dioxide released from the RBC diffuses into the alveolus and is excreted.

Dissociation Curves of Carbon Dioxide

Figure 9.2 shows the classic form of the dissociation curve of carbon dioxide relating blood content to partial pressure. For decades there has been great interest in curves that relate any pair of the following: (1) plasma bicarbonate concentration, (2) $P\text{co}_2$ and (3) pH. These three quantities are related by the Henderson–Hasselbalch equation (Equation 7), and therefore the third variable can always be derived from the other two. The most famous is the Siggaard–Andersen plot, which relates $P\text{co}_2$ on a logarithmic scale to pH (Fig. 9.5). These graphs can be used to explore the effects of changes in respiratory and metabolic acid–base balance, but care must be taken in using these in vitro data in intact subjects. For example, if the $P\text{co}_2$ of an entire patient is altered, the pH changes are not the same as those of a blood sample of which the $P\text{co}_2$ is altered in vitro. This is because the blood of a patient is in continuity with the extracellular fluid (of very low buffering capacity) and also with intracellular fluid (of high buffering capacity). Bicarbonate ions pass rapidly and freely across the various interfaces. As a result, the in vivo change in pH is normally greater than the in vitro change in the patient's blood when subjected to the same change in $P\text{co}_2$.

Factors Influencing the $P\text{co}_2$ in the Steady State

In common with other catabolites, the level of carbon dioxide in the body fluids depends on the balance between production and elimination. There is a continuous gradient of $P\text{co}_2$ from the mitochondria to the expired air and thence to ambient air. The $P\text{co}_2$ in all cells is not identical, but is lowest in tissues with the lowest metabolic activity and the highest perfusion (e.g., skin) and highest in tissues with the highest metabolic activity for their perfusion (e.g., the myocardium). Therefore the $P\text{co}_2$ of venous blood differs substantially from one tissue to another.

In the pulmonary capillaries, carbon dioxide passes into the alveolar gas, and this causes the alveolar $P\text{co}_2$ to rise

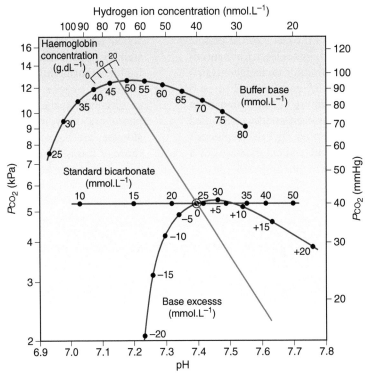

• **Fig. 9.5** The Siggaard–Andersen nomogram. The blue line shows the normal in vitro relationship between pH and log$P\text{co}_2$, and is derived by varying the $P\text{co}_2$ of a blood sample and measuring its pH. The slope is that of a line joining the normal arterial point (*shown by a small circle*) and the relevant point on the haemoglobin scale. Intersections of this line indicate three other indices of metabolic acid–base state: buffer base, standard bicarbonate and base excess. If both pH and $P\text{co}_2$ are measured in vivo, a single point may be plotted on the graph and a line parallel to the in vitro one is drawn that passes through this point. All three acid–base indices can then be read from the nomogram. This process is now routinely performed mathematically by blood-gas analysers. (From Siggaard-Andersen O. The pH, log $P\text{co}_2$ blood acid–base nomogram revisited. *Scand J Clin Lab Invest.* 1962;14:598-604. With permission of Taylor & Francis AS).

steadily during expiration. During inspiration, the inspired gas dilutes the alveolar gas, and the $P\text{CO}_2$ falls by about 0.4 kPa, imparting a sawtooth curve to the alveolar $P\text{CO}_2$ when it is plotted against time (Fig. 9.6).

Blood leaving the pulmonary capillaries has a $P\text{CO}_2$ that is very close to that of the alveolar gas and, therefore, varies with time in the same manner as the alveolar $P\text{CO}_2$. These oscillations in arterial $P\text{CO}_2$ with respiratory rate may be involved in respiratory control, particularly during exercise (page 188) and at altitude. There is also a regional variation, with $P\text{CO}_2$ inversely related to the ventilation/perfusion ratio of different parts of the lung (Fig. 7.14). The mixed arterial $P\text{CO}_2$ is the integrated mean of blood from different parts of the lung, and a sample drawn over several seconds will average out the cyclical variations.

It is more convenient to consider partial pressure than content, because carbon dioxide always moves in accord with partial pressure gradients, even if they are in the opposite direction to concentration gradients. Also, the concept of partial pressure may be applied with equal significance to gas and liquid phases, with content having a rather different connotation in the two phases. Furthermore, the effects of carbon dioxide (e.g., upon respiration) are a function of partial pressure rather than content. Finally, it is easier to measure blood $P\text{CO}_2$ than carbon dioxide content. Normal values for partial pressure and content are shown in Figure 9.7.

Each factor that influences the $P\text{CO}_2$ has already been mentioned in this book, and in this chapter they will be drawn together, illustrating their relationship to one another. It is convenient first to summarize the factors influencing the alveolar $P\text{CO}_2$, and then to consider the factors that influence the relationship between the alveolar and the arterial $P\text{CO}_2$ (Fig. 9.8).

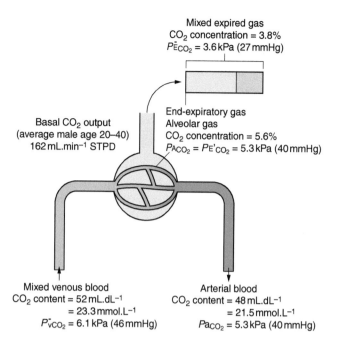

• **Fig. 9.7** Normal values of carbon dioxide levels. These normal values are rounded off and ignore the small difference in $P\text{CO}_2$ between end-expiratory gas, alveolar gas and arterial blood. Actual values of $P\text{CO}_2$ depend mainly on alveolar ventilation, but the differences depend on maldistribution; the alveolar/end-expiratory $P\text{CO}_2$ difference depends on alveolar dead space and the very small arterial/alveolar $P\text{CO}_2$ difference on shunt. Scatter of ventilation/perfusion ratios makes a small contribution to both alveolar/end-expiratory and arterial/alveolar $P\text{CO}_2$ gradients. The arterial/mixed venous CO_2 content difference is directly proportional to CO_2 output and inversely proportional to cardiac output. Secondary symbols: A, alveolar; a, arterial; Ē, mixed expired; E′, end-expiratory; v̄, mixed venous.

Alveolar $P\text{CO}_2$ ($P\text{ACO}_2$)

Carbon dioxide is constantly being added to the alveolar gas from the pulmonary arterial blood and removed from it by the alveolar ventilation. Therefore, ignoring inspired carbon dioxide, it follows that

$$\text{Alveolar } CO_2 \text{ concentration} = \frac{\text{Carbon dioxide output}}{\text{Alveolar ventilation}}.$$

This axiomatic relationship is the basis for prediction of the alveolar concentration of any gas that enters or leaves the body. With inclusion of the inspired concentration, it may be written as a form of alveolar air equation (page 107), for which the version for carbon dioxide is as follows:

$$\text{Alveolar } P_{CO_2} = \text{dry barometric pressure} \left(\begin{array}{c} \text{mean inspired } CO_2 \\ \text{concentration} \end{array} + \frac{CO_2 \text{ output}}{\text{alveolar ventilation}} \right).$$

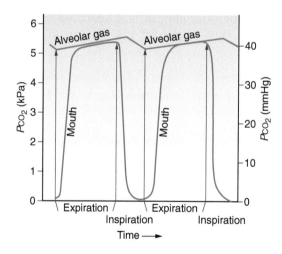

• **Fig. 9.6** Changes in alveolar and mouth $P\text{CO}_2$ during the respiratory cycle. The alveolar $P\text{CO}_2$ is shown by the blue curve, and the mouth $P\text{CO}_2$ by the green curve. The mouth $P\text{CO}_2$ falls at the commencement of inspiration, but does not rise during expiration until the anatomical dead space gas is washed out. The alveolar $P\text{CO}_2$ rises during expiration and also during the early part of inspiration until fresh gas penetrates the alveoli after the anatomical dead space is washed out. The alveolar $P\text{CO}_2$ then falls until expiration commences. This imparts a sawtooth curve to the alveolar $P\text{CO}_2$.

This equation includes all of the more important factors influencing P_{CO_2} (Fig. 9.8), and examples of the hyperbolic relationship between P_{CO_2} and alveolar ventilation are shown in Figure 9.9. Individual factors will now be considered.

Dry barometric pressure is not a very important factor in the determination of alveolar P_{CO_2}, and normal variations of barometric pressure at sea level are unlikely to influence the P_{CO_2} by more than 0.3 kPa (2 mmHg).

The mean inspired carbon dioxide concentration. The effect of inspired carbon dioxide on the alveolar P_{CO_2} is additive. If, for example, a patient breathes gas containing 4.2% carbon dioxide (P_{CO_2} = 4.0 kPa or 30 mmHg), the alveolar P_{CO_2} will be raised 4.0 kPa above the level that it would be if there were no carbon dioxide in the inspired gas, and other factors, including ventilation, remained the same.

It is carbon dioxide output, and not production, that directly influences the alveolar P_{CO_2}. Output equals production in a steady state, but it may be quite different during unsteady states. During acute hypoventilation, much of the carbon dioxide production is diverted into the body stores so that the output may temporarily fall to very low figures until the alveolar carbon dioxide concentration has risen to its new level. Conversely, acute hyperventilation results in a transient increase in carbon dioxide output. A sudden fall in cardiac output decreases the carbon dioxide output until the carbon dioxide concentration in the mixed venous blood rises. The unsteady state is considered in more detail later in this chapter.

Alveolar ventilation, for present purposes, means the product of the respiratory frequency and the difference between the tidal volume and the physiological dead space (page 99). It can change over very wide limits, and is the most important factor influencing alveolar P_{CO_2}. Factors governing ventilation are considered in Chapter 4, and dead space in Chapter 7.

Apart from the factors shown in the previous equation and in Figure 9.9, the alveolar P_{CO_2} may be temporarily influenced by net transfer of soluble inert gases across the alveolar/capillary membrane. Rapid uptake of an inert gas increases the concentration (and partial pressure) of carbon dioxide (and oxygen) in the alveolar gas, a phenomenon referred to as the concentration effect. This occurs, for example, at the beginning of an anaesthetic when large quantities of nitrous oxide are passing from the alveolar gas into the body stores, and a much smaller quantity of nitrogen is passing from the body into the alveolar gas. The converse occurs during elimination of the inert gas, and results in transient reduction of alveolar P_{CO_2} and P_{O_2}.

End-Expiratory P_{CO_2} (PE'_{CO_2})

In the normal, healthy conscious subject, the end-expiratory gas consists almost entirely of alveolar gas. If, however, appreciable parts of the lung are ventilated but not perfused, they will contribute a significant quantity of carbon dioxide–free gas from the alveolar dead space to the end-expiratory gas (see Fig. 7.11). As a result, the end-expiratory P_{CO_2} will have a lower P_{CO_2} than that of the alveoli which are perfused. Gas cannot be sampled selectively from the perfused alveoli. However, because arterial P_{CO_2} usually approximates closely to P_{CO_2} of the perfused alveoli (see later), it is possible to compare arterial and end-expiratory P_{CO_2} to demonstrate the existence of an appreciable proportion of underperfused alveoli.

Alveolar/Arterial P_{CO_2} Gradient

For reasons that have been discussed in Chapter 8, we may discount the possibility of any significant gradient between the P_{CO_2} of alveolar gas and that of pulmonary

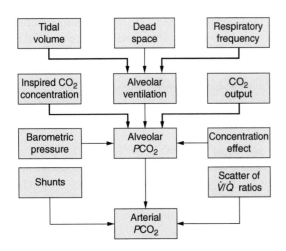

• **Fig. 9.8** Summary of factors that influence P_{CO_2}; the more important ones are indicated with the thicker arrows. In the steady state, the CO_2 output of a resting subject usually lies within the range of 150 to 200 mL.min⁻¹, and the alveolar P_{CO_2} is largely governed by the alveolar ventilation, provided that the inspired CO_2 concentration is zero. See text for explanation of the concentration effect.

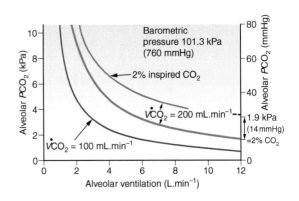

• **Fig. 9.9** The effect of CO_2 output, alveolar ventilation and inspired CO_2 concentration on alveolar P_{CO_2}. The purple curve shows the relationship between ventilation and alveolar P_{CO_2} for a CO_2 output of 100 mL.min⁻¹. The blue curve shows the normal relationship when the CO_2 output is 200 mL.min⁻¹. The orange curve represents the relationship when the CO_2 output is 200 mL.min⁻¹ and there is an inspired CO_2 concentration of 2%. CO_2 at 2% is equivalent to about 1.9 kPa (14 mmHg), and each point on the orange curve is 1.9 kPa above the blue curve.

end-capillary blood (page 115). Arterial P_{CO_2} may, however, be slightly greater than the mean alveolar P_{CO_2} because of shunting or scatter of ventilation/perfusion ratios. Factors governing the magnitude of the gradient were considered in Chapter 7, where it was shown that a shunt of 10% will cause an alveolar/arterial P_{CO_2} gradient of only about 0.1 kPa (0.7 mmHg; see Fig. 7.12). Because the normal degree of ventilation/perfusion ratio scatter causes a gradient of the same order, neither has much significance for carbon dioxide (in contrast to oxygen), and there is an established convention by which the arterial and ideal alveolar P_{CO_2} values are identical. It is only in exceptional patients with, for example, a shunt in excess of 30% that the gradient is likely to exceed 0.3 kPa (2 mmHg).

Arterial P_{CO_2} (Pa_{CO_2})

Pooled results for the normal arterial P_{CO_2} reported by various authors show a mean of 5.1 kPa (38.3 mmHg) with 95% confidence limits of ± 1.0 kPa (7.5 mmHg). This means that 5% of normal subjects will lie outside these limits, and it is therefore preferable to call it the reference range rather than the normal range. There is no evidence that P_{CO_2} is influenced by age in the healthy subject.

Carbon Dioxide Stores and the Unsteady State

The quantity of carbon dioxide and bicarbonate ion in the body is very large, about 120 L, which is almost 100 times greater than the volume of oxygen. Therefore, when ventilation is altered out of accord with metabolic activity, carbon dioxide levels change only slowly, and new equilibrium levels are only attained after about 20 to 30 minutes. In contrast, corresponding changes in oxygen levels are very rapid.

Figure 9.10 shows a three-compartment hydraulic model in which depth of water represents P_{CO_2}, and the volume in the various compartments corresponds to volume of carbon dioxide. The metabolic production of carbon dioxide is represented by the variable flow of water from the supply tank. The outflow corresponds to alveolar ventilation, and the controller watching the P_{CO_2} represents the central chemoreceptors. The rapid compartment represents circulating blood, brain, kidneys and other well-perfused tissues. The medium compartment represents skeletal muscle (resting) and other tissues with a moderate blood flow. The slow compartment includes bone, fat and other tissues with a large capacity for carbon dioxide. Each compartment has its own time constant (see Appendix E), and the long time constants of the medium and slow compartments buffer changes in the rapid compartment.

Hyperventilation is represented by a wide opening of the outflow valve with subsequent exponential decline in the levels in all three compartments, the rapid compartment

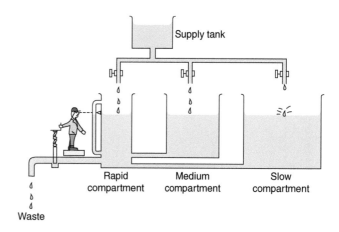

• **Fig. 9.10** A hydrostatic analogy of the elimination of carbon dioxide. See text for full description.

falling most quickly. The rate of decrease of P_{CO_2} is governed primarily by ventilation and the capacity of the stores. Hypoventilation is fundamentally different. The rate of increase of P_{CO_2} is now limited by the metabolic production of carbon dioxide, which is the only factor directly increasing the quantity of carbon dioxide in the body compartments. Therefore the time course of the increase of P_{CO_2} following step decrease of ventilation is not the mirror image of the time course of decrease of P_{CO_2} when ventilation is increased. The rate of rise is much slower than the rate of fall, which is fortunate for patients in asphyxial situations.

When all metabolically produced carbon dioxide is retained, the rate of rise of arterial P_{CO_2} is of the order of 0.4 to 0.8 kPa.min^{-1} (3–6 mmHg.min^{-1}). This is the result of the rate of production of carbon dioxide and the capacity of the body stores for carbon dioxide. During hypoventilation, the rate of increase in P_{CO_2} will be less than this, and Figure 9.11 shows typical curves for P_{CO_2} increase and decrease following step changes in ventilation of anaesthetized patients. The time course of rise of P_{CO_2} after step reduction of ventilation is faster when the previous level of ventilation has been of short duration.

The difference in the rate of change of P_{CO_2} and P_{O_2} after a step change in ventilation (see Fig. 10.18) has two important implications for monitoring and measurement. First, changes in P_{O_2} (or oxygen saturation) will often provide an earlier warning of acute hypoventilation than will the capnogram, provided that the alveolar P_{O_2} is not much higher than the normal range. However, in the steady state P_{CO_2} gives the best indication of the adequacy of ventilation, because oxygenation is so heavily influenced by intrapulmonary shunting and the inspired oxygen concentration. Second, step changes in ventilation are followed by temporary changes in the respiratory exchange ratio because, in the unsteady state, carbon dioxide output changes more than oxygen uptake. However, if the ventilation is held constant at its new level, the respiratory exchange ratio must eventually return to the value determined by the metabolic process of the body.

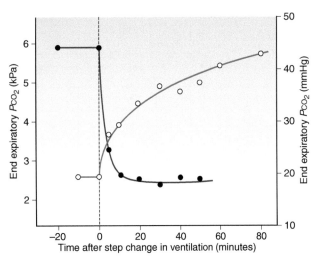

• **Fig. 9.11** Time course of changes in end-expiratory P_{CO_2} after step changes in ventilation. The solid circles and purple line indicate the changes in end-expiratory P_{CO_2} that follow a change in ventilation from 3.3 to 14 $L.min^{-1}$. The open circles and blue line show the change after a reduction in ventilation from 14 to 3.3 $L.min^{-1}$ in the same patient. During the fall in P_{CO_2}, half the total change is completed in about 3 minutes; during the rise in P_{CO_2}, half-change takes approximately 16 minutes.

Cardiac Output and Carbon Dioxide Transport

In the normal subject, fluctuations in cardiac output have little effect on arterial, alveolar or end-expiratory P_{CO_2} because of the efficiency of the chemical control of breathing. However, with a constant level of artificial ventilation, for example, during anaesthesia or cardiopulmonary resuscitation, the situation is quite different. In the extreme circumstance of a total cessation of cardiac output, alveolar and end-expiratory P_{CO_2} will fall dramatically as the delivery of blood containing carbon dioxide to the lung also ceases. In a similar fashion, a sudden reduction in cardiac output during anaesthesia causes an abrupt reduction in end-expiratory P_{CO_2}. This almost certainly results from increased alveolar dead space caused by an increase in the number of nonperfused but ventilated alveoli (zone 1, page 78). If low cardiac output is sustained for more than a few minutes, blood P_{CO_2} will rise, and the expired P_{CO_2} returns towards normal as the blood passing through the still-perfused lung regions releases more carbon dioxide into the expired gas. Apart from being a useful early warning of cardiovascular catastrophe during anaesthesia, the measurement of expired carbon dioxide has also been advocated during cardiopulmonary resuscitation, both as a method of monitoring the efficacy of chest compressions and as an indicator of the return of spontaneous cardiac output.

Apnoea

When a patient becomes apnoeic while breathing air, alveolar gas reaches equilibrium with mixed venous blood within a few minutes. Assuming normal starting conditions and ignoring changes in the composition of the recirculated mixed venous blood, this would entail a rise of alveolar P_{CO_2} from 5.3 to 6.1 kPa (40–46 mmHg) and a fall of P_{O_2} from 14 to 5.3 kPa (105–40 mmHg). These changes correspond to the uptake of 230 mL of oxygen, but the output of only 21 mL of carbon dioxide. Carbon dioxide appears to reach equilibrium within about 10 seconds,[10] whereas oxygen would take about a minute, being limited by the ability of the cardiac output and the arterial/mixed venous oxygen content difference to remove about two-thirds of the oxygen in the alveolar gas (normally about 450 mL).

These calculations assume that alveolar gas is not replenished from outside the patient. What actually happens to the arterial blood gases in apnoea depends on the patency of the airway and the composition of the ambient gas if the airway is patent.

With Airway Occlusion

As described previously, there is rapid attainment of equilibrium between alveolar and mixed-venous P_{CO_2}. Thereafter, arterial, alveolar and mixed venous P_{CO_2} values remain close, and, with recirculation of the blood, increase together at a rate of about 0.4 to 0.8 $kPa.min^{-1}$ (3–6 mmHg.min^{-1}), more than 90% of the metabolically produced carbon dioxide passing into the body stores. Alveolar P_{O_2} decreases close to the mixed venous P_{O_2} within about a minute, and then decreases further as recirculation continues. The lung volume falls by the difference between the oxygen uptake and the carbon dioxide output. Initially the rate would be $230 − 21 = 209$ mL.min^{-1}. The change in alveolar P_{O_2} may be calculated, and gross hypoxia supervenes after about 90 seconds if apnoea with airway occlusion follows air breathing at functional residual capacity.

With Patent Airway and Air as Ambient Gas

The initial changes are as described earlier. However, instead of the lung volume falling by the net gas exchange rate (initially 209 mL.min^{-1}), this volume of ambient gas is drawn in by mass movement down the trachea. If the ambient gas is air, the oxygen in it will be removed, but the nitrogen will accumulate and rise above its normal concentration until gross hypoxia supervenes after about 2 minutes. This is likely to occur when the accumulated nitrogen has reached 90%, because the alveolar carbon dioxide concentration will then have reached about 8%. Carbon dioxide elimination cannot occur, as there is mass movement of air down the trachea, preventing loss of carbon dioxide by either convection or diffusion.

With Patent Airway and Oxygen as the Ambient Gas

Oxygen is continuously removed from the alveolar gas as previously described but is replaced by oxygen drawn in by mass movement. No nitrogen is added to the alveolar gas, and the alveolar P_{O_2} only falls as fast as the P_{CO_2} rises (approximately 0.4–0.8 kPa.min^{-1} or 3–6 mmHg.min^{-1}).

Therefore the patient will not become seriously hypoxic for several minutes. If the patient has been breathing 100% oxygen before the respiratory arrest, the starting alveolar Po_2 would be of the order of 88 kPa (660 mmHg); therefore the patient could theoretically survive about 100 minutes of apnoea provided that his or her airway remained clear and he or she remained connected to a supply of 100% oxygen. This does, in fact, happen, and has been demonstrated in both animals and humans, and is referred to as apnoeic mass-movement oxygenation or diffusion respiration. The phenomenon was in vogue briefly in anaesthetic practice as a way of maintaining oxygenation during apnoea, particularly for airway surgery or bronchoscopy (page 399), and remains a widely used method for oxygenation of the nonventilated lung during one-lung ventilation (page 406). Application of high flows of oxygen to the upper airway during apnoea facilitates very prolonged periods of apnoea by providing a reliable oxygen supply to the airway and increasing carbon dioxide removal by a variety of mechanisms (page 293).

In clinical practice there are many other factors affecting the rate of change of both Po_2 and Pco_2 during apnoea, such as variations in oxygen consumption and carbon dioxide production, the inspired oxygen before apnoea occurs, lung volume, shunt fraction, obesity, and so on. These can now be investigated by physiological modelling to avoid the ethical difficulties of in vivo studies.[11]

Carbon Dioxide Carriage During Hypothermia

Understanding the carriage of carbon dioxide during hypothermia is important both to clinicians involved in the care of hypothermic patients and to the comparative physiologist studying differences between homeothermic and poikilothermic animals (page 302). These two diverse areas of physiology have over recent years converged to produce two alternative theories regarding the optimal system for carbon dioxide carriage at low temperature.

In common with most gases, carbon dioxide becomes more soluble in water as temperature decreases (Table 9.1) such that, in plasma, maintenance of the same Pco_2 under hypothermic conditions will require a greater total carbon dioxide content. In addition, decreasing temperature reduces the ionization of water into H^+ and OH^- ions, so pH increases by approximately 0.016 per degree Celsius fall in temperature.[12] If carbon dioxide production and excretion remain constant, hypothermia would therefore be expected to result in alkalotic conditions in both the intracellular and extracellular spaces. Different animals are believed to respond to these changes in two ways.

The pH-stat hypothesis,[13] as the name suggests, involves the animal responding to hypothermia by maintaining the same blood pH regardless of its body temperature. This is achieved by hypoventilation, which increases the Pco_2 to maintain pH at close to 7.4, and is seen in hibernating mammals. Indeed it is thought possible that the high Pco_2,

and the resulting intracellular acidosis, may contribute to the hypothermic 'sleep' state.

The alpha-stat hypothesis is more complex.[12] In this situation, the pH of the animal is allowed to change in keeping with the physical chemistry laws described earlier. As temperature falls, the blood pH, again measured at the animal's body temperature, increases. Studies of protein function and acid–base disturbances have revealed the importance of the α-imidazole moiety of histidine in buffering changes in pH, and that the state of dissociation of these α-imidazole groups is crucial to protein function. The pK of α-imidazole is unique among amino acids in that it changes with temperature to a similar degree as the dissociation of water. Thus as temperature decreases, blood and tissue pH rise, but the dissociative state of α-imidazole, and thus protein function, remains close to normal. Most poikilothermic animals use an α-stat system and can function well through a broad range of temperatures.

There is controversy about whether the blood gases of hypothermic humans (e.g., during cardiac surgery or following cardiac arrest) should be managed by the α-stat or pH-stat techniques.[13,14] In the former case, arterial blood drawn from the cold patient is warmed to 37°C before measurement of Pco_2, and the cardiopulmonary bypass adjusted to achieve normal values. For pH-stat control, Pco_2 is again measured at 37°C but mathematically corrected to the patient's temperature, and then carbon dioxide is administered to the patient to achieve a pH of 7.4. Increased arterial Pco_2 during pH-stat will, in theory, improve cerebral perfusion, and possibly improve cerebral function. However, there remains little evidence that the two forms of blood gas management result in differences in patient wellbeing during or after hypothermic surgery except at very low temperatures, when pH-stat may be superior.

Outline of Methods of Measurement of Carbon Dioxide

Blood Partial Pressure

The Pco_2-sensitive electrode technique was first described by Severinghaus and Bradley in 1958.[15] It allows the Pco_2 of any gas or liquid to be determined directly. The Pco_2 of a film of bicarbonate solution is allowed to come into equilibrium with the Pco_2 of a sample on the other side of a membrane that is permeable to carbon dioxide but not to hydrogen ions. The pH of the bicarbonate solution is constantly monitored by a glass electrode, and the log of the Pco_2 is inversely proportional to the recorded pH. Analysis is easily performed by untrained staff as a point-of-care test with results available within 2 minutes.

While handling blood samples, it is important that they are preserved from contact with air, including bubbles and froth in the syringe, to which they may lose carbon dioxide and either lose or gain oxygen depending on the relative Po_2 of the sample and the air. Dilution with excessive volumes of heparin or 'dead space' fluids from indwelling arterial cannulae should be avoided. Analysis should be undertaken quickly because the P_{CO_2} of blood in vitro rises by approximately 0.013 kPa per minute (0.1 mmHg per minute) at 37°C, whereas P_{O_2} declines at 0.07 to 0.3 kPa (0.5–2.3 mmHg) per minute, depending on the P_{O_2}. If rapid analysis is not possible (within 10 minutes), the specimen should be stored on ice, which reduces this carbon dioxide production and oxygen consumption by about 90%. Blood gas analysers invariably work at 37°C, so for patients with abnormal body temperature a correction factor should be applied.

Continuous measurement of arterial P_{CO_2} using indwelling arterial catheters is a realistic, but rarely used, clinical technique.[16] The method uses a 'photochemical optode', which consists of a small optical fibre (140 μm in diameter) along which light of a specific wavelength is passed to impinge on a dye incorporated into the tip of the fibre, which lies within the patient's artery. The dye may either absorb the light or fluoresce (give off light of a different wavelength) in a pH-sensitive fashion, and these changes are transmitted back to the analyser via the same or a second optical fibre. For analysis of P_{aCO_2}, the pH-sensitive optode is again enclosed within a carbon dioxide-permeable membrane with a bicarbonate buffer, as for the P_{CO_2}-sensitive electrode but on a very small scale.

Fractional Concentration in Gas Mixtures[17]

Infrared Analysis

This is the most widely used method for rapid breath-to-breath analysis and is also convenient for analysis of discrete gas samples. Most diatomic gases absorb infrared radiation, and errors may arise because of overlap of absorption bands and collision broadening. Infrared analysers are available with a response time of less than 300 microseconds, and will adequately follow the respiratory cycle provided the respiratory frequency is not too high. Breathe-through cells (placed near the patient's airway) have a better frequency response than systems which draw gas from the airway for analysis in a distant machine, as mixing of the inspired and expired gases occurs along the sampling tube.

Capnography[17,18]

Capnograms consist of plots of carbon dioxide concentration in airway gas against either time or expired volume. Despite the curves being of similar shape (Figs 7.18 and 9.12), they contain quite different information; for example, time capnography has both inspiratory and expiratory phases, whereas carbon dioxide against volume plots only involve expiration. Plots of carbon dioxide and expired volume allow calculation of anatomical dead space (see Fig. 7.18), physiological dead space and tidal volume, but this form of capnography is not commonly used clinically. Current generations of capnometer allow the carbon dioxide concentration to be displayed as either volume %, kPa or mmHg. Infrared analysers measure the partial pressure of carbon dioxide, and so conversion to

fractional concentration will be affected by the atmospheric pressure, for example by the altitude at which the capnometer is being used. Current technical specifications for capnometers therefore require that the equipment must automatically compensate for barometric pressure when converting the measured units into the displayed units.[17]

The nomenclature of a normal time capnogram is shown in Figure 9.12, *A*. There is an inspiratory phase (0), and expiration is divided into three phases: phase I represents carbon dioxide–free gas from the apparatus and anatomical dead space; phase II a rapidly changing mixture of alveolar and dead space gas; and phase III the alveolar plateau, the peak of which represents end-expiratory P_{CO_2} (PE'_{CO_2}). The alpha and beta angles allow quantification of abnormalities of the capnogram. Much information may be obtained from a time capnogram:

1. Inspiratory carbon dioxide concentration.
2. Respiratory rate.
3. Demonstration of the capnogram is a reliable indication of the correct placement of a tracheal tube.
4. PE'_{CO_2} is related to arterial P_{CO_2} (see next).
5. Lung elastance and resistance affect the shape of the capnogram in early expiration, and can be assessed from

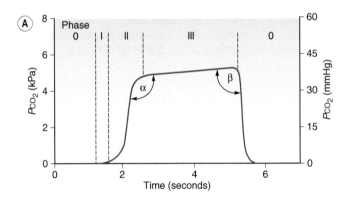

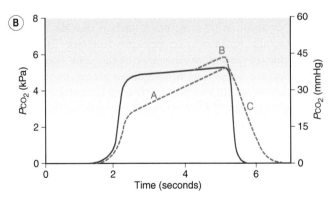

• **Fig. 9.12** Time capnography. **(A)** Normal trace showing the phases of the respiratory cycle and the angles used to quantify the shape of the capnogram. See text for details. **(B)** Dashed lines show abnormalities of the trace, which may occur separately or together. *A*, varying alveolar time constants (page 90) such as asthma; *B*, phase IV terminal upswing seen in pregnancy or obesity; *C*, rebreathing of expired gases.

the slopes of phases II and III and the transition between these two phases.[19]

6. Sudden decrease in $P_E'_{CO_2}$ at a fixed level of ventilation is a valuable indication of a sudden reduction in cardiac output (page 132) or a pulmonary embolus (Chapter 29).

7. Cardiac arrest during artificial ventilation will cause $P_E'_{CO_2}$ to fall to zero within a few breaths.

There are three principal abnormalities of a capnogram,[17] which may occur separately or together, and are shown in Figure 9.12, *B*. Line A, with an increased α-angle and phase III slope, results from increased ventilation perfusion mismatch. Almost any lung pathology may result in a sloping phase III, and a common clinical cause is acute asthma: line A is typical of a patient with bronchospasm. Line B, sometimes referred to as phase IV, is occasionally seen in pregnancy or severe obesity, but more commonly results from a leak between the sampling tube and analyser in an artificially ventilated patient. Line C and an increase in the β-angle occur with rebreathing from either excessive apparatus dead space or a malfunctioning anaesthetic breathing system.

Technical considerations should always be borne in mind when considering abnormalities of a capnogram. The response time of the analyser, excessive lengths of sampling tube and inadequate sampling rates will all tend to 'blunt' the normal capnogram trace because of increased mixing of gases along the sample tube. This is a particular problem when the tidal volume is low, for example in children or tachypneic patients.

Arterial to End-Expiratory P$_{CO_2}$ Gradient

Arterial to end-expiratory P_{CO_2} gradient has already been mentioned (page 130) and occurs to some extent in almost all subjects, but particularly in elderly patients, smokers, those with lung disease or during anaesthesia.[20] The magnitude of the difference is greatest in patients with significant alveolar dead space (page 99). Use of $P_E'_{CO_2}$ see above as a monitor of absolute arterial P_{CO_2} is therefore unhelpful, but the assessment remains useful for following changes within a subject.

References

1. Esbaugh AJ, Tufts BL. The structure and function of carbonic anhydrase isozymes in the respiratory system of vertebrates. *Respir Physiol Neurobiol.* 2006;154:185-198.
2. Teppema LJ. Multifaceted clinical effects of acetazolamide: will the underlying mechanisms please stand up? *J Appl Physiol.* 2014;116:713-714.
3. Hasselbalch KA. Die Berechnung der Wasserstoffzahl des Blutes usw. *Biochem Z.* 1916;78:112-144.
4. Teboul JL, Scheeren T. Understanding the Haldane effect. *Intensive Care Med.* 2017;43:91-93.
5. Christiansen J, Douglas CG, Haldane JS. The adsorption and dissociation of carbon dioxide by human blood. *J Physiol.* 1914;48:244-271.
6. Hamburger HJ. Anionenwander-ungen in serum und Blutunterdem Einfluss von CO_2. Säure und Alkali. *Biochem Z.* 1918;86:309.
7. Tanner MJ. Band 3 anion exchanger and its involvement in erythrocyte and kidney disorders. *Curr Opin Hematol.* 2002;9:133-139.
8. Zhang D, Kiyatkin A, Bolin JT, et al. Crystallographic structure and functional interpretation of the cytoplasmic domain of erythrocyte membrane band 3. *Blood.* 2000;96:2925-2933.
9. Perrotta S, Gallagher PG, Mohandas N. Hereditary spherocytosis. *Lancet.* 2008;372:1411-1426.
10. Stock MC, Downs JB, McDonald JS, et al. The carbon dioxide rate of rise in awake apneic humans. *J Clin Anesth.* 1988;1:96-99.
11. Farmery AD. Simulating hypoxia and modelling the airway. *Anaesthesia.* 2011;66(suppl 2):11-18.
12. Nattie EE. The alpha-stat hypothesis in respiratory control and acid-base balance. *J Appl Physiol.* 1990;69:1201-1207.
13. Burrows FA. Con: pH-stat management of blood gases is preferable to alpha-stat in patients undergoing brain cooling for cardiac surgery. *J Cardiothorac Vasc Anesth.* 1995;9:219-221.
14. Hoedemaekers C, van der Hoeven JG. Is α-stat or pH-stat the best strategy during hypothermia after cardiac arrest? *Crit Care Med.* 2014;42:1950-1951.
15. Severinghaus JW, Bradley AF. Electrodes for blood P_{O_2} and P_{CO_2} determination. *J Appl Physiol.* 1958;13:515-520.
16. Ganter M, Zollinger A. Continuous intravascular blood gas monitoring: development, current techniques, and clinical use of a commercial device. *Br J Anaesth.* 2003;91:397-407.
*17. **Gravenstein JS, Jaffe MB, Paulus DA. Capnography: *Clinical Aspects*. Cambridge, UK: Cambridge University Press; 2004.**
18. Ortega R, Connor C, Kim S, et al. Monitoring ventilation with capnography. *N Engl J Med.* 2012;367:e27.
19. Csorba Z, Petak F, Nevery K, et al. Capnographic parameters in ventilated patients: correspondence with airway and lung tissue mechanics. *Anesth Analg.* 2016;122:1412-1420.
20. Wahba RW, Tessler MJ. Misleading end-tidal CO_2 tensions. *Can J Anaesth.* 1996;43:862-866.

KEY POINTS

- Oxygen moves down a partial pressure gradient between the inspired gas and its point of use in the mitochondria, where the oxygen partial pressure may be only 0.13 kPa (1 mmHg).
- Significant barriers to oxygen transfer are between inspired and alveolar gas, between alveolar and arterial oxygen partial pressures and on diffusion from the capillary to the mitochondria.
- Each 100 mL of arterial blood carries 0.3 mL of oxygen in physical solution and around 20 mL of oxygen bound to haemoglobin, which reduces to about 15 mL.dL^{-1} in venous blood.

- Oxygen carriage by haemoglobin is influenced by carbon dioxide, pH, temperature and red blood cell 2,3-diphosphoglycerate; the molecular mechanism of haemoglobin is now well elucidated.
- Glucose and other substrates are used to produce energy in the form of adenosine triphosphate (ATP), each glucose molecule yielding 38 molecules of ATP in the presence of oxygen, compared with only two molecules in anaerobic conditions.
- Oxygen delivery is the total amount of oxygen leaving the heart per minute, and is about 1000 mL.min^{-1}, compared with oxygen consumption of around 250 mL.min^{-1}.

The appearance of oxygen in the atmosphere of the Earth has played a crucial role in the development of life (see Chapter 34, *The Atmosphere*). The whole animal kingdom is totally dependent on oxygen, not only for function but also for survival. This is notwithstanding the fact that oxygen is extremely toxic in the absence of elaborate defence mechanisms at a cellular level (see Chapter 25). Before considering the role of oxygen within the cell, it is necessary to bring together many strands from previous chapters and outline the transport of oxygen all the way from the atmosphere to the mitochondria.

Oxygen Cascade

The P_{O_2} of dry air at sea level is 21.2 kPa (159 mmHg). Oxygen moves by mass transport (ventilation and blood movement) and down partial pressure gradients from the inspired air, through the respiratory tract, the alveolar gas, the arterial blood, the systemic capillaries, the tissues and the cell. It finally reaches its lowest level in the mitochondria, where it is consumed (Fig. 10.1). At this point, the P_{O_2} is probably within the range of 0.5 to 3 kPa (3.8–22.5 mmHg), varying from one tissue to another, from one cell to another and from one region of a cell to another.

The steps by which the P_{O_2} decreases from air to the mitochondria are known as the oxygen cascade, and are of great practical importance. Any one step in the cascade may be increased under pathological circumstances, and this may result in hypoxia. The steps will now be considered *seriatim*.

Dilution of Inspired Oxygen by Water Vapour

The normally quoted value for the concentration of atmospheric oxygen (20.94% or 0.2094 fractional concentration) indicates the concentration of oxygen in dry gas. As gas is inhaled through the respiratory tract, it becomes humidified at body temperature, and the added water vapour dilutes the oxygen, reducing the P_{O_2} below its level in the ambient air. When dry gas at normal barometric pressure becomes fully saturated with water vapour at 37°C, 100 volumes of the dry gas take up about 6 volumes of water vapour, which gives a total gas volume of 106 units but containing the same number of molecules of oxygen. The P_{O_2} is thus reduced by the fraction 6/106. It follows from Boyle's law that P_{O_2} after humidification is indicated by the following expression:

$$\begin{pmatrix} \text{fractional} \\ \text{concentration} \\ \text{of oxygen in} \\ \text{the dry gas phase} \end{pmatrix} \times \begin{pmatrix} \text{barometric} \\ \text{pressure} \end{pmatrix} - \begin{pmatrix} \text{saturated} \\ \text{water} \\ \text{vapour} \\ \text{pressure} \end{pmatrix}$$

(the quantity in parentheses is known as the dry barometric pressure). Therefore the effective P_{O_2} of inspired air at a body temperature of 37°C is

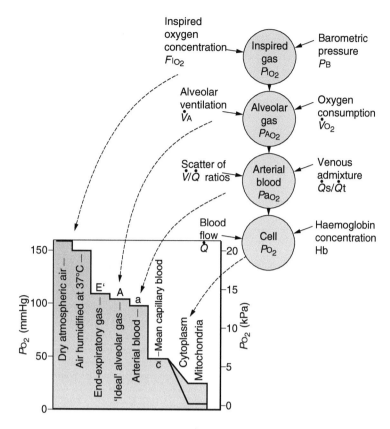

• **Fig. 10.1** On the left is shown the oxygen cascade with P_{O_2} falling from the level in the ambient air down to the level in mitochondria. On the right is a summary of the factors influencing oxygenation at different levels in the cascade.

$$0.2094 \times (101.3 - 6.3) = 0.2094 \times 95 = 19.9 \text{ kPa,}$$

or, in mmHg,

$$0.2094 \times (760 - 47) = 0.2094 \times 713 = 149 \text{ mm Hg.}$$

Primary Factors Influencing Alveolar Oxygen Partial Pressure

Dry Barometric Pressure

If other factors remain constant, the alveolar P_{O_2} will be directly proportional to the dry barometric pressure. Thus with increasing altitude, alveolar P_{O_2} falls progressively to become zero at 19 km, where the actual barometric pressure equals the saturated vapour pressure of water at body temperature (see Table 16.1). The effect of increased pressure is complex (see Chapter 17); for example, a pressure of 10 atm (absolute) increases the alveolar P_{O_2} by a factor of about 15 if other factors remain constant (see Table 17.1).

Inspired Oxygen Concentration

The alveolar P_{O_2} will be raised or lowered by an amount equal to the change in the inspired gas P_{O_2}, provided that other factors remain constant. Because the concentration of oxygen in the inspired gas should always be under control,

it is a most important therapeutic tool that may be used to counteract a number of different factors that may impair oxygenation. Figure 10.2 shows the effect of an increase in the inspired oxygen concentration from 21% to 30% on the relationship between alveolar P_{O_2} and alveolar ventilation. For any alveolar ventilation, the improvement of alveolar P_{O_2} will be 8.5 kPa (64 mmHg). This will be of great importance if, for example, hypoventilation while breathing air has reduced the alveolar P_{O_2} to 4 kPa (30 mmHg), a value that presents a significant threat to life. Oxygen enrichment of inspired gas to 30% will then increase the alveolar P_{O_2} to 12.5 kPa (94 mmHg), which is almost within the normal range. However, at this level of hypoventilation, arterial P_{CO_2} would be about 13 kPa (98 mmHg), and might well have risen further on withdrawal of the hypoxic drive to ventilation. In fact, 30% is the maximum concentration of oxygen in the inspired gas that should be required to correct the alveolar P_{O_2} of a patient breathing air, who has become hypoxaemic purely as a result of hypoventilation. This problem is discussed further on page 322.

An entirely different problem is hypoxaemia from venous admixture. This results in an increased alveolar/arterial P_{O_2} difference, which, within limits, can be offset by increasing the alveolar P_{O_2}. Quantitative aspects are quite different from the problem of hypoventilation and are considered later in this chapter.

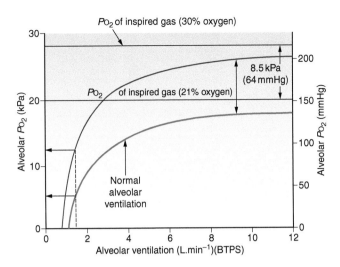

• **Fig. 10.2** The effect on alveolar Po_2 of increasing the inspired oxygen concentration from 21% (*blue curve*) to 30% (*red curve*). In this example, the alveolar Po_2 is reduced to a dangerously low level when breathing air at an alveolar minute ventilation of 1.5 L.min⁻¹. In this situation, oxygen enrichment of the inspired gas to 30% is sufficient to raise the alveolar Po_2 almost to within the normal range. Oxygen consumption is assumed to be 200 mL.min⁻¹ (standard temperature and pressure, dry). *BTPS*, Body temperature and pressure, saturated.

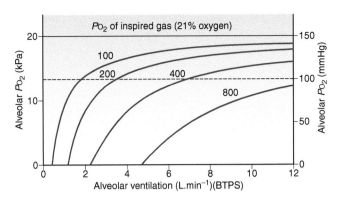

• **Fig. 10.3** The relationship between alveolar ventilation and alveolar Po_2 for different values of oxygen consumption for a patient breathing air at normal barometric pressure. The figures on the curves indicate the oxygen consumption in mL.min⁻¹ (standard temperature and pressure, dry). A value of 100 mL.min⁻¹ is typical of a hypothermic patient at 30°C; 200 mL.min⁻¹ a normal subject at rest or during anaesthesia; and higher values result from exercise or fever. Note that the alveolar ventilation required for maintaining any particular alveolar Po_2 is directly proportional to the oxygen consumption. (In calculations of this type it is important to make the correction required by the fact that oxygen consumption and alveolar ventilation values are commonly expressed at different temperatures and pressures; see Appendix C.) *BTPS*, Body temperature and pressure, saturated.

Oxygen Consumption

In the past there has been an unfortunate tendency to consider that all patients consume 250 mL of oxygen per minute under all circumstances. Oxygen consumption must, of course, be raised by exercise, but is often well above basal in a patient supposedly 'at rest'. This may be from restlessness, pain, increased work of breathing, shivering or fever. These factors may well coexist with failure of other factors controlling the arterial Po_2. Thus, for example, a patient may be caught by the pincers of a falling ventilatory capacity and a rising ventilatory requirement (see Fig. 27.4).

Figure 10.3 shows the effect of different values for oxygen consumption on the relationship between alveolar ventilation and alveolar Po_2 for a patient breathing air, and clearly shows the potential for an increase in oxygen consumption to cause hypoxia. Altered oxygen consumption is very common in patients, and is substantially increased with sepsis, thyrotoxicosis or convulsions, the first of which may lead to difficulties with weaning patients from artificial ventilation (page 385). Oxygen consumption is reduced with general anaesthesia, hypothyroidism or hypothermia, the last of which causes a marked reduction in oxygen consumption, with values of about 50% of normal at 31°C.

Alveolar Ventilation

The alveolar air equation (page 107) implies a hyperbolic relationship between alveolar Po_2 and alveolar ventilation. This relationship, which is considered in Appendix E, is clinically very important. As ventilation is increased, the alveolar Po_2 rises asymptomatically towards (but never reaches) the Po_2 of the inspired gas (Fig. 10.2). From the shape of the curves, changes in ventilation above the normal level have comparatively little effect on alveolar Po_2. In contrast, changes in ventilation below the normal level may have a marked effect. At very low levels of ventilation, the alveolar ventilation becomes critical, and small changes may precipitate severe hypoxia. Note that there is a finite alveolar ventilation at which alveolar Po_2 becomes zero.

Secondary Factors Influencing Alveolar Oxygen Partial Pressure

Cardiac Output

In the short term, cardiac output can influence the alveolar Po_2. For example, if other factors remain constant, a sudden reduction in cardiac output will temporarily increase the alveolar Po_2 because less blood passes through the lungs to remove oxygen from the alveolar gas. However, the reduced cardiac output also causes increased oxygen extraction in the tissues supplied by the systemic circulation, and the mixed venous oxygen level soon decreases. When that has happened, the removal of oxygen from the alveolar gas returns to its original level, as the reduction in blood flow rate is compensated by the greater amount of oxygen that is taken up per unit volume of blood flowing through the lungs. In the long term, cardiac output does not directly influence the alveolar Po_2; thus it does not appear in the alveolar air equation.

'Concentration', Third Gas or Fink Effect

The diagrams and equations previously discussed have ignored nitrous oxide, a factor that influences alveolar Po_2 during exchanges of large quantities of soluble gases. This effect was mentioned briefly in connection with carbon dioxide on page 130, but its effect on oxygen is probably more important. During the early part of the administration of nitrous oxide, large quantities of the more soluble gas replace smaller quantities of the less soluble nitrogen previously dissolved in body fluids. Then there is a net transfer of 'inert' gas from the alveoli into the body, causing a temporary increase in the alveolar concentration of both oxygen and carbon dioxide, which will temporarily exert a higher partial pressure than would otherwise be expected. Conversely, during recovery from nitrous oxide anaesthesia, large quantities of nitrous oxide leave the body to be replaced with smaller quantities of nitrogen. There is thus a net outpouring of 'inert' gas from the body into the alveoli, causing dilution of oxygen and carbon dioxide, both of which will temporarily exert a lower partial pressure than would otherwise be expected. There may then be temporary hypoxia, the direct reduction of alveolar P_{O_2} sometimes exacerbated by ventilatory depression from decreased alveolar P_{CO_2}. Fortunately such effects last only a few minutes, and hypoxia can easily be avoided by small increases in the inspired oxygen concentration when nitrous oxide administration is stopped.

Alveolar/Arterial P_{O_2} Difference

The next step in the oxygen cascade is of great clinical relevance. In the healthy young adult breathing air, the alveolar/arterial P_{O_2} difference does not exceed 2 kPa (15 mmHg), but it may rise to greater than 5 kPa (37.5 mmHg) in aged but healthy subjects. These values may be exceeded in a patient with any lung disease that causes shunting or mismatching of ventilation to perfusion. An increased alveolar/arterial P_{O_2} difference is the commonest cause of arterial hypoxaemia in clinical practice; therefore it is a very important step in the oxygen cascade.

Unlike the alveolar P_{O_2}, the alveolar/arterial P_{O_2} difference cannot be predicted from other more easily measured quantities. There is no simple way of knowing the magnitude of the alveolar/arterial P_{O_2} difference in a particular patient other than by measurement of the arterial blood gas partial pressure and calculation of alveolar P_{O_2}. Thus it is particularly important to understand the factors that influence the difference and the principles of restoration of arterial P_{O_2} by increasing the inspired oxygen concentration when hypoxia is from an increased alveolar/arterial P_{O_2} difference.

Factors Influencing the Magnitude of the Alveolar/Arterial P_{O_2} Difference

In Chapter 7 it was explained how the alveolar/arterial P_{O_2} difference results from venous admixture (or physiological shunt), which consists of two components: (1) shunted venous blood that mixes with the oxygenated blood leaving the pulmonary capillaries and (2) a component because of scatter of ventilation/perfusion ratios in different parts of the lungs. Any component from impaired diffusion across the

alveolar/capillary membrane is likely to be very small, and in most circumstances can probably be ignored.

Figure 7.12 shows the derivation of the following axiomatic relationship for the first component, shunted venous blood:

$$\frac{\dot{Q}s}{\dot{Q}t} = \frac{Cc'_{O_2} - Ca_{O_2}}{Cc'_{O_2} - C\bar{v}_{O_2}}.$$

Two points should be noted:
1. The equation gives a slightly false impression of precision, because it assumes that all the shunted blood has the same oxygen content as mixed venous blood; but this is not the case, as Thebesian and bronchial venous blood are exceptions (see Fig. 6.1).
2. Oxygen content of pulmonary end-capillary blood (Cc'_{O_2}) is, in practice, calculated on the basis of the end-capillary oxygen partial pressure (Pc'_{O_2}) being equal to the 'ideal' alveolar P_{O_2} which is derived by means of the alveolar air equation (see page 107).

The equation may be cleared and solved for the pulmonary end-capillary/arterial oxygen content difference as follows:

$$Cc'_{O_2} - Ca_{O_2} = \frac{\frac{\dot{Q}s}{\dot{Q}t}\left(Ca_{O_2} - C\bar{v}_{O_2}\right)}{1 - \frac{\dot{Q}s}{\dot{Q}t}} \quad \text{[Eq. 10.1]}$$

(scaling factors are required to correct for the inconsistency of the units which are customarily used for the quantities in this equation).

$Ca_{O_2} - C\bar{v}_{O_2}$ is the arterial/mixed venous oxygen content difference, and is a function of the oxygen consumption and the cardiac output, thus

$$\dot{Q}t\left(Ca_{O_2} - C\bar{v}_{O_2}\right) = \dot{V}_{O_2}. \quad \text{[Eq. 10.2]}$$

Substituting for $Ca_{O_2} - C\bar{v}_{O_2}$ in Equation 10.1, we have

$$Cc'_{O_2} - Ca_{O_2} = \frac{\dot{V}_{O_2}\frac{\dot{Q}s}{\dot{Q}t}}{\dot{Q}t\left(1 - \frac{\dot{Q}s}{\dot{Q}t}\right)}. \quad \text{[Eq. 10.3]}$$

This equation shows the content difference in terms of oxygen consumption ($\dot{V}_{O_2}$), the venous admixture ($\dot{Q}s/\dot{Q}t$) and the cardiac output ($\dot{Q}t$).

The final stage in the calculation is to convert the end-capillary/arterial oxygen content difference to the partial pressure difference. The oxygen content of blood is the sum of the oxygen in physical solution and that which is combined with haemoglobin:

$$\text{Oxygen content of blood} = \alpha P_{O_2} + (S_{O_2} \times [Hb] \times 1.39)$$

where α is the solubility coefficient of oxygen in blood (not plasma); S_{O_2} is the haemoglobin saturation and varies with P_{O_2} according to the oxygen dissociation curve, which itself is influenced by temperature, pH and base excess (Bohr effect); [Hb] is the haemoglobin concentration (g.dL^{-1}); and 1.39 is the volume of oxygen (mL) that has been found to combine with 1 g of haemoglobin (page 144).

Derivation of the oxygen content from the P_{O_2} requires account to be taken of pH, base excess, temperature and haemoglobin concentration. Derivation of P_{O_2} from content is even more laborious, as an iterative approach is required to convert S_{O_2} to P_{O_2}, a procedure previously done using tables of values but now more conveniently achieved using mathematical formulae that represent the oxyhaemoglobin dissociation curve (page 145).

The principal factors influencing the magnitude of the alveolar/arterial P_{O_2} difference caused by venous admixture may be summarized as follows.

The magnitude of the venous admixture increases the alveolar/arterial P_{O_2} difference with direct proportionality for small shunts, although this is lost with larger shunts (Fig. 10.4). The resultant effect on arterial P_{O_2} is shown in Figure 7.13. Different forms of venous admixture are considered on pages 101 *et seq.*

It was explained in Chapter 7 that scatter in ventilation/perfusion ratios ($\dot{V}/\dot{Q}$ scatter) produces an alveolar/arterial P_{O_2} difference for the following reasons:

1. More blood flows through the underventilated overperfused alveoli, and the mixed arterial blood is therefore heavily weighted in the direction of the poorly oxygenated blood from areas of low $\dot{V}/\dot{Q}$ ratio. The smaller amount of blood flowing through areas of high $\dot{V}/\dot{Q}$ ratio cannot compensate for this (see Fig. 7.14).
2. Because of the bend in the dissociation curve around a P_{O_2} of 8 kPa, the fall in saturation of blood from areas of low $\dot{V}/\dot{Q}$ ratio tends to be greater than the rise in saturation of blood from areas of correspondingly high $\dot{V}/\dot{Q}$ (see Fig. 7.15).

These two reasons in combination explain why blood from alveoli with high $\dot{V}/\dot{Q}$ ratios cannot compensate for blood from alveoli with low $\dot{V}/\dot{Q}$ ratios.

The actual alveolar P_{O_2} has a profound but complex and nonlinear effect on the alveolar/arterial P_{O_2} gradient (see Fig. 10.4). The alveolar/arterial oxygen content difference for a given shunt is uninfluenced by the alveolar P_{O_2} (Eq. 10.3), and the effect on the partial pressure difference arises entirely in conversion from content to partial pressure: it is thus a function of the slope of the dissociation curve at the P_{O_2} of the alveolar gas. For example, a loss of 1 mL per 100 mL of oxygen from blood with a P_{O_2} of 93 kPa (700 mmHg) causes a fall of P_{O_2} of about 43 kPa (325 mmHg), and most of the oxygen is lost from physical solution. However, if the initial P_{O_2} were 13 kPa (100 mmHg), then a loss of 1 mL

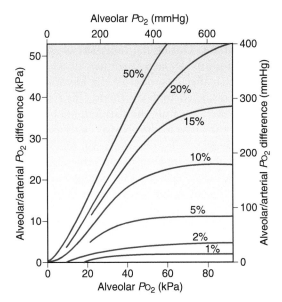

• **Fig. 10.4** Influence of shunt on alveolar/arterial P_{O_2} difference at different levels of alveolar P_{O_2}. Numbers in the graph indicate shunt as percentage of total pulmonary blood flow. For small shunts, the difference (at constant alveolar P_{O_2}) is roughly proportional to the magnitude of the shunt. For a given shunt, the alveolar/arterial P_{O_2} difference increases with alveolar P_{O_2} in a nonlinear manner governed by the oxygen dissociation curve. At high alveolar P_{O_2}, a plateau of alveolar/arterial P_{O_2} difference is reached, but the alveolar P_{O_2} at which the plateau is reached is higher with larger shunts. Note that, with a 50% shunt, an increase in alveolar P_{O_2} produces an almost equal increase in alveolar/arterial P_{O_2} difference. Therefore the arterial P_{O_2} is virtually independent of changes in alveolar P_{O_2}, if other factors remain constant. Constants incorporated into the diagram: arterial/venous oxygen content difference, 5 mL.dL^{-1}; Hb concentration 14 g.dL^{-1}; temperature of blood, 37°C; pH of blood, 7.40; base excess, zero.

per 100 mL would cause a fall of P_{O_2} of only 4.6 kPa (35 mmHg), and most of the oxygen is lost from combination with haemoglobin. If the initial P_{O_2} is only 6.7 kPa (50 mmHg), a loss of 1 mL per 100 mL would cause a very small change in P_{O_2} of the order of 0.7 kPa (5 mmHg), drawn almost entirely from combination with haemoglobin at a point where the dissociation curve is steep.

The quantitative considerations outlined in the previous paragraph have most important clinical implications. Figure 10.4 clearly shows that, for the same degree of shunt, the alveolar/arterial P_{O_2} difference will be greatest when the alveolar P_{O_2} is highest. If the alveolar P_{O_2} is reduced (e.g., by underventilation), the alveolar/arterial P_{O_2} gradient will also be diminished if other factors remain the same. The arterial P_{O_2} thus falls less than the alveolar P_{O_2}. This is fortunate and may be considered as one of the many benefits deriving from the shape of the oxyhaemoglobin dissociation curve. With a 50% venous admixture, changes in the alveolar P_{O_2} are almost exactly equal to the resultant changes in the alveolar/arterial P_{O_2} difference (Fig. 10.4). Therefore the arterial P_{O_2} is almost independent of changes in alveolar P_{O_2}, and administration of oxygen will do little to relieve hypoxia (see Fig. 7.13).

Cardiac output changes have extremely complex effects on the alveolar/arterial P_{O_2} difference. The Fick relationship

(Eq. 10.2; page 139) tells us that a reduced cardiac output per se must increase the arterial/mixed venous oxygen content difference if the oxygen consumption remains the same. This means that the shunted blood will be more desaturated, causing a greater decrease in the arterial oxygen level than would less desaturated blood flowing through a shunt of the same magnitude. Equation 10.3 showed an inverse relationship between the cardiac output and the alveolar/arterial oxygen content difference if the venous admixture is constant (Fig. 10.5, *B*). However, when the content difference is converted to partial pressure difference, the relationship to cardiac output is no longer truly inverse, but assumes a complex nonlinear form in consequence of the shape of the oxyhaemoglobin dissociation curve. An example of the relationship between cardiac output and alveolar/arterial P_{O_2} difference is shown in Figure 10.5, *A*, but this applies only to the conditions specified, with an alveolar P_{O_2} of 24 kPa (180 mmHg).

Unfortunately the influence of cardiac output is even more complicated, because it has been observed that a reduction in cardiac output is almost always associated with a reduction in the shunt fraction. Conversely, an increase in cardiac output usually results in an increased shunt fraction. This approximately counteracts the effect on mixed venous desaturation so that arterial P_{O_2} tends to be relatively little influenced by changes in cardiac output (see page 103). Nevertheless, it must be remembered that, even if the

arterial P_{O_2} is unchanged, the oxygen delivery will be reduced in proportion to the change in cardiac output.

Temperature, pH and base excess of the patient's blood influence the oxyhaemoglobin dissociation curve (page 146). In addition, temperature affects the solubility coefficient of oxygen in blood. Thus all three factors influence the relationship between partial pressure and content (see Table 10.1), and therefore the effect of venous admixture on the alveolar/arterial P_{O_2} difference, although the effect is not usually important except in extreme deviations from normal.

Haemoglobin concentration influences the partition of oxygen between physical solution and chemical combination. Although the haemoglobin concentration does not influence the pulmonary end-capillary/arterial oxygen *content* difference (Eq. 10.3), it does alter the partial pressure difference. An increased haemoglobin concentration causes a small decrease in the alveolar/arterial P_{O_2} difference. Table 10.1 shows an example with a cardiac output of 5 L.min^{-1}, oxygen consumption of 200 mL.min^{-1} and a venous admixture of 20%. This would result in a pulmonary end-capillary/arterial oxygen content difference of 0.5 mL per 100 mL. Assuming an alveolar P_{O_2} of 24 kPa (180 mmHg), the alveolar/arterial P_{O_2} difference is influenced by haemoglobin concentration, as shown in Table 10.1. (Different figures would be obtained by selection of a different value for alveolar P_{O_2}.)

The overall effect of changes in *alveolar ventilation* on the arterial P_{O_2} presents an interesting problem, and serves to illustrate the integration of the separate aspects of the factors previously discussed. An increase in the alveolar ventilation may be expected to have the following results:

1. The alveolar P_{O_2} must be raised, provided the barometric pressure, inspired oxygen concentration and oxygen consumption remain the same (Fig. 10.2).
2. The alveolar/arterial P_{O_2} difference is increased for the following reasons:
   - The increase in the alveolar P_{O_2} will increase the alveolar/arterial P_{O_2} difference by the same proportion if other factors remain the same (Fig. 10.4).
   - Under many conditions it has been demonstrated that a fall of P_{CO_2} (resulting from an increase in alveolar

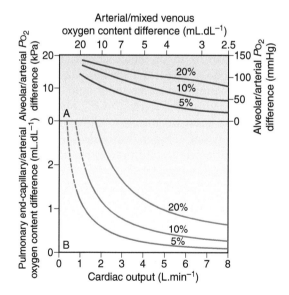

• **Fig. 10.5** Influence of cardiac output on the alveolar/arterial P_{O_2} difference in the presence of shunts (values indicated for each curve). In this example, it is assumed that the patient has an oxygen consumption of 200 mL.min^{-1} and an alveolar P_{O_2} of 24 kPa (180 mmHg). Changes in cardiac output produce an inverse change in the pulmonary end-capillary/arterial oxygen content difference **(B)**. When converted to partial pressure differences, the inverse relationship is distorted by the effect of the oxygen dissociation curve in a manner that is applicable only to the particular alveolar P_{O_2} of the patient **(A)**. (Alveolar P_{O_2} is assumed to equal pulmonary end-capillary P_{O_2}.)

TABLE 10.1	Effect of Different Haemoglobin Concentrations on the Arterial P_{O_2} under Venous Admixture Conditions Defined in the Text			
Haemoglobin Concentration	Alveolar/Arterial P_{O_2} Difference		Arterial P_{O_2}	
g.L^{-1}	kPa	mmHg	kPa	mmHg
80	15.0	113	9.0	67
100	14.5	109	9.5	71
120	14.0	105	10.0	75
140	13.5	101	10.5	79
160	13.0	98	10.0	82

ventilation) reduces the cardiac output, with the consequent changes that were outlined earlier.

- The change in arterial pH resulting from the reduction in $P\text{CO}_2$ causes a small, unimportant increase in alveolar/arterial $P\text{O}_2$ difference.

Thus an increase in alveolar ventilation may be expected to increase both the alveolar $P\text{O}_2$ and the alveolar/arterial $P\text{O}_2$ difference. The resultant change in arterial $P\text{O}_2$ will depend on the relative magnitude of the two changes. Figure 10.6 shows the changes in arterial $P\text{O}_2$ caused by variations of alveolar ventilation at an inspired oxygen concentration of 30% in the presence of varying degrees of venous admixture, assuming that cardiac output is influenced by $P\text{CO}_2$ as described in the legend. Up to an alveolar ventilation of 1.5 L.min^{-1}, an increase in ventilation will always raise the arterial $P\text{O}_2$. Beyond that, in the example cited, further increases in alveolar ventilation will increase the arterial $P\text{O}_2$ only if the venous admixture is less than 3%. For larger values of venous admixture, the increase in the alveolar/arterial $P\text{O}_2$ difference exceeds the increase in the alveolar $P\text{O}_2$, and the arterial $P\text{O}_2$ is thus decreased.

Compensation for Increased Alveolar/Arterial $P\text{O}_2$ Difference by Raising the Inspired Oxygen Concentration

Many patients with severe respiratory dysfunction are hypoxaemic while breathing air. The main objective of treatment is clearly to remove the cause of the hypoxaemia,

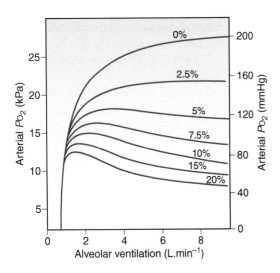

- **Fig. 10.6** The effect of alveolar ventilation on arterial $P\text{O}_2$ is the algebraic sum of the effect upon the alveolar $P\text{O}_2$ (Fig. 10.2) and the consequent change in alveolar/arterial $P\text{O}_2$ difference (Fig. 10.4). When the increase in the latter exceeds the increase in the former, the arterial $P\text{O}_2$ will be diminished. The figures in the diagram indicate the percentage venous admixture. The curve corresponding to 0% venous admixture will indicate alveolar $P\text{O}_2$. Constants incorporated in the design of this figure: inspired oxygen concentration, 30%; oxygen consumption, 200 mL.min^{-1}; and respiratory exchange ratio, 0.8. (From Kelman GR, Nunn JF, Prys-Roberts C, et al. The influence of cardiac output on arterial oxygenation. *Br J Anaesth*. 1967;39:450-458, with permission of the Editor of *British Journal of Anaesthesia* and Oxford University Press.)

but, when this is not immediately feasible, it is often possible to relieve the hypoxaemia by increasing the inspired oxygen concentration. The principles for doing this depend on the cause of the hypoxaemia. As a broad classification, hypoxaemia may be from hypoventilation, venous admixture or a combination of the two. When hypoxaemia is primarily from hypoventilation, and when it is not appropriate or possible to restore normal alveolar ventilation, the arterial $P\text{O}_2$ can usually be restored by elevation of the inspired oxygen within the range of 21% to 30%, as explained earlier (page 137 and Fig. 10.2) and also in Chapter 27.

Quantitatively, the situation is entirely different when hypoxaemia is primarily because of venous admixture. It is then only possible to restore the arterial $P\text{O}_2$ by oxygen enrichment of the inspired gas when the venous admixture does not exceed the equivalent of a shunt of 30% of the cardiac output, and at this level it may require up to 100% inspired oxygen (page 103). The quantitative aspects of the relationship are best considered in relation to the iso-shunt diagram (see Fig. 7.13).

Carriage of Oxygen in the Blood

The preceding section has considered in detail the factors that influence the $P\text{O}_2$ of the arterial blood. It is now necessary to consider how oxygen is carried in the blood and, in particular, the relationship between the $P\text{O}_2$ and the quantity of oxygen that is carried. The latter is crucially important to the delivery of oxygen, and is no less important than the partial pressure at which it becomes available to the tissue.

Oxygen is carried in the blood in two forms. Much of the greater part is in reversible chemical combination with haemoglobin, whereas a smaller part is in physical solution in plasma and intracellular fluid. The ability to carry large quantities of oxygen in the blood is of great importance to most organisms in the animal kingdom, and a variety of oxygen carrying molecules exist (page 309), all based around protein chains containing a metal atom (iron or copper).

Physical Solution of Oxygen in Blood

Oxygen is carried in physical solution in both red blood cells (RBCs) and plasma. The amount carried in normal blood in solution at 37°C is about 0.0232 mL.dL^{-1}.kPa^{-1}, or 0.00314 mL.dL^{-1}.mmHg^{-1}. At normal arterial $P\text{O}_2$, the oxygen in physical solution is thus about 0.25 to 0.3 mL.dL^{-1}, or rather more than 1% of the total oxygen carried in all forms. However, when breathing 100% oxygen, the level rises to about 2 mL.dL^{-1}. Breathing 100% oxygen at 3 atm pressure absolute (303 kPa), the amount of oxygen in physical solution rises to about 6 mL.dL^{-1}, which is sufficient for the normal resting arteriovenous extraction. The amount of oxygen in physical solution rises with decreasing temperature for the same $P\text{O}_2$ (see Table 26.2).

Haemoglobin

The haemoglobin molecule consists of four protein chains, each of which carries a haem group (Fig. 10.7, *A*), and the total molecular weight is 64 458. In the most common type of adult human haemoglobin (HbA), there are two types of chain, two of each occurring in each molecule. The two α-chains each have 141 amino acid residues, with the haem attached to a histidine residue occupying position 87. The two β-chains each have 146 amino acid residues, with the haem attached to a histidine residue occupying position 92. Figure 10.7, *B*, shows details of the point of attachment of the haem in the α-chain.

Molecular Mechanisms of Oxygen Binding[1]

The four chains of the haemoglobin molecule lie in a ball, like a crumpled necklace. However, the form is not random,

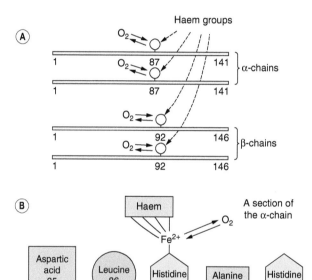

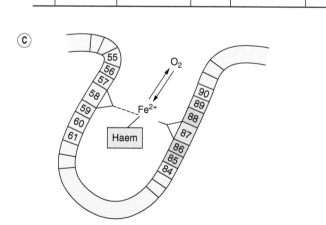

• **Fig. 10.7** The haemoglobin molecule consists of four amino acid chains, each carrying a haem group. **(A)** There are two pairs of identical chains: α-chains with 141 amino acid residues each and β-chains with 146 amino acid residues each. **(B)** The attachment of the haem group to the α-chain. **(C)** The crevice that contains the haem group.

and the actual shape (the quaternary structure) is of critical importance and governs the reaction with oxygen. The shape is maintained by loose (electrostatic) bonds between specific amino acids on different chains, and also between some amino acids on the same chain. One consequence of these bonds is that the haem groups lie in crevices formed by electrostatic bonds between the haem groups and histidine residues, other than those to which they are attached by normal valency linkages. For example, Figure 10.7, *C*, shows a section of an α-chain with the haem group attached to the iron atom, which is bound to the histidine residue in position 87. However, the haem group is also attached by an electrostatic bond to the histidine residue in position 58 and also by nonpolar bonds to many other amino acids. This forms a loop and places the haem group in a crevice, the shape of which controls the ease of access for oxygen molecules.

In deoxyhaemoglobin, the electrostatic bonds within and between the protein chains are strong, holding the haemoglobin molecule in a tense (T) conformation, in which the molecule has a relatively low affinity for oxygen. In oxyhaemoglobin the electrostatic bonds are weaker, and the haemoglobin adopts its relaxed (R) state, in which the crevices containing the haem groups can open and bind oxygen, and the molecule's affinity for oxygen becomes 500 times greater than in the T state. Binding of oxygen to just one of the four protein chains induces a conformational change in the whole haemoglobin molecule, which increases the affinity of the other protein chains for oxygen. This 'cooperativity' between oxygen-binding sites is fundamental to the physiological role of haemoglobin, and affects the kinetics of the reaction between haemoglobin and oxygen, which are described later. The conformational state (R or T) of the haemoglobin molecule is also altered by other factors that influence the strength of the electrostatic bonds; such factors include carbon dioxide, pH and temperature.

The Bohr effect describes the alteration in haemoglobin oxygen affinity that arises from changes in hydrogen ion or carbon dioxide concentrations, and is generally considered in terms of its influence upon the dissociation curve (Fig. 10.10). Changes in pH affect the numerous electrostatic bonds that maintain the quaternary structure of haemoglobin, and so stabilize the molecule in the T conformation, reducing its affinity for oxygen. Similarly, carbon dioxide binds to the N-terminal amino acid residues of the α-chain to form carbaminohaemoglobin (page 124), and this small alteration in the function of the protein chains stabilizes the T conformation and facilitates release of the oxygen molecule from haemoglobin.

Conversely, the Haldane effect describes the smaller amount of carbon dioxide that can be carried in oxygenated blood compared with deoxygenated blood (page 125). Crystallographic studies have shown that in deoxyhaemoglobin the histidine in position 146 of the β-chain is loosely bonded to the aspartine residue at position 94, and that when haemoglobin binds oxygen and changes to the R conformation histidine 146 moves 10 Å further away from the aspartine residue, which is sufficient distance to change its pK value.[2] Once again, this small change in one area of the β-chains has widespread effects on electrostatic bonds throughout the molecule, changing the quaternary structure of the entire molecule and altering its ability to buffer hydrogen ions and form carbamino compounds with carbon dioxide.

Oxygen-Binding Capacity of Haemoglobin (Bo$_2$) or Hüfner Constant

Following the determination of the molecular weight of haemoglobin, the theoretical value for its oxygen-binding capacity (Bo$_2$) of 1.39 mL.g^{-1} was easily derived (4 moles of oxygen of 22 414 mL (at standard temperature and pressure, dry) each bind to 1 mol of haemoglobin with molecular mass 64 458 g) and passed into general use. However, it gradually became clear that this value was not obtained when direct measurements of haemoglobin concentration and oxygen capacity were compared, with values between 1.306 and 1.36 mL.g^{-1} being reported. The difference between the theoretical and in vivo values results from the presence of dyshaemoglobins,[3] which include any form of haemoglobin that lacks oxygen-binding capacity; the most common are methaemoglobin (metHb) and carboxyhaemoglobin (COHb). If the dyshaemoglobins are taken into account, then the theoretical value for the Hüfner constant may be used, and the Bo$_2$ calculated as:

$$Bo_2 = 1.39 \times (tHb - (metHb + COHb)),$$

where tHb = total haemoglobin present in the sample.

Current blood gas analysers routinely measure all four forms of haemoglobin that make up the majority of tHb in blood that is, oxyhaemoglobin (O$_2$Hb), deoxyhaemoglobin (HHb), metHb and COHb. If the first two of these have been measured, then the dyshaemoglobins can be excluded completely, and the calculation of Bo$_2$ becomes even simpler:

$$Bo_2 = 1.39 \times (HHb + O_2Hb).$$

Kinetics of the Reaction of Oxygen with Haemoglobin

Adair first proposed in 1925 that the binding of oxygen to haemoglobin proceeds in four separate stages:[4]

$$Hb + 4O_2 \underset{}{\overset{K_1}{\rightleftharpoons}} HbO_2 + 3O_2$$
$$\overset{K_2}{\rightleftharpoons} Hb(O_2)_2 + 2O_2$$
$$\overset{K_3}{\rightleftharpoons} Hb(O_2)_3 + O_2 \overset{K_4}{\rightleftharpoons} Hb(O_2)_4.$$

For each of the four reactions there are two velocity constants, with small k indicating the reverse reaction (towards deoxyhaemoglobin) and small k prime (k') indicating the forward reaction. Large K is used to represent the ratio of the forward and reverse reactions, for example: $K_1 = k'_1/k_1$. In this way, the dissociation between deoxyhaemoglobin and oxyhaemoglobin may be represented by the four velocity constants K_1–K_4.

The Adair equation described assumes that the α- and β-chains of haemoglobin behave identically in their chemical reactions with oxygen, which is unlikely in vivo. When α-and β-chains are taken into account, there are many different reaction routes that may be followed between deoxyhaemoglobin and oxyhaemoglobin, in theory giving rise to 16 different reversible reactions (Fig. 10.8).[5] However, the

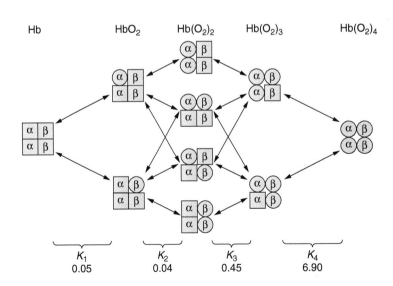

• **Fig. 10.8** Oxygenation of tetrameric haemoglobin. If chemical interactions with oxygen differ between α- and β-chains, then the transition from deoxyhaemoglobin to fully oxygenated haemoglobin can take a variety of routes, as shown. Arrows indicate the 16 possible separate dissociation equilibria, which must be combined to derive the four Adair constants K_1 to K_4, the values of which are indicated. It can be clearly seen that the final stage of oxygenation is considerably faster than the previous three.

multiple separate forward and reverse reactions can again be combined to give a single value for K, which does not differ significantly from those obtained using the simpler Adair equation.

In both cases, the separate velocity constants have been measured,[5] and values for K_1 to K_4 are shown in Figure 10.8. It can be seen that the last reaction has a forward velocity that is many times higher than that of the other reactions. During the oxygenation of the final 25% of deoxyhaemoglobin, the last reaction will predominate, and the high velocity constant counteracts the effect of the ever-diminishing number of oxygen-binding sites that would otherwise slow the reaction rate by the law of mass action. The magnitude of the forward reaction for K_4 also explains why the dissociation of oxyhaemoglobin is somewhat slower than its formation.

The velocity constant of the combination of carbon monoxide with haemoglobin is of the same order, but the rate of dissociation of COHb is extremely slow by comparison.

Oxyhaemoglobin Dissociation Curve

As a result of the complex kinetics of the chemical reaction between oxygen and haemoglobin, the relationship between Po_2 and percentage saturation of haemoglobin is nonlinear, and the precise form of the nonlinearity is of fundamental biological importance. It is shown, under standard conditions, in graphic form for adult and foetal haemoglobin (HbF), and also for myoglobin and COHb, in Figure 10.9.

An 'S'-shaped oxyhaemoglobin dissociation curve was first described by Bohr in 1904 (see Fig. 35.11). Adair[4] and Kelman[6] subsequently developed equations that would reproduce the observed oxygen dissociation curve, using a variety of coefficients. The Kelman equation, which uses seven coefficients, generates a curve indistinguishable from the true curve above a Po_2 of about 1 kPa (7.5 mmHg). Calculation of Po_2 from saturation requires an iterative approach, but saturation may be conveniently determined from Po_2 by computer, a calculation that is automatically performed by most blood gas analysers in clinical use. The following simplified version of the Kelman equation is convenient to use, and yields similar results at Po_2 values greater than 4 kPa (30 mmHg)[7] (Po_2 values here are in kPa; So_2 is a percentage):

$$So_2 = \frac{100\left(Po_2^3 + 2.667 \times Po_2\right)}{Po_2^3 + 2.667 \times Po_2 + 55.47}$$

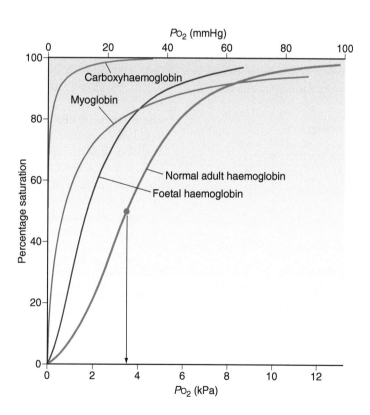

• **Fig. 10.9** Dissociation curves of normal adult and foetal haemoglobins. Curves for myoglobin and carboxyhaemoglobin are shown for comparison. The arrow shows the P_{50} for this curve, which is the oxygen partial pressure at which the Hb saturation is 50%. Note: (1) Foetal haemoglobin is adapted to operate at a lower Po_2 than adult blood. (2) Myoglobin approaches full saturation at Po_2 levels normally found in voluntary muscle (2–4 kPa, 15–30 mmHg); the bulk of its oxygen can only be released at very low Po_2 during exercise. (3) Carboxyhaemoglobin can be dissociated only by the maintenance of very low levels of Pco.

This equation takes no account of the position of the dissociation curve, as described in the next section, so it must be used with caution in clinical situations.

Factors Causing Displacement of the Dissociation Curve

Several physiological and pathological changes to blood chemistry cause the normal dissociation curve to be displaced in either direction along its x-axis. A convenient approach to quantifying a shift of the dissociation curve is to indicate the P_{O_2} required for 50% saturation, and, under the standard conditions shown in Figure 10.9, this is 3.5 kPa (26.3 mmHg). Referred to as the P_{50}, this is the usual method of reporting a shift of the dissociation curve.

The Bohr effect, as a result of changes in blood pH, is shown in Figure 10.10. Shifts may be defined as the ratio of the P_{O_2} that produces a particular saturation under standard conditions to the P_{O_2} that produces the same saturation with a particular shift of the curve. Standard conditions include pH 7.4, temperature 37°C and zero base excess. In Figure 10.10, a saturation of 80% is produced by P_{O_2} 6 kPa (45 mmHg) at pH 7.4 (standard). At pH 7.0 the P_{O_2} required for 80% saturation is 9.4 kPa (70.5 mmHg). The ratio is 0.64, and this applies to all saturations at pH 7.0.

The Bohr effect has an influence on oxygen carriage under normal physiological conditions. As blood moves along a capillary, either pulmonary or systemic, the transfer of carbon dioxide alters the pH of the blood, and the dissociation curve is shifted. Although the effect may seem to be small (e.g., the arteriovenous pH difference is only about 0.033),

the effect on oxygen saturation at the venous point, where the dissociation curve is steep, will be significant. It has been suggested that 25% of oxygen release and uptake by haemoglobin as it traverses systemic and pulmonary capillaries, respectively, is because of the Bohr effect.

Temperature has a large influence on the dissociation curve, with a left shift in hypothermia and a right shift in hyperthermia.

Base excess is a parameter derived from blood pH and P_{CO_2} to quantify the metabolic (as opposed to respiratory) component of an observed change in blood pH. Compared with pH itself, alterations in base excess have only a small effect on the position of the dissociation curve, but must be taken into account for accurate results.

Quantifying Displacement of the Haemoglobin Dissociation Curve

Estimation of haemoglobin saturation from P_{O_2} using the modified Kelman equation was shown in an earlier section. However, this equation assumes a normal P_{50}, yielding erroneous results in all but the most 'normal' physiological circumstances. In clinical practice, the type of patient who requires blood gas measurement invariably also has abnormalities of pH, temperature and base excess. Automated calculation of saturation from P_{O_2} by blood gas analysers routinely takes these factors into account, using a variety of equations to correct for dissociation curve displacement, of which one example is:[8]

$$\text{Corrected } P_{O_2} = P_{O_2} \times 10^{\left[0.48(pH-7.4)-0.024(T-37)-0.0013\times\text{Base Excess}\right]},$$

where P_{O_2} is in kPa and temperature (T) in °C. The corrected P_{O_2} may then be entered into any version of the haemoglobin dissociation curve equation as shown earlier (page 145). For even more accurate calculation of oxygen saturation under a wider range of conditions, as may be required for physiological modelling, more complex computational formulae are available that also incorporate the effects of P_{CO_2} and 2,3-diphosphoglycerate (DPG) levels.[9]

Clinical Significance of Displacement of the Haemoglobin Dissociation Curve

The important effect is on tissue P_{O_2}, and the consequences of a shift in the dissociation curve are not intuitively obvious. It is essential to think quantitatively. For example, a shift to the right (caused by low pH or high temperature) impairs oxygenation in the lungs but aids release of oxygen in the tissues. Do these effects in combination increase or decrease tissue P_{O_2}? An illustrative example is shown in Figure 10.10. The arterial P_{O_2} is assumed to be 13.3 kPa (100 mmHg), and there is a decrease in arterial saturation with a reduction of pH. At normal arterial P_{O_2} the effect on arterial saturation is relatively small, but at the venous point the position is quite different, and the examples in Figure 10.10 show the venous oxygen partial pressures to be

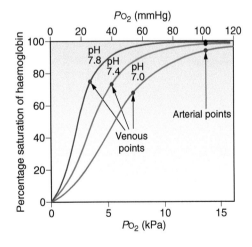

• **Fig. 10.10** The Bohr effect and its effect upon oxygen partial pressure. The centre (*green*) curve is the normal curve under standard conditions; the other two curves show the displacement caused by differing blood pH as indicated, other factors remaining constant. The venous points have been determined on the basis of a fixed arterial/mixed venous oxygen saturation difference of 25%. They are thus 25% less saturated than the corresponding arterial saturation, which is equivalent to a P_{O_2} of 13.3 kPa (100 mmHg) in each case. Under the conditions shown, alkalosis lowers venous P_{O_2}, and acidosis raises venous P_{O_2}. Temperature, 37°C; base excess, zero.

very markedly affected. Assuming that the arterial/venous oxygen saturation difference is constant at 25%, it will be seen that at low pH the venous Po_2 is raised to 6.9 kPa (52 mmHg), whereas at high pH the venous Po_2 is reduced to 3.5 kPa (26 mmHg). This is important because the tissue Po_2 equates more closely to the venous Po_2 than to the arterial Po_2 (page 120). Thus in the example shown, the shift to the right is beneficial for tissue oxygenation.

It is a general rule that a shift to the right (increased P_{50}) will benefit venous Po_2, provided that the arterial Po_2 is not critically reduced. At an arterial Po_2 of less than 5 kPa (38 mmHg), the arterial point is on the steep part of the dissociation curve, and the deficiency in oxygenation of the arterial blood would outweigh the improved off-loading of oxygen in the tissues. Thus, with severe arterial hypoxaemia, the venous Po_2 would tend to be reduced by a shift to the right, and a *leftward* shift would then be advantageous. It is therefore of great interest that a spontaneous leftward shift occurs at extreme altitude when arterial Po_2 is critically reduced (see later).

Orally active drugs which can alter P_{50} are now under development.[10] These bind reversibly to the terminal valine of the α-chain, altering the structure of the molecule and leading to a dramatic fall in P_{50} from 5.7 to 1.1 kPa (43 to 8 mmHg). This increase in oxygen affinity may prove to be a hugely beneficial contributor to survival in diseases resulting in severe tissue hypoxia.

2,3-Diphosphoglycerate

For many years it has been known that the presence of certain organic phosphates in RBCs has a pronounced effect on the P_{50}. The most important of these compounds is DPG, one molecule of which becomes bound by electrostatic bonds between the two β-chains, stabilizing the T conformation of haemoglobin, reducing its oxygen affinity, thus displacing the dissociation curve to the right. The percentage of haemoglobin molecules containing a DPG molecule governs the overall P_{50} of a blood sample within the range of 2 to 4.5 kPa (15–34 mmHg). DPG is formed in the Rapoport–Luebering shunt off the glycolytic pathway, and its level is determined by the balance between synthesis and degradation. Activities of the enzymes which produce and metabolize DPG are both pH-sensitive.

The relationship between DPG levels and P_{50} suggested that DPG levels would have a most important bearing on clinical practice. Much research effort was devoted to this topic, which mostly failed to substantiate the theoretical importance of DPG for oxygen delivery. In fact, the likely effects of changes in P_{50} mediated by DPG seem to be of marginal significance in comparison with changes in arterial Po_2, acid–base balance and tissue perfusion.

DPG levels with blood storage and transfusion remain the only area where RBC DPG levels may have significant effects in clinical practice.[11] Storage of blood for transfusion at less than 6°C reduces glycolysis to less than 5% of normal rates, reducing DPG production by a similar amount. Thus

after 1 to 2 weeks of storage, RBC DPG levels are effectively zero. Blood preservation solutions have evolved through the years to include the addition of dextrose to encourage glycolytic activity, citrate to buffer the resulting lactic acid and adenine or phosphate to help maintain ATP levels, but DPG levels still become negligible within a few weeks.

Once transfused, the RBCs are quickly warmed and provided with all required substrates, and the limiting factor for return to normal DPG levels will be reactivation of the DPG synthetic enzyme DPG mutase. In vivo studies in healthy volunteers indicate that RBC DPG levels in transfused RBCs are approximately 50% of normal 7 hours after transfusion, and pretransfusion levels are not achieved until 48 hours (Fig. 10.11).[12] This ingenious study involved the administration of 35-day-old type O blood to type A volunteers, and then in repeated venous samples RBCs were separated according to their blood group before measuring DPG levels. In this way, DPG levels of both the recipients own cells and the transfused cells could be monitored separately (Fig. 10.11).

The clinical significance of the slow return to normal DPG levels is uncertain, and in most cases likely to be minimal, as the proportion of the patient's haemoglobin that consists of transfused blood will usually be small, and poorly functioning haemoglobin will still carry more oxygen than no haemoglobin. This is confirmed in studies of critically ill patients in whom the duration of blood storage before being transfused did not affect clinical outcomes.[13] However, rapid transfusion of large volumes of DPG-depleted blood does result in a reduced P_{50}, which will in theory impair tissue oxygenation (page 146).

Other causes of altered DPG levels include anaemia, which results in a raised DPG level, with P_{50} of the order of 0.5 kPa (3.8 mmHg) higher than control levels. The problem of oxygen delivery in anaemia is considered in Chapter 24.

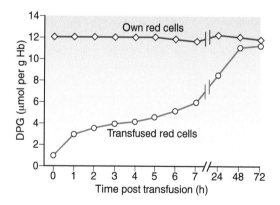

• **Fig. 10.11** Restoration of red cell 2,3-diphosphoglycerate (DPG) levels following blood transfusion. The type O transfused red blood cells were stored for 35 days in CPD-A, preservative solution, before being given to type A volunteers. Red blood cells were subsequently separated into the transfused cells and the volunteer's own cells before analysis. The clinical implications of this slow return to normal DPG levels are unclear; see text for details. (From reference 12, with permission of the authors and the publishers of *British Journal of Haematology*.)

Normal Arterial P_{O_2}

In contrast to the arterial P_{CO_2}, the arterial P_{O_2} shows a progressive decrease with age. Using the pooled results from 12 studies of healthy subjects, one review suggested the following relationship in subjects breathing air:[14]

$$\text{Arterial } P_{O_2} = 13.6 - 0.044 \times \text{age in years (kPa)}$$
$$\text{or} \qquad = 102 - 0.33 \times \text{age in years (mm Hg)}.$$

About this regression line there are 95% confidence limits of $\pm$ 1.33 kPa (10 mmHg; Table 10.2), so 5% of normal patients will lie outside these limits, and it is therefore preferable to refer to this as the reference range rather than the normal range.

Nitric Oxide and Haemoglobin[15]

It has been known for some time that nitric oxide binds to haemoglobin very rapidly, and this observation is fundamental to its therapeutic use when inhaled nitric oxide exerts its effects in the pulmonary vasculature but is inactivated by binding to haemoglobin before it reaches the systemic circulation (page 84). There are two quite separate chemical reactions between nitric oxide and the haemoglobin molecule:

1. Nitric oxide binds to the haem moiety of each haemoglobin chain, but the resulting reaction differs with the state of oxygenation. For deoxyhaemoglobin, in the T conformation, a fairly stable nitric oxide haemoglobin (NO-Hb) complex is rapidly formed, which has little vasodilator activity, whereas for oxyhaemoglobin, in the R conformation, the oxygen is displaced by nitric oxide, the iron atom is oxidized to metHb, and a nitrate ion produced:

$$Hb\left[Fe^{2+}\right] + NO \rightarrow Hb\left[Fe^{2+}\right]NO$$
$$\text{or } Hb\left[Fe^{2+}\right]O_2 + NO \rightarrow Hb\left[Fe^{3+}\right] + NO_3^-.$$

TABLE 10.2	Normal Values for Arterial P_{O_2}	
	Mean (95% Confidence Intervals)	
Age (Years)	kPa	mmHg
20–29	12.5 (10.2–13.8)	94 (84–104)
30–39	12.1 (10.7–13.4)	90 (80–100)
40–49	10.6 (10.3–13.0)	87 (77–97)
50–59	10.2 (9.9–12.5)	84 (74–94)
60–69	10.7 (9.4–12.1)	81 (71–91)
70–79	10.3 (9.0–10.6)	77 (67–87)
80–89	9.9 (8.5–10.2)	74 (64–84)

(From reference 14.)

These reactions are so rapid that there is doubt that endogenous nitric oxide itself can exert any effects within blood (e.g., on platelets) before being bound by haemoglobin, and must therefore act via an intermediate molecule.

2. Nitric oxide is also known to form stable compounds with sulphydryl groups termed S-nitrosothiols, with the general formula R-S-NO, where the R group may be glutathione- or sulphur-containing amino acid residues within proteins.[15,16] Nitrosothiols retain biological activity as vasodilators and can survive for longer than free nitric oxide within the blood vessels. Nitric oxide forms a nitrosothiol group with the cysteine residue at position 93 on the β-chains, producing S-nitrosohaemoglobin (SNO-Hb). As a result of conformational changes in haemoglobin, the reaction is faster with R-state oxyhaemoglobin and under alkaline conditions.

Thus in vivo, nitric oxide in arterial blood is predominantly in the form of SNO-Hb, whereas in venous blood haem-bound NO-Hb predominates. It has been proposed that, as haemoglobin passes through the pulmonary capillary, changes in oxygenation, P_{CO_2} and pH drive the change from the deoxygenated T conformation to the oxygenated R conformation, and this change in quaternary structure of haemoglobin causes the intramolecular transfer of nitric oxide from the haem to cysteine-bound positions. In the systemic capillaries, the opposite sequence of events occurs, which encourages release of nitric oxide from the R-S-NO group, where it may again bind to the haem group, or be released from the RBC to act as a local vasodilator, effectively improving flow to vessels with the greatest demand for oxygen. Export of nitric oxide activity from the RBC is believed to occur via a complex mechanism. Deoxygenated T conformation haemoglobin binds to one of the cytoplasmic domains of the RBC transmembrane band 3 protein (see Fig. 9.4),[17] which may act as a metabolon (page 127) and directly transfer the nitric oxide via a series of nitrosothiol reactions to the outside of the cell membrane, where it can exert its vasodilator activity. The biological implications of this series of events are yet to be determined. The suggestion that haemoglobin is acting as a nitric oxide carrier to regulate capillary blood flow and oxygen release from the RBC represents a fundamental advance in our understanding of the delivery of oxygen to tissues.[18] One role postulated for these interactions between haemoglobin and nitric oxide is to modulate the vascular response to changes in oxygen availability, for example during haemorrhage when nitric oxide activity from RBCs may be involved in overcoming the catecholamine-mediated vasoconstriction in vital organs.[18]

Abnormal Forms of Haemoglobin

There are a large number of alternative amino acid sequences in the haemoglobin molecule. Most animal species have their own peculiar haemoglobins (page 309), whereas in humans γ- and δ-chains occur in addition to the α- and β-chains already described. The γ- and δ-chains occur normally in combination with α-chains. The combination of two γ-chains with two α-chains constitutes HbF, which has a dissociation curve well to the left of adult haemoglobin (Fig. 10.9). The combination of two δ-chains with two α-chains constitutes A_2 haemoglobin (HbA_2), which forms 2% of the total haemoglobin in normal adults. Other variations in the amino acid chains can be considered abnormal, and, although over 600 have been reported and named, only one-third of these have any clinical effects. Some abnormal haemoglobins (such as San Diego and Chesapeake) have a high P_{50}, but it is more common for the P_{50} to be lower than normal (such as Sickle and Kansas). In the long term, a reduced P_{50} results in excessive production of RBCs (erythrocytosis), presumed to result from cellular hypoxia in the kidney leading to erythropoietin production.[19] However, many abnormal haemoglobins also have deranged quaternary protein structure and are unstable, a situation that leads to haemoglobin chains becoming free within the RBC cytoplasm and membrane causing cell lysis.[19] These patients therefore have a higher than normal rate of RBC production, but are generally anaemic because of even greater degrees of RBC destruction. This combination of abnormalities results in severe long-term problems with body iron metabolism.

Sickle cell disease[20] is caused by the presence of sickle haemoglobin (HbS), in which valine replaces glutamic acid in position 6 on the β-chains. This apparently trivial substitution is sufficient to cause critical loss of solubility of reduced haemoglobin, resulting in polymerization of HbS within the RBC causing RBCs to take on the characteristic 'sickle' shape and be more prone to haemolysis. It is a hereditary condition, and in the homozygous state is a grave abnormality, with sickling occurring at an arterial Po_2 of less than 5.5 kPa (40 mmHg), which is close to the normal venous Po_2. Thus any condition that increases the arteriovenous oxygen difference, such as infection, risks precipitating a sickle 'crisis'. Sickle cells cause damage in two ways. First, the sickled cells are crescent-shaped and rigid, so can more easily occlude small blood vessels, usually venules. Second, haemolysis releases free haemoglobin into the circulation, where it binds nitric oxide released from the vascular endothelium, causing vasoconstriction, further impairing the ability of the sickle cells to pass through the microcirculation. In the long term these effects cause widespread microvascular damage, including pulmonary hypertension.[21]

The intracellular concentration of HbS does not affect the rate at which polymerization occurs, but rather the lag time an RBC spends in hypoxic conditions before sickling occurs.[22] Thus, with a higher HbS concentration, sickling is more likely to occur under physiological conditions. In patients homozygous for sickle cell disease, two factors affect RBC HbS concentration: (1) intracellular dehydration, which is dependent on the functioning of the various ion channels on the RBC membrane, which may also be abnormal in sickle cell disease;[22] and (2) the levels of HbF in the RBC, which vary widely in patients and are inversely related to the severity of clinical symptoms of sickle cell disease. Thus most therapies in recent years have focussed

on increasing HbF synthesis by the bone marrow with drugs such as hydroxyurea.[23] The only potential cure for sickle cell disease remains haematopoietic stem cell transplantation, which sadly remains too high risk and expensive to be an option for most patients with the disease.[24]

Heterozygous carriers of the disease only sickle below an arterial Po_2 of less than 2.7 kPa (20 mmHg), and so are usually asymptomatic.

Thalassaemia is another hereditary disorder of haemoglobin.[25] It consists of a suppression of formation of HbA, again with a compensatory production of HbF, which persists throughout life instead of falling to low levels after birth. The functional disorder thus includes a shift of the dissociation curve to the left (Fig. 10.9).

MetHb is haemoglobin in which the iron has been oxidized and assumes the trivalent ferric form. One way in which metHb forms is when oxyhaemoglobin acts as a nitric oxide scavenger, a process that occurs physiologically to limit the biological activity of endogenous nitric oxide, or pharmacologically during treatment with inhaled nitric oxide. Other drugs may cause methaemoglobinaemia, most notably some local anaesthetics[26] (prilocaine, benzocaine), but also nitrites and dapsone. MetHb is unable to combine with oxygen, but is slowly reconverted to haemoglobin in the normal subject by the action of four different systems:

1. A metHb reductase enzyme is present in RBCs and uses nicotinamide adenine dinucleotide (NADH) generated by glycolysis to reduce metHb. This system is by far the most important in normal subjects, accounting for over two-thirds of metHb reducing activity, and is deficient in familial methaemoglobinaemia.
2. Ascorbic acid may also bring about the reduction of metHb by a direct chemical effect, though the rate of this reaction is slow.
3. Glutathione-based reductive enzymes have a small amount of metHb reductase activity.
4. The NADPH-dehydrogenase enzyme in RBCs can reduce metHb using NADPH generated from the pentose phosphate pathway. Under physiological conditions, this system has almost no effect, and is regarded as the 'reserve' metHb reductase.

Elevated metHb levels of whatever cause may be treated by the administration of either ascorbic acid or methylene blue.[26] The latter is extremely effective, and brings about metHb reduction by activation of NADPH-dehydrogenase.

Abnormal Ligands

The iron in haemoglobin is able to combine with other inorganic molecules apart from oxygen. Compounds so formed are, in general, more stable than oxyhaemoglobin, and therefore block the combination of haemoglobin with oxygen. The most important of these abnormal compounds is COHb, but ligands may also be formed with nitric oxide (see previous discussion), cyanide, sulphur and ammonia. In addition to the loss of oxygen-carrying power, there is also often a shift of the dissociation curve to the left.

Carboxyhaemoglobin

Carbon monoxide is known to displace oxygen from combination with haemoglobin, and its affinity is approximately 300 times greater than the affinity for oxygen. Thus, in a subject with 20% of their haemoglobin bound to carbon monoxide, blood oxygen content will be reduced by a similar amount (the small contribution from dissolved oxygen will be unchanged). However, the presence of COHb also causes a leftward shift of the dissociation curve of the remaining oxyhaemoglobin, partly mediated by reduced DPG levels. Tissue oxygenation is therefore impaired to an even greater extent than simply reducing the amount of haemoglobin available for oxygen carriage. This situation contrasts with that of anaemia, where P_{50} is increased, so the reduced oxygen-carrying capacity is partially alleviated by an improved unloading of oxygen in the tissues (page 146).

Blood Substitutes

There are obvious advantages in the provision of an artificial oxygen-carrying solution that would avoid the infectious and antigenic complications seen with transfusion of another individual's RBCs. The search for a blood substitute has followed two quite different parallel paths.

Perfluorocarbons[27]

Oxygen is highly soluble in these hydrophobic compounds, which, with an 8 to 10 carbon chain, are above the critical molecular size to act as anaesthetics. Perfluorooctyl bromide (Perflubron) is a 60% emulsion, which will carry about 50 mL of oxygen per 100 mL on equilibration with 100% oxygen at normal atmospheric pressure. Because oxygen is in physical solution in fluorocarbons, its 'dissociation curve' is a straight line, with the quantity of dissolved oxygen directly proportional to Po_2. Because of the requirement to maintain adequate blood constituents apart from RBCs (e.g., platelets, clotting factors, blood chemistry and oncotic pressure), the proportion of blood that may be replaced by Perflubron is small, so that even when breathing 100% oxygen the additional oxygen-carrying capacity is limited. Even so, clinical uses for intravenous Perflubron were extensively investigated, for example by intravenous administration to delay the need for blood transfusion[28] or as a rescue therapy during coronary angioplasty[29] or by instillation into the lungs for partial liquid ventilation in adults (page 372), but none of these proved successful enough for widespread clinical use.

Haemoglobin-Based Oxygen Carriers[30,31]

Early attempts at using RBC haemolysates resulted in acute renal failure because of the stroma from the RBC rather than the free haemoglobin. Development of stroma-free haemoglobin solutions failed to solve the problem because, although relatively stable in vitro, the haemoglobin tetramer dissociates in the body into dimers, which are excreted in the urine within a few hours. Other problems include the absence of DPG resulting in a low P_{50} and a high colloid oncotic pressure, limiting the amount that can be used. The short half-life and high oncotic pressure can be improved by either polymerization or cross-linking of haemoglobin molecules. The P_{50} of the solution can be improved by using recombinant human haemoglobin rather than animal haemoglobin, and by choosing a specific variant of human haemoglobin (Presbyterian Hb) which has a naturally higher P_{50}.[32] Unfortunately, despite these advances, haemoglobin-based oxygen carriers all have significant drawbacks in clinical use,[31] mostly from the haemoglobin-scavenging nitric oxide which causes vasoconstriction, release of inflammatory mediators and inhibition of platelet function. These effects are not theoretical: clinical studies of a variety of products show haemoglobin-based blood substitutes cause increased occurrences of death, myocardial infarction, cardiac arrhythmia and renal injury.[31]

Strategies currently being investigated to counteract the vasoconstrictor effects include co-administration of endothelin receptor antagonists (page 84) or nitric oxide donors such as nitroglycerin.[33] It may soon be possible to encapsulate haemoglobin within liposomes or artificial cell membranes, for example by incorporating the haemoglobin into a lipid vesicle, sometimes even including reducing agents and oxygen-affinity modifiers to produce a more functional oxygen carrying unit.[30] Animal studies show these solutions have the potential to deliver useful quantities of oxygen to hypoxic tissues.[34]

The latest attempt at producing a haemoglobin-based oxygen carrier without relying on blood donation uses stem cell technology.[35] With the application of suitable growth factors human stem cells can be developed in vitro to produce mature RBCs with all the physiological characteristics of a normal RBC.

Role of Oxygen in the Cell

Dissolved molecular oxygen (dioxygen) enters into many metabolic processes in the mammalian body. Quantitatively the most important is the cytochrome *c* oxidase system, which is responsible for about 90% of the total oxygen consumption of the body. However, cytochrome *c* oxidase is only one of more than 200 oxidases, which may be classified as follows.

Electron transfer oxidases. As a group, these oxidases involve the reduction of oxygen to superoxide anion, hydrogen peroxide or water; the last is the fully reduced state (see Chapter 25, Fig. 25.2). The most familiar of this group of enzymes is cytochrome *c* oxidase. It is located in the mitochondria and is concerned in the production of the high-energy phosphate bond in ATP, which is the main source of biological energy. This process is described in greater detail later.

Oxygen transferases (dioxygenases). This group of oxygenases incorporates oxygen into substrates without the formation of any reduced oxygen product. Familiar examples are cyclooxygenase and lipoxygenase, which are concerned in the first stage of conversion of arachidonic acid into prostaglandins and leukotrienes (see Chapter 11).

Mixed function oxidases. These oxidases result in oxidation of both a substrate and a cosubstrate, which is most commonly NADPH. The best-known examples are the cytochrome P-450 hydroxylases, which play an important role in detoxification.

Energy Production

Most of the energy deployed in animals is derived from the oxidation of food fuels, of which the most important is glucose:

$$C_6H_{12}O_6 + 6O_2 \rightarrow 6CO_2 + 6H_2O + energy.$$

This equation accurately describes the combustion of glucose in vitro, but is only a crude overall representation of the oxidation of glucose in the body. The direct reaction would not produce energy in a form in which it could be used by the body, so biological oxidation proceeds by a large number of stages with a phased production of energy. This energy is not immediately released, and is stored mainly by means of the reaction of adenosine diphosphate (ADP) with inorganic phosphate ion to form ATP. The third phosphate group in ATP is held by a high-energy bond that releases its energy when ATP is split back into ADP and inorganic phosphate ion during any of the myriad of biological reactions requiring energy input. ADP is thus recycled indefinitely, with ATP acting as a short-term store of energy, available in a form that may be used directly for work such as muscle contraction, ion pumping, protein synthesis and secretion.

There is no large store of ATP in the body, and it must be synthesized continuously as it is being used. The ATP/ADP ratio is an indication of the level of energy that is currently carried in the ADP/ATP system, and the ratio is normally related to the state of oxidation of the cell. The ADP/ATP system is not the only short-term energy store in the body, but it is the most important.

Complete oxidation of glucose requires a three-stage process, the first of which, glycolysis, is independent of oxygen supply.

Glycolysis and Anaerobic Energy Production

Figure 10.12 shows detail of the glycolytic (Embden–Meyerhof) pathway for the conversion of glucose to lactic acid. Glycolysis occurs entirely within the cytoplasm, and under normal conditions proceeds only as far as pyruvic acid, which then enters the citric acid cycle (see below). In RBCs, where there is an absence of the respiratory enzymes located in the mitochondria, or in other cells when cellular Po_2 falls below its critical level, lactic acid is produced. Figure 10.12 shows that, overall, four molecules of ATP are produced, but two of these are consumed in the priming stages before the formation of fructose-1,6-diphosphate. The conversion of glyceraldehyde-3-phosphate to 3-phosphoglyceric acid produces a hydrogen ion, which becomes bound to extramitochondrial nicotinamide adenine dinucleotide (NAD). This hydrogen cannot enter the mitochondria for further oxidative metabolism, so is taken up lower down the pathway by the reduction of pyruvic acid to lactic acid.

This series of changes is therefore associated with the net formation of only two molecules of ATP from one of glucose:

$$Glucose + 2Pi + 2ADP \rightarrow 2Lactic\ acid \\ + 2ATP + 2H_2O$$

(Pi = inorganic phosphate)

However, considerable chemical energy remains in the lactic acid, which, in the presence of oxygen, can be reconverted to pyruvic acid and then oxidized in the citric acid cycle, producing a further 36 molecules of ATP. Alternatively, lactic acid may be converted into liver glycogen to await more favourable conditions for oxidation.

Despite its inefficiency for ATP production, anaerobic metabolism is of great biological importance, and was universal before the atmospheric Po_2 was sufficiently high for aerobic pathways (Chapter 34, *The Atmosphere*). Anaerobic metabolism is still the rule in anaerobic bacteria and also in the mammalian body whenever energy requirements outstrip oxygen supply.

Aerobic Energy Production

The aerobic pathway permits the release of far greater quantities of energy from the same amount of substrate, and is therefore used whenever possible. Under aerobic conditions, most reactions of the glycolytic pathway remain unchanged, with two very important exceptions. The conversion of glyceraldehyde-3-phosphate to 3-phosphoglyceric acid occurs in the mitochondrion, when the two NADH molecules formed may enter oxidative phosphorylation (see later discussion) rather than producing lactic acid. Similarly, pyruvate does not continue along the pathway to lactic acid but diffuses into the mitochondria and enters the next stage of oxidative metabolism.

The citric acid (Krebs) cycle occurs within the mitochondria, as shown in Figure 10.13. It consists of a series of reactions to reduce the length of the carbon chain of the molecules before adding a new two-carbon chain (acetyl CoA) derived from glycolysis. During these reactions, six molecules of carbon dioxide are produced (for each molecule of glucose), along with a further eight molecules of NADH and one molecule of FADH$_2$. Therefore in total, each glucose molecule yields 12 hydrogen ions bound to either NAD or FAD carrier molecules.

The scheme shown in Figure 10.13 also accounts for the consumption of oxygen in the metabolism of fat. After hydrolysis, glycerol is converted into pyruvic acid, while the fatty acids shed a series of two-carbon molecules in the form of acetyl CoA. Pyruvic acid and acetyl CoA enter the citric acid cycle and are then degraded in the same manner as

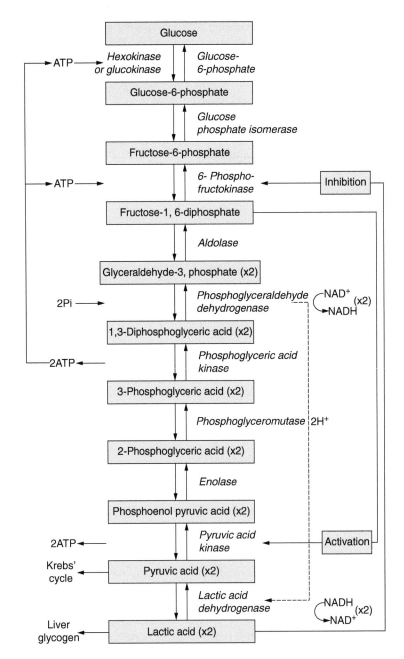

• **Fig. 10.12** The glycolytic (Embden–Meyerhof) pathway for anaerobic metabolism of glucose. From glyceraldehyde-3-phosphate downwards, two molecules of each intermediate are formed from one of glucose. Note the consumption of two molecules of adenosine triphosphate (ATP) in the first three steps. These must be set against the total production of four molecules of ATP, leaving a net gain of only two molecules of ATP from each molecule of glucose. All the acids are largely ionized at tissue pH. NAD, nicotinamide adenine dinucleotide; Pi, inorganic phosphate.

though they had been derived from glucose. Amino acids are dealt with in similar manner after deamination.

Oxidative phosphorylation is the final stage of energy production, and again occurs in the mitochondria.[36] Hydrogen ions are forced to move along a chain of enzymes, arranged in rows along the cristae of the mitochondria, against their concentration gradient. This process, called chemiosmosis, involves the electron donor molecules NADH or $FADH_2$, generated from the citric acid cycle and other metabolic pathways, modifying the electrical charge of the mitochondrial enzymes. This forces the positively charged protons across the mitochondrial membrane. At the end of the mitochondrial chain the protons reach a high enough energy level to combine with molecular oxygen at cytochrome a_3, forming water. Figure 10.14 shows the transport of electrons along the chain, forcing the hydrogen ions to move against their concentration gradient. Three molecules of ATP are formed at various stages of the chain during the transfer of each hydrogen ion. The process is not associated directly with the production of carbon dioxide, which is formed only in the citric acid cycle.

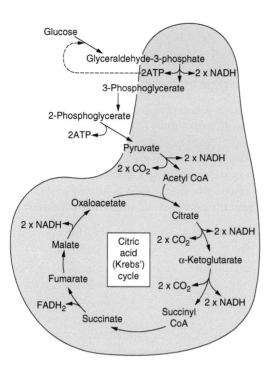

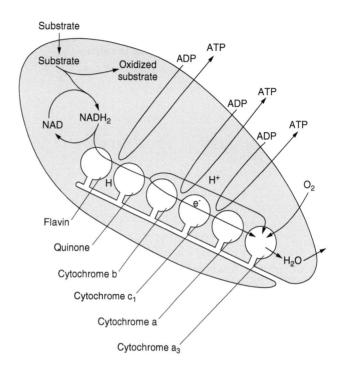

• **Fig. 10.13** Oxidative metabolic pathway of glucose by the citric acid cycle. The shaded area represents the mitochondria and indicates the reactions that can take place only within them. Substances shown straddling the shaded area are capable of diffusion across the mitochondrial membrane. Many stages of the glycolytic pathway (Fig. 10.12) have been omitted for clarity. Note that one molecule of glucose will produce two molecules of all the other intermediate substances. Only two molecules of adenosine triphosphate (ATP) are produced, along with 12 molecules of NADPH$_2$, each of which enters oxidative phosphorylation within the mitochondria, producing three molecules of ATP (Fig. 10.14). NAD, nicotinamide adenine dinucleotide; FAD, flavin adenine dinucleotide; uccinyl CoA, succinyl coenzyme A.

• **Fig. 10.14** Diagrammatic representation of oxidative phosphorylation within the mitochondrion. Intramitochondrial nicotinamide adenine dinucleotide (NAD)H$_2$ produced from glycolysis and the citric acid cycle provides hydrogen to the first of a chain of hydrogen carriers that are attached to the cristae of the mitochondria. When the hydrogen reaches the cytochromes, ionization occurs; the proton passes into the lumen of the mitochondrion, while the electron is passed along the cytochromes, where it converts ferric iron to the ferrous form. The final stage is at cytochrome a$_3$, where the proton and the electron combine with oxygen to form water. Three molecules of adenosine diphosphate (ADP) are converted to adenosine triphosphate (ATP) at the stages shown in the diagram. ADP and ATP can cross the mitochondrial membrane freely, whereas there are separate pools of intramitochondrial and extramitochondrial NAD that cannot interchange.

Cytochromes have a structure similar to haemoglobin, with an iron-containing haem complex bound within a large protein. Their activity is controlled by the availability of oxygen and hydrogen ions and the local concentrations of ATP relative to ADP and phosphate.[36,37] Different cytochromes have different values for P$_{50}$, and may act as oxygen sensors in several areas of the body. There is evidence for an interaction between nitric oxide and several cytochromes, with nitric oxide forming nitrosyl complexes in a similar fashion to its reaction with haemoglobin (page 148).[38] It is postulated that nitric oxide or nitric oxide–derived nitrosyl compounds may play an important role in controlling oxygen consumption at a mitochondrial level. High levels of endogenous nitric oxide, for example during sepsis, may produce sufficient inhibition of cytochrome activity, and therefore oxygen consumption, to contribute to the impaired tissue function seen in vital organs such as the heart.[38] The reduction of oxygen to water by cytochrome a$_3$ is inhibited by cyanide.

Significance of Aerobic Metabolism

Glycolysis under aerobic conditions and the citric acid cycle yields a total of 12 hydrogen atoms for each glucose molecule used. In turn, each hydrogen molecule enters oxidative

phosphorylation to yield three ATP molecules. These, along with the two produced during glycolysis, result in a total production of 38 ATP molecules (Table 10.3).

In vitro combustion of glucose liberates 2820 kJ.mol^{-1} as heat. Thus, under conditions of oxidative metabolism, 45% of the total energy is made available for biological work, which compares favourably with most machines.

Use of anaerobic pathways must therefore either consume much larger quantities of glucose or, alternatively, yield less ATP. In high energy-consuming organs such as brain, kidney and liver, it is not possible to transfer the increased quantities of glucose; therefore these organs suffer ATP depletion under hypoxic conditions. In contrast, voluntary muscle is able to function satisfactorily on anaerobic metabolism during short periods of time, and this is normal in the diving mammals.

Critical Oxygen Partial Pressure for Aerobic Metabolism

When the mitochondrial Po_2 is reduced, oxidative phosphorylation continues normally down to a level of about 0.3 kPa (2 mmHg). Below this level, oxygen consumption falls,

TABLE 10.3	Comparison of Energy Produced by the Two Pathways for Glucose Metabolism	
Anaerobic Pathway	**Aerobic Pathway**	
Glucose ↓ Pyruvic acid ↓ Lactic acid + 2 ATP (67 kJ of energy)	Glucose ↓ Pyruvic acid ↓ CO_2 + H_2O + 38 ATP (1270 kJ of energy)	

and the various members of the electron transport chain tend to revert to the reduced state. Reduced to oxidised nicotinamide adenine dinucleotide ($NADH/NAD^+$) and lactate/pyruvate ratios rise, and the ATP/ADP ratio falls. The critical Po_2 varies between different organs and different species, but, as an approximation, a mitochondrial Po_2 of about 0.13 kPa (1 mmHg) may be taken as the level below which there is serious impairment of oxidative phosphorylation and a switch to anaerobic metabolism. Tissue hypoxia is discussed further on page 277. The critical Po_2 for oxidative phosphorylation is also known as the Pasteur point, and has applications beyond the pathophysiology of hypoxia in man. In particular, it has a powerful bearing on putrefaction, many forms of which are anaerobic metabolism resulting from a fall of Po_2 below the Pasteur point in, for example, polluted rivers.

Tissue Po_2

It is almost impossible to quantify tissue Po_2. It is evident that there are differences between different organs, with the tissue Po_2 influenced not only by arterial Po_2 but also by the ratio of tissue oxygen consumption to perfusion.[39] However, even greater difficulties arise from the regional variations in tissue Po_2 in different parts of the same organ, which are again presumably caused by regional variations in tissue perfusion and oxygen consumption. But this is not the whole story. As described on page 119, movement of oxygen from capillaries into the tissue is by simple diffusion, with complex radial and longitudinal gradients in Po_2 around individual capillaries (see Fig. 8.4). For a single cell, the capillary Po_2 will be that of the nearest section of capillary, and so anywhere between the local arterial and venous values, and the final tissue Po_2 will also depend on the distance between the capillary and the cell, which may be up to 200 μm. These factors explain why the largest drop in Po_2 of the oxygen cascade is the final stage between capillary and mitochondrial Po_2 (Fig. 10.1). In spite of this sometimes-long diffusion path and low value for mitochondrial Po_2, oxygen supply is extremely efficient, and it is believed to be the supply of metabolic substrates (fatty acids and glucose) that normally limit cellular energy production. Tissue Po_2 is thus an unsatisfactory quantitative index of the state of oxygenation of an organ, and indirect assessments must be made (page 160).

Transport of Oxygen from the Lungs to the Cell

The Concept of Oxygen Delivery

The most important function of the respiratory and circulatory systems is the supply of oxygen to the cells of the body in adequate quantity and at a satisfactory partial pressure. The quantity of oxygen made available to the body in 1 minute is known as oxygen delivery ($\dot{D}o_2$) or oxygen flux and is equal to cardiac output × arterial oxygen content.

At rest, the numerical values are approximately:

$$\begin{array}{c}\text{5000 mL blood} \times \text{20 mL } O_2 \text{ per 100 mL}\\ \text{per min} \qquad \text{blood (arterial}\\ \text{(cardiac output)} \quad \text{oxygen content)}\\ = \text{1000 mL } O_2 \text{ per min}\\ \text{(oxygen delivery).}\end{array}$$

Of this 1000 mL.min^{-1}, approximately 250 mL.min^{-1} are used by a conscious resting subject. The circulating blood thus loses 25% of its oxygen, and the mixed venous blood is approximately 70% saturated (i.e., 95 − 25). The 70% of unextracted oxygen forms an important reserve that may be drawn upon under the stress of such conditions as exercise, to which additional extraction forms one of the integrated adaptations (see Fig. 13.3).

Oxygen consumption must clearly depend on delivery, but the relationship is nonlinear. Modest reduction of oxygen delivery is well-tolerated by the body, which is, within limits, able to draw on the reserve of unextracted venous oxygen without reduction of oxygen consumption. However, below a critical value for delivery, consumption is decreased, and the subject shows signs of hypoxia.

Quantification of Oxygen Delivery

The arterial oxygen content consists predominantly of oxygen in combination with haemoglobin, and this fraction is given by the following expression:

$$Ca_{O_2} = Sa_{O_2} \times [\text{Hb}] \times 1.39,$$

where Ca_{O_2} is the arterial oxygen content, Sa_{O_2} is the arterial oxygen saturation (as a fraction), [Hb] is the haemoglobin concentration of the blood, and 1.39 is the volume of oxygen (mL) which has been found to combine with 1 g of haemoglobin (excluding dyshaemoglobins: see page 144).

To the combined oxygen must be added the oxygen in physical solution, which will be of the order of 0.3 mL.dL^{-1}, and the expression for total arterial oxygen concentration may now be expanded thus:

$$\begin{array}{cccc} Ca_{O_2} & = (Sa_{O_2} \times [\text{Hb}] \times 1.39) & + & 0.3\\ \text{e.g., mL.dL}^{-1} & \% / 100 \text{ g.dL}^{-1} \text{ mL.g}^{-1} & & \text{mL.dL}^{-1}.\\ 19 & = (0.97 \times 14 \times 1.39) & + & 0.3 \end{array}$$

$$\text{(Eq. 10.4)}$$

Because oxygen delivery is the product of cardiac output and arterial oxygen content:

$$\dot{D}o_2 = \dot{Q} \times Ca_{o_2}$$

e.g. $\quad$ mL.min^{-1} $\qquad$ L.min^{-1} $\qquad$ mL.dL^{-1},

$$1000 = 5.25 \times 19$$

(Eq. 10.5)

$\dot{Q}$ is cardiac output (right-hand side is multiplied by a scaling factor of 10).

By combining Equations 10.4 and 10.5, the full expression for oxygen delivery is as follows:

$$\dot{D}o_2 = \dot{Q} \times \left\{ \left(Sa_{o_2} \times [Hb] \times 1.39 \right) + 0.3 \right\}$$

e.g.mL.min^{-1} $\quad$ L.min^{-1} $\quad$ %/100 $\quad$ g.dL^{-1} $\quad$ mL.g^{-1} $\quad$ mL.dL^{-1}

$$1000 = 5.25 \times \left\{ (0.97 \times 14 \times 1.39) + 0.3 \right\}$$

(Eq. 10.6)

(right-hand side is multiplied by a scaling factor of 10).

For comparison between subjects, values for oxygen delivery must be related to body size, which is done by relating the value to body surface area. Oxygen delivery divided by surface area is known as the oxygen delivery index, and has units of mL.min^{-1}.m^{-2}.

Interaction of the Factors Governing Oxygen Delivery

Equation 10.6 contains, on the right-hand side, three variable factors that determine oxygen delivery:
1. Cardiac output (or, for a particular organ, the regional blood flow). Failure of this factor has been termed 'stagnant anoxia'.
2. Arterial oxygen saturation. Failure of this (for whatever reason) has been termed 'anoxic anoxia'.
3. Haemoglobin concentration. Reduced haemoglobin, as a cause of tissue hypoxia, has been termed 'anaemic anoxia'.

The classification of anoxia into stagnant, anoxic and anaemic was proposed by Barcroft in 1920[40] and has stood the test of time. The three types of anoxia may be conveniently displayed on a Venn diagram (Fig. 10.15), which shows the possibility of combinations of any two types of anoxia or all three together. For example, the combination of anaemia and low cardiac output, which occurs in untreated haemorrhage, would be indicated by the overlapping area of the stagnant and anaemic circles (indicated by ×). If the patient also suffered from lung injury, he or she might then move into the central area, indicating the addition of anoxic anoxia. On a more cheerful note, compensations are more usual. Patients with anaemia normally have a high cardiac output; subjects resident at altitude have polycythaemia, and so on.

Relationship Between Oxygen Delivery and Consumption

The relationship between $\dot{D}o_2$ and oxygen consumption ($\dot{V}o_2$) is best illustrated on the coordinates shown in

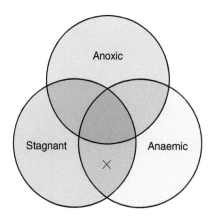

• **Fig. 10.15** Barcroft's classification of causes of hypoxia displayed on a Venn diagram to illustrate the possibility of combinations of more than one type of hypoxia. The lowest overlap, marked with a cross, shows coexistent anaemia and low cardiac output. The central area illustrates a combination of all three types of hypoxia (e.g., a patient with sepsis resulting in anaemia, circulatory failure and lung injury).

Figure 10.16. The abscissa shows oxygen delivery as previously defined, whereas consumption is shown on the ordinate. The fan of lines originating from the zero point indicates different values for oxygen extraction ($\dot{V}o_2/\dot{D}o_2$) expressed as a percentage. Because the mixed venous oxygen saturation is the arterial saturation less the extraction, it is a simple matter to indicate the mixed venous saturation, which corresponds to a particular value for extraction. The black dot indicates a typical normal resting point, with $\dot{D}o_2$ of 1000 mL.min^{-1}, $\dot{V}o_2$ of 250 mL.min^{-1} and extraction of 25%.

When oxygen delivery is moderately reduced, for whatever reason, oxygen consumption tends to be maintained at its normal value by increasing oxygen extraction and therefore decreasing mixed venous saturation. There should be no evidence of additional anaerobic metabolism, such as increased lactate production. This is termed *supply-independent oxygenation*, a condition that applies provided that delivery remains above a critical value. This is shown by the horizontal line in Figure 10.17. Below the critical level of oxygen delivery, oxygen consumption decreases as a linear function of delivery. This is termed *supply-dependent oxygenation*, and is usually accompanied by evidence of hypoxia, such as increased blood lactate and organ failure. Pathological supply dependency of oxygen consumption has been a source of controversy for many years.[41] In critically ill patients, the transition between supply-dependent and supply-independent oxygen consumption (critical oxygen delivery, see Fig. 10.17) was thought to move to the right, such that increasing oxygen delivery continued to increase oxygen consumption even at levels greater than those seen in normal healthy subjects. Early work in critical care units claimed better survival in patients in whom oxygen delivery, and therefore consumption, was increased above normal values,[41] but this was never confirmed in larger randomized studies.[42]

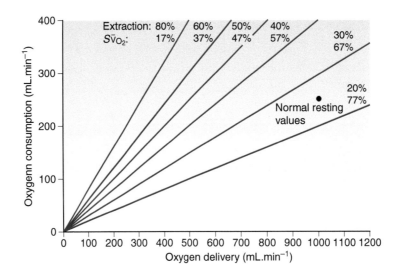

• **Fig. 10.16** Grid relating oxygen delivery and consumption to extraction and mixed venous oxygen saturation, on the assumption of 97% saturation for arterial blood. The spot marks the normal resting values. $S\bar{v}O_2$, oxygen saturation of mixed venous blood.

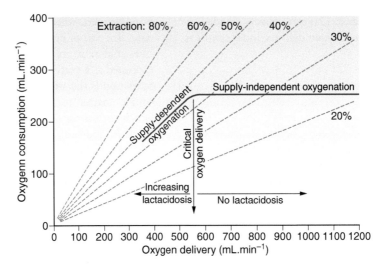

• **Fig. 10.17** This diagram is based on the grid shown in Figure 10.16. For an otherwise healthy subject, the thick horizontal line shows the extent to which oxygen delivery can be reduced without reducing oxygen consumption and causing signs of cellular hypoxia (supply-independent oxygenation). Below the postulated critical delivery, oxygen consumption becomes supply-dependent, and there are signs of hypoxia. There is uncertainty of the exact values for critical delivery in otherwise healthy subjects.

It is therefore possible that the value for critical oxygen delivery is unchanged in critically ill patients, and that pathological supply dependency may not exist at all. Current advice is to concentrate more closely on achieving normal values for cardiac output, haemoglobin and blood volume, rather than pursuing supranormal targets.

Oxygen Stores

Despite its great physiological importance, oxygen is a very difficult gas to store in a biological system. There is no satisfactory method of physical storage in the body. Haemoglobin is the most efficient chemical carrier, but more than 0.5 kg is required to carry 1 g of oxygen. The concentration of haemoglobin in blood far exceeds the concentration of any other protein in any body fluid. Even so, the quantity of oxygen in the blood is barely sufficient for 3 minutes of metabolism in the resting state. It is a fact of great clinical importance that the body oxygen stores are so small, and, if replenishment ceases, they are normally insufficient to sustain life for more than a few minutes. The principal stores are shown in Table 10.4.

TABLE 10.4	Principal Stores of Body Oxygen	
	While Breathing Air (mL)	While Breathing 100% Oxygen (mL)
In the lungs (FRC)	450	3000
In the blood	850	950
Dissolved in tissue fluids	50	?100
Combined with myoglobin	?200	?200
Total	1550	4250

FRC, Functional residual capacity.

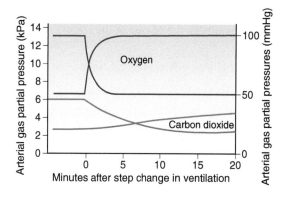

• **Fig. 10.18** The upper pair of red curves indicates the rate of change of arterial Po_2 following a step change in ventilation. Half of the total change occurs in about 30 seconds. The rising curve could be produced by an increase of alveolar ventilation from 2 to 4 L.min^{-1} while breathing air (see Fig. 10.2). The falling curve could result from the corresponding reduction of alveolar ventilation from 4 to 2 L.min^{-1}. The lower pair of blue curves indicates the time course of changes in Pco_2, which are much slower than for oxygen (these changes are shown in greater detail in Fig. 9.11).

While breathing air, not only are the total oxygen stores very small, but also, to make matters worse, only part of the stores can be released without an unacceptable reduction in Po_2. Half of the oxygen in blood is still retained when the Po_2 is reduced to 3.5 kPa (26 mmHg). Myoglobin is even more reluctant to part with its oxygen, and very little can be released above a Po_2 of 2.7 kPa (20 mmHg).

Breathing oxygen causes a substantial increase in total oxygen stores. Most of the additional oxygen is accommodated in the alveolar gas, from which 80% may be withdrawn without causing the Po_2 to fall below the normal value. With 2400 mL of easily available oxygen after breathing oxygen, there is no difficulty in breath holding for several minutes without becoming hypoxic.

The small size of the oxygen stores means that changes in factors affecting the alveolar or arterial Po_2 will produce their full effects very quickly after the change. This is in contrast to carbon dioxide, where the size of the stores buffers the body against rapid changes (page 131). Figure 10.18 compares the time course of changes in Po_2 and Pco_2 produced by the same changes in ventilation. Figure 9.11 showed how the time course of changes of Pco_2 is different for falling and rising Pco_2.

Factors that reduce the Po_2 always act rapidly, but two examples of changes that produce anoxia illustrate different degrees of 'rapid':

Circulatory arrest. When the circulation is arrested, hypoxia supervenes as soon as the oxygen in the tissues and stagnant capillaries has been exhausted. In the case of the brain, with its high rate of oxygen consumption, there is only about 10 seconds before consciousness is lost. Circulatory arrest also differs from other forms of hypoxia in the failure of clearance of products of anaerobic metabolism (e.g., lactic acid), which should not occur in arterial hypoxaemia.

Apnoea. The rate of onset of anoxia depends on many factors—the initial alveolar Po_2, the lung volume and the rate of oxygen consumption are the most important—with lesser contributions made by the initial arterial oxygen saturation, pulmonary shunt fraction and cardiac output.[43] It is, for example, more rapid while swimming underwater than while breath holding at rest in the laboratory. Generally speaking, after breathing air, 90 seconds of apnoea results in a substantial fall of Po_2 to a level that threatens loss of consciousness. If a patient has previously inhaled a few breaths of oxygen, the arterial Po_2 should remain above 13.3 kPa (100 mmHg) for at least 3 minutes of apnoea; this is the basis of the usual method of protection against hypoxia during any deliberate interference with ventilation, as, for example, during tracheal intubation.

In view of the rapid changes shown in Figure 10.18, it follows that, for a patient breathing air, a pulse oximeter will probably give an earlier indication of underventilation than will a capnogram. However, if the patient is protected from hypoxia by the inhalation of a gas mixture enriched with oxygen, then the carbon dioxide will give the earlier indication of hypoventilation. It should be remembered that oxygen levels change quickly and are potentially much more dangerous. Carbon dioxide levels change only slowly (in response to a change in ventilation) and are usually less dangerous.

Cyanosis

Cyanosis describes a blue discoloration of a subject's skin and mucous membranes and is almost universally caused by arterial hypoxaemia. Although now regarded as a sign of rather advanced hypoxia, there must have been countless occasions in which the appearance of cyanosis has given warning of hypoventilation, pulmonary shunting, stagnant circulation or decreased oxygen concentration of inspired gas. Indeed, it is interesting to speculate on the additional hazards to life if gross arterial hypoxaemia could occur without overt changes in the colour of the blood.

Central and Peripheral Cyanosis

If shed arterial blood is seen to be purple, this is a reliable indication of arterial desaturation. However, when skin or mucous membrane is inspected, most of the blood which colours the tissue is lying in veins (i.e., subpapillary venous plexuses), and its oxygen content is related to the arterial oxygen content as follows:

$$\text{venous oxygen content} = \text{arterial oxygen content} - \text{arterial/venous oxygen content difference}.$$

The last term may be expanded in terms of the tissue metabolism and perfusion:

$$\text{venous oxygen content} = \text{arterial oxygen content} - \frac{\text{tissue oxygen consumption}}{\text{tissue blood flow}}.$$

In normal circumstances, oxygen consumption by the skin is low in relation to its circulation, so the second term on the right-hand side of the second equation is generally small. Therefore the cutaneous venous oxygen content is close to that of the arterial blood, and inspection of the skin usually gives a reasonable indication of arterial oxygen content. However, when circulation is reduced in relation to skin oxygen consumption, cyanosis may occur in the presence of normal arterial oxygen levels. This occurs typically in patients with low cardiac output or in cold weather. Vigorous coughing, particularly when lying flat, or placing a patient in the Trendelenburg position causes the skin capillaries of the upper body to become engorged with venous blood, once again causing the appearance of cyanosis with normal arterial oxygen saturation.

Sensitivity of Cyanosis as an Indication of Hypoxaemia

Two factors may affect the ability to detect cyanosis. Anaemia will inevitably make cyanosis less likely to occur, and it is now generally accepted that cyanosis can be detected when arterial blood contains greater than 1.5 g.dL^{-1} of reduced haemoglobin,[44] or at an arterial oxygen saturation of 85% to 90%, although there is much variation. Such levels would probably correspond to a 'capillary' reduced haemoglobin concentration of about 3 g.dL^{-1}. The source of illumination can also affect the perceived colour of a patient's skin, with some types of fluorescent tube tending to make the patient look pinker, whereas others impart a bluer tinge.

Thus the appearance of cyanosis is considerably influenced by the circulation, patient position, haemoglobin concentration and lighting conditions. Even when all these are optimal, cyanosis is by no means a precise indication of the arterial oxygen level, and it should be regarded as a warning sign rather than a measurement. Cyanosis is detected in about half of patients who have an arterial saturation of 93%, and about 95% of patients with a saturation of 89%. In other words, cyanosis is not seen in 5% of patients at or below a saturation of 89% (arterial $P_{O_2} \approx 7.5$ kPa or 56 mmHg). It is quite clear that absence of cyanosis does not necessarily mean normal arterial oxygen levels.

Nonhypoxic cyanosis has several causes, all of which are rare but worth considering in a patient who appears cyanosed but displays no other evidence of hypoxia. Sulphhaemoglobin, and more importantly metHb (at concentrations of 1.5 g.dL^{-1}), cause a blue-grey appearance, and chronic use of drugs or remedies that include gold or silver has been reported to cause 'pseudocyanosis'.[45]

Principles of Measurement of Oxygen Levels

Oxygen Concentration in Gas Samples

Paramagnetic analysers rely on the fact that oxygen will influence an electrically generated magnetic field in direct proportion to its concentration in a mixture of gases. A particularly attractive feature of the method for physiological use is the complete lack of interference by other gases likely to be present, as significant paramagnetic properties are unique to oxygen. Measurement of breath-to-breath changes in oxygen concentrations of respired gases requires an instrument with a response time of less than about 300 ms, and current paramagnetic analysers are easily capable of this.

Fuel cells have similarities to the polarographic electrode described later. An oxygen-permeable membrane covers a cell made up of a gold cathode and lead anode separated by potassium hydroxide, which generates a current in proportion to the oxygen concentration. The response time is many seconds, so these analysers are not suitable for measuring inspired and expired oxygen concentrations. No electrical input is needed, because the fuel cell acts like a battery, generating its own power from the absorption of oxygen. However, the cell therefore also has a limited life span, depending on the total amount of oxygen to which it is exposed over time, but in normal clinical use, fuel cells last several months.

Blood P_{O_2}

This is measured by polarography, first described by Clark in 1956.[46] The technique is based on a cell comprised of a silver anode and a platinum cathode, both in contact with an electrolyte in dilute solution. If a potential difference of about 700 mV is applied to the cell, a current is passed that is directly proportional to the P_{O_2} of the electrolyte in the region of the cathode. In use, the electrolyte is separated from the sample by a thin membrane that is permeable to oxygen. The electrolyte rapidly attains the same P_{O_2} as the sample, and the current passed by the cell is proportional to the Po_2 of the sample, which may be gas, blood or other liquids. Polarographic electrodes may now be made small enough to facilitate continuous intra-arterial monitoring of Po_2, and a photochemical Po_2 sensor with a response time suitable for clinical use is also under development.[47]

Errors in Measuring Oxygen Levels

Errors arising from the handling of samples for blood gas analysis are considered on page 133. Temperature has a marked effect on Po_2 measurement. If blood Po_2 is measured at a lower temperature than the patient's Po_2, the measured Po_2 will be less than the Po_2 of the blood while it was in the patient. It is usual to maintain the measuring apparatus at 37°C, and, if the patient's body temperature differs from this by more than 1°C, then a significant error will result. Automated blood gas machines correct for this automatically, provided the patient's temperature is entered.

Transcutaneous Po_2

Cutaneous venous or capillary blood Po_2 may, under ideal conditions, be close to the arterial Po_2, but a modest reduction in skin perfusion will cause a substantial fall in Po_2, because the oxygen is consumed at the flat part of the dissociation curve, where small changes in content correspond to large changes in Po_2. Heating of the skin to 44°C minimizes differences between arterial and capillary/skin Po_2, which can be measured by a directly applied polarographic electrode.

Oxygen Saturation[3,48]

Blood oxygen saturation is measured photometrically. Near-infrared absorption spectra for different forms of haemoglobin are shown in Figure 10.19. Methods are based on the fact that the absorption of monochromatic light of certain wavelengths is the same (isosbestic) for deoxygenated and oxygenated haemoglobin (800 nm). At other wavelengths there is a marked difference between the absorption of transmitted or reflected light by the two forms of haemoglobin. Use of a greater number of different wavelengths also allows the detection and quantification of other commonly present haemoglobins. For example, current generations of cooximeter measure absorption at 128 different wavelengths, and from the spectra obtained can calculate the quantities of O_2Hb, HHb, COHb and metHb.

Pulse Oximetry

Saturation may be measured photometrically in vivo as well as in vitro. Light at two different wavelengths is either transmitted through a finger or an ear lobe or else is reflected from the skin, usually on the forehead. The usual wavelengths used are 660 nm, where there is a large difference between the oxyhaemoglobin and deoxyhaemoglobin spectra (Fig. 10.19), and 940 nm, close to the isosbestic point. With the original techniques, most of the blood that was visualized was venous or capillary rather than arterial, and the result depended on a brisk cutaneous blood flow to minimize the arterial/venous oxygen difference. The older techniques have now been completely replaced by pulse oximeters, which relate the optical densities at the two wavelengths to the pulse wave detected by the same sensor. The signal between the pulse waves is subtracted from the signal at the height of the pulse wave; the difference is because of the inflowing arterial blood reflecting the saturation of the arterial blood.

Similar to the measurement of the Hüfner constant (page 144), the presence of dyshaemoglobins (COHb and metHb) has caused controversy regarding the terminology used when discussing pulse oximetry.[3] Oxygen saturation, as originally defined by Christian Bohr, is the ratio

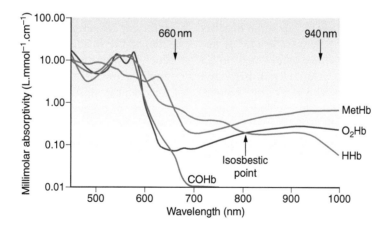

• **Fig. 10.19** Near-infrared absorption spectra for the four common types of haemoglobin seen in vivo. The isosbestic point for oxyhaemoglobin (O_2Hb) and deoxyhaemoglobin (HHb) is shown. To measure oxygen saturation, pulse oximeters use two wavelengths at around 660 and 940 nm, where the absorptivities of O_2Hb and HHb differ significantly. If measurement of carboxyhaemoglobin (COHb) and methaemoglobin (metHb) is also required, a greater number of wavelengths must be used, and current generations of cooximeter use over 100 different wavelengths. (From Zijlstra WG, Buursma A, Meeuwsen-van der Roest WP. Absorption spectra of human fetal and adult oxyhemoglobin, de-oxyhemoglobin, carboxyhemoglobin, and methemoglobin. *Clin Chem.* 1991;37:1633-1638.)

of O_2Hb to active, oxygen-binding Hb (= O_2Hb + HHb), rather than the more commonly used definition of the ratio of O_2Hb to total Hb. The original definition is the more relevant, as COHb and metHb do not carry oxygen and do not affect pulse oximeter readings.[9] Pulse oximeter So_2 values are therefore a good assessment of pulmonary oxygenation, but not necessarily of oxygen carriage. Provided the dyshaemoglobins are only present in small quantities, as is usually the case, this distinction is of minor clinical importance. However, when larger quantities of dyshaemoglobins are present, particularly with carbon monoxide poisoning, the pulse oximeter will give falsely reassuring readings. For example, if 30% of the total haemoglobin present is bound to carbon monoxide and Po_2 is normal, the pulse oximeter will read normal values despite the oxygen content of the blood being reduced by 30%. With metHb a more complex situation results, because its absorption spectrum is more similar to those of O_2Hb and HHb than that of COHb (Fig. 10.19), so it causes a slight reduction in So_2 readings up to about 20% metHb. At higher levels of metHb, pulse oximeter readings tend to become fixed at about 85%. A pulse co-oximeter is now available that uses eight different wavelengths of light, which allows noninvasive measurement of dyshaemoglobins, achieving an accuracy that makes it a useful screening tool for patients at risk of carboxyhaemoglobinaemia.[49]

There are many other sources of error with pulse oximetry. Currently available pulse oximeters continue to function even in the presence of arterial hypotension, although there may be a delayed indication of changes in So_2, and readings become less accurate below a systolic blood pressure of 80 mmHg.[50] Anaemia tends to exaggerate desaturation readings: at a haemoglobin concentration of 80 g.L^{-1} normal saturations were correctly recorded, but there was a mean bias of −15% at a true So_2 of 53.6%.[51] Patients with dark skin were previously reported to have accurate readings with pulse oximetry, but some bias has been demonstrated at lower So_2 values (<80%).[52] If fingers or toes are used for pulse oximetry, then nail polish should be removed, as different coloured polishes cause variable decreases in So_2 values, with red/purple colours having less effect and darker or green/blue colours causing an average of between 1.6% and 5.5% fall in So_2 values.[53] Acrylic nails have also been shown to cause minor inaccuracies in pulse oximeter readings with some, but not all, instruments.[54] Finally, technical problems with pulse oximetry such as degradation of the light-emitting diode over time and 'wear and tear' of cables in the clinical environment can potentially cause inaccurate readings in a large proportion of oximeters.[55]

Calibration of pulse oximeters presents a problem. Optical filters may be used for routine calibration, but the gold standard is calibration against arterial blood Po_2 or saturation, which is seldom undertaken. When oxygenation is critical, there is no substitute for direct measurement of arterial Po_2.

Tissue Po_2

Clearly the tissue Po_2 is of greater significance than the Po_2 at various intermediate stages higher in the oxygen cascade. It would therefore appear logical to attempt the measurement of Po_2 in the tissues, but this has proved difficult both in technique and in interpretation. For experimental procedures, needle electrodes may be inserted directly into tissue and Po_2 measured on the tip of a needle. Difficulties of interpretation arise from the fact that Po_2 varies immensely within the tissue, so even if a mean tissue Po_2 can be measured, this may not represent Po_2 in the more relevant 'lethal corner' region (page 120).

Tissue Surface Electrodes

Miniaturized oxygen monitors may be placed on or attached to the surface of an organ to indicate the Po_2. The device may simply be a small polarographic electrode, but more recently developed techniques use fluorophores,[39] which are molecules that emit light energy when illuminated with light of a different wavelength. Several fluorophores exist which are responsive to oxygen levels, and these can either be used on the tip of probes for insertion into the tissue or even administered systemically. Interpretation of the reading is subject to many of the same limitations as with the needle electrode. Nevertheless, tissue surface Po_2 may provide the surgeon with useful information regarding perfusion and viability in cases of organ ischaemia.

Near-Infrared Spectroscopy[56]

In tissues that are relatively translucent the biochemical state of tissue oxidation may be determined using transmission spectroscopy in the near-infrared range (700–1000 nm). The state of relative oxidation of haemoglobin, myoglobin and cytochrome a_3 may be determined within this wave band. At present it is feasible to study transmission spectroscopy over a path length up to about 9 cm, which is sufficient to permit monitoring of the brain of newborn infants. Use in adults requires reflectance spectroscopy, and does allow assessment of oxygenation in, for example, an area of a few cubic centimetres of brain tissue. This is useful, for example, during surgery on the carotid arteries, when changes in oxygenation in the area supplied by the artery concerned can be followed. However, the technique has failed to gain widespread acceptance because of interference from extracranial tissue,[57] particularly scalp blood flow, and difficulties with calibrating the readings and defining any 'normal' values.

Indirect Assessment of Tissue Oxygenation

Such are the difficulties of measurements of tissue Po_2 that in clinical practice it is more usual simply to seek evidence of anaerobic tissue metabolism. In the absence of this, tissue perfusion and oxygenation can be assumed to be acceptable. Indirect methods that assess global (i.e., whole body) tissue perfusion include mixed venous oxygen saturation, measured either by sampling pulmonary arterial blood or using a fibreoptic catheter to measure oxygen saturation continuously in the pulmonary artery. Blood lactate levels also provide a global indication of tissue perfusion. However, acceptable global tissue oxygenation provides no reassurance about function either of regions in an individual organ or in an entire organ. Methods of assessing oxygenation in a specific tissue have focused on the gut, because of ease of access and the observation that gut blood flow is often the first to be reduced when oxygen delivery is inadequate. Gastric intramucosal pH measurement allows an assessment to be made of cellular pH within the stomach mucosa, which has been shown to correlate with other assessments of tissue oxygenation and patient well-being during critical illness.

Measurement of Oxygen Consumption and Delivery

Oxygen Consumption

There are three main methods for the measurement of oxygen consumption:
1. Oxygen loss from (or replacement into) a closed breathing system
2. Subtraction of the expired from the inspired volume of oxygen
3. Multiplication of cardiac output by arterial/mixed venous oxygen content difference

Oxygen Loss from a Closed Breathing System

Probably the simplest method of measuring oxygen consumption is by observing the loss of volume from a closed-circuit spirometer, with expired carbon dioxide absorbed by soda lime. It is essential that the spirometer should initially contain an oxygen-enriched mixture so that the inspired oxygen concentration does not fall to a level that is dangerous for the subject or patient. Alternatively, a known flow rate of oxygen may be added to maintain the volume of the spirometer and its oxygen concentration constant: under these conditions, the oxygen inflow rate must equal the oxygen consumption.

Subtraction of Expired from Inspired Volume of Oxygen

The essence of the technique is subtraction of the volume of oxygen breathed out (expired minute volume × mixed expired oxygen concentration) from the volume of oxygen breathed in (inspired minute volume × inspired oxygen concentration). The difference between the inspired and expired minute volumes is a very important factor in achieving accuracy with the method, particularly when a high concentration of oxygen is inhaled. Inspired and expired minute volumes differ as a result of the respiratory exchange ratio, and also any exchange of inert gas (e.g., nitrogen) that might occur. On the assumption that the patient is in equilibrium for nitrogen, and the mass of nitrogen inspired is the same as that expired, it follows that the ratio of inspired/expired minute volumes is inversely proportional to the respective ratios of nitrogen concentrations. Therefore:

Inspired minute volume
$$= \text{expired minute volume} \times \frac{\text{Expired nitrogen concentration}}{\text{Inspired nitrogen concentration}}.$$

This is the basis of the classical Douglas bag technique, in which expired gas is measured for volume and analysed for oxygen and carbon dioxide concentrations. The expired nitrogen concentration is determined by subtraction, and the inspired minute volume derived.

Multiplication of Cardiac Output by Arterial/Mixed Venous Oxygen Content Difference

This approach is the reverse of using the Fick principle for measurement of cardiac output (see page 85), and is commonly known as the reversed Fick technique:

$$\dot{V}_{O_2} = \dot{Q}\left(Ca_{O_2} - C\bar{v}_{O_2}\right),$$

where $\dot{V}_{O_2}$ is the oxygen consumption, $\dot{Q}$ is the cardiac output, Ca_{O_2} is the arterial oxygen content and $C\bar{v}_{O_2}$ is the mixed venous oxygen content.

The technique is essentially invasive, as the cardiac output must be measured by an independent method (usually thermodilution), and it is also necessary to sample arterial and mixed venous blood, the latter preferably from the pulmonary artery. Nevertheless, it is convenient in the critical care situation where the necessary vascular lines may be in place.

The method has a larger random error than the gasometric techniques previously described, but also has a systematic error as it excludes the oxygen consumption of the lungs. Studies comparing the two methods in humans show wide variations between different patient groups. The necessity for invasive monitoring prevents the study of normal awake subjects, but results from patients in intensive care (with presumed lung pathology) do not seem to differ from patients with normal lungs undergoing routine surgery.[58]

Oxygen Delivery

Oxygen delivery is measured as the product of cardiac output and arterial oxygen content. This excludes oxygen delivered for consumption within the lung. In the intensive care situation, cardiac output is now commonly measured by thermal dilution, and simultaneously an arterial sample is drawn for measurement of oxygen content by any of the methods described earlier. If oxygen delivery is determined at the same time as oxygen consumption is measured by the reversed Fick technique, it should be remembered that two of the variables (cardiac output and arterial oxygen content) are common to both measurements. This linking of data is a potential source of error in inferring the consequences of changes in one product on the other (see page 155).[59]

References

1. Russo R, Benazzi L, Perrella M. The Bohr effect of hemoglobin intermediates and the role of salt bridges in the tertiary/quaternary transitions. *J Biol Chem.* 2001;276:13628-13634.
2. Ho C. Perussi JR. Proton nuclear magnetic resonance studies of haemoglobin. *Methods Enzymol.* 1994;232:97-139.
3. Toffaletti J, Zijlstra WG. Misconceptions in reporting oxygen saturation. *Anesth Analg.* 2007;105:S5-S9.
4. Adair GS. The hemoglobin system. VI. The oxygen dissociation curve of hemoglobin. *J Biol Chem.* 1925;63:529-545.
5. Imai K. Adair fitting to oxygen equilibration curves of hemoglobin. *Methods Enzymol.* 1994;232:559-576.
6. Kelman GR. Digital computer subroutine for the conversion of oxygen tension into saturation. *J Appl Physiol.* 1966;21:1375-1376.
7. Severinghaus JW, Stafford M, Thunstrom AM. Estimation of skin metabolism and blood flow with tcPO2 and tcPCO2 electrodes by cuff occlusion of the circulation. *Acta Anaesthesiol Scand Supp.* 1978;68:9-15.
8. Thomas LJ. Algorithms for selected blood acid-base and blood gas calculations. *J Appl Physiol.* 1972;33:154-158.
9. Dash RK, Korman B, Bassingthwaighte JB. Simple accurate mathematical models of blood HbO2 and HbCO2 dissociation curves at varied physiological conditions: evaluation and comparison with other models. *Eur J Appl Physiol.* 2016;116:97-113.
10. Dufu K, Yalcin O, Ao-Ieong ESY, et al. GBT1118, a potent allosteric modifier of hemoglobin O2 affinity, increases tolerance to severe hypoxia in mice. *Am J Physiol Heart Circ Physiol.* 2017;313:H381-H391.
11. Orlov D, Karkouti K. The pathophysiology and consequences of red blood cell storage. *Anaesthesia.* 2015;70(suppl 1):29-37.
12. Heaton A, Keegan T, Holme S. In vivo regeneration of red cell 2, 3-diphosphoglycerate following transfusion of DPG-depleted AS-1, AS-3 and CPDA-1 red cells. *Br J Haematol.* 1989;71:131-136.
13. Rygård SL, Jonsson AB, Madsen MB, et al. Effects of shorter versus longer storage time of transfused red blood cells in adult ICU patients: a systematic review with meta-analysis and trial sequential analysis. *Intensive Care Med.* 2018;44:204-217.
14. Marshall BE, Whyche MQ. Hypoxemia during and after anesthesia. *Anesthesiology.* 1972;37:178-209.
15. Gaston B, Singel D, Doctor A, et al. S-Nitrosothiol signaling in respiratory biology. *Am J Respir Crit Care Med.* 2006;173:1186-1193.
16. Hogg N. The biochemistry and physiology of S-nitrosothiols. *Annu Rev Pharmacol Toxicol.* 2002;42:585-600.
17. Pawloski JR, Hess DT, Stamler JS. Export by red blood cells of nitric oxide bioactivity. *Nature.* 2001;409:622-626.
18. Atkins JL, Day BW, Handrigan MT, et al. Brisk production of nitric oxide and associated formation of S-nitrosothiols in early hemorrhage. *J Appl Physiol.* 2006;100:1267-1277.
19. Wajcman H, Galacteros F. Abnormal haemoglobins with high oxygen affinity and erythrocytosis. *Hematol Cell Ther.* 1996;38:305-312.
*20. Piel FB, Steinberg MH, Rees DC. Sickle cell disease. *N Engl J Med.* 2017;376:1561-1573.
21. Mehari A, Klings ES. Chronic pulmonary complications of sickle cell disease. *Chest.* 2016;149:1313-1324.
22. Alper SL. Harnessing red cell membrane pathophysiology towards point-of-care diagnosis for sickle cell disease. *J Physiol.* 2013;591(6):1403-1404.
23. Lettre G, Bauer DE. Fetal haemoglobin in sickle-cell disease: from genetic epidemiology to new therapeutic strategies. *Lancet.* 2016;387:2554-2564.
24. de Montalembert M, Brousse V, Chakravorty S, et al. Are the risks of treatment to cure a child with severe sickle cell disease too high? *BMJ.* 2017;359:j5250.

25. Taher AT, Weatherall DJ, Cappellini MD. Thalassaemia. *Lancet.* 2018;391:155-167.
26. Guay J. Methemoglobinemia related to local anesthetics: a summary of 242 episodes. *Anesth Analg.* 2009;108:837-845.
27. Spiess BD. Perflurocarbon emulsions: one approach to intravenous artificial respiratory gas transport. *Int Anesthesiol Clin.* 1995;33:103-113.
28. Spahn DR, van Brempt R, Theilmeier G, et al. Perflubron emulsion delays blood transfusions in orthopaedic surgery. European Perflubron emulsion study group. *Anesthesiology.* 1999;91:1195-1208.
29. Tobias MD, Longnecker DE. Recombinant haemoglobin and other blood substitutes. *Baillières Clin Anaesth.* 1995;9:165-179.
30. Chang TMS. Future generations of red blood cell substitutes. *J Intern Med.* 2003;253:527-535.
31. Weiskopf RB. Hemoglobin-based oxygen carriers: disclosed history and the way ahead: the relativity of safety. *Anesth Analg.* 2014;119:758-760.
32. Looker D, Abbott-Brown D, Kozart P, et al. A human recombinant hemoglobin designed for use as a blood substitute. *Nature.* 1992;356:258-260.
33. Taverne YJ, de Wijs-Meijler D, te Lintel Hekkert M, et al. Normalization of hemoglobin-based oxygen carrier-201 induced vasoconstriction: targeting nitric oxide and endothelin. *J Appl Physiol.* 2017;122:1227-1237.
34. Awasthi V, Yee S-H, Jerabek P, et al. Cerebral oxygen delivery by liposome- encapsulated hemoglobin: a positron-emission tomographic evaluation in a rat model of hemorrhagic shock. *J Appl Physiol.* 2007;103:28-38.
35. Lu SJ, Feng Q, Park JS. Biologic properties and enucleation of red blood cells from human embryonic stem cells. *Blood.* 2008;112:4475-4484.
*36. Wilson DF. Oxidative phosphorylation: regulation and role in cellular and tissue metabolism. *J Physiol.* 2017;595:7023-7038.
37. Wilson DF, Harrison DK, Vinogradov SA. Oxygen, pH, and mitochondrial oxidative phosphorylation. *J Appl Physiol.* 2012;113:1838-1845.
38. Shen W, Hintze TH, Wolin MS. Nitric oxide: an important signaling mechanism between vascular endothelium and parenchymal cells in the regulation of oxygen consumption. *Circulation.* 1995;92:3505-3512.
39. De Santis V, Singer M. Tissue oxygen tension monitoring of organ perfusion: rationale, methodologies, and literature review. *Br J Anaesth.* 2015;115:357-365.
40. Barcroft J. Physiological effects of insufficient oxygen supply. *Nature.* 1920;106:125-129.
41. Hinds C, Watson D. Manipulating hemodynamics and oxygen transport in critically ill patients. *N Engl J Med.* 1995;333:1074-1075.
42. Kem JW, Shoemaker WC. Meta-analysis of haemodynamic optimization in high-risk patients. *Crit Care Med.* 2002;30:1686-1692.
43. Farmery AD. Simulating hypoxia and modelling the airway. *Anaesthesia.* 2011;66(suppl 2):11-18.
44. Goss GA, Hayes JA, Burdon JAW. Deoxyhaemoglobin in the detection of central cyanosis. *Thorax.* 1988;43:212-213.
45. Timmins AC, Morgan GAR. Argyria or cyanosis. *Anaesthesia.* 1988;43:755-756.
46. Clark LC. Monitor and control of tissue oxygen tensions. *Trans Am Soc Artif Intern Organs.* 1956;2:41-48.
47. Formenti F, Farmery AD. Intravascular oxygen sensors with novel applications for bedside respiratory monitoring. *Anaesthesia.* 2017;72(suppl 1):95-104.
48. Severinghaus JW. Monitoring oxygenation. *J Clin Monit Comput.* 2011;25:155-161.
49. Zaoutera C, Zavorsky GS. The measurement of carboxyhemoglobin and methemoglobin using a non-invasive pulse CO-oximeter. *Respir Physiol Neurobiol.* 2012;182:88-92.

50. Hinkelbein J, Genzwuerker HV, Fiedler F. Detection of a systolic pressure threshold for reliable readings in pulse oximetry. *Resuscitation*. 2005;64:315-319.

51. Severinghaus JW, Koh SO. Effect of anemia on pulse oximeter accuracy at low saturation. *J Clin Monit*. 1990;6:85-88.

52. Feiner JR, Severinghaus JW, Bickler PE. Dark skin decreases the accuracy of pulse oximeters at low oxygen saturation: the effects of oximeter probe. *Anesth Analg*. 2007;105:S18-S23.

53. Hinkelbein J, Genzwuerker HV, Sogl R, et al. Effect of nail polish on oxygen saturation determined by pulse oximetry in critically ill patients. *Resuscitation*. 2007;72:82-91.

54. Hinkelbein J, Koehler H, Genzwuerker HV, et al. Artificial acrylic finger nails may alter pulse oximetry measurement. *Resuscitation*. 2007;74:75-82.

55. Milner QJW, Mathews GR. An assessment of the accuracy of pulse oximeters. *Anaesthesia*. 2012;67:396-401.

56. Davis ML, Barstow TJ. Estimated contribution of hemoglobin and myoglobin to near infrared spectroscopy. *Respir Physiol Neurobiol*. 2013;186:180-187.

57. Caccioppola A, Carbonara M, Macrì M, et al. Ultrasound-tagged near-infrared spectroscopy does not disclose absent cerebral circulation in brain-dead adults. *Br J Anaesth*. 2018;121:588-594.

58. Saito H, Minamiya Y, Kawai H, et al. Estimation of pulmonary oxygen consumption in the early postoperative period after thoracic surgery. *Anaesthesia*. 2007;62:648-653.

59. Walsh TS, Lee A. Mathematical coupling in medical research: lessons from studies of oxygen kinetics. *Br J Anaesth*. 1998;81:118-120.

11

Nonrespiratory Functions of the Lung

KEY POINTS

- The entire cardiac output passes through the pulmonary circulation, so the lungs act as a filter, preventing emboli from passing to the left side of the circulation.
- The lungs constitute a huge interface between the outside environment and the body, requiring the presence of

multiple systems for defence against inhaled biological and chemical hazards.
- In the pulmonary circulation there is active uptake and metabolism of many endogenous compounds, including amines, peptides and eicosanoids.

The lungs' primary purpose is gas exchange, and to achieve this with such efficiency almost the entire blood volume passes through the lungs during each circulation. This characteristic makes the lungs ideally suited to undertake many other important functions. The location of the lungs within the circulatory system is ideal for its role as a filter to protect the systemic circulation, not only from particulate matter but also from a wide range of chemical substances that undergo removal or biotransformation in the pulmonary circulation. The pulmonary arterial tree is well adapted for the reception of emboli without resultant infarction, and the very large area of vascular endothelium gives the lung a metabolic role out of proportion to its total mass. This large interface between the external atmosphere and the circulation is not without its own hazards, and the lung must protect the circulation from many potentially harmful inhaled substances.

Filtration

Sitting astride the whole output of the right ventricle, the lung is ideally situated to filter out particulate matter from the systemic venous return. Without such a filter, there would be a constant risk of particulate matter entering the arterial system, where the coronary and cerebral circulations are particularly vulnerable to damaging emboli. The vast majority of emboli are thrombus, but nonthrombotic emboli also occur and may be organic (e.g., air, tumour, fat, amniotic fluid) or inorganic (e.g., catheter tips or radiotherapy seeds).[1]

Pulmonary capillaries have a diameter of approximately 7 μm, but this does not appear to be the effective pore size of the pulmonary circulation when considered as a filter. For

example, it is well known that small quantities of gas and fat emboli may gain access to the systemic circulation in patients without obvious intracardiac shunting. Emboli may bypass the alveoli via some of the precapillary anastomoses that are known to exist in the pulmonary circulation, either between the bronchial and pulmonary circulations (page 73) or through the intrapulmonary arteriovenous anastomoses. The last of these are much larger than normal capillaries, at 25 to 50 μm diameter, but fortunately remain closed most of the time (page 12), most commonly opening during hypoxic conditions. Despite this, in one-third of normal healthy subjects echocardiography demonstrates transpulmonary passage of microbubble contrast, and this is reduced by breathing 100% oxygen.[2] More extensive invasion of the systemic circulation may occur in the presence of a right-to-left intracardiac shunt, which is now known to be quite common. Postmortem studies show that over 25% of the population have a 'probe-patent' foramen ovale, usually in the form of a slit-like defect that acts as a valve, and which is therefore normally kept closed by the left atrial pressure being slightly greater than the right.[3] In 10% of normal subjects, a simple Valsalva manoeuvre or cough results in easily demonstrable blood flow between the right and left atria. Paradoxical embolism may therefore result from a relative increase in right atrial pressure caused by physiological events or pulmonary embolism (Chapter 29).

As far as the survival of the lung is concerned, the geometry of the pulmonary microcirculation is particularly well adapted to maintaining alveolar perfusion in the face of quite large degrees of embolization. However, a significant degree of embolization inevitably blocks the circulation to parts of the lung, disturbing the balance between ventilation and perfusion. This situation is considered in Chapter 29.

Pulmonary microembolism with small clumps of fibrin and/or platelets will not have a direct effect on gas exchange until it is very extensive. Plugging of pulmonary capillaries by microemboli does, however, initiate neutrophil activation in the area, leading to an increase in endothelial permeability and alveolar oedema, and has been implicated in the aetiology of acute lung injury (Chapter 31).

Thrombi are cleared more rapidly from the lungs than from other organs. The lung possesses well-developed proteolytic systems not confined to the removal of fibrin. Pulmonary endothelium is known to be rich in plasmin activator, which converts plasminogen into plasmin, which in turn converts fibrin into fibrin degradation products. However, the lung is also rich in thromboplastin, which converts prothrombin to thrombin. To complicate the position further, the lung is a particularly rich source of heparin, and bovine lung is used in its commercial preparation. The lung can thus produce high concentrations of substances necessary for promoting or delaying blood clotting, and also for fibrinolysis. Apart from the lung's ability to clear itself of thromboemboli, these substances may play a role in controlling the overall coagulability of the blood.

Defence Against Inhaled Substances

The skin, gastrointestinal tract and lungs form the major interfaces between the outside world and the carefully controlled internal body systems. Efficient gas exchange in the lung requires a physically very thin interface between air and blood, which leaves the lung vulnerable to invasion by many airborne hazards, both chemical and biological. These are almost entirely prevented from reaching the distal airways by the airway lining fluid found throughout the tracheobronchial tree.

Airway Lining Fluid

Within the airway lining fluid there are two distinct layers, a periciliary or 'sol' layer which is of low viscosity containing water and solutes and in which the cilia are embedded, and a mucous or 'gel' layer above.[4,5]

Mucous Layer[5]

Large airways are completely lined by a mucous layer, whereas in smaller, more distal airways the mucus is found in 'islands', and a mucous layer is absent in small bronchioles and beyond. Mucus is 97% water, and about one-third of the remaining 3% is glycoproteins called mucins,[6] which determine the viscoelastic and other properties of the mucus. The human genome encodes 17 mucins, of which only seven are secreted, while the remainder are membrane-bound mucins.[4] Mucin is released by rapid (<150 ms) exocytosis from the mucous-secreting goblet cells in response to a range of stimuli, including direct chemical irritation, inflammatory cytokines and neuronal stimulation, predominantly by cholinergic nerves. Mucins have a core composed of glycoprotein subunits joined by disulphide

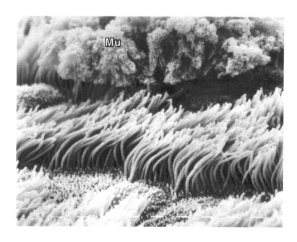

• **Fig. 11.1** Scanning electron micrograph of ciliated epithelial cells beneath the mucous *(Mu)* lining the larger airways. (From Dr P. K. Jeffery, Imperial College School of Science, Technology and Medicine, London and the publishers of Brewis RAL, Corrin B, Geddes DM, et al., eds. *Respiratory Medicine.* London: WB Saunders; 1995:54-72. With permission.)

bonds, and their length may extend up to 6 μm. The core is 80% glycosylated, with side chains attached via *O*-glycosidic bonds. Almost all terminate in sialic acid and possess microorganism binding sites. Mucus plays a vital role in pathogen entrapment and removal, and also has a variety of antimicrobial actions (see later).

Ciliary Function[7,8]

The mucous layer is propelled cephalad by the ciliated epithelial cells (Fig. 11.1) at an average rate of 4 mm. min^{-1}, to be passed through the posterior commissure of the larynx between the vocal folds into the oesophagus and swallowed, or removed by expectoration.[4] The cilia beat mostly within the low-viscosity periciliary layer of airway lining fluid, with the cilia tips intermittently gripping the underside of the mucous layer, propelling the mucous layer along the airway wall.

Cilial beat frequency is 12 to 14 beats per second, but this may speed up in response to increased extracellular adenosine triphosphate (ATP) levels,[9] and is affected by pollutants, tobacco smoke, anaesthetic agents and infection. There is a general slowing of ciliary activity with increasing age.[8] Two phases occur for each beat (Fig. 11.2). First is the recovery stroke, which occupies 75% of the time of each cycle and involves a slow bowing movement away from the resting position by a sideways action of the cilium. Then follows the power stroke, in which the cilium extends to its full height, gripping the mucous layer above with claws on its tip, before moving forward in a plane perpendicular to the cell below and returning to its resting position. Adjacent cilia somehow coordinate their strokes to produce waves of activity that move the mucous layer along, probably by a physical effect of cilia stimulating adjacent cilia during the sideways sweep of the recovery stroke.

Periciliary Layer

For this propulsion system to work effectively, it is crucial that the depth of the periciliary fluid layer be closely

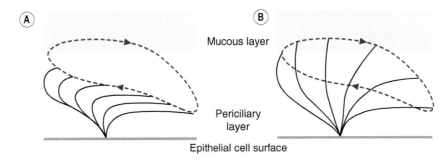

• **Fig. 11.2** Mechanism of action of a single cilium on the respiratory epithelium. **(A)** Recovery stroke in which the cilium bows backwards and sideways within the low-viscosity periciliary layer. **(B)** Power stroke in which the cilium extends perpendicular to the epithelial cell into the mucous layer and propels it forwards. The red dashed line shows the trajectory of the cilium tip.

controlled to 7 μm deep, particularly considering the increasing amount of mucus that will occur each time two smaller airways converge into one larger airway. The depth of both layers of the airway lining fluid is controlled by changes in the volume of secretions and the speed of their reabsorption, with both processes occurring simultaneously in different regions of airways.[10] If the periciliary layer reduces in depth, the gel layer will compensate for this by donating liquid to the periciliary layer to maintain the correct depth of fluid, an effect probably mediated by simple osmotic gradients between the two layers. The mucous layer may donate fluid to the periciliary layer until its volume is diminished by 70%. The reverse happens as the mucus converges on the larger airways, with the mucous layer absorbing excess periciliary water. Airway epithelium is freely permeable to water, so the volume of periciliary fluid is therefore determined by its salt concentration, which is in turn controlled by active ion transport on the surface of the epithelial cells. Several ion channels are responsible for this active control,[11] the most important of which are amiloride-sensitive epithelial sodium channels and the chloride channel better known as the cystic fibrosis transmembrane regulator (CFTR) protein. CFTR is likely to be partially active at rest but is stimulated when sodium channels are inhibited. The factors responsible for controlling this system are incompletely understood, but a critical component is the various adenine nucleotides released from ciliated cells in response to mechanical stress, acting on the same cells to influence the ion channels controlling fluid transfer into the periciliary layer.[4,12]

Dysfunction of this mucociliary system causes severe lung disease from an early age. In patients with both cystic fibrosis, an inherited defect of CFTR which adversely affects the regulation of airway lining fluid homeostasis (Chapter 28), and the rare inherited condition primary ciliary dyskinesia,[13] lung disease occurs soon after birth in many cases.

Humidification

The airway lining fluid acts as a heat and moisture exchanger to humidify and warm inspired gas. During inspiration, relatively cool, dry air causes evaporation of surface water and cooling of the airway lining, then on expiration moisture condenses on the surface of the mucus and warming occurs. Thus only about one-half of the heat and moisture needed to condition (fully warm and saturate) each breath is lost to the atmosphere. With quiet nasal breathing, air is conditioned before reaching the trachea, but as ventilation increases smaller airways are recruited until, at minute volumes of over 50 L.min^{-1}, airways of 1 mm in diameter are involved in humidification.

Inhaled Particles

Where in the respiratory tract inhaled particles are deposited depends on both their size and the breathing pattern during inhalation. Three mechanisms cause deposition:

1. Inertial impaction occurs with large particles (>3 μm). Particles greater than 8 μm rarely reach further than the pharynx before impaction, whereas smaller particles penetrate further into the respiratory tract. Inertial impaction is greatly influenced by the velocity of the particles, so a greater inspiratory flow rate and tidal volume will increase the penetration into the lungs of large particles.

2. Sedimentation occurs with particles of 1 to 3 μm, and occurs in the smaller airways or alveoli where slow gas velocity allows the particles to fall out of suspension and be deposited on lung tissue. Breath holding after inhalation of particles encourages sedimentation. Particles of this size pass easily into the alveoli, and may either diffuse back out of the alveolus to be exhaled or be deposited on the alveolar walls, where they will be absorbed into the tissue or ingested by alveolar macrophages. After deposition, different dust types have variable persistence in the lung; some are rapidly cleared, and others persist within the pulmonary macrophage for many years. Differing particle types activate the macrophage to varying extents, but may stimulate cytokine release and cause lung inflammation that then proceeds to lung tissue repair, the deposition of collagen and pulmonary fibrosis.

3. Diffusion, caused by Brownian motion of particles, occurs with particles less than 1 μm in size. These particles should simply be inhaled and exhaled with minimal contact with the airway or alveolar walls, although modelling studies suggest some very small particles (0.1 μm) will be deposited near alveolar openings.[14]

Aiding all these mechanisms is the high humidity within the respiratory tract. Absorption of water by the particle during its journey along the airways will increase the particle's mass, and so encourage both inertial impaction and sedimentation to occur. Naturally this affects hygroscopic particles to a greater degree. Any particles which are not trapped by the airway lining fluid and deposited in the alveoli are cleared by alveolar macrophages.[5]

Defence Against Inhaled Pathogens[15]

As an interface with the outside environment, the lung is exposed to a great many organisms carried by the approximately 10 000 L of air breathed each day. Pulmonary defence mechanisms have evolved to protect the respiratory tract from invasion by microorganisms. They can be subdivided into direct removal of the pathogen, chemical inactivation of the invading organism and, if these fail, immune defences.

Direct Removal of Pathogens

With normal nasal breathing, a majority of inhaled pathogens impact on the nasal mucous which is swept backwards by the ciliated nasal epithelium and swallowed. At higher inspiratory flow rates, for example when a subject is dyspnoeic, pathogens will penetrate deeper into the airways and be trapped by the sticky mucous layer of the airway lining fluid before being removed.

Chemical Inactivation of Pathogens

Airway lining fluid is more than a simple transport mechanism for impacted microorganisms. Some smaller particles will penetrate far into the bronchial tree and take some time to be transported out of the respiratory tract. To prevent these organisms from causing damage during this time, the airway lining fluid contains multiple systems for killing pathogens. Surfactant proteins are part of a larger protein family referred to as collectins. In addition to their role in reducing lung compliance (page 16), they also act as part of the innate defences in the lung. Surfactant proteins A and D are the most active in pulmonary defence, responding to specific molecular patterns on common respiratory pathogens to opsonize or neutralize the pathogen directly and stimulate macrophage migration and release of other inflammatory cytokines. Lysozyme is also present in airway lining fluid. This enzyme, secreted by neutrophils, is capable of destroying microbial cell walls, causing bacterial lysis, particularly of grampositive bacteria.

Finally, airway lining fluid contains a range of natural antimicrobial peptides, broadly divided into cathelicidins, human β-defensins (HBDs) and neutrophil α-defensins.[16] These are small molecular weight (3- to 5-kD) peptides with a broad antimicrobial range, acting either directly on the bacterial cell wall or indirectly by stimulating respiratory epithelial cells to release chemokines to recruit inflammatory cells. α-Defensins are released from neutrophils, and

have activity against a range of bacteria and the herpes simplex virus. HBDs originate from the epithelial cells, and at least four have been identified. HBD-1 is found in lung secretions in normal individuals, whereas HBD-2 is found in secretions of patients with cystic fibrosis, as well as those with inflammatory lung disease. These small peptides contribute to inflammation and repair. Defective functioning of HBDs in the airway lining fluid is believed to be a major contributor to chronic airway infection in cystic fibrosis (Chapter 28).[17]

Control of these systems rests mostly with the epithelial cells, which express on their surface several types of toll-like receptors (TLRs)[18] which recognize various molecular components of respiratory pathogens such as viral RNA, nonmammalian DNA and bacterial lipopolysaccharide or lipopeptides. Activation of TLRs initiates a chain of responses such as increased secretion of defensins, activation of the cathelicidins (a reaction requiring vitamin D), generation of inflammatory cytokines and changes to the cell-to-cell junctions between epithelial cells to impede inward migration of pathogens and allow external migration of phagocytic cells.[15]

Protease–Antiprotease System

The human genome includes 565 proteases, many of which occur in the lung (Table 11.1).[19] Lung protease enzymes are normally released in the lung following activation of neutrophils or macrophages in response to pathogens or tobacco smoke. These enzymes are powerful antimicrobial molecules in the airway lining fluid, but if left unchecked, they will damage lung tissue. There are at least two mechanisms that protect the lung from damage by its own protease enzymes. First, the proteases are mostly confined to the mucous layer of the airway surface liquid, avoiding close contact with underlying epithelial cells whilst being in close proximity to inhaled microorganisms. Second, they are inactivated by conjugation with antiprotease enzymes present in the lung. Antiprotease enzymes active in the lung include α_1-antitrypsin, α_2-macroglobulin and α_1-chymotrypsin. α_1-Antitrypsin is manufactured in the liver and transported to the lung. It constitutes a major proportion of antiprotease activity in the alveoli and is the most active inhibitor of neutrophil elastase.

Inactivation of such powerful protease enzymes presents a significant biochemical challenge. The α_1-antitrypsin molecule exists in a semistable state, held together by a loop of amino acids that projects from the molecule with a pair of methionine-serine residues at its tip, which acts as a 'bait' for protease enzymes. When a protease binds the peptide loop, the α_1-antitrypsin structure becomes unstable and rapidly flips the bound protease onto the other side of the molecule, an action that has been likened to a mousetrap. Once flipped to the other side of the molecule, the protease becomes bound so tightly within a β-sheet of the α_1-antitrypsin that it is effectively crushed, preventing the conformational changes required for its function.

Protease Enzymes in the Lung and Their Physiological and Pathophysiological Roles[19]

Group	Examples	Molecular Target in Lung Tissue	Potential Role in Lung Disease
Cysteine proteases	Cathepsins	Collagens	Linked to IPF
Serine proteases	Neutrophil elastase Proteinase-3	Elastin	Risk factor for bronchiectasis in CF
Metalloproteases	ADAM MMP	Collagen Collagen types IV and V Serpins	ADAM-33 linked to asthma (page 329) Possible marker of IPF Smoking and COPD

ADAM, A disintegrin and metalloproteinase; *MMP*, matrix metalloproteinase; *CF*, cystic fibrosis; *IPF*, idiopathic pulmonary fibrosis; *COPD*, chronic obstructive pulmonary disease.

In 1963 a group of patients were described whose plasma proteins were deficient in α_1-antitrypsin and who had developed emphysema.[20] The enzyme deficiency is inherited as an autosomal recessive gene, with 7.7% of people of European descent being carriers for one of the two common mutations of the gene encoding α_1-antitrypsin. Lower plasma levels of α_1-antitrypsin in homozygous patients result not from failed production of α_1-antitrypsin, but from failure to secrete the protein from hepatocytes. The retained α_1-antitrypsin protein polymerizes within the cell and leads to hepatic damage. About 1:4500 members of the population are believed to be homozygous for the more severe Z mutation of the α_1-antitrypsin gene,[21] although many of these may succumb to pulmonary and liver disease before the α_1-antitrypsin deficiency is ever found. Homozygotes do form a higher proportion of patients with emphysema, and tend to have basal emphysema, onset at a younger age and a severe form of the disease. It thus appears that α_1-antitrypsin deficiency is an aetiological factor in a small proportion of patients with emphysema (page 332). Smoking, which increases neutrophil protease production (page 239), is associated with more severe lung disease in patients with a deficiency of α_1-antitrypsin. Disturbances of the less well understood protease–antiprotease systems, such as the matrix metalloproteases group of enzymes, are now also believed to be involved in pathogenesis of a variety of inflammatory lung diseases (Table 11.1).[19,22]

Immune Systems

Humoral immunity is provided in the lung by immunoglobulins found in the airway lining fluid. IgA is the major type present in the nasopharyngeal area and large bronchi. Its role seems to be to prevent the binding of bacteria to the nasal mucosa, and specific IgA has the ability to act as an opsonin and induce complement. Further down the respiratory tract IgG is present in larger amounts, becoming the most prevalent immunoglobulin in the alveoli.

Cellular immunity involves the immunologically active epithelial cells and macrophages that are present in normal airways. In response to the variety of stimuli previously described, activation of TLRs in airway epithelial cells initiates an inflammatory response, and these cells are probably also responsible for terminating the response and initiating tissue repair. This is done by secretion of numerous molecules:

- Adhesion molecules such as intercellular adhesion molecule 1 (ICAM-1) to induce margination of inflammatory cells in nearby pulmonary capillaries
- Chemokines such as interleukins (IL) (e.g., IL-8) to recruit inflammatory cells into the lung tissue
- Cytokines (e.g., IL-1, IL-6, tumour necrosis factor) to amplify the inflammatory response by further stimulation of inflammatory cells
- Growth factors, such as transforming growth factor beta (TGF-β) and epidermal growth factor (EGF), to stimulate the cells responsible for tissue repair such as fibroblasts
- Extracellular matrix proteins (e.g., collagen, hyaluronan) to begin the tissue repair process.

Once initiated, this response causes large numbers of phagocytic cells to enter the lung tissue. The presence of immunoglobulins complement, and other opsonins enhance, the phagocytic cells' recognition process. In severe infections, the reactive oxygen species used in the killing of microorganisms by phagocytic cells may spill out of the lysosome and into the lung tissue, exacerbating the tissue injury.

Chemical Hazards

Many factors will influence the fate of inhaled chemicals:

Particle size. As with biological particles described earlier, this will affect where in the lung deposition occurs.

Water solubility. Once incorporated into the lung tissue, water solubility affects the rate at which chemicals are cleared from the lung, with water-soluble substances taking longer than lipid-soluble ones to be absorbed into the blood for disposal elsewhere.

Concentration. The concentration of inhaled chemicals is important because metabolic activity within the lung is easily saturated.

Metabolism. The metabolism of inhaled chemicals is poorly understood in the human lung, and, although it has been extensively investigated in animals, there are known to be large species differences. Metabolic activity is found in all cell types of the respiratory mucosa, but in animals is particularly well-developed in club cells and type II alveolar cells (page 11). As in the liver, metabolism of toxic chemicals involves two stages:

1. Phase I metabolism, in which the toxic molecule is converted into a different compound, usually by oxidative reactions. This is achieved in the lung by the cytochrome P-450 monooxygenase and, to a much lesser extent, flavin-based monooxygenase systems. The lung is one of the major extrahepatic sites of mixed function oxidation by the cytochrome P-450 systems, but, gram for gram, remains considerably less active than the liver.

2. Phase II metabolism involves conjugation of the resulting compounds to 'carrier' molecules, which render them less biologically active and more water soluble, and therefore easier to excrete. In the lung, phase II metabolism is normally by conjugation with glucuronide or glutathione.

Metabolic changes to inhaled chemicals may not be beneficial, especially with many synthetic organic compounds and several chemicals in cigarette smoke (page 236). Bioactivation by phase I metabolism converts some quite innocuous compounds into potent carcinogens, whereas slightly different metabolic conversions may do the reverse. The balance between activating and inactivating pathways varies between species. What little data are available on human lungs indicates that we are fortunate in having a very favourable ratio, with the inactivation of potential carcinogens 100-fold greater than in rodents. Presumably, without this evolutionary advantage, the history of cigarette smoking would have been different.

Processing of Endogenous Compounds By the Pulmonary Vasculature

Some hormones may pass through the lung unchanged, others may be almost entirely removed from the blood during a single pass and some may be activated during transit (Table 11.2).

Of the many types of cell in the lungs, it is endothelial cells that are most active metabolically. The most important location is the pulmonary capillary, but it must be stressed that endothelium from a range of vessels throughout the body has been shown to possess a similar repertoire of metabolic processes. The extensive metabolic actions of the pulmonary endothelium take place in spite of the paucity of organelles that are normally associated with metabolic activity, in particular mitochondria and smooth endoplasmic reticulum or microsomes. Nevertheless, the caveolae result in a major increase in the already extensive surface area of these cells ($\sim$126 m^2), which is particularly advantageous for membrane-bound enzymes.

Catecholamines and Acetylcholine

Noradrenaline (Norepinephrine)

There is a striking difference in the handling of noradrenaline and adrenaline. Although each catecholamine has a half-life of about 20 seconds in blood, about 30% of noradrenaline is removed in a single pass through the lungs, whereas adrenaline (and isoprenaline and dopamine) is unaffected. Monoamine oxidase and catechol-O-methyl transferase within the endothelial cells will metabolize all amine derivatives with equal efficiency. The specificity of pulmonary endothelium for noradrenaline therefore lies with the cell membrane, which selectively takes up only

TABLE 11.2 **Summary of Metabolic Changes to Hormones on Passing Through the Pulmonary Circulation***

Group	Effect of Passing Through Pulmonary Circulation		
	Activated	No change	Inactivated
Amines		Dopamine Adrenaline Histamine	5-Hydroxy-tryptamine Noradrenaline
Peptides	Angiotensin I	Angiotensin II ANP Oxytocin Vasopressin	Bradykinin Endothelins
Arachidonic acid derivatives	Arachidonic acid	PGI$_2$ (prostacyclin) PGA$_2$	PGD$_2$ PGE$_2$
			PGF$_2\alpha$
			Leukotrienes
Purine derivatives			Adenosine ATP, ADP, AMP

*ANP, atrial natriuretic peptide; PG, prostaglandin; ATP, ADP and AMP, adenosine triphosphate, diphosphate and monophosphate respectively.

noradrenaline and 5-hydroxytryptamine (5-HT, serotonin). Extraneuronal uptake of noradrenaline is not confined to the endothelium of the lungs, but uptake by the pulmonary circulation (uptake 1) differs from extraneuronal uptake (uptake 2) in other tissues, which is less specific for noradrenaline.

5-HT is removed very effectively by the lungs, with up to 98% removed in a single pass. There are considerable similarities to the processing of noradrenaline. 5-HT is taken up by the endothelium, mainly in the capillaries, and is then rapidly metabolized by monoamine oxidase. The half-life of 5-HT in blood is about 1 to 2 min, and pulmonary clearance plays the major role in the prevention of its recirculation.

Histamine, dopamine and adrenaline (epinephrine) are not removed from blood on passing through the pulmonary circulation, in spite of the high concentrations of monoamine oxidase in lung tissue. Their removal from the circulation is limited by the lack of a transport mechanism across the endothelium.

Acetylcholine is rapidly hydrolysed in blood, where it has a half-life of less than 2 seconds. This tends to overshadow any changes attributable to the lung, which nevertheless does contain acetylcholinesterases and pseudocholinesterases.

Peptides

Angiotensin

It has long been known that angiotensin I, a decapeptide formed by the action of renin on a plasma α_2-globulin (angiotensinogen), is converted into the vasoactive octapeptide angiotensin II by incubation with plasma. Angiotensin-converting enzyme (ACE) is found free in the plasma but is also bound to the surface of endothelium. This appears to be a general property of endothelium, but ACE is present in abundance on the vascular surface of pulmonary endothelial cells, also lining the inside of the caveolae and extending onto the projections into the lumen. About 80% of angiotensin I passing through the lungs is converted to angiotensin II in a single pass. ACE is a zinc-containing carboxypeptidase with two active sites, each located within a deep groove in the side of the protein.[23] Binding sites in the groove attach the substrate firmly to the protein, and the zinc moiety then cleaves either a phenylalanine-histidine bond (angiotensin I) or a phenylalanine-arginine bond (bradykinin). Drugs that inhibit ACE (see later) do so by becoming buried deep within the protein groove, simply covering the active site.[23]

Bradykinin

Bradykinin is a vasoactive nonapeptide, and is very effectively removed during passage through the lung and other vascular beds. The half-life in blood is about 17 seconds, but is less than 4 seconds in various vascular beds. Like angiotensin I, ACE is the enzyme responsible for metabolism of bradykinin.

By its effects on bradykinin and angiotensin, ACE plays a crucial role in controlling arterial blood pressure. Bradykinin, which promotes blood vessel dilation and a lowering of blood pressure, is inactivated. Conversely, angiotensin II production results in a host of events that increase blood pressure, such as renal sodium retention, vasoconstriction and release of noradrenaline. Drugs that inhibit ACE are now widely used in the treatment of cardiovascular disease. However, this also decreases the degradation of bradykinin by ACE, although other enzymes are capable of metabolizing bradykinin, allowing ACE inhibitors to exert their hypotensive effects. Angiotensin II itself passes through the lung unchanged, as do vasopressin and oxytocin.

Atrial Natriuretic Peptide

Atrial natriuretic peptide (ANP) is largely removed by the lung in many animal species. Methodological problems caused by the secretion of ANP from both left and right atria in humans led to uncertainty about the ability of human lungs to metabolize ANP. Studies using radiolabelled ANP have now shown that, in humans, ANP is not metabolized by the lung to any significant extent.

Endothelins

Endothelins are a group of 21-amino acid peptides with diverse biological activity (page 82) that have a plasma half-life of just a few minutes and are cleared by the kidney, liver and lungs. The pulmonary enzymes responsible are not clearly defined, but there are believed to be several different types in humans.

Arachidonic Acid Derivatives

The lung is a major site of synthesis, metabolism, uptake and release of arachidonic acid metabolites. The group as a whole are 20-carbon carboxylic acids, generically known as eicosanoids. The initial stages of eicosanoid synthesis involve the conversion, by phospholipase A_2, of membrane phospholipids into arachidonic acid. Metabolism of arachidonic acid involves its oxygenation by two main pathways, for which the enzymes are cyclooxygenase (COX) and lipoxygenase (Figs 11.3 and 3.10, respectively). Oxygenation and cyclization of arachidonic acid by COX produces the prostaglandin PGG_2 (the subscript 2 indicates two double bonds in the carbon chain). A nonspecific peroxidase then converts PGG_2 to prostaglandin PGH_2, which is the parent compound for synthesis of the many important derivatives shown in Figure 11.3.

Eicosanoids are not stored preformed but are synthesized as required by many cell types in the lung, including endothelium, airway smooth muscle, mast cells, epithelial cells and vascular muscle. Activation of phospholipase initiates the pathway, and results from a variety of stimuli such as inflammatory cytokines, complement activation, hormones, allergens or mechanical stimuli. The enzyme for the next step of the pathway, COX, exists in multiple isoforms, including COX-1, which is a constitutive enzyme present at low concentrations, and COX-2, which is induced by inflammatory cytokines. In the normal lung, the physiological role of these COX isoforms is uncertain, but in some

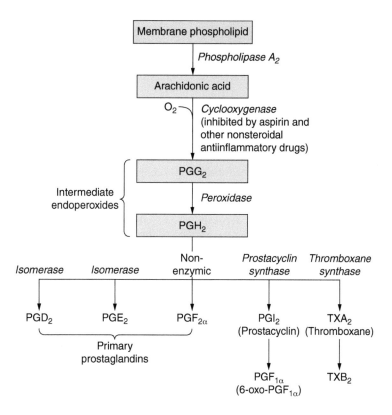

• **Fig. 11.3** The cyclooxygenase pathway for the production of arachidonic acid, and its subsequent conversion to form the prostaglandins (PG) and thromboxanes (TX). See text for metabolism taking place in the lungs.

patients with asthma, inhibition of COX-1 by aspirin induces bronchospasm, whereas inhibition of COX-2 does not (page 330).

Prostaglandins $PGF_{2\alpha}$, PGD_2, PGG_2, PGH_2 and thromboxane are bronchial and tracheal constrictors, and $PGF_{2\alpha}$ and PGD_2 are much more potent in asthmatic patients compared with normal subjects. PGE_1 and PGE_2 are bronchodilators, particularly when administered by aerosol. Prostaglandins in the lung are generally antiinflammatory, for example, PGD_2 and PGE_2 have a role in suppressing the development of T-helper cells (Th9) which contribute to some allergic lung diseases.[24] Prostacyclin (PGI_2) has different effects in different species. In humans, it has no effect on airway calibre in doses that have profound cardiovascular effects. PGI_2 and PGE_1 are pulmonary vasodilators. PGH_2 and $PGF_2\alpha$ are pulmonary vasoconstrictors.

Various specific enzymes in the lung are responsible for extensive metabolism of PGE_2, PGE_1 and $PGF_{2\alpha}$, but PGA_2 and PGI_2 pass through the lung unchanged. As for catecholamine metabolism, specificity for pulmonary prostaglandin metabolism is in the uptake pathways, rather than with the intracellular enzymes.

Leukotrienes[25] are also eicosanoids derived from arachidonic acid but by the lipoxygenase pathway (see Fig. 3.10). The leukotrienes LTC_4 and LTD_4 are mainly responsible for the bronchoconstrictor effects of what was formerly known as slow-reacting substance A (SRS-A). SRS-A also contains LTB_4, which is a less powerful bronchoconstrictor but

increases vascular permeability. These compounds, which are synthesized by the mast cell, have an important role in asthma, and the mechanism of their release is discussed in Chapter 28, whereas drugs that inhibit leukotrienes are described on page 36.

Purine Derivatives

Specific enzymes exist on the surface of pulmonary endothelial cells for the degradation of adenosine monophophate (AMP), adenosine diphosphate and adenosine triphosphate to adenosine. Adenosine itself has potent effects on the circulation, but is also inactivated in the lungs by rapid uptake into the endothelial cells, where it is either phosphorylated into AMP or deaminated to produce inosine and ultimately uric acid for excretion.

Pharmacokinetics and the Lung

Drug Delivery[26,27]

Inhalation of drugs to treat lung disease may be considered as topical administration of the drug to the respiratory tract, although systemic absorption of the drug is likely to be greater than other topical routes. Pulmonary administration of a drug that is intended to work systemically offers many advantages over other routes, such as very rapid delivery into the circulation and avoidance of first pass metabolism in the liver.

For delivery to the alveoli, particles around 3 μm are the optimal size, as larger particles tend to deposit in the airways, and smaller particles tend to be inhaled and exhaled without being deposited in lung tissue (page 166). Targeted delivery of drugs to specific regions of the respiratory tract should be possible by, for example, modifying the particle size, the timing of their addition to the breath or the breathing pattern during inhalation.[27] In the future even more specific targeting of inhaled drugs may be possible, as demonstrated by a study in which magnetic iron oxide nanoparticles were added to aerosol solutions and a magnetic field used to modify where in the lung the aerosol was deposited.[28] Most delivery devices in clinical use produce aerosols containing a wide range of particle sizes, commonly generating particles between 1 and 35 μm. Three main types of inhaled drug delivery systems are used in practice:[27]

1. Metered dose inhalers (MDIs) deliver a known quantity of drug into the inspired gas, and may be activated manually by the patient or automatically based on inspiratory flow (breath actuated). With modern MDIs, 40% to 50% of the drug released is deposited in the lungs, although this is reduced further if only those particles small enough to reach the small airways (<4.7 μm) are considered. For many years the propellants in MDIs were chlorofluorocarbon molecules, but the environmental effects of these has led to them now being replaced with hydrofluoroalkanes, requiring a redesign of the delivery system resulting in changes to the distribution of particle size produced for some drugs. Use of a spacer device with an MDI reduces the requirement for the patient to coordinate their breathing with activating the MDI, and allows the largest particles to fall out of the aerosol before inhalation, improving drug delivery and reducing side effects from large particles impacting on the pharynx.

2. Dry powder inhalers do not use propellants and deliver a similar proportion of drug to the lungs, but still require patient coordination to use and require a faster inspiration to ensure all the powdered drug is aerosolized.

3. Nebulizers use a variety of techniques to convert a liquid solution of the drug into a fine mist, which again contains a wide range of particle sizes. The continuous flow of drug particles means no patient coordination is required, and a large dose of drug is therefore delivered to the airways, making this the ideal technique for emergency situations. However, the large dose of drugs delivered also makes side effects more common, and the equipment required to deliver a nebulizer is complex and expensive.

Drug Elimination

The wide range of mechanisms present in the lung for the processing of endogenous and inhaled substances makes an effect on drug disposition almost inevitable.

Inhaled drugs will be subjected to the same metabolic activity in the airway and alveolar cells as the other toxic chemicals previously described. Mixed function oxidase and cytochrome P-450 systems are active in the lung, and so are presumed to metabolize drugs in the same way as in hepatocytes. Steroids are known to be metabolized in lung airway tissue, as is isoprenaline.

Pulmonary Circulation[29]

Many drugs are removed from the circulation on passing through the lungs. However, in the majority of cases this occurs by retention of the drug in lung tissue rather than actual metabolism. This low activity of metabolic enzymes found in the lung occurs for two reasons. First, access to the metabolic enzymes in endothelial cells is closely controlled by highly specific uptake mechanisms that are vital to allow the highly selective metabolism of endogenous compounds. Second, it is possible that the oxidative systems responsible for drug metabolism elsewhere in the body are located mostly in the airways, thus preventing bloodborne drugs gaining access to them. Drugs that are basic (pKa >8) and lipophilic tend to be taken up in the pulmonary circulation, whereas acidic drugs preferentially bind to plasma proteins. Drug binding in the pulmonary circulation may act as a first pass filter for any drug administered intravenously. This drug reservoir within the lung may then be released slowly, or even give rise to rapid changes in plasma drug levels either when the binding sites become saturated or when one drug is displaced by a different drug with greater affinity for the same binding site.

Pulmonary Toxicity of Drugs

Accumulation of some drugs and other toxic substances in the lung may cause dangerous local toxicity. Paraquat is an outstanding example: it is slowly taken up into alveolar epithelial cells, where it promotes the production of reactive oxygen species (page 285), with resulting lung damage. Some drugs cause pulmonary toxicity by a similar mechanism, including nitrofurantoin and bleomycin. Toxicity from the latter is strongly associated with exposure to high oxygen concentrations (page 294). Amiodarone, a highly effective and commonly used antiarrhythmic agent, is also associated with pulmonary toxicity, which occurs in 6% of patients given the drug. When toxicity occurs it may be severe and is fatal in up to 10% of cases. The cause is unknown, but formation of reactive oxygen species, immunologic activation and direct cellular toxicity are all believed to contribute.

The Endocrine Lung

To qualify as a true endocrine organ, the lung must secrete a substance into the blood which brings about a useful physiological response in a distant tissue. In spite of its wide-ranging metabolic activities already described, the endocrine functions of the lung remain ill-defined. Contenders for lung-secreted endocrine effectors include the following:

Inflammatory mediators. Histamine, endothelin and eicosanoids are released from the lung following immunologic activation by inhaled allergens (Chapter 28). These mediators are undoubtedly responsible for cardiovascular and other physiological changes in the rest of the body, such as a rash, peripheral vasodilation and a reduction in blood pressure. However, it is doubtful if this can really be regarded as a desirable physiological effect.

Hypoxic endocrine responses.[30] Animal studies have demonstrated the presence of clusters of peptide- and amine-secreting cells in lung tissue. These cells degranulate in the presence of acute hypoxia, but the substances secreted, and their effects are not known. The cells belong to the 'diffuse endocrine system,' and are present in humans, but their role is extremely unclear.

Nitric oxide (NO). This plays an important role in the regulation of airway smooth muscle (page 34) and pulmonary vascular resistance (page 80), and is well known for its effects on platelet function and the systemic vasculature elsewhere in the body. There is no evidence that pulmonary endothelium secretes NO into the blood to exert an effect elsewhere, mainly because of the rapid uptake of NO by haemoglobin (page 148). However, this does not rule out an indirect effect of pulmonary NO production in influencing peripheral blood flow, which may be controlled by the balance between different forms of NO–haemoglobin complexes (page 148).

References

1. Asah D, Raju S, Ghosh S, et al. Nonthrombotic pulmonary embolism from inorganic particulate matter and foreign bodies. *Chest.* 2018;153:1249-1265.

2. Elliott JE, Nigama SM, Lauriea SS, et al. Prevalence of left heart contrast in healthy, young, asymptomatic humans at rest breathing room air. *Respir Physiol Neurobiol.* 2013;188:71-78.

3. Kerut EK, Norfleet WT, Plotnick GD, et al. Patent foramen ovale: a review of associated conditions and the impact of physiological size. *J Am Coll Cardiol.* 2001;38:613-623.

4. Fahy JV, Dickey BF. Airway mucus function and dysfunction. *N Engl J Med.* 2010;363:2233-2247.

5. Janssen WJ, Stefanski AL, Bochner BS, et al. Control of lung defence by mucins and macrophages: ancient defence mechanisms with modern functions. *Eur Respir J.* 2016;48:1201-1214.

6. Hattrup CL, Gendler SJ. Structure and function of the cell surface (tethered) mucins. *Annu Rev Physiol.* 2008;70:431-457.

7. Tilley AE, Walters MS, Shaykhiev R, et al. Cilia dysfunction in lung disease. *Annu Rev Physiol.* 2015;77:379-406.

8. Bartoszewski R, Matalon S, Collawn JF. Ion channels of the lung and their role in disease pathogenesis. *Am J Physiol Lung Cell Mol Physiol.* 2017;313:L859–L872.

9. Tilley AE, Walters MS, Shaykhiev R, et al. Cilia dysfunction in lung disease. *Annu Rev Physiol.* 2015;77:379-406.

10. de Jonge HR, Sheppard DN. The small airways accordion: concurrent or alternating fluid absorption and secretion? *J Physiol.* 2012;590(15):3409-3410.

*11. **Widdicombe JH, Wine JJ. Airway gland structure and function. *Physiol Rev.* 2015;95:1241-1319.**

12. Button B, Picher M, Boucher RC. Differential effects of cyclic and constant stress on ATP release and mucociliary transport by human airway epithelia. *J Physiol.* 2007;580:577-592.

13. Knowles MR, Daniels LA, Davis SD, et al. Primary ciliary dyskinesia. Recent advances in diagnostics, genetics, and characterization of clinical disease. *Am J Respir Crit Care Med.* 2013;188:913-922.

14. Hofemeier P, Sznitman J. Revisiting pulmonary acinar particle transport: convection, sedimentation, diffusion, and their interplay. *J Appl Physiol.* 2015;118:1375-1385.

15. Evans SE, Xu Y, Tuvim MJ, et al. Inducible innate resistance of lung epithelium to infection. *Annu Rev Physiol.* 2010;72:413-435.

*16. **Hiemstra PS, Amatngalim GD, van der Does AM, et al. Antimicrobial peptides and innate lung defenses. Role in infectious and noninfectious lung diseases and therapeutic applications. *Chest.* 2016;149:545-551.**

17. Hiemstra PS. Antimicrobial peptides in the real world: implications for cystic fibrosis. *Eur Respir J.* 2007;29:617-618.

18. Baral P, Batra S, Zemans RL, et al. Divergent functions of toll-like receptors during bacterial lung infections. *Am J Respir Crit Care Med.* 2014;190:722-732.

19. Droguett K, Rios M, Carreño DV, et al. An autocrine ATP release mechanism regulates basal ciliary activity in airway epithelium. *J Physiol.* 2017;595:4755-4767.

20. Stockley RA. α1-Antitrypsin deficiency. What has it ever done for us? *Chest.* 2013;144:1923-1929.

21. Stoller JK, Aboussouan LS. A review of α1-antitrypsin deficiency. *Am J Respir Crit Care Med.* 2012;185:246-259.

*22. **Greenlee KJ, Werb Z, Kheradmand F. Matrix metalloproteinases in lung: multiple, multifarious, and multifaceted. *Physiol Rev.* 2007;87:69-98.**

23. Brew K. Structure of human ACE gives new insights into inhibitor binding and design. *Trends Pharmacol Sci.* 2003;24:391-394.

24. Boyce JA, Peebles RS. Regulation of Th9-type pulmonary immune responses. A new role for COX-2. *Am J Respir Crit Care Med.* 2013;187:785-786.

25. Peters-Golden M, Henderson WR. Leukotrienes. *N Engl J Med.* 2007;357:1841-1854.

26. Sims MW. Aerosol therapy for obstructive lung diseases. Device selection and practice management issues. *Chest.* 2011;140:781-788.

*27. **Dolovich MB, Dhand R. Aerosol drug delivery: developments in device design and clinical use. *Lancet.* 2011;377:1032-1045.**

28. Coates AL. Guiding aerosol deposition in the lung. *N Engl J Med.* 2008;358:304-305.

29. Boer F. Drug handling by the lungs. *Br J Anaesth.* 2003;91:50-60.

30. Gosney JR. The endocrine lung and its response to hypoxia. *Thorax.* 1994;49:S25-S26.

PART II

Applied Physiology

12

Pregnancy, Neonates and Children

KEY POINTS

- Hormonal changes of pregnancy stimulate breathing, causing an increase in tidal volume and hypocapnia.
- In late pregnancy the enlarged uterus reduces lung volume, particularly in the supine position.
- Human lung development is incomplete at birth, with new alveoli continuing to form until around 3 years of age.

- Compared with adults, the respiratory system of a neonate has a very low compliance and a high resistance.
- In children, most measures of lung function are the same as adults, provided the values are related to lung volume or height.

Respiratory Function in Pregnancy

Several physiological changes occur during pregnancy that affect respiratory function. Fluid retention resulting from increasing oestrogen levels causes oedema throughout the airway mucosa and increases blood volume, substantially increasing oxygen delivery. Progesterone levels rise six-fold through pregnancy and have significant effects on the control of respiration, and therefore arterial blood gases. Finally, in the last trimester of pregnancy, the enlarging uterus has a direct impact on respiratory mechanics. A summary of the changes for common respiratory measurements is shown in Table 12.1.

Lung volumes. During the last third of pregnancy the diaphragm becomes displaced cephalad by the expansion of the uterus into the abdomen. This reduces both the residual volume (by about 20%) and expiratory reserve volume, such that functional residual capacity (FRC) is greatly reduced (Table 12.1). This is particularly true in the supine position, and effectively removes one of the largest stores of oxygen available to the body, making pregnant women very susceptible to hypoxia during anaesthesia or if they have respiratory disease. Vital capacity, forced expiratory volume in one second and maximal breathing capacity are normally unchanged during pregnancy.

Oxygen consumption. Oxygen consumption increases throughout pregnancy, peaking at between 15% and 30% above normal at full term. The increase is mainly attributable to the demands of the fetus, uterus and placenta, such that when oxygen consumption is expressed per kilogram of body weight there is little change.

Ventilation. Respiratory rate remains unchanged, whereas tidal volume, and therefore the minute volume of ventilation, increases by up to 40% above normal at full term. The increase in ventilation is beyond the requirements of the enhanced oxygen uptake or carbon dioxide production, so alveolar and arterial P_{CO_2} are reduced to about 4 kPa (30 mmHg). There is also an increase in alveolar and arterial P_{O_2} of about 1 kPa (7.5 mmHg). Both these changes will facilitate blood gas exchange across the placenta.

Hyperventilation is attributable to progesterone, and the mechanism is assumed to be a sensitization of the central chemoreceptors. Pregnancy gives rise to a threefold increase in the slope of a P_{CO_2}/ventilation response curve. The hypoxic ventilatory response is increased twofold, with most of the change occurring before the midpoint of gestation, at which time oxygen consumption has hardly begun to increase.

Dyspnoea occurs in more than half of pregnant women, often beginning early in pregnancy, before the mass effect of the uterus becomes apparent. Dyspnoeic pregnant women, compared with nondyspnoeic controls, show a greater degree of hyperventilation in spite of having similar plasma progesterone levels. Dyspnoea early in pregnancy therefore seems to arise from a greater sensitivity of the chemoreceptors to the increase in progesterone levels. In the third trimester, when dyspnoea on mild exercise is almost universal, the extra effort required by the respiratory muscles to increase tidal volume is believed to be responsible for breathlessness, rather than an altered perception of respiratory discomfort.[1]

TABLE 12.1	Respiratory Function Throughout Pregnancy			
			Pregnant	
Variable	Nonpregnant	1st Trimester	2nd Trimester	3rd Trimester
Tidal volume (L)	0.52	0.60	0.65	0.72
Respiratory rate (breaths per minute)	18	18	18	18
Minute volume (L.min^{-1})	9.3	11.0	11.8	13.1
Residual volume (L)	1.37	1.27	1.26	1.01
Functional residual capacity (L)	2.69	2.52	2.48	1.95
Vital capacity (L)	3.50	3.45	3.58	3.0
Oxygen consumption (mL.min^{-1})	194	211	242	258
Arterial P_{O_2} (kPa)	12.6	14.2	13.7	13.6
(mmHg)	95	106	103	102
Arterial P_{CO_2} (kPa)	4.70	3.92	3.93	4.05
(mmHg)	35	29	29	31
Carbon dioxide response slope (L.min^{-1}.kPa^{-1})	11.6	15.0	17.3	19.8
Oxygen saturation response slope (L.min^{-1}.%$^{-1}$)	0.64	1.04	1.13	1.33

Nonpregnant figures refer to normal subjects with an average body weight of 60 kg; pregnant figures refer to the end of each trimester of pregnancy.

The Lungs Before Birth

Embryology

The lungs develop in four stages, under the control of a host of transcriptional factors:[2,3]

1. *Pseudoglandular stage (5–17 weeks' gestation).* A ventral outgrowth from the foregut first appears about 24 days after fertilization, and at around week 5 of gestation this begins to form the basic airway and vascular architecture. The branching patterns of the adult airways and vasculature are believed to develop by a common process of branching morphogenesis, ensuring the two components remain closely related in the lung tissue.[4] Dividing epithelial cells lengthen the airways, and their ability to do this is influenced by physical factors relating to the lung liquid (LL) and fetal breathing described next.
2. *Canalicular stage (16–26 weeks' gestation).* The primitive pulmonary capillaries now become more closely associated with the airway epithelium, and the connective tissue architecture of the lung is formed. Fibroblasts and other cells involved in morphogenesis of the lung undergo apoptosis, reducing the wall thickness of the embryonic lung structures.
3. *Saccular stage (24 weeks' gestation to term).* Distal airways now develop primitive alveoli in their walls to become respiratory bronchi (see Fig. 1.6). Saccules form at the termination of airways, these being primitive pulmonary acini.
4. *Alveolar stage.* Saccules on embryonic bronchioles now expand, and septation occurs to form the groups of alveoli seen in adult pulmonary acini. This phase of development begins at 36 weeks' gestation, and in humans is believed to be mostly complete around 2 years of age, although there is some evidence the process may continue throughout childhood, particularly in infants born prematurely.[5] In humans at full term all major elements of the lungs are therefore fully formed, but the number of alveoli present is only about 15% of that in the adult lung. This postnatal maturation of lung structure is only seen in altricial mammals (humans, mice and rabbits) that have the luxury of being able to remain 'helpless' after birth. Precocial species such as range animals are born with a structurally mature lung, ready for immediate activity. Once alveolarization is complete, further lung growth is dimensional, that is, simple enlargement of existing structures.

The lungs begin to contain surfactant and are first capable of function by approximately 24 to 28 weeks, this being a major contributor to the viability of premature infants, although the factors influencing surfactant development, particularly of the surfactant proteins, are poorly understood.[6]

Lung Liquid

Fetal lungs contain LL which is secreted by the pulmonary epithelial cells and flows out through the developing airway into the amniotic fluid or gastrointestinal tract, flushing debris from the airways as it does so. A more important function of LL seems to be to prevent the developing lung tissues from collapsing. It is thought that LL maintains the lung at a slight positive pressure relative to the amniotic fluid, and that this expansion is responsible for stimulating cell division and lung growth, particularly with respect to airway branching.[2] The respiratory tract in late pregnancy contains about 40 mL of LL, but its turnover is rapid, believed to be of the order of 500 mL per day. Its volume corresponds approximately with the FRC after breathing is established.

Fetal breathing movements also contribute to lung development. In humans they begin in the middle trimester of pregnancy, and are present for over 20 minutes per hour in the last trimester, normally during periods of general fetal activity. During episodes of breathing, the frequency is about 45 breaths per minute, and the diaphragm seems to be the main muscle concerned, producing an estimated fluid shift of about 2 mL at each 'breath'.

Maintenance of a positive pressure in the developing lung requires the upper airway to offer some resistance to the outflow of LL. During apnoea, elastic recoil of the lung tissue and continuous production of LL are both opposed by intrinsic laryngeal resistance and a collapsed pharynx. Fetal inspiratory activity, as in the adult, includes dilation of the upper airway. With quiet breathing this would allow increased efflux of LL from the airway, but simultaneous diaphragmatic contraction opposes this. During vigorous breathing movements with the mouth open, pharyngeal fluid may be 'sucked' into the airway, thus contributing to the expansion of the lungs. Thus fetal breathing movements are believed to contribute to maintaining lung expansion, and their abolition is known to impair lung development.

Lung Development and Lung Function Later in Life

As the lungs develop in utero, they face a variety of environmental challenges associated with the pregnancy that can affect their development and influence the individual's lung function in both childhood and adult life. Adverse effects on lung function arising during pregnancy include a greater likelihood of developing childhood wheeze (which may or may not be asthma), developing asthma or having lower lung volumes as an adult. The more well-studied factors contributing to these lung problems include:

- *Low birth weight.* This is associated with lower lung volumes as both a child and adult, with the greatest effect seen when aged 21 years,[7] and results in a greater likelihood of developing asthma[8] and requiring hospitalization for respiratory disease as an adult. The cause of these effects remains uncertain, but it most likely results from poor fetal lung growth in the first trimester, although early postnatal growth also influences future lung health.[8]
- *Prematurity.* Birth at less than 37 weeks' gestation leads to lower lung volumes in childhood,[9] with values

lower still in neonates who develop and survive bronchopulmonary dysplasia (page 180). Pulmonary gas transfer remains lower than control subjects at 21 years of age, although this does not adversely affect exercise capacity.[10]
- *Maternal tobacco smoking.*[11] This leads to lower birth weight and earlier birth, meaning these babies will therefore have poorer lung function. Babies whose mothers smoked during pregnancy also have a higher incidence of childhood wheeze and asthma, with smoking during the first trimester having the greatest effect; of course postnatal passive smoking also plays a role (page 239). Nicotine is believed to play a major role in the effects of smoking on in utero lung development, leading to concern that use of e-cigarettes (page 239) may be similarly harmful to the fetus.[12] In utero smoke exposure also causes epigenetic changes in the fetus (resulting from changes to DNA by its methylation) that mean a susceptibility to respiratory disease may be passed down to subsequent generations.[11]
- *Maternal stress during pregnancy.* Stress, particularly in overweight mothers, leads to children being more likely to develop wheeze at 2 to 3 years old.[13] Raised maternal cortisol levels may directly influence early lung development, but maternal stress also has much broader effects on fetal well-being relating to placental function and immune system development.[14]
- *Indoor air pollution* (page 242). Prenatal exposure to indoor carbon monoxide is associated with impaired lung function for the child in the first year of life.[15]

Fetal Circulation

The fetal circulation differs radically from the postnatal circulation (Fig. 12.1). Blood from the right heart is deflected away from the lungs, partly through the foramen ovale and partly through the ductus arteriosus. Less than 10% of the output of the right ventricle reaches the lungs, the remainder passing to the systemic circulation and the placenta. Right atrial pressure exceeds left atrial pressure, and this maintains the patency of the foramen ovale. Finally, because the vascular resistance of the pulmonary circulation exceeds that of the systemic circulation before birth, pressure in the right ventricle exceeds that in the left ventricle, and these factors control the direction of flow through the ductus arteriosus.

The umbilical veins drain via the ductus venosus into the inferior vena cava, which contains better-oxygenated blood than the superior vena cava. The anatomy of the atria and the foramen ovale is such that the better-oxygenated blood from the inferior vena cava passes preferentially into the left atrium, and then to the left ventricle, and so to the brain. (This is not shown in Fig. 12.1). Overall gas tensions in the fetus are of the order of 6.4 kPa (48 mmHg) for $P\mathrm{CO_2}$ and 4 kPa (30 mmHg) for $P\mathrm{O_2}$. The fact that the fetus remains apnoeic for much of the time in utero with these blood-gas

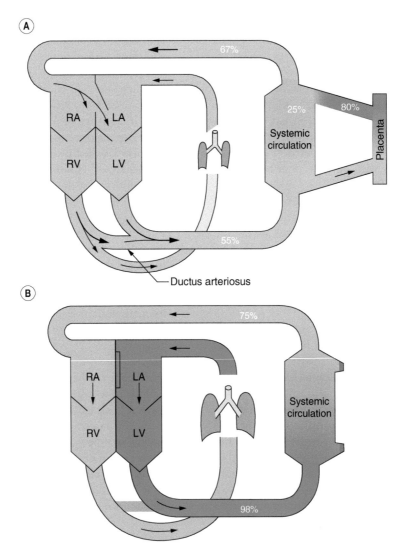

• **Fig. 12.1** Fetal circulation **(A)** compared with adult circulation **(B)**. The foramen ovale is between the right atrium (*RA*) and left atrium (*LA*). *LV*, Left ventricle; *RV*, right ventricle.

levels is probably in part attributable to central hypoxic ventilatory depression (page 53).

Events at Birth

Oxygen stores in the fetus are small, and it is therefore essential that air breathing and oxygen uptake be established within a few minutes of birth. This requires radical changes in the function of both lungs and circulation.

Factors in the Initiation of Breathing

Most infants take their first breath within 20 seconds of delivery, and rhythmic respiration is usually established within 90 seconds. Thoracic compression during vaginal delivery followed by recoil of the rib cage causes air to be drawn passively into the lungs. However, the major stimuli to breathing are probably the cooling of the skin and mechanical stimulation, both acting via the respiratory centre. Without this, babies born via Caesarean section would suffer greatly from immediate respiratory difficulties, which is not the case in practice. Hypoxaemia, resulting from apnoea or clamping of the cord, is unlikely to be a reliable respiratory stimulus at this time because of central hypoxic ventilatory depression (see previous discussion).

Fate of the Fetal Lung Liquid

The volume of LL decreases just before and during labour. Some of the residual fluid may be expressed during a vaginal delivery, but this is not thought to be a major factor. During in utero life, the pulmonary epithelium actively secretes LL, but at birth this process reverses, and the epithelial cells switch to absorption of fluid from the airway. Absorption of fluid from airways and alveoli is an active process facilitated by a sodium channel (page 341) and aquaporin, a transmembrane protein that facilitates water transport across membranes. The sodium channels are primed during the third trimester by thyroid and steroid hormones, and at birth, fetal adrenaline and oxygen trigger the channels to become active.

Changes in the Circulation

The geometry of the circulation changes radically and quickly at birth. The establishment of spontaneous breathing causes a massive decrease in the vascular resistance of the pulmonary circulation, due partly to mechanical factors and partly to changes in blood gases. Simultaneously there is an increase in the resistance of the systemic circulation, due partly to vasoconstriction and partly to cessation of the placental circulation. As a result, the right atrial pressure falls below the left atrial pressure, to give the relationship that is then maintained throughout life. This normally results in closure of the foramen ovale (Fig. 12.1), which is followed by closure of the ductus arteriosus as a result of active vasoconstriction of its smooth muscle layer in response to increased Po_2. The circulation is thus converted from the fetal mode, in which the lungs and the systemic circulation are essentially in parallel, to the adult mode in which they are in series.

Mechanism of Reduced Pulmonary Vascular Resistance at Birth

Pulmonary vascular resistance declines because of a combination of ventilation of the lung, the circulatory reconfiguration and changes in blood gases. Removal of LL from the lung establishes an air–liquid interface that is responsible for a rapid increase in lung recoil pressure, which, possibly along with changes in chest wall compliance, results in a negative intrapleural pressure as in adult lungs. This creates the transmural pressure gradient between the alveoli and pleura, which physically dilates the pulmonary capillaries (page 77). These mechanical forces leading to a reduction in pulmonary vascular resistance are believed to account for over half of the observed changes at birth. Loss of the placental circulation and closure of the ductus arteriosus increases systemic vascular resistance and so raises left heart pressures, leading to foramen ovale closure and a rapid increase in pulmonary blood flow, facilitated by recruitment and distension of pulmonary capillaries. This distension of pulmonary blood vessels may contribute to further vasodilatation by increased shear stress on endothelial cells stimulating the release of vasodilator mediators.

Further reductions in pulmonary vascular resistance occur as a result of increased Po_2 and decreased Pco_2. Hypoxic pulmonary vasoconstriction (HPV) (page 80), which is active in utero, is reduced by the high alveolar Po_2 with the first breath of air. In the first few hours and days after birth active attenuation of HPV occurs, most likely by increased release of both prostacyclin and nitric oxide from endothelial cells. Within a few weeks functional changes to potassium channels in the airway cells and gradual loss of pulmonary artery smooth muscle cells lead to the permanently low pulmonary vascular resistance seen in adults.

Neonatal Lung Function

Mechanics of Breathing

FRC is about 30 mL.kg^{-1}, and total respiratory compliance 50 mL.kPa^{-1} (5 mL.cmH$_2$O^{-1}). Most of the impedance to expansion is because of the lung and depends primarily on the presence of surfactant in the alveoli. The chest wall of the neonate is highly compliant. This contrasts with the adult, in whom compliance of lung and chest wall are approximately equal. Total respiratory resistance is of the order of 7 kPa.L^{-1}.s (70 cmH$_2$O.L^{-1}.s), most of which is in the bronchial tree. Compliance is about one-twentieth that of an adult, and resistance about 15 times greater. At the first breath the infant is capable of generating a subatmospheric intrathoracic pressure of the order of 7 kPa (70 cmH$_2$O).

Ventilation and Gas Exchange

For a 3-kg neonate, the minute volume is about 0.6 L.min^{-1}, with a high respiratory frequency of 25 to 40 breaths per minute. Dead space is close to half of the tidal volume, giving a mean alveolar ventilation of about 0.3 L.min^{-1} for a neonate of average size. There is a shunt of about 10% immediately after birth. However, distribution of gas is better than in the adult, and there is, of course, a negligible hydrostatic pressure gradient in the vertical axis of the tiny lungs of an infant.

Oxygen consumption is of the order of 20 to 30 mL. min^{-1}, depending on weight in the range of 2 to 4 kg. Arterial Pco_2 is close to 4.5 kPa (34 mmHg), and Po_2 9 kPa (68 mmHg). Because of the shunt of 10%, there is an alveolar/arterial Po_2 gradient of about 3.3 kPa (25 mmHg) compared with less than half of this in a young adult. Arterial pH is within the normal adult range.

Control of Breathing

Animal studies have shown that, in the fetus, carotid chemoreceptors are active but at a much lower Po_2 than in adults; the ventilatory response curve is displaced far to the left compared with adults. Prolonged periods of apnoea seen in utero in spite of this carotid sinus activity occur because of brainstem inhibition of the respiratory centre. In contrast to this, cardiovascular responses to hypoxia are well developed in the fetus, bradycardia and vasoconstriction being well-recognized responses to hypoxia in neonates. After birth, there is a very rapid transition towards the adult pattern of respiratory control. Brainstem hypoxic ventilatory depression ceases, and the carotid chemoreceptors 're-set' to adult values within a few weeks. Ventilatory response to carbon dioxide appears to be similar to that in the adult if allowance is made for body size, and the apnoeic threshold (page 50) may be closer to the normal Pco_2 in neonates, resulting in a susceptibility to apnoea.

At birth, changes in respiratory pattern must, by necessity, be substantial, as the long periods of apnoea seen in utero are incompatible with life in the outside world. Although most changes occur shortly after birth, complete transition to 'adult' respiration may take some weeks to complete, particularly in premature and small babies, and in those with other respiratory problems that cause repeated periods of hypoxia.[16] In the meantime, newborn infants have a variety of breathing patterns. For example, 'periodic breathing' consists of slowly oscillating changes in respiratory rate and tidal volume size; 'periodic apnoea' consists of a series of respiratory pauses of over 4 seconds with a few normal breaths in between. In normal babies under 2 months of age, there may be in excess of 200 apnoeic episodes and 50 minutes of periodic breathing per day, and these may be associated with short-lived reductions in saturation. The proportion of time spent with regular breathing increases with age, such that, beyond 3 months old, periodic breathing and apnoeas are significantly less. Moderate reductions in inspired oxygen (15%), similar to that seen during flying or at altitude (Chapter 16), cause a dramatic increase in the amount of time 3-month-old infants spend with periodic apnoea, indicating that adult hypoxic ventilatory responses are not fully developed.[17]

In babies born prematurely these abnormal breathing patterns are more severe, with prolonged periods of apnoea and periodic breathing which threaten oxygenation.[18] This, coupled with immature lungs making oxygenation difficult, gives rise to a cycle of chronic intermittent hypoxia that contributes to long-term morbidity in premature babies.[19]

Haemoglobin

Children are normally born polycythaemic, with a mean haemoglobin of about 180 g.L^{-1} and a haematocrit (packed cell volume) of 53%. About 70% of the haemoglobin is fetal haemoglobin (HbF), and the resultant P_{50} is well below the normal adult value (see Fig. 10.9). Arterial oxygen content is close to the normal adult value in spite of the low arterial Po_2. The haemoglobin concentration decreases rapidly to become less than the normal adult value by 3 weeks of life. HbF gradually disappears from the circulation to reach negligible values by 6 months, by which time the P_{50} has already attained the normal adult value.

Premature Birth and the Lungs

Respiratory Distress Syndrome

Respiratory distress syndrome (RDS) comprises respiratory distress within a few hours of birth, and occurs in 2% of all live births, but with a greatly increased incidence in premature infants. The essential lesion is a deficiency of surfactant, which is first detectable in the fetal lung at about 24 weeks' gestation, but the concentration increases rapidly after the 30th week. Therefore prematurity is a major factor in the aetiology of RDS, although male babies, Caesarean delivery, perinatal stress, birth asphyxia and maternal diabetes are all additional risk factors for its development.

There is believed to be a genetic susceptibility to developing RDS, possibly resulting from inherited variations in surfactant proteins A and B (page 16).

The disease presents with difficulty in inspiration against the decreased compliance because of the high surface tension of the surfactant-deficient alveolar lining fluid. This progresses to ventilatory failure, alveolar collapse, hyaline membrane deposit, pulmonary oedema leading to denaturing of surfactant and ultimately interference with gas exchange, resulting in hypoxaemia. Increased pulmonary vascular resistance may raise right atrial pressure and reopen the foramen ovale, increasing shunt.

The physiological basis of therapy is to supplement surfactant activity and use artificial ventilation as a temporary expedient to spare the infant the excessive work of breathing against stiff lungs.[20]

Surfactant replacement therapy is difficult because endogenous surfactant is complex, consisting of phospholipids and protein components (page 16). Exogenous surfactants may be either synthetic, consisting mostly of phospholipids, or natural surfactant preparations, obtained from mammalian lungs which contain both phospholipid and some of the surfactant proteins, although not necessarily of the same type and proportion as in humans. Surfactant proteins are important to facilitate spreading of the surfactant around the lung following administration by intratracheal instillation, and natural surfactants may therefore be more effective as therapeutic agents. Surfactant replacement therapy has now been conclusively shown to improve survival and reduce complication rates in RDS.[21]

Artificial ventilation is considered in Chapter 32. A high respiratory frequency is required, such that inspiratory and expiratory durations may be as little as 0.3 seconds, but inflation pressures are similar to those used in adults and do not usually exceed 3 kPa (30 cmH$_2$O). Both the compressible volume of the ventilator circuit and the apparatus dead space tend to be large in relation to the size of very small children, so pressure generators are preferable to volume generators. As in adults, current trends in artificial ventilation are moving away from tracheal intubation and ventilation towards noninvasive ventilation with nasal continuous positive airway pressure or high-flow nasal therapy (page 292).[21]

Bronchopulmonary Dysplasia[21]

Bronchopulmonary dysplasia describes a condition in which a neonate requires oxygen therapy for more than 28 days because of poor lung function. It is a common complication of RDS, and may simply be a form of pulmonary barotrauma (page 392) in the ventilated neonate, or may represent abnormal lung development as a result of prematurity. Airway damage, including smooth muscle hypertrophy, inflammation and fibrosis all occur, and the alveolar stage of lung development (page 176) may be abnormal. Long-term impairment of lung function results, at least into childhood and possibly throughout the patient's whole life, although numbers of alveoli in the lung at 10 to 14 years of age may be normal.[22] Improvements in neonatal care balanced by survival of ever more prematurely born babies means that the overall incidence of BPD remains unchanged, although the disease pattern is changing.[21]

Sudden Infant Death Syndrome[23]

Sudden infant death syndrome (SIDS) is defined simply as the sudden death of an infant younger than 1 year of age that remains unexplained after review of the clinical history, examination of the circumstances of the death and post-mortem examination. The peak incidence is at 2 to 4 months of age, and there remains a multitude of theories regarding the aetiology, although the respiratory system is implicated in most. A triple risk model is proposed, which suggests that an infant must be vulnerable to SIDS, must be at a critical stage of development of homeostatic control and must receive a stressor such as an infection, parental smoking or sleeping in the prone position.

Abnormal homeostatic control may include respiratory disturbances.[24] The apnoea hypothesis remains popular, mainly because of the frequent periods of apnoea and desaturation observed in almost all babies under 3 months old (see earlier discussion). The peak incidence of SIDS corresponds to the period of development when the fetal and adult systems for ventilatory control are swapping over, and it is believed that this may make the infant susceptible to respiratory disturbances. Normal patterns of arousal from sleep are altered in babies who subsequently become SIDS victims. Despite the popularity of the apnoea hypothesis, evidence that these episodes of periodic breathing or apnoeas contribute directly to SIDS is lacking. Postmortem studies have found decreased binding of serotonin in several areas of the brain, including an area which, in adults, is believed to be crucial in controlling arousal from sleep. Furthermore, animal studies have demonstrated that maternal diet when pregnant may affect serotonergic responses in their offspring, including those affecting respiratory control, providing a potential mechanism for the link in humans between SIDS and poverty.[25]

There is a substantial body of agreement that the prone sleeping position is more common in infants dying of SIDS, although the mechanism remains uncertain.[23] In the late 1980s and early 1990s many countries introduced national health educational policies to encourage the avoidance of the prone sleeping position, and the incidence of SIDS was reduced by 50% to 90%.

Development of Lung Function During Childhood

The lungs continue to develop during childhood. Chest wall compliance, which is very high at birth, decreases rapidly for the first 2 years of life, when it becomes approximately equal to lung compliance as in the adult. Below the age of 8 years, measurement of lung volumes is difficult, but beyond this age many studies of normal lung function are available. Because of large variations in the rate at which children grow, reference values are usually related to height rather than age or weight. Equations relating lung volumes to height are available,[26] and some are shown in graphical form in Figure 12.2.

Various indices of respiratory function are independent of age and body size, so adult values can be used. These include forced expiratory volume (1 second) as a fraction of vital capacity, FRC and peak expiratory flow rate as a fraction of total lung capacity, specific airway conductance and specific compliance (page 21) and probably dead space/tidal volume ratio.[26]

Lung growth in childhood is affected by environmental factors, particularly in the first few years of life, such as air pollution, exposure to allergens and lower respiratory tract infections.[27,28] In many individuals these effects result in lower adult lung volumes than other individuals of the same stature, and this is associated with an increased life-long susceptibility to respiratory disease.

Blood gases and the control of breathing are also important. Arterial P_{CO_2} and alveolar P_{O_2} do not change appreciably during childhood, but arterial P_{O_2} increases from the neonatal value to reach a maximum of about 13 kPa (98 mmHg) at young adulthood. Much of this increase occurs during the first year of life. There are obvious difficulties in determining the normal arterial P_{O_2} in children. Ventilatory responses to both hypercapnia and hypoxia are at their highest in early childhood and decrease progressively into adulthood. The changes are small for hypoxic responses, but quite marked for hypercapnia, and are believed to relate to the higher metabolic rate in children.

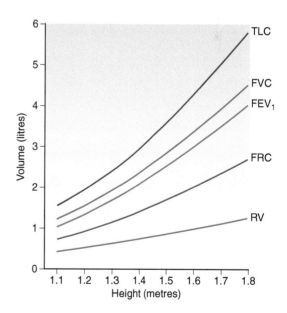

• **Fig. 12.2** Changes in lung volumes as a function of stature. When considering reference values for children, height in metres is used in preference to age to allow for large differences in growth rate. Each graph represents the mean for both boys and girls, although boys generally have greater values at equivalent heights. *FEV₁*, Forced expiratory volume in 1 second; *FRC*, functional residual capacity; *FVC*, forced vital capacity; *RV*, residual volume; *TLC*, total lung capacity.

References

1. Jensen D, Webb KA, Davies GAL, et al. Mechanical ventilatory constraints during incremental cycle exercise in human pregnancy: implications for respiratory sensation. *J Physiol.* 2008;586:4735-4750.
2. Shi W, Bellusci S, Warburton D. Lung development and adult lung diseases. *Chest.* 2007;132:651-656.
3. Surate Solaligue DE, Rodríguez-Castillo JA, Ahlbrecht K, et al. Recent advances in our understanding of the mechanisms of late lung development and bronchopulmonary dysplasia. *Am J Physiol Lung Cell Mol Physiol.* 2017;313:L1101-L1153.
4. Glenny RW. Emergence of matched airway and vascular trees from fractal rules. *J Appl Physiol.* 2011;110:1119-1129.
5. Merkus PJFM. Catch-up alveolar development into adulthood: also in those born prematurely? *Eur Respir J.* 2016;47:710-713.
6. Orgeig S, Morrison JL, Daniels CB. Prenatal development of the pulmonary surfactant system and the influence of hypoxia. *Respir Physiol Neurobiol.* 2011;178:129-145.
7. Suresh S, Mamun AM, O'Callaghan M, et al. The impact of birth weight on peak lung function in young adults. *Chest.* 2012;142:1603-1610.
8. Turner SW, Devereux G. Fetal ultrasound: shedding light or casting shadows on the fetal origins of airway disease. *Am J Respir Crit Care Med.* 2012;185:694-695.
*9. **Kotecha SJ, Edwards MO, Watkins WJ, et al. Effect of preterm birth on later FEV1: a systematic review and meta-analysis. *Thorax.* 2013;68:760-766.**
10. Narang I, Bush A, Rosenthal M. Gas transfer and pulmonary blood flow at rest and during exercise in adults 21 years after preterm birth. *Am J Respir Crit Care Med.* 2009;180:339-345.
*11. **Gibbs K, Collaco JM, McGrath-Morrow SA. Impact of tobacco smoke and nicotine exposure on lung development. *Chest.* 2016;149:552-561.**
12. Spindel ER, McEvoy CT. The role of nicotine in the effects of maternal smoking during pregnancy on lung development and childhood respiratory disease implications for dangers of E-cigarettes. *Am J Respir Crit Care Med.* 2016;193:486-494.
13. Kozyrskyj AL, Pawlowski AN. Maternal distress and childhood wheeze: mechanisms and context. *Am J Respir Crit Care Med.* 2013;187:1160-1162.
14. Quon BS, Goss CH. Maternal stress: a cause of childhood asthma? *Am J Respir Crit Care Med.* 2012;186:116-124.
15. Lee AG, Kaali S, Quinn A, et al. Prenatal household air pollution is associated with impaired infant lung function with sex-specific effects. Evidence from Graphs, a cluster randomized cookstove intervention trial. *Am J Respir Crit Care Med.* 2019;199:738-746.
16. Greer J. Development of respiratory rhythm generation. *J Appl Physiol.* 2008;104:1211-1212.
17. Parkins KJ, Poets CF, O'Brien LM, et al. Effect of exposure to 15% oxygen on breathing patterns and oxygen saturation in infants: interventional study. *BMJ.* 1998;316:887-894.
18. Mohr MA, Vergales BD, Lee H, et al. Very long apnea events in preterm infants. *J Appl Physiol.* 2015;118:558-568.
19. Di Fiore JM, Martin RJ, Gauda EB. Apnea of prematurity–perfect storm. *Respir Physiol Neurobiol.* 2013;189:213-222.
20. Stevens TP, Sinkin RA. Surfactant replacement therapy. *Chest.* 2007;131:1577-1582.
*21. **Owen LS, Manley BJ, Davis PG, et al. The evolution of modern respiratory care for preterm infants. *Lancet.* 2017;389:1649-1659.**
22. Jobe AH. Good news for lung repair in preterm infants. *Am J Respir Crit Care Med.* 2013;187:1043-1044.
*23. **Kinney HC, Thach BT. The sudden infant death syndrome. *N Engl J Med.* 2009;361:795-805.**
24. Porzionato A, Macchi V, De Caro R. Central and peripheral chemoreceptors in sudden infant death syndrome. *J Physiol.* 2018;596(15):3007-3019.
25. Bavis RW. Poor diets, abnormal breathing, and SIDS risk. *J Appl Physiol.* 2011;110:303-304.
26. Cotes JE, Chinn DJ, Miller MR. *Lung function. Physiology, measurement and application in medicine.* Oxford: Blackwell Publishing; 2006.
27. Belgrave DCM, Granell R, Turner SW, et al. Lung function trajectories from preschool age to adulthood and their associations with early life factors: a retrospective analysis of three population-based birth cohort studies. *Lancet Respir Med.* 2018;6:526-534.
28. Litonjua AA, Gold DR. Early-life exposures and later lung function. Add pollutants to the mix. *Am J Respir Crit Care Med.* 2016;193:110-111.

13

Exercise

KEY POINTS

- Oxygen consumption increases linearly with the power expended during exercise.
- The extra tissue oxygen requirement is provided by increases in cardiac output and blood oxygen extraction.
- To accommodate these changes ventilation also increases linearly with exercise—this response occurs the moment exercise begins.

- With increasing exercise intensity, lactate is produced from anaerobic muscle metabolism, and blood lactate levels increase, initially reaching a steady state but continuing to rise in severe exercise.

The respiratory response to exercise depends on the level of exercise performed, which can be conveniently divided into three grades:

1. *Moderate exercise* is below the subject's anaerobic threshold (AT; see later), and the arterial blood lactate is not raised. The subject is able to transport all the oxygen required and remain in a steady state.
2. *Heavy exercise* is above the AT. The arterial blood lactate is elevated but remains constant. This too may be regarded as a steady state.
3. *Severe exercise* is well above the AT, and the arterial blood lactate continues to rise. This is an unsteady state, and the level of work cannot be sustained for long.

Oxygen Consumption During Exercise

There is a close relationship between the external power that is produced and the oxygen consumption of the subject (Fig. 13.1). The oxygen consumption at rest (the basal metabolic rate) is of the order of 200 to 250 mL.min^{-1}. As work is done, the oxygen consumption increases by approximately 12 mL.min^{-1} per watt. Exercise intensity is commonly described in terms of metabolic equivalents (METs), which refer to the number of multiples of the normal resting oxygen consumption for that subject. For example, walking briskly on the level requires an oxygen consumption of about 1 L.min^{-1}, or 4 METs, whereas running at 12 km/h (7.5 mph) requires about 3 L.min^{-1} of

oxygen and is rated as 12 METs of activity. Further examples are shown in Figure 13.1.

Time Course of the Increase in Oxygen Consumption

Oxygen consumption rises rapidly at the onset of a period of exercise, with an accompanying increase in carbon dioxide production and a small increase in blood lactate. With moderate exercise (Fig. 13.2, *A*) a plateau is quickly reached, and the lactate level remains well below the normal maximum resting level (<3.5 mmol.L^{-1}). With heavy exercise $\dot{V}_{O_2}$ (oxygen consumption), $\dot{V}_{CO_2}$ (carbon dioxide production) and lactate all increase more quickly, again reaching constant levels within a few minutes, the magnitude of which relates to the power generated and the fitness of the subject (Fig. 13.2, *B*). If the level of exercise exceeds approximately 60% of the subject's maximal exercise ability (see later), there is usually a secondary 'slow component' to the increase in oxygen consumption, associated with a continuing increase in blood lactate level, which ultimately prevents the exercise from continuing (Fig. 13.2, *C*). There have been many explanations proposed for this slow component of $\dot{V}_{O_2}$, including increased temperature, the oxygen cost of breathing, lactic acidosis and changes in muscle metabolism secondary to the use of differing fibre types with prolonged exercise.[1] The physiological mechanism underlying the linkage between oxygen requirement by

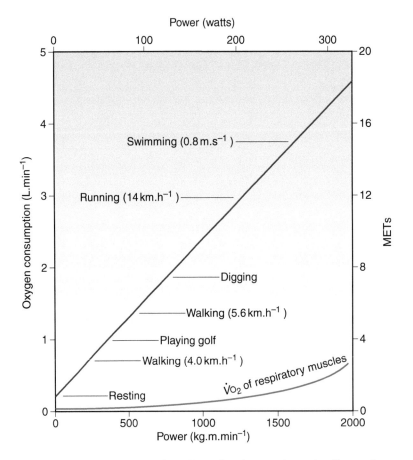

Power (watts)

Oxygen consumption (L.min^{-1})

METs

Swimming (0.8 m.s^{-1})

Running (14 km.h^{-1})

Digging

Walking (5.6 km.h^{-1})

Playing golf

Walking (4.0 km.h^{-1})

$\dot{V}_{O_2}$ of respiratory muscles

Resting

Power (kg.m.min^{-1})

• **Fig. 13.1** Steady-state oxygen consumption with varying degrees of exercise. The continuous red line denotes whole-body oxygen consumption as a function of the level of power developed. The blue curve is an estimate of the oxygen cost of breathing for the increasing hyperventilation of exercise. *METs*, Metabolic equivalents, which is the number of multiples of basal oxygen consumption required for different activities.

muscles and its delivery during exercise, and the time course of this response, remain incompletely explained.[2]

Maximal Oxygen Uptake

$\dot{V}_{O_2max}$ is the maximum rate of oxygen uptake possible for that subject. A fit and healthy young adult should be able to achieve a $\dot{V}_{O_2max}$ of about 40 mL.min^{-1}.kg^{-1} for female subjects and 48 mL.min^{-1}.kg^{-1} for males, which equates to using over 3 L of oxygen per minute for a 70-kg man.[3] However, the type of exercise evoking $\dot{V}_{O_2max}$ varies between subjects, so that where only a single graded exercise test is used, the highest $\dot{V}_{O_2}$ recorded represents a peak response, $\dot{V}_{O_2peak}$. $\dot{V}_{O_2max}$ represents *the* upper functional limit for that subject, whereas $\dot{V}_{O_2peak}$ represents *an* upper functional limit for that subject during a single test and is the preferred term here.[4] Normal values for $\dot{V}_{O_2peak}$ decrease at approximately 8% per decade beyond 30 years of age. A sedentary existence without exercise can reduce $\dot{V}_{O_2peak}$ to 50% of the expected value. Conversely, $\dot{V}_{O_2peak}$ can be increased by regular exercise, and athletes commonly achieve values of

5 L.min^{-1}. The highest levels (>6 L.min^{-1}) are attained in rowers, who use a greater muscle mass than other athletes, and require an impressive respiratory effort such as a minute volume of 200 L.min^{-1} (tidal volume 3.29 L at a frequency of 62 breaths per minute).

$\dot{V}_{O_2peak}$ is commonly used in exercise physiology as a measure of cardiorespiratory fitness. Subjects undertake a period of graduated exercise, whereas $\dot{V}_{O_2}$ is measured continuously by a spirometric method (page 161). In all but severe exercise, within a few minutes $\dot{V}_{O_2}$ reaches a plateau (Fig. 13.2), which is the subject's $\dot{V}_{O_2peak}$. At higher levels of exercise, as seen in athletes, defining when maximal oxygen uptake is reached may be difficult because of the slow component of oxygen consumption. Elite athletes rarely reach a satisfactory plateau in $\dot{V}_{O_2peak}$, and secondary criteria such as high plasma lactate levels or a raised respiratory exchange ratio may be used to define $\dot{V}_{O_2peak}$. At $\dot{V}_{O_2peak}$ in trained athletes, approximately 80% of the oxygen consumed is used by locomotor muscles. With the high minute volumes seen during exercise, the oxygen consumption of respiratory muscles also becomes significant, and is around 5% of total $\dot{V}_{O_2}$ with moderate exercise and 10% at $\dot{V}_{O_2peak}$ (Fig. 13.1).

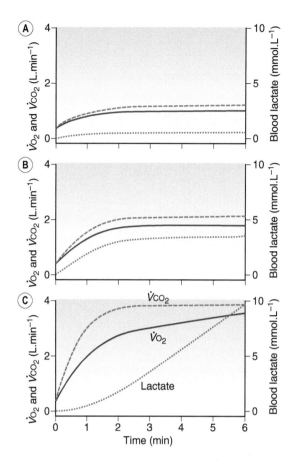

• **Fig. 13.2** Changes in oxygen consumption ($\dot{V}O_2$, *solid red line*), carbon dioxide production ($\dot{V}CO_2$, *blue dashed line*) and blood lactate (*dotted orange line*) with the onset of varying levels of exercise. **(A)** Light to moderate exercise with little or no increase in lactate; **(B)** heavy exercise with an increase in lactate to an increased, but steady, level; **(C)** severe exercise, above the anaerobic threshold when levels continue to rise as exercise proceeds. Note that, with severe exercise **(C)**, the increase in oxygen consumption is biphasic, with a second 'slow' component.

Response of the Oxygen Delivery System

A 10- or 20-fold increase in oxygen consumption requires a complex adaptation of both circulatory and respiratory systems.

Oxygen Delivery

Oxygen delivery is the product of cardiac output and arterial oxygen content (page 155). The latter cannot be significantly increased, so an increase in cardiac output is essential. However, the cardiac output does not, and indeed could not, increase in proportion to the oxygen consumption. For example, an oxygen consumption of 4 L.min^{-1} is a 16-fold increase compared with the resting state. A typical cardiac output at this level of exercise would be only 25 L.min^{-1} (Fig. 13.3), which is only five times the resting value. Therefore there must also be increased extraction of oxygen from the blood. Figure 13.3 shows that the largest relative increase in cardiac output occurs at mild levels of

exercise. At an oxygen consumption of 1 L.min^{-1} cardiac output is already close to 50% of its maximal value.

Oxygen Extraction

In the resting state, blood returns to the right heart with haemoglobin 70% saturated. This provides a substantial reserve of available oxygen, and the arterial/mixed venous oxygen content difference increases progressively as oxygen consumption is increased, particularly in heavy exercise when the mixed venous saturation may be as low as 20% (Fig. 13.3). This decrease in mixed venous saturation covers the steep part of the oxygen dissociation curve (see Fig. 10.9), and therefore the decrease in P_{O_2} is relatively less (5–2 kPa, or 37.5–15 mmHg). High levels of blood lactate seen during heavy exercise may contribute to the increase in oxygen extraction by shifting the dissociation curve to the right at a capillary level.

The increasingly desaturated blood returning to the lungs and the greater flow of blood require that the respiratory system transports a larger quantity of oxygen to the alveoli. If there were no increased oxygen transport to the alveoli, the reserve oxygen in the mixed venous blood would be exhausted in one or two circulation times. Fortunately the respiratory system normally responds rapidly to this requirement.

Anaerobic Metabolism

During heavy exercise, the total work exceeds the capacity for aerobic work, which is limited by oxygen transport (see later). The difference is made up by anaerobic metabolism, of which the principal product is lactic acid (see Fig. 10.12), which is almost entirely ionized to lactate and hydrogen ions. The AT may be defined as the highest intensity of exercise at which measured oxygen uptake can account for the entire energy requirement.[5] Exercise intensity at the AT depends not only on the power produced, but also on many other factors, including environmental temperature, the degree of training undertaken by the subject and altitude. An additional factor is the muscle groups that are used to accomplish the work, as different skeletal muscle fibres, and therefore muscle groups, have different metabolic products.

During severe exercise the lactate level continues to rise (Fig. 13.2, *C*) and begins to cause distress at levels greater than 11 mmol.L^{-1}, 10 times the normal resting level. Lactate accumulation seems to be the limiting factor for sustained heavy work, and the progressive increase in blood lactate results in the level of work being inversely related to the time for which it can be maintained. Thus there is a reciprocal relationship between the record time for various distances and the speed at which they are run.

Oxygen Debt

The difference between the total work and the aerobic work is achieved by anaerobic metabolism of carbohydrates to lactate, which is ultimately converted to citrate, enters the citric acid cycle and is then fully oxidized (page 153). Like glucose, lactate has a respiratory quotient of 1.0. Although

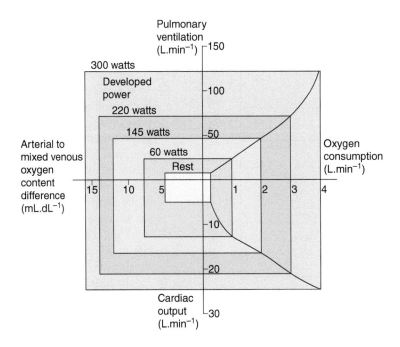

• **Fig. 13.3** Changes in ventilation, oxygen consumption, cardiac output and oxygen extraction at different levels of power developed.

this process continues during heavy exercise, lactate accumulates, and the excess is oxidized in the early stages of recovery. Oxygen consumption remains above the resting level during recovery for this purpose. This constitutes the 'repayment of the oxygen debt', and is related to the lactate level attained by the end of exercise.

Repayment of the oxygen debt is especially well developed in diving mammals such as seals and whales (page 311). During a dive, their circulation is largely diverted to the heart and brain, and the metabolism of the skeletal muscles is almost entirely anaerobic. On regaining the surface, very large quantities of lactate are suddenly released into the circulation and are rapidly metabolized while the animal is on the surface between dives.

Excess Post-Exercise Oxygen Consumption

Sustained heavy exercise results in an increased $\dot{V}_{O_2}$ even when the subject's blood lactate remains only mildly elevated. Excess oxygen consumption may occur for several hours, and is related to both the intensity and duration of exercise undertaken. Previous hypotheses put forward to explain the excess $\dot{V}_{O_2}$ included an increase in body temperature and increased fat metabolism, although proof of these is lacking. Exercise at around 75% of $\dot{V}_{O_{2peak}}$ raises levels of catabolic hormones such as cortisol and catecholamines, which may explain the excess $\dot{V}_{O_2}$.[6]

Ventilatory Response to Exercise

Time Course[7]

In the previous section it was seen that exercise without a rapid ventilatory response would be dangerous, if not fatal.

In fact, the respiratory system does respond with great rapidity (Fig. 13.4). There is an instant increase in ventilation at, if not slightly before, the start of exercise (phase I). During moderate exercise, there is then a further increase (phase II) to reach an equilibrium level of ventilation (phase III) within about 3 minutes. With heavy exercise there is a secondary increase in ventilation that may reach a plateau, but ventilation continues to rise in severe work. At the end of exercise, the minute volume falls to resting levels within a few minutes. After heavy and severe exercise, return to the resting level of ventilation takes longer, as the oxygen debt is repaid and lactate levels return to normal.

Ventilation Equivalent for Oxygen

The respiratory minute volume is normally very well matched to the increased oxygen consumption, and the relationship between minute volume and oxygen consumption is approximately linear up to an oxygen consumption of about 2 L.min^{-1} in the untrained subject, and more after training (Fig. 13.5). The slope of the linear part is the ventilation equivalent for oxygen, and is within the range of 20 to 30 L.min^{-1} ventilation per L.min^{-1} of oxygen consumption. The slope does not appear to change with training.

In heavy exercise, above a critical level of oxygen consumption (Owles point), the ventilation increases above the level predicted by an extrapolation of the linear part of the ventilation/oxygen consumption relationship (Fig. 13.5). This is surplus to the requirement for gas exchange, and is accompanied by hypocapnia with arterial P_{CO_2} decreasing by levels of the order of 1 kPa (7.5 mmHg). The excess ventilation is probably driven by lactic acidosis. In the trained athlete, the break from linearity occurs at higher

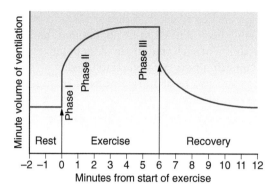

• **Fig. 13.4** The time course of changes in ventilation in relation to a short period of moderate exercise. Note the instant increase in ventilation at the start of exercise before the metabolic consequences of exercise have had time to develop.

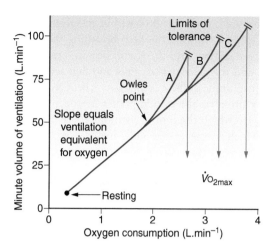

• **Fig. 13.5** Changes in minute volume of ventilation in response to the increased oxygen consumption of exercise. The break from linearity (Owles point) occurs at higher levels of oxygen consumption in trained athletes, who can also tolerate higher minute volumes. A to C show progressive levels of training. Both mechanisms combine to enable the trained athlete to increase his or her maximum oxygen consumption.

levels of oxygen consumption. This, together with improved tolerance of high minute volumes, allows the trained athlete to increase his $\dot{V}_{O_{2peak}}$, as shown in Figure 13.5.

Minute Volume and Dyspnoea

It is generally believed that the ventilatory system does not limit exercise in normal subjects. Approximately 50% to 60% of maximal breathing capacity (MBC) is required for work at 80% of aerobic capacity. However, the breaking point of exercise is usually determined by breathlessness, which occurs when the exercise ventilation uses a high proportion of the MBC. There is a close correlation between MBC and $\dot{V}_{O_{2peak}}$.

Minute volumes as great as 200 L.min^{-1} have been recorded during exercise, although the normal subject cannot maintain a minute volume approaching MBC for more than a very short period. Tidal volume during maximal exercise is about half vital capacity, and 70% to 80% of MBC can normally be maintained, with difficulty, for 15 minutes by fit young subjects. Ventilation approximates to 60% of MBC at maximal oxygen consumption. The usable fraction of the MBC can, however, be increased by training.

Control of Ventilation

Elucidation of the mechanisms that underlie the remarkably efficient adaptation of ventilation to the demands of exercise has remained a challenge to generations of physiologists, and a complete explanation remains elusive.[7,8]

Neural Factors

It has long been evident that neural factors play an important role, particularly as ventilation normally increases at or even before the start of exercise (phase I), when no other physiological variable has changed except cardiac output (Fig. 13.4). These neural factors may involve afferent input from the exercising muscles and the higher centres of the brain. Evidence for the former is found by interrupting the peripheral afferent input by spinal anaesthesia, which decreases the ventilatory response to exercise. Evidence for the latter includes the observation that the phase I ventilatory response may be in part a 'learned' response to the onset of exercise. Simply imagining exercising in an otherwise relaxed subject causes an increase in ventilation. Under these conditions, positron emission tomography shows activation of several areas of the cerebral cortex, again indicating that the early increase in ventilation with exercise is a behavioural response.[8]

Arterial Blood Gas Partial Pressures and the Chemoreceptors

There is ample evidence that, during exercise at sea level with oxygen consumption up to about 3 L.min^{-1}, in the majority of subjects there is no significant change in either the P_{CO_2} or the P_{O_2} of arterial blood. In one study, even at the point of exhaustion (oxygen consumption 3.5 L.min^{-1}), the arterial P_{O_2} was the same as the resting value, and P_{CO_2} was reduced. Therefore in healthy subjects, blood gas partial pressures do not seem at first sight to be the main factor governing the increased minute volume. There is a caveat to this conclusion.

The P_{O_2}/ventilation response curve is known to be steeper during exercise (see Fig. 4.8), so ventilation will respond to small fluctuations in normal arterial P_{O_2} under these circumstances. Carotid body resection or administration of dopamine to inhibit carotid body activity reduces the ventilatory response to exercise, particularly phase II (Fig. 13.4). Thus it seems likely that the peripheral chemoreceptors contribute to exercise-induced hyperpnoea, particularly during the non-steady state.[7] This response may not result from changes in P_{O_2}, but from oscillations in arterial P_{CO_2}.[9] Unlike in the resting state, when gas flow within the alveolus is by diffusion (page 7), during the deep breathing that accompanies exercise, air flow into the alveoli becomes more tidal in nature, and the arterial $P\text{CO}_2$ rises and falls with each breath. The magnitude of these oscillations is believed to affect respiratory drive via the carotid bodies irrespective of the mean $P\text{CO}_2$ (to which the central chemoreceptors respond), an effect which is exaggerated under hypoxic conditions.

Humoral Mechanisms

Humoral factors play a comparatively minor role in moderate exercise but are more important in heavy and severe exercise when metabolic acidosis is an important factor. Lactic acidosis contributes to excess ventilation during heavy and severe exercise (Fig. 13.5), causing a slight reduction in arterial $P\text{CO}_2$. Slight additional respiratory drive may result from hyperthermia.

Fitness and Training

The definitions of moderate, heavy and severe exercise at the beginning of this chapter are not transferable between individuals. A given amount of energy expenditure that constitutes severe exercise to a sedentary unfit subject is likely to represent less than moderate exercise to a trained athlete. The linear relationship between power generated and $\dot{V}\text{O}_2$ (Fig. 13.1) is remarkably consistent irrespective of fitness and training, but the distance a subject may progress along this line, that is their $\dot{V}\text{O}_{2\text{peak}}$, is extremely variable.

In healthy untrained subjects, rapidly increasing lactate levels normally limit exercise tolerance. Intracellular lactic acidosis in muscles gives rise to weakness and cramp, the respiratory stimulation rapidly takes the subject towards an intolerable minute ventilation, and exhaustion occurs. Training changes many aspects of exercise physiology. For example, improved cardiovascular fitness results in improved oxygen delivery, such that the $\dot{V}\text{O}_2$ at which lactate rises is greatly increased. Muscle in trained athletes releases less lactate than in untrained subjects (see later), and animal studies indicate that training may improve the ability of the liver to remove circulating lactate. Finally, trained athletes can tolerate much higher blood lactate levels, up to 20 mmol.L^{-1}, or twice that of untrained subjects.

Maximizing physiological and performance adaptations through training is well recognized, and there has been recent interest in identifying the optimal exercise 'prescription.' Aerobic training is broadly divided into chronic endurance training and higher intensity training, the latter involving bursts of exercise interspersed with rest periods. Higher intensity training may be further categorized as either sprint interval training (SIT) involving short bursts (<30 seconds) of supra-maximal, usually anaerobic, exercise or high-intensity interval training (HIIT) with longer periods (1–4 minutes) of less intense, usually aerobic, exercise. The higher intensity types have been promoted as time-efficient alternatives to endurance training, and enhanced $\dot{V}\text{O}_2$ kinetics and skeletal muscle mitochondrial

function are described.[10] Studies of SIT and HIIT have so far mainly been limited to fit populations, and the effects or suitability of such training in older populations or those with comorbidity is less well established.[11]

There are two respiratory aspects of training that merit further consideration.

Minute Volume of Ventilation

Maximal expiratory flow rate is limited by flow-dependent airway closure (page 32), and is relatively unaffected by training. However, within the limits of MBC, it is possible to increase the strength and endurance of the respiratory muscles. It is therefore possible to improve the fraction of the MBC that can be sustained during exercise. Highly trained athletes may be able to maintain ventilations as much as 90% of their MBC. Age and sex have significant effects on work of breathing, operating lung volumes, expiratory flow limitation and dyspnea during maximal exercise. Women and older subjects have a higher work of breathing for a given minute ventilation during maximal exercise, although this was not significant at submaximal minute ventilation.[12]

Ventilation Equivalent for Oxygen

There is no evidence that training can alter the slope of the plot of ventilation against oxygen consumption (Fig. 13.5). However, the upward inflection of the curve (Owles point) is further to the right in the trained subject. This permits the attainment of a higher oxygen consumption for the same minute volume. Prolongation of the straight part of the curve is achieved by improving metabolic processes in skeletal muscle to minimize the stimulant effect of lactic acid. There is ample evidence that training can improve the aerobic performance of muscles by many adaptations, including, for example, the increased density of the capillary network in the muscles. The consequent reduction in lactic acidosis and therefore the excess ventilation, together with an increase in the tolerable minute volume, combine to increase the $\dot{V}\text{O}_2$, as shown in Figure 13.5. It would seem that the major factor in increasing the $\dot{V}\text{O}_{2\text{peak}}$ is improved performance of skeletal muscle and the cardiovascular system, rather than any specific change in respiratory function.

Exercise-Induced Arterial Hypoxaemia

In contrast to cardiac and skeletal muscle, the lungs do not undergo structural or morphological changes in response to training. This is not usually a problem as healthy individuals exercising at or near to sea level are able to maintain normal arterial oxygen levels. There is some evidence that individuals with a high $\dot{V}\text{O}_{2\text{peak}}$ have a greater pulmonary capillary blood volume at rest, and in some cases lung diffusing capacity is also greater. Despite these factors, in approximately half of highly trained male athletes and in a slightly greater proportion of females, arterial hypoxaemia develops just before maximal exercise is achieved.[13] Many possible causes have been proposed, including the development of a diffusion barrier when large quantities of oxygen are being absorbed (page 119), maldistribution of pulmonary ventilation/perfusion and mechanical constraints such as expiratory airflow limitation. The last of these can be improved by breathing helium–oxygen mixtures (page 30), which reduces resistance to turbulent gas flow and attenuates exercise-induced arterial hypoxaemia (EIAH). In thoroughbred racehorses EIAH is a significant problem, as horses are unable to mount a large enough ventilatory response to match their enormous exercise capacity (page 310).

Cardiorespiratory Disease

Patients with cardiovascular or respiratory disease have poor exercise tolerance for three main reasons. First, the ventilatory response to exercise is more rapid, so a greater minute volume is required to achieve a given $\dot{V}_{O_2}$. Second, the proportion of MBC that a patient can tolerate is reduced, and when combined with the previous observation this results in an extreme limitation of exercise tolerance before shortness of breath intervenes. Hypoxia or hypercapnia occur more commonly during exercise in patients with respiratory disease. Third, a limited increase in cardiac output in response to exercise means that mixed venous oxygen levels will fall to low levels more quickly, and also causes inadequate muscle blood flow, impairing the function of respiratory and other muscles. Anaerobic metabolism therefore occurs much more quickly, leading to extra ventilatory requirements and exhaustion.

Exercise Testing

The limited respiratory response to exercise seen in patients with cardiorespiratory disease has led to the use of exercise testing as a means of quantifying the extent of their disease or assessing their ability to withstand physiological stresses such as major surgery. A variety of exercise tests exist in which the patient is observed and monitored performing exercise. A shuttle test involves the subject walking between two points 9 m apart with the required speed determined by auditory signals, the outcome being the number of shuttles achieved before stopping because of tiredness or other symptoms. The 6-minute walk test (6MWT) simply measures the distance walked in the fixed time. Both tests are useful measures of respiratory disease severity, but are partly subjective; for example, the 6MWT distance is influenced by the verbal instructions given to the patient during the test.[14] A more complex test is cardiopulmonary exercise testing (CPET). During a progressively increasing workload, a variety of measures may be made, including $\dot{V}_{O_{2peak}}$, AT,[5] ventilation equivalent for oxygen ($\dot{V}/\dot{V}_{O_2}$) and ventilation equivalent for carbon dioxide ($\dot{V}/\dot{V}_{CO_2}$). These measures are reduced in patients with cardiac and/or respiratory disease, and have been shown to be predictive of poor outcomes in patients undergoing major, high-risk surgery.[15] Variation in measured parameters exists between

institutions, along with a lack of consensus regarding their interpretation, for example the AT level that leads to a patient being considered 'high risk'. Recent guidelines have been produced on the organization, conduct and interpretation of CPET[16] which seek to improve the performance of, and evidence for, CPET. Scores have been developed based on patient-reported exercise status, for example, the Duke Activity Status Index which has been shown to predict perioperative death or myocardial infarction.[17] All the above scores and measures should however only be regarded as additional data which may be used to inform complex clinical decisions about perioperative management. A relatively new area of study is 'respiratory prehabilitation' where, in addition to preoperative testing of cardiorespiratory function, individuals undertake training preoperatively to seek to improve outcomes.[18]

References

1. Poole DC, Barstow TJ, Gaesser GA, et al. $\dot{V}_{O_2}$ slow component: physiological and functional significance. *Med Sci Sports Exerc.* 1994;26:1354-1358.
2. Poole DC. Oxygen's double-edged sword: balancing muscle O_2 supply and use during exercise. *J Physiol.* 2011;589:457-458.
3. Edvardsen E, Hansen BH, Holme IM, et al. Reference values for cardiorespiratory response and fitness on the treadmill in a 20- to 85-year-old population. *Chest.* 2013;144:241-248.
4. Green S, Askew C. $\dot{V}_{O_{2peak}}$ is an acceptable estimate of cardiorespiratory fitness but not $\dot{V}_{O_{2max}}$. *J Appl Physiol.* 2018;125:229-232.
*5. **Hopker JG, Jobson SA, Pandit JJ. Controversies in the physiological basis of the 'anaerobic threshold' and their implications for clinical cardiopulmonary exercise testing. *Anaesthesia.* 2011;66:111-123.**
6. Quinn TJ, Vroman NB, Kertzer R. Postexercise oxygen consumption in trained females: effect of exercise duration. *Med Sci Sports Exerc.* 1994;26:908-913.
7. Whipp BJ. Peripheral chemoreceptor control of exercise hyperpnea in humans. *Med Sci Sports Exerc.* 1994;26:337-347.
8. Asahara R, Matsukawa K, Ishii K, et al. The prefrontal oxygenation and ventilatory responses at start of one-legged cycling exercise have relation to central command. *J Appl Physiol.* 2016;121:1115-1126.
*9. **Collier DJ, Nickol AH, Milledge JS, et al. Alveolar P_{CO_2} oscillations and ventilation at sea level and at high altitude. *J Appl Physiol.* 2008;104:404-415.**
10. Christensen PM, Jacobs RA, Bonne T. A short period of high-intensity interval training improves skeletal muscle mitochondrial function and pulmonary oxygen uptake kinetics. *J Appl Physiol.* 2016;120:1319-1327.
11. Holloway TM, Spriet LL. Crosstalk opposing view: High intensity interval training does not have a role in risk reduction or treatment of disease. *J Physiol.* 2015;594:5219-5221.
12. Molgat-Seon Y, Dominelli PB, Ramsook AH, et al. The effects of age and sex on mechanical ventilatory constraint and dyspnea during exercise in healthy humans. *J Appl Physiol.* 2018;124:1092-1106.
*13. **Olfert IM. Exercise and the lungs: nature or nurture? *J Physiol.* 2016;594:5037-5038.**
14. Weir NA, Brown AW, Shlobin OA, et al. The influence of alternative instruction on 6-min walk test distance. *Chest.* 2013;144:1900-1905.

15. Carlisle J, Swart M. Mid-term survival after abdominal aortic aneurysm surgery predicted by cardiopulmonary exercise testing. *Br J Surg*. 2007;94:966-969.

16. Levett DZH, Jack S, Swart M, et al. Perioperative cardiopulmonary exercise testing (CPET): consensus clinical guidelines on indications, organization, conduct, and physiological interpretation. *Br J Anaesth*. 2018;120:484-500.

17. Wijeysundera DN, Pearse RM, Shulman MA, et al. Assessment of functional capacity before major non-cardiac surgery; an international prospective cohort study. *Lancet*. 2018;391:2631-2640.

18. Lumb AB. Pre-operative respiratory optimisation: an expert review. *Anaesthesia*. 2019;74(suppl 1):43-48.

14

Sleep

KEY POINTS

- During normal sleep tidal volume is reduced, with maximal reduction in ventilation occurring during rapid eye movement sleep when breathing also becomes irregular.
- Reduction in the speed and strength of pharyngeal muscle reflexes causes increased airways resistance, leading to snoring in many normal individuals.

- Sleep-disordered breathing describes a continuum of abnormalities ranging from occasional snoring to frequent periods of airway obstruction and hypoxia during sleep.

Normal Sleep

Sleep is classified on the basis of the electroencephalogram (EEG) and electro-oculogram (EOG) into rapid eye movement (REM) and non-REM (stages N1–N4) sleep.

Stage N1 is dozing, from which arousal easily takes place. The EEG is low voltage, and the frequency is mixed but predominantly fast. This progresses to stage N2 in which the background EEG is similar to stage N1 but with episodic sleep spindles (frequency 12–14 Hz) and K complexes (large biphasic waves of characteristic appearance). Slow, large-amplitude (delta) waves start to appear in stage N2, but become more dominant in stage N3 in which spindles are less conspicuous and K complexes become difficult to distinguish. In stage N4, which is often referred to as deep sleep, the EEG is mainly high voltage (more than 75 μV) and more than 50% slow (delta) frequency.

REM sleep has quite different characteristics. The EEG pattern is the same as in stage N1, but the EOG shows frequent rapid eye movements that are easily distinguished from the rolling eye movements of non-REM sleep. Skeletal muscle tone generally decreases, and dreaming occurs during REM sleep.

The stage of sleep changes frequently during the night, and the pattern varies between different individuals and on different nights for the same individual (Fig. 14.1). Sleep is entered in stage N1 and usually progresses through stage N2 to N3 and sometimes into stage N4. Episodes of REM sleep alternate with non-REM sleep throughout the night. On average there are four or five episodes of REM sleep per night, with a tendency for the duration of the episodes to increase towards morning. Conversely, stages N3 and N4 predominate in the early part of the night.

Respiratory Changes

Ventilation[1]

Tidal volume decreases with deepening levels of non-REM sleep and is minimal in REM sleep, when it is about 25% less than in the awake state. Respiratory frequency is generally unchanged, although breathing is normally irregular during REM sleep. Minute volume is progressively reduced in parallel with the tidal volume. These changes in ventilation are brought about by the same neurochemical changes that cause sleep. Increased activity of gamma aminobutyric acid (GABA)-secreting neurones during sleep has a direct depressant effect on the respiratory centre (see Fig. 4.4), and activation of cholinergic neurones is thought to be responsible for the respiratory patterns seen during non-REM sleep.[1]

Arterial P_{CO_2} is usually slightly elevated by about 0.4 kPa (3 mmHg). In the young healthy adult, arterial P_{O_2} decreases by about the same amount as the P_{CO_2} is increased, therefore the oxygen saturation remains reasonably normal. The rib cage contribution to breathing (page 63) is close to the normal awake supine position value of 29% during REM sleep, but increases during non-REM stages.

Chemosensitivity

In humans, the slopes of the hypercapnic and hypoxic ventilatory responses are markedly reduced during sleep. In both cases, the slope is reduced by approximately one-third during non-REM sleep, and even further reduced during

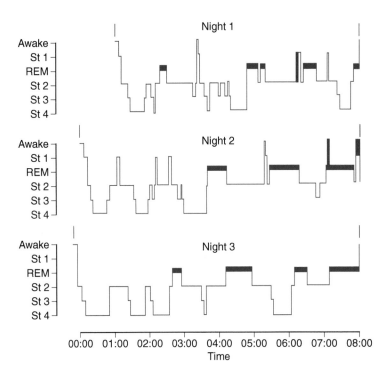

• **Fig. 14.1** Patterns of sleep on three consecutive nights in a 20-year-old fit man. The thick horizontal bars indicate rapid eye movement (REM) sleep.

REM sleep, but fortunately the responses are never abolished completely.

Effect of Age

Compared with young subjects, the elderly have more variable ventilatory patterns when awake, which seems to result in more episodes of breathing instability and apnoea when asleep.[2] Elderly subjects also have significant oscillations in upper airway resistance during sleep (see later), which may contribute to the observed variations in ventilation. Thus as age advances, episodes of transient hypoxaemia occur in subjects who are otherwise healthy, with saturations commonly falling to as low as 75% during sleep. Such changes must be regarded as a normal part of the ageing process.

Pharyngeal Airway Resistance

Air flow through the sharp bends of the upper airway is normally laminar, but is believed to be very close to becoming turbulent even in normal subjects.[3] Pharyngeal muscles may play a crucial role in maintaining the optimum shape of the airway to maintain laminar flow, and the speed at which these control mechanisms can respond to changes in pharyngeal pressure (page 59) may be critical. Any condition that attenuates or delays these reflexes even slightly, such as sleep or alcohol ingestion, will then have a major effect on air flow in the pharynx, causing breakdown of the normally laminar flow.

The nasal airway is normally used during sleep, and upper airway resistance is consistently increased, especially during inspiration and in REM sleep. The main sites of increase are across the soft palate and in the hypopharynx.

Changes in pharyngeal muscle activity with sleep are complex. Muscles with predominantly tonic activity, such as the tensor palati, show a progressive decrease in activity with deepening non-REM sleep, reaching only 20% to 30% of awake activity in stage N4 sleep. This loss of tonic activity correlates with increased upper airway resistance. Unlike in the awake state, the tensor palati also fails to respond to an inspiratory resistive load. The activity of muscles with predominantly phasic inspiratory activity (e.g., geniohyoid and genioglossus) is influenced little by non-REM sleep. In spite of maintained phasic activity during non-REM sleep, tonic activity of geniohyoid is reduced, whereas that of genioglossus is well-preserved and responds appropriately to resistive loading.[4] It thus appears that the major effect is upon the tonic activity of nasopharyngeal muscles, and the increase in hypopharyngeal resistance seems to be because of secondary downstream collapse.

The ventilatory response to increased airway resistance is important in normal sleep because of the increased pharyngeal resistance and is generally well preserved. There are substantial and rapid increases in both diaphragmatic and genioglossal inspiratory activity following nasal occlusion in normal sleeping adults.[5]

Snoring

Snoring may occur at any age, but the incidence is bimodal, peaking in the first and the fifth to sixth decades of life. It occurs more frequently in males than females, is linked to obesity and is common in the third trimester of pregnancy.[6] It may occur in any stage of sleep, becoming more pronounced as non-REM sleep deepens, although usually attenuated in REM sleep. As may be expected, snoring is less severe when sleeping in the lateral rather than supine position.[7] About one-quarter of the population are habitual snorers, but these vary from the occasional snorer (e.g., after alcohol or with an upper respiratory tract infection) to the habitual, persistent and heavy snorer.

Snoring originates in the oropharynx, and in its mildest form is because of vibration of the soft palate and posterior pillars of the fauces. However, in its more severe forms, during inspiration the walls of the oropharynx collapse and the tongue is drawn back as a result of the subatmospheric pressure generated during inspiration against more upstream airway obstruction. This may be at the level of the palate, as previously described, or may be the result of nasal polyps, nasal infection or enlarged adenoids, which are the commonest cause of snoring in children.[8] As obstruction develops, the inspiratory muscles greatly augment their action, and intrathoracic pressure may fall as low as -7 kPa (-70 cmH$_2$O).

'Normal' snoring is not associated with frequent arousal from sleep, frequent apnoea or changes in blood gases, but is believed to precede the development of more serious sleep-related breathing disorders, with both increasing age and obesity making this progression more likely.

Sleep-Disordered Breathing

This term is used to describe a continuum of respiratory abnormalities seen during sleep, ranging from simple snoring to life-threatening obstructive sleep apnoea, and affecting almost one-fifth of those aged 30 to 49 years and around one-third of people aged 50 to 70 years.[9] All are characterized by periods of apnoea, with or without episodes of airway narrowing or obstruction, that lead to repeated episodes of subcortical arousal from sleep and arterial hypoxia, the latter occurring more frequently in obese patients.[10] Repeated arousals throughout the night give rise to excessive daytime sleepiness. Four syndromes are described, but there is considerable overlap between them:

Upper airway resistance syndrome[8] in which tidal volume and arterial oxygen saturation (Sa_{O2}) remain normal, but at the expense of extensive respiratory effort, which causes over 15 arousals per hour.

Obstructive sleep hypopnoea involves frequent (>15 per hour) episodes of airway obstruction of sufficient severity to reduce tidal volume to less than 50% of normal for over 10 seconds. There may be small decreases in Sa_{O2}.

Obstructive sleep apnoea is characterized by more than five episodes per hour of obstructive apnoeas lasting over 10 seconds and associated with severe decreases in Sa_{O2}. In fact, durations of apnoea may be as long as 90 seconds, and the frequency of the episodes as high as 160 per hour. In severe cases, 50% of sleep time may be spent without tidal exchange.

The last two syndromes are commonly grouped together as sleep apnoea/hypopnoea syndrome (SAHS). Severity is quantified by recording the apnoea/hypopnoea index (AHI), which is simply the number of occurrences per hour of apnoea or hypopnoea lasting longer than 10 seconds. Milder forms of sleep-disordered breathing tend to progress to more severe forms as patients grow older and fatter. In the United States population, based solely on an AHI of over 5, the prevalence of SAHS is around a quarter of men and 1 in 10 women, but when daytime sleepiness is added into the definition these prevalences fall to 4% and 2%, respectively.[11,12]

Apnoea or hypopnoea may be central or obstructive. Differentiation between central and obstructive apnoea is conveniently made by recording rib cage and abdominal movements continuously during sleep (Fig. 14.2). If, as a result of upper airway obstruction, abdominal and rib cage movements become uncoordinated (Fig. 14.2, C), then hypopnoea results. When these movements are equal but opposite in phase, there is obstructive apnoea (Fig. 14.2, D). Obstructive apnoea may occur in REM or non-REM sleep, but the longest periods of apnoea tend to occur in REM sleep. As for snoring, airway obstruction is less frequent when sleeping in the lateral, rather than supine, position.[7]

Central apnoeas are more common in elderly subjects. Patients with heart failure have a high prevalence of sleep-disordered breathing, often manifesting as central apnoeas which become cyclical and lead to Cheyne–Stokes respiration (page 54). The repeated swings in intrathoracic pressure and episodes of hypoxaemia have mostly adverse effects on the patient's already poor cardiac function.[13] Sadly, treatment of sleep-disordered breathing in these patients does not improve, and may even worsen survival, possibly because of the adverse effects of positive pressure ventilation on cardiac function (page 389).[14]

Obesity hypoventilation syndrome is specific to subjects with severe obesity, and is described on page 203.

Sleep-disordered breathing, including snoring, is common in children, and SAHS affects 4% of children, with a higher prevalence in some conditions such as Down syndrome.[15] Aetiology in children normally involves enlarged tonsils and adenoids. Instead of daytime sleepiness, disturbed sleep in children with SAHS leads to behavioural and neurocognitive problems, which can be improved with treatment.

The Mechanism of Airway Obstruction[9]

There are four components contributing to airway obstruction during sleep-disordered breathing: an anatomically narrow airway, inadequate control of airway muscles, the ease of arousal during apnoea (the arousal threshold) and instability of the respiratory control system.

Anatomically Narrow Airway

On average, patients with SAHS have anatomically narrower airways than controls, and the airway shape differs. Anatomical airway narrowing is believed to relate to three main factors.

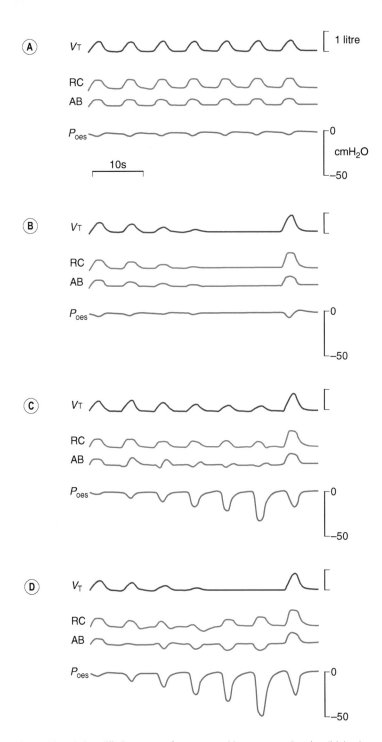

• **Fig. 14.2** Continuous records of breathing during differing types of apnoea and hypopnoea showing tidal volume (V_T), rib cage *(RC)* and abdominal *(AB)* contributions to breathing, and oesophageal pressure (P_{oes}). **(A)** Normal; **(B)** central apnoea; **(C)** obstructive hypopnoea; **(D)** obstructive apnoea.

First, obesity influences pharyngeal airway size in the retropalatal region.[16] A central pattern of obesity, commonly seen in males, includes extensive fat deposition in the neck tissues. This accounts for the association between SAHS and neck circumference.[17] Adipose tissue is best visualized using magnetic resonance imaging, and in patients with SAHS collections of fat are invariably seen lateral to the pharynx, between the pterygoid muscles and the carotid artery (Fig. 14.3). Pharyngeal fat is increased above normal levels even in nonobese patients with SAHS (Fig. 14.3, *C*). In addition, the quantity of adipose tissue seen correlates with the AHI, and weight loss predictably reduces both.

Second, some patients with SAHS may exhibit different facial structure, including micrognathia (small mandible) or retrognathia (posterior positioned mandible), both of which

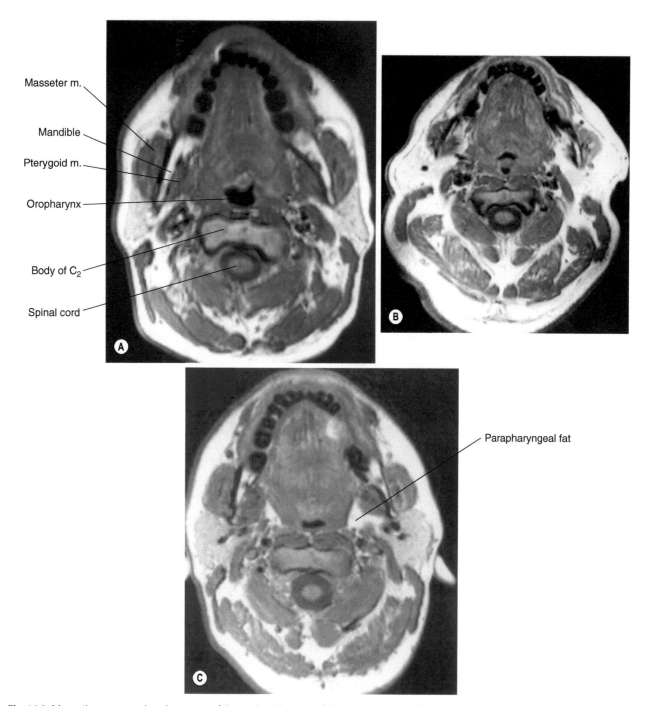

Masseter m.

Mandible

Pterygoid m.

Oropharynx

Body of C₂

Spinal cord

Parapharyngeal fat

• **Fig. 14.3** Magnetic resonance imaging scans of the neck at the level of the oropharynx. In this type of scan fat tissue appears white. **(A)** Normal, nonobese subject. **(B)** Obese patient with obstructive sleep apnoea, showing deposits of adipose tissue throughout the neck (the uvula is seen in the pharynx). **(C)** Nonobese patient with sleep apnoea, showing fat deposits lateral to the pharynx with normal amounts of adipose tissue elsewhere. (Parts **(A)** and **(C)** from Mortimore IL, Marshall I, Wraith PK, et al. Neck and total body fat deposition in nonobese and obese patients with sleep apnea compared with that in control subjects. *Am J Respir Crit Care Med.* 1998;157:280-283. With permission of the publishers of *American Journal of Respiratory and Critical Care Medicine.*)

will tend to displace the tongue backwards, requiring extra genioglossus activity to maintain a normal-sized airway. This hypothesis raises the interesting possibility that SAHS may begin in early childhood, when mouth breathing attributed to atopy or enlarged adenoids and tonsils can influence facial bone development, and may also explain familial 'aggregations' of SAHS and snoring.[18]

Finally, nocturnal rostral fluid shifts from the legs to the head and neck may occur when adopting the recumbent position at night, causing swelling of pharyngeal tissues and so worsening SAHS.[19] The most compelling evidence for this is the higher prevalence of SAHS in patients with diseases which cause fluid retention such as heart or renal failure, but the same mechanism is likely to contribute to

SAHS in pregnancy,[6] and potentially in the perioperative period.[20]

Inadequate Control of Respiratory Muscles

Pharyngeal dilator muscles are more active in awake subjects with SAHS compared with controls, presumably as a physiological response to the anatomically abnormal airway. The activity is believed to originate from the usual reflex, stimulated by a negative pharyngeal pressure (page 59), which may be present to a greater extent in subjects with SAHS even when awake. This requirement for increased pharyngeal muscle activity to maintain airway size may become impossible to maintain during sleep. In obese subjects, the extent to which muscle activity can be further increased during sleep determines which individuals develop SAHS.[21]

Airway collapse occurs only in obstructive sleep apnoea, and normally results from increased upstream resistance behind the soft palate leading to secondary downstream collapse. The ease with which this collapse occurs is a function of the compliance (collapsibility) of the hypopharyngeal walls, opposed by the action of the pharyngeal dilator muscles. Collapse is more likely to occur when pharyngeal compliance is high, and particularly when there is increased submucosal fat in the pharynx, a situation that seems to occur more commonly in men than women. Collapse of the hypopharynx occurs with the combination of upstream obstruction, enhanced diaphragmatic contraction and depressed or asynchronous pharyngeal dilator muscle activity.[22]

Arousal

Apnoea and hypopnoea are normally terminated when the patient is aroused from sleep, although this arousal is usually subcortical; that is, the patient does not return to full consciousness. Arousal is followed by a rapid increase in pharyngeal dilator muscle activity and opening of the pharyngeal airway. Despite the depressed ventilatory response curves, hypoxia and hypercapnia do contribute to airway opening, probably alongside increasing afferent input from pressure-sensitive pharyngeal receptors. Current opinion suggests that a combination of all these factors results in increased respiratory drive, which brings about pharyngeal opening, although not all of these events are associated with arousal from sleep.[23] Whatever the mechanism, arousal is often accompanied by significant sympathetic discharge.

The threshold for arousal varies widely between patients with SAHS, and is probably the main determinant of clinical severity, alongside the time taken after an arousal for sleep stage to again deepen and lead to the next apnoea.[24]

Respiratory Instability

Instability of the respiratory control system also contributes to the pattern of respiration seen with SAHS.[25] Multiple feedback loops are involved in controlling breathing (Chapter 4), such as the responses to Pco_2, Po_2 and mechanical pharyngeal reflexes. A small alteration in the rate at which a feedback loop detects a physiological change, or responds to that change, will lead to instability of the overall system. Sleep is believed to cause sufficient disturbance of the feedback loops to cause this type of instability, and repetitive respiratory cycles are established involving cyclical over-stimulation of breathing (immediately before arousal) followed by rebound under-stimulation. The simplest example is the normal periodic breathing (page 54) seen in old age, a more dramatic example is severe SAHS with long periods of apnoea, hypoxia and hypercarbia.

Drug Effects in Sleep Apnoea/Hypopnoea Syndrome

Considering the delicate balance that exists in SAHS between airway muscle activity, sleep state and the chemical control of breathing, it is unsurprising that almost any sedative drug can exacerbate the situation. The most widely administered sedative, alcohol, increases the number and duration of apnoeas and the degree of hypoxaemia associated with them. There is some evidence that benzodiazepines and opioids have a similar effect, but the mechanism of this exacerbation of SAHS remains uncertain.[26] Most of these drugs have multiple physiological effects, including on the chemical control of breathing (page 55), maintenance of airway patency and sleep patterns, all of which are likely to contribute to their effects in SAHS. Children with SAHS seem to be particularly sensitive to the adverse effects of opioids, which is believed to have led to a number of postoperative deaths following tonsillectomy.[27]

Despite these mostly adverse effects of drugs on SAHS, pharmacological intervention may also have a place in treating the disease. In a specific and small subgroup of SAHS patients sedative drugs may actually improve AHI by changing sleep pattern, for example by reducing REM sleep: in patients whose apnoeas occur predominantly during REM (around one-third of patients) this will reduce the overall AHI.[28] Desipramine, a tricyclic antidepressant drug with central noradrenergic and cholinergic stimulant effects, has been shown to abolish the normal attenuation of genioglossus activity occurring during sleep, providing a potential treatment for a large proportion of SAHS patients.[29]

Effects of Sleep Apnoea/Hypopnoea Syndrome

The effects of the SAHS are not trivial, and, over a period of years, morbidity and mortality in patients with SAHS are considerably higher than in controls. There has been difficulty proving that this observation relates to SAHS itself rather than the associated smoking, obesity and alcohol consumption, although the link with cardiovascular disease is now believed to be independent of these confounding variables, particularly with more severe forms of sleep-disordered breathing.[30] There are two main causes of increased morbidity and mortality:

Sleep deprivation. A night's sleep that is disturbed hundreds of times, even subconsciously, leaves the individual with severe daytime sleepiness, with decrement of performance in many fields. The ability to drive is impaired, such that patients with SAHS have a greater incidence of accidents than control subjects, with some studies finding a direct association between the AHI and likelihood of an accident.[31] Treatment with nasal continuous positive airway pressure (nCPAP, see later discussion) reverses this observation.

Medical effects. Each arousal, particularly if associated with hypoxaemia, causes significant sympathetic activation.[32,33] These events, occurring many times each night, cause multiple adverse effects on the cardiovascular system by initiation and amplification of inflammatory processes.[34] It is therefore unsurprising that SAHS is strongly implicated in the development of hypertension,[32] and also believed to contribute to the development of heart failure, ischaemic strokes, metabolic syndrome,[35] hypercholesterolaemia, chronic kidney disease[36] and cognitive deficits.[30,37]

Principles of Therapy[12,38,39]

Conservative Treatment

Avoidance of alcohol, sedative drugs and the supine position during sleep will all improve the AHI. Weight loss is effective at reducing the AHI in obese patients with SAHS, and is believed to act by reducing peripharyngeal fat, increasing airway diameter and reducing the tendency of the airway to collapse. Some studies show weight loss to be associated with large reductions in AHI, but few patients with SAHS are 'cured' by weight loss.[40,41] Drugs continue to be developed for treatment of the daytime sleepiness associated with SAHS, including the general central nervous system stimulant modafinil or, more recently, the centrally-acting dopamine and noradrenaline reuptake inhibitor solriamfetol.[42,43]

nCPAP[44] aims to avoid the development of a subatmospheric pharyngeal pressure sufficient to cause downstream pharyngeal collapse. It requires a well-fitting nasal mask or soft plastic tubes that fit inside the external nares. Compressed air must then be provided at the requisite gas flow, preferably with humidification. nCPAP serves no useful purpose during expiration, and systems have been developed to return airway pressure to atmospheric during expiration. In effect this provides a low level of intermittent positive pressure ventilation. Compliance with nCPAP is the only major limitation to its use, and the technique is now widely accepted as the most effective treatment for SAHS, including for the reduction of the daytime somnolence that has such a detrimental effect on the patient's life.

Oral appliances are available that can be maintained in the mouth at night to move the tongue and mandible forward (mandibular advancement devices), increasing the size of the airway. They are a noninvasive form of SAHS treatment that is less intrusive than nCPAP, reducing AHI by 26% in one study.[45] Although less efficacious than nCPAP, patients are more likely to be compliant with the device, and so the two therapies may have comparable overall effectiveness.[46]

Surgical Relief of Obstruction

For snoring alone, the first approach is the removal of any pathological obstruction such as nasal polyps that cause downstream collapse, although this may not improve patients with SAHS. A variety of more radical operations have been tried in the past, including uvulopalatopharyngoplasty, which aimed to dampen palatal oscillations and collapse by reducing the size of the soft palate. Nonobese patients with SAHS who have facial bone abnormalities may benefit from maxillofacial corrective surgery, usually involving advancement of the anterior mandible and/or maxilla. Tracheotomy (opened only at night) has been used in some cases as a last resort. The benefits of surgical treatment of SAHS remain uncertain, and these treatments are now usually reserved for patients who have a specific and identified anatomical area of collapse in their airway as part of their SAHS.[38,47]

Upper Airway Stimulation

A rather invasive treatment option is surgical implantation of a hypoglossal nerve stimulator, activation of which causes a small degree of tongue protrusion, and so relief of airway obstruction and improvement in both AHI and symptoms. The procedure also includes implanting a sensing electrode in the intercostal muscles so the device can then be active only during inspiration. A much less invasive option using transcutaneous stimulation is currently being developed, with promising early results.[48]

References

1. Joseph V, Pequignot JM, Van Reeth O. Neurochemical perspectives on the control of breathing during sleep. *Respir Physiol Neurobiol.* 2002;130:253-263.
2. Chowdhuri S, Pranathiageswaran S, Loomis-King H, et al. Aging is associated with increased propensity for central apnea during NREM sleep. *J Appl Physiol.* 2018;124:83-90.
3. Shome B, Wang L-P, Prasad AK, et al. Modeling of airflow in the nasopharynx with applications to sleep apnea. *J Biomech Eng.* 1998;120:416-422.
4. Henke KG. Upper airway muscle activity and upper airway resistance in young adults during sleep. *J Appl Physiol.* 1998;84:486-491.
5. Kuna ST, Smickley J. Response of genioglossus muscle activity to nasal airway occlusion in normal sleeping adults. *J Appl Physiol.* 1988;64:347-353.
6. Pamidi S, Kimoff RJ. Maternal sleep-disordered breathing. *Chest.* 2018;153:1052-1066.
7. Nakano H, Ikeda T, Hayashi M, et al. Effects of body position on snoring in apneic and nonapneic snorers. *Sleep.* 2003;2:169-172.
8. Rappai M, Colop N, Kemp S, et al. The nose and sleep disordered breathing. *What we know and what we do not know. Chest.* 2003;124:2309-2323.
*9. Subramani Y, Singh M, Wong J, et al. **Understanding phenotypes of obstructive sleep apnea: applications in anesthesia, surgery, and perioperative medicine.** *Anesth Analg.* 2017;124:179-191.
10. Peppard PE, Ward NR, Morrell MJ. The impact of obesity on oxygen desaturation during sleep-disordered breathing. *Am J Respir Crit Care Med.* 2009;180:788-793.

11. Memtsoudis SG, Besculides MC, Mazumdar M. A rude awakening—the perioperative sleep apnea epidemic. *N Engl J Med.* 2013;368:2352-2353.

*12. **Greenstone M, Hack M. Obstructive sleep apnoea. *BMJ.* 2014;348:g3745.**

13. Cao M, Guilleminault C, Lin C. Central sleep apnea: effects on stroke volume in heart failure. *Am J Respir Crit Care Med.* 2013;187:340-341.

14. Magalang UJ, Pack AI. Heart failure and sleep-disordered breathing — the plot thickens. *N Engl J Med.* 2015;373:1166-1167.

15. Horne RSC, Davey MJ, Nixon GM. Investing in the future: the benefits of continuous positive airway pressure for childhood obstructive sleep apnea. *Am J Respir Crit Care Med.* 2012;185:908-909.

16. Feng Y, Keenan BT, Wang S, et al. Dynamic upper airway imaging during wakefulness in obese subjects with and without sleep apnea. *Am J Respir Crit Care Med.* 2018;198:1435-1443.

17. Crummy F, Piper AJ, Naughton MT. Obesity and the lung: 2. Obesity and sleep disordered breathing. *Thorax.* 2008;63:738-746.

18. Sullivan SS, Guilleminault C. Can we avoid development of a narrow upper airway and secondary abnormal breathing during sleep? *Lancet Respir Med.* 2017;5:P843-P844.

19. Kent BD, Steier J. A brief history of fluid and sleep. *Am J Respir Crit Care Med.* 2015;191:1219-1220.

20. Lam T, Singh M, Yadollahi A, et al. Is perioperative fluid and salt balance a contributing factor in postoperative worsening of obstructive sleep apnea? *Anesth Analg.* 2016;122:1335-1339.

21. Sands SA, Eckert DJ, Jordan AS, et al. Enhanced upper-airway muscle responsiveness is a distinct feature of overweight/obese individuals without sleep apnea. *Am J Respir Crit Care Med.* 2014;190:930-937.

22. Oliven R, Cohen G, Dotan Y, et al. Alteration in upper airway dilator muscle coactivation during sleep: comparison of patients with obstructive sleep apnea and healthy subjects. *J Appl Physiol.* 2018;124:421-429.

23. Rapoport DM. To breathe, perchance not to wake? *J Appl Physiol.* 2012;112:247-248.

24. Younes M, Hanly PJ. Immediate postarousal sleep dynamics: an important determinant of sleep stability in obstructive sleep apnea. *J Appl Physiol.* 2016;120:801-808.

25. Pham LV, Schwartz AR, Polotsky VY. Integrating loop gain into the understanding of obstructive sleep apnoea mechanisms. *J Physiol.* 2018;596:3819-3820.

26. Wang D, Eckert DJ, Grunstein RR. Drug effects on ventilatory control and upper airway physiology related to sleep apnea. *Respir Physiol Neurobiol.* 2013;188:257-266.

27. Coté CJ, Posner KL, Domino KB. Death or neurologic injury after tonsillectomy in children with a focus on obstructive sleep apnea: Houston, we have a problem! *Anesth Analg.* 2014;118:1276-1283.

28. Jordan AS, O'Donoghue FJ, Cori JM, et al. Physiology of arousal in obstructive sleep apnea and potential impacts for sedative treatment. *Am J Respir Crit Care Med.* 2017;196:814-821.

29. Taranto-Montemurro L, Edwards BA, Sands SA, et al. Desipramine increases genioglossus activity and reduces upper airway collapsibility during non-REM sleep in healthy subjects. *Am J Respir Crit Care Med.* 2016;194:878-885.

30. Bradley TD, Floras JS. Obstructive sleep apnoea and its cardiovascular consequences. *Lancet.* 2009;373:82-93.

31. Stradling J. Driving and obstructive sleep apnoea. *Thorax.* 2008;63:481-483.

*32. **Kohler M, Stradling JR. OSA and hypertension. Do we know all the answers? *Chest.* 2013;144:1433-1435.**

33. Weiss JW, Tamisier R, Liu Y. Sympathoexcitation and arterial hypertension associated with obstructive sleep apnea and cyclic intermittent hypoxia. *J Appl Physiol.* 2015;119:1449-1454.

34. Bäck M, Stanke-Labesque F. Obstructive sleep apnoea and cardiovascular calcification. *Thorax.* 2015;70:815-816.

35. Ryan S. Adipose tissue inflammation by intermittent hypoxia: mechanistic link between obstructive sleep apnoea and metabolic dysfunction. *J Physiol.* 2017;595(8):2423-2430.

36. Phillips CL, Laher I, Yee BJ. Is the kidney yet another potential end-organ casualty of obstructive sleep apnea? *Am J Respir Crit Care Med.* 2015;192:779-781.

37. Twigg GL, Papaioannou I, Jackson M, et al. Obstructive sleep apnea syndrome is associated with deficits in verbal but not visual memory. *Am J Respir Crit Care Med.* 2010;182:98-103.

38. Ryan CF. Sleep 9: an approach to treatment of obstructive sleep apnoea/hypopnoea syndrome including upper airway surgery. *Thorax.* 2005;60:595-604.

39. Veasey SC, Rosen IM. Obstructive sleep apnea in adults. *N Engl J Med.* 2019;380:1442-1449.

40. Joosten SA, Hamilton GS, Naughton MT. Impact of weight loss management in OSA. *Chest.* 2017;152:194-203.

41. Hudge DW, Patel SR, Ahasic AM, et al. The role of weight management in the treatment of adult obstructive sleep apnea. An official American Thoracic Society Clinical Practice Guideline. *Am J Respir Crit Care Med.* 2018;198:e70-e87.

42. Chapman JL, Kempler L, Chang CL, et al. Modafinil improves daytime sleepiness in patients with mild to moderate obstructive sleep apnoea not using standard treatments: a randomised placebo-controlled crossover trial. *Thorax.* 2014;69:274-279.

43. Schweitzer PK, Rosenberg R, Zammit GK, et al. Solriamfetol for excessive sleepiness in obstructive sleep apnea (TONES 3). A randomized controlled trial. *Am J Respir Crit Care Med.* 2019;199:1421-1431.

44. Gordon P, Sanders MH. Sleep 7: Positive airway pressure therapy for obstructive sleep apnoea/hypopnoea syndrome. *Thorax.* 2005;60:68-75.

45. Quinnell TG, Bennett M, Jordan J, et al. A crossover randomised controlled trial of oral mandibular advancement devices for obstructive sleep apnoea-hypopnoea (TOMADO). *Thorax.* 2014;69:938-945.

46. Hamoda MM, Kohzuka Y, Almeida FR. Oral appliances for the management of OSA. An updated review of the literature. *Chest.* 2018;153:544-553.

47. Smith DF, Cohen AP, Ishman SL. Surgical management of OSA in adults. *Chest.* 2015;147:1681-1690.

48. Pengo MF, Xiao S, Ratneswaran C, et al. Randomised sham-controlled trial of transcutaneous electrical stimulation in obstructive sleep apnoea. *Thorax.* 2016;71:923-931.

15

Obesity

KEY POINTS

- Obese subjects have reduced static and dynamic lung volumes because of compression of the chest cavity by the mass of the chest wall and abdominal contents.
- Chest wall compliance is reduced by obesity, and the lower lung volume leads to a decrease in lung compliance and an increase in airway resistance, making airway closure more frequent.
- Hormonal changes in obesity such as increased leptin levels affect respiratory control and help to maintain adequate respiration despite a greater oxygen requirement, such that most obese subjects have normal arterial oxygen and carbon dioxide levels.
- These changes can cause or exacerbate obstructive respiratory diseases, and in children may even affect lung development, causing a greater susceptibility to respiratory disease and symptoms later in life.

The word obesity derives from the Latin *obesus,* meaning 'portly', and has been used to describe overweight individuals for 400 years.[1] Other meanings of *obesus* in Latin include 'coarse' or 'gross', so for many centuries the gentler description of 'corpulent' was common.

Obesity is quantified in various ways. The most common variable used is body mass index (BMI) – the subject's weight in kilograms divided by their height in metres squared. The BMI obtained is widely used to define clinical obesity, and its severity as shown in Table 15.1, although this is a rather poor measure because it does not take into account muscle mass in athletic individuals or the distribution of body fat. The latter is better recorded as waist circumference or waist-to-hip ratio, which identify centrally distributed obesity: a more common finding in males and associated with greater health risks.

Obesity prevalence has been increasing for centuries, and obesity as a disease is now accepted to be a global epidemic. The rate of increase is also accelerating, with estimates suggesting global prevalence has doubled between 1980 and 2017, now being approximately 5% of children and 12% of all adults.[3] There are wide variations between different countries, with obesity prevalence in both adults and children being generally higher in areas with a higher sociodemographic index (SDI), which incorporates, among other factors, per capita income and educational attainment.[3] However, in some demographic groups, for example young men, the most rapid increase in obesity is occurring in countries with low-middle SDI, and in most areas the rate of increase of obesity prevalence in children is greater than in adults. The burden of disease associated with these changes is massive, accounting for an estimated 4 million deaths globally in 2015.[3] Cardiovascular disease and diabetes account for the majority of obesity-related deaths, but its contribution to respiratory disease is also important. Obesity increases the likelihood of developing several respiratory diseases, for the multiple reasons described below. Respiratory symptoms such as dyspnoea and a reduced breath-hold time[4] are also more common in obese subjects, even in the absence of respiratory disease, as a result of the physiological challenges of severe obesity.

Respiratory Physiology of Obesity

Mild and moderate obesity have minimal effects on the respiratory system, but once the condition becomes severe the main physiological effect is the mass of the chest wall tissues. Figure 15.1 shows a computerized tomography (CT) scan of the lungs in an individual with severe obesity, clearly showing that the relative size of lungs and chest wall means that expansion of the lungs will require much more work than in a nonobese individual.

Lung Volumes and Respiratory Mechanics

There is an increase in pleural pressure as a result of compression by the weight of the chest wall. Respiratory system compliance (page 21) is reduced, with both lung and chest wall components contributing to the change.[2] Chest wall and mediastinal fat deposits explain the changes in chest wall compliance, whereas reduced lung compliance most likely results from decreased lung volume. Airway resistance

199

TABLE 15.1	**Classification of Clinical Obesity in Adults and its Effects on Functional Residual Capacity[2]**	
Body Mass Index (kg.m⁻²)	**Classification**	**Change in Functional Residual Capacity Relative to Non-obese Subjects**
<18.5	Underweight	
18.5–24.9	Healthy	
25–29.9	Overweight	–10%
30–34.9	Obese—class I	–22%
35–39.9	Obese—class II	
≥40	Obese—class III (morbid obesity)	–33%

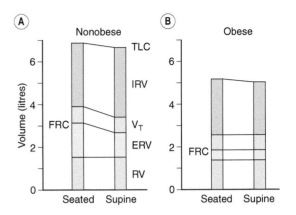

• **Fig. 15.2** Effects of position and obesity on static lung volumes. **(A)** Nonobese subjects with a mean body mass index (BMI) of 23.2. Note the reduction in expiratory reserve volume (ERV), and so functional residual capacity (FRC), when supine because of the weight of the abdominal contents displacing the diaphragm in a cephalad direction. **(B)** Severely obese subjects with a mean BMI of 46.8, in whom intra-abdominal pressure is increased irrespective of body position, causing an even greater reduction in ERV and FRC. IRV, Inspiratory reserve volume; RV, residual volume; TLC, total lung capacity; Vt, tidal volume. (From reference 5 with permission from BMJ Publishing Group Ltd.)

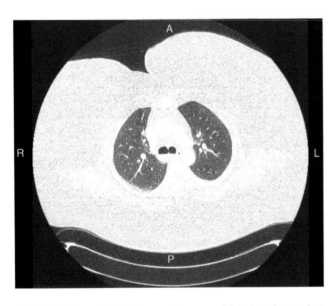

• **Fig. 15.1** Computerized tomography scan of the chest in a patient with severe obesity showing a single slice at the level of the carina. The thickness of the chest wall relative to the size of the lungs can be easily seen.

is increased, again resulting from reduced lung volume (page 31) and causing a greater likelihood of airway closure and risk of developing airway disease (see below). The work of breathing (page 67) and the oxygen cost of breathing are both greatly increased in obese individuals.

Static Lung Volumes

As a result of these changes, most lung volumes are affected, particularly in the supine position when increased pressure from the abdominal contents displaces the diaphragm in a cephalad direction, reducing thoracic volume. Figure 15.2 shows a summary of the changes in static lung volumes between the upright (seated) and supine positions in non-obese and obese subjects. With the exception of tidal

volume, obesity causes a reduction in all static lung volumes, particularly expiratory reserve volume (ERV), and so functional residual capacity (FRC) (Fig. 15.2).[5] In obese and nonobese subjects static compliance is similar when measured at normal lung volume, but is reduced at both high and low lung volume in the obese. As a result of their low FRC obese subjects are therefore breathing at a less favourable part of their compliance curve, which contributes to an increased work of breathing.

Closing capacity (page 31) seems to be independent of body position and unaffected by obesity,[6] but the reduced FRC relative to normal closing capacity will still cause increased airway closure.

Dynamic Lung Volumes

There is an inverse relationship between BMI and forced expiratory volume in one second (FEV_1).[7] This effect is thought to be insignificant until obesity becomes severe,[8] is more marked in male subjects and is reversible if the individual loses weight.[9] Central or 'abdominal' obesity is more common in males, and is more strongly associated with reductions in FEV_1 and forced vital capacity (FVC) than either weight or BMI,[10] in keeping with the mechanism already described of abdominal mass impairing respiratory mechanics. In one study, each cm increase in waist circumference was associated with a 13 mL decrease in FVC and a 11 mL decrease in FEV_1.[11] Other measures of lung fitness such as maximum voluntary ventilation (page 71) are also reduced in severe obesity.[8]

Respiratory Muscles

Upper airway resistance is increased in obese individuals, and the contribution of this to sleep-disordered breathing is described in Chapter 14.

In obese individuals there is increased absolute strength of antigravity muscles because of the greater loading, but not so in other muscles, including the diaphragm. Contractile performance of the diaphragm is impaired in obesity, with animal studies suggesting reductions in both maximal power output and fatigue resistance for diaphragm muscle in obese versus nonobese animals.[12] There is no change in the ratio of fast and slow fibre types (page 66), and the mechanism of the diaphragm dysfunction remains uncertain, but most likely begins with lipid accumulation within skeletal muscle tissue.

Ventilation Perfusion Relationships

Considering the changes in lung volume and increased airway resistance in obese subjects, it would be expected that ventilation/perfusion ($\dot{V}/\dot{Q}$) relationships would also be abnormal. In subjects with mild-moderate grades of obesity, arterial blood gases remain normal, suggesting good $\dot{V}/\dot{Q}$ matching. Early studies with radioactive tracers (^{133}Xe, page 106) found a shift of ventilation towards upper lung regions, but only in severe obesity when ERV was significantly reduced, that is when the subject is breathing almost at residual volume. In subjects whose obesity is not severe, an increase in lung recoil is believed to counteract the effects of low lung volume on small airway resistance, maintaining homogenous ventilation until FRC is less than two-thirds of normal.[13] A different method of assessing regional ventilation involves measuring lung tissue density from CT scans. This technique shows a direct association between increasing BMI and greater heterogeneity of lung tissue density, strongly suggesting greater variation in ventilation of different lung regions.[14] Thus in severe obesity there may be increased ventilation of nondependent areas, increasing regions of lung with $\dot{V}/\dot{Q}$ greater than 1, resulting in some alveolar dead space (page 99).

Respiratory Control

Maintenance of normal blood gas partial pressures in severe obesity is a physiological challenge. The metabolic rate of the extra tissue mass may be similar to that of a nonobese individual, or lower in the case of adipose tissue, but overall O_2 requirement and CO_2 production will inevitably be raised. This may be exacerbated by the chronically elevated activity of the sympathetic nervous system and low-grade inflammatory processes that occur in many obese individuals. There is also an increased oxygen requirement by respiratory muscles.[15] Obese subjects must therefore maintain a higher than normal respiratory drive and minute ventilation despite their adverse respiratory mechanics. Fortunately, the extra oxygen requirement is normally easily accommodated by the acceptably maintained $\dot{V}/\dot{Q}$ relationships and the finding from multiple studies that lung diffusing capacity is normal in obesity.

Acceptable excretion of CO_2 is less easily achieved. CO_2 production is high in severely obese subjects, although normal if corrected for body surface area,[16] and contributes to a high prevalence of nocturnal, and in some cases daytime, hypercapnia. Despite these challenges to gas exchange in obese individuals, blood gases remain normal in most, including half of those with very severe obesity (BMI >50 kg.m^{-2}).

The reasons why only some obese subjects develop hypercapnia is poorly understood and multifactorial (Fig. 15.3). Although increased CO_2 production and alveolar dead space undoubtedly contribute to hypercapnia, this

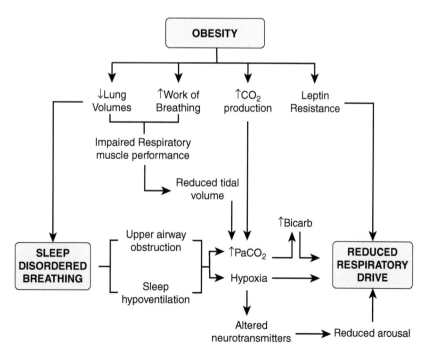

• **Fig. 15.3** Summary of the physiological changes in obese subjects contributing to the development of hypercapnia. (From reference 17.)

does not explain why only a minority of obese patients retain CO_2, suggesting an abnormality of CO_2 regulation. In hypercapnic severely obese patients, the slope of the hypercapnic ventilatory response (page 49) is reduced compared with eucapnic obese subjects.[16] It is unclear whether this difference causes the hypercapnia or is an effect of prolonged hypercapnia. The former is unlikely because there is no known genetic predisposition to developing hypercapnia in obese individuals, and the latter is quite possible as long-term hypercapnia in other situations, for example in submarines (page 226), is known to attenuate the hypercapnic ventilatory response. The mechanism of this change probably involves both biochemical effects such as an increased extracellular fluid bicarbonate concentration and the plasticity of the central CO_2 chemoreflex. Compared with when awake, episodes of hypercapnia and hypoxia are more frequent and severe in obese subjects when asleep, as part of their sleep-disordered breathing. These nocturnal changes are believed to exacerbate the increase in bicarbonate concentration and blunt the ventilatory response to CO_2 even during the day.[17]

Endocrine changes may also contribute to altered respiratory control in obesity. Leptin is a hormone produced by adipocytes that enters the central nervous system and regulates both food intake and energy expenditure.[18,19] Leptin is also a respiratory stimulant, exerting its effects in multiple areas of the respiratory centre (page 42), including on the nucleus tractus solitarius and in the chemosensitive retrotrapezoid nucleus.[18] Leptin may also stimulate breathing by a peripheral action, with increased activity from the carotid sinus nerve in the carotid body, particularly in the initial stages of obesity.[19,20] Serum leptin concentration increases with increasing mass of body fat,[15] and this is believed to be the source of the 'normal' increased respiratory drive seen in obesity. An attenuated response to leptin in some obese individuals or in severe obesity could explain their development of hypercapnia. Many possible mechanisms for this have been proposed. Animal models of advanced obesity and the metabolic syndrome show resistance to leptin signalling in the carotid body.[21] Central leptin resistance also occurs in severe obesity, from a combination of impaired transfer of leptin across the blood–brain barrier and altered leptin receptor responses.[15]

Impact of Obesity on Lung Disease

The contribution of obesity to sleep-disordered breathing is described in Chapter 14.

Lung Development in Childhood

Children born to obese mothers are at greater risk of neonatal respiratory problems and are more likely to develop wheeze symptoms during childhood. Type 2 diabetes and premature birth are both more common in obese mothers, and are associated with poor neonatal lung function, but this does not explain all the cases seen. There are plausible mechanisms by which obesity may affect intrauterine lung development and perinatal lung function. Animal studies have found that overfeeding during pregnancy affects gene expression and so impairs the development of type II alveolar epithelial cells, which produce surfactant (page 16), and the enzymes responsible for generating some of the molecular components of surfactant.[22] Surfactant deficiency in late pregnancy is a major factor in the development of neonatal respiratory distress syndrome (page 180). Leptin is also implicated, as its receptors are present in fetal lungs, and maternal leptin levels have been shown to affect fetal adipose tissue formation. Finally, leptin has immune-modulatory functions[23] and can affect in vitro growth of tracheal epithelial cells.[24]

Dysanapsis

Human lungs at birth are not fully developed, with new alveoli continuing to form until around 3 years of age, after which lungs continue to increase in size until adulthood (Chapter 12). As lungs grow, the relative size of the airways and lung parenchyma may not remain constant. A disparity in the growth of these two functional parts of a lung is termed dysanapsis,[25] and is regarded as a normal between-individual physiological variance. Some subjects will therefore have narrow airways relative to the volume of lung tissue they supply. Girls seem to have wider or shorter airways (less dysanapsis) in childhood than boys, but adult men have larger airways relative to lung size than adult women. Dysanapsis is easy to quantify; it is simply the ratio of a measure of airway resistance (usually FEV_1 to FVC ratio) to a measure of lung volume (usually FEV_1 or FVC). A large study has found that around a quarter of children have dysanapsis, and that it is significantly more likely to occur in overweight or obese children.[26] Furthermore, children with asthma and dysanapsis had more severe symptoms, such as exacerbations and a requirement for steroids. Even in children without asthma, dysanapsis led to more expiratory flow limitation, which resulted in exertional dyspnoea.[27]

The mechanism of this association between dysanapsis and obesity is unknown, but a similar pattern of lung growth is seen in children in the hypoxic conditions found at altitude (page 210), providing a possible link. It is also unknown whether the dysanapsis developed in early life results in a lifetime of greater susceptibility to respiratory symptoms and disease, but, considering the rising prevalence of childhood obesity, if this were the case it could lead to a considerable respiratory disease burden in the long term.

Asthma Obesity Phenotype

In both adults and children obesity is a risk factor for developing asthma, particularly in adult females, and is associated with poor control of symptoms.[28] These observations can be partly explained by the effect of obesity on lung volumes described above. Similarly, the changes in respiratory mechanics also lead to dynamic hyperinflation (page 333) during exercise in obese patients with asthma, contributing to their poor exercise capacity.[29] These effects may explain why symptoms of asthma are worse in obese patients, but not why asthma occurs more frequently in obesity. Hormonal changes with obesity are becoming increasingly recognized as potential contributors to developing asthma. Obese patients with asthma have reduced levels of the antiinflammatory hormone adiponectin, and high levels of leptin, which, in addition to its effects already described, is a proinflammatory hormone.[28] Furthermore, the effect of these hormones on asthma symptoms may be greater in women because of an interaction with reproductive hormones.[30]

Most of these interactions between obesity and asthma are reversible with weight loss.[31] For example, weight loss after bariatric surgery leads to improved forced expiratory volumes because of reduced resistance in peripheral airways, and also reduced systemic and bronchial inflammation.[32]

Chronic Obstructive Pulmonary Disease

There is an association between obesity and chronic obstructive pulmonary disease (COPD), with a greater proportion of patients with mild COPD being obese than in the healthy population, whereas there are fewer obese patients in the severe COPD group.[33] The link between obesity and COPD severity may involve altered inflammatory responses,[34] possibly mediated by adipose tissue hormones such as adiponectin,[35] or effects on respiratory muscle strength.

The Obesity Paradox

One possible explanation for the higher prevalence of obesity in patients with mild COPD could be that obese patients have less severe COPD symptoms, and indeed there is some evidence of a survival benefit for obese patients with COPD.[36] This is referred to as the 'obesity paradox', and is also seen in critically ill patients, although in the latter group nutritional requirements may contribute to the observation.[37,38] There is also an intriguing explanation for better survival in COPD patients involving lung mechanics during exercise. Dynamic hyperinflation is a common occurrence during exercise in COPD, and leads to an increase in lung volumes, including FRC. In obese patients FRC is low (Fig. 15.2), and it may be that the increase in FRC seen with dynamic hyperinflation during exercise returns the lungs to a more favourable part of their compliance curve, reducing the severity of dyspnoea in comparison to a nonobese patient with the same degree of COPD.[39] As described earlier, the same pathophysiology occurs in obese patients with asthma and causes dyspnoea on exertion, presumably, in these patients, because of hyperinflation to lung volumes well above normal FRC.

Obesity Hypoventilation Syndrome

Obesity hypoventilation syndrome (Pickwickian syndrome) describes a combination of obesity, daytime hypercapnia and sleep-disordered breathing, usually severe obstructive sleep apnoea.[17,40] Why some individuals develop this extreme type of sleep-disordered breathing is unknown, but severe obesity is a factor. Another possible explanation is that obstructive episodes are so frequent and the respiratory system during sleep so impeded that ventilation between apnoeas becomes inadequate, leading to severe nocturnal hypercapnia. Compensatory metabolic alkalosis develops during the night, which then attenuates the normal CO_2-mediated respiratory control during the day. As discussed, why some severely obese individuals develop daytime hypercapnia and others do not is unknown. The syndrome has a poor prognosis without treatment. Although early diagnosis and commencement of noninvasive ventilation remain important, a more holistic approach is now recommended to manage the inflammatory and metabolic problems which also contribute to mortality.[17]

References

1. Barnett F. Obesity. *The Lancet.* 2017;389:591.
*2. Peters U, Suratt BT, Bates JHT, et al. **Obesity and lung disease. *Chest.* 2018;153:702-709.**
3. The GBD Obesity Collaborators. Health effects of overweight and obesity in 195 countries over 25 years. *N Engl J Med.* 2017;377:13-27.
4. Trembach NV, Zabolotskikh IB. Voluntary breath-holding duration in healthy subjects with obesity: Role of peripheral chemosensitivity to carbon dioxide. *Respir Physiol Neurobiol.* 2018;249:7-10.
*5. Steier J, Lunt A, Hart N, et al. **Observational study of the effect of obesity on lung volumes. *Thorax.* 2014;69:752-759.**
6. Mahadeva S, Salome CM, Berend N, et al. The effect of low lung volume on airway function in obesity. *Respir Physiol Neurobiol.* 2013;188:192-199.
7. McClean KM, Kee F, Young IS, et al. Obesity and the lung: 1. Epidemiology. *Thorax.* 2008;63:649-654.
8. Biring MS, Lewis MI, Liu JT, et al. Pulmonary physiologic changes of morbid obesity. *Am J Med Sci.* 1999;318:293-297.
9. Bottai M, Pistelli F, Di Pede F, et al. Longitudinal changes of body mass index, spirometry and diffusion in a general population. *Eur Respir J.* 2002;20:665-673.
10. Ochs-Balcom HM, Grant BJB, Muti P, et al. Pulmonary function and abdominal adiposity in the general population. *Chest.* 2006;129:853-862.
11. Chen Y, Rennie D, Cormier YF, et al. Waist circumference is associated with pulmonary function in normal-weight, overweight, and obese subjects. *Am J Clin Nutr.* 2007;85:35-39.
12. Tallis J, Hill C, James RS, et al. The effect of obesity on the contractile performance of isolated mouse soleus, EDL, and diaphragm muscles. *J Appl Physiol.* 2017;122:170-181.
13. Pellegrino R, Gobbi A, Antonelli A, et al. Ventilation heterogeneity in obesity. *J Appl Physiol.* 2014;116:1175-1181.
14. Subramaniam K, Clark AR, Hoffman EA, et al. Metrics of lung tissue heterogeneity depend on BMI but not age. *J Appl Physiol.* 2018;125:328-339.
15. Lin C-K, Lin C-C. Work of breathing and respiratory drive in obesity. *Respirol.* 2012;17:402-411.
16. Javaheri S, Simbart LA. Respiratory determinants of diurnal hypercapnia in obesity hypoventilation syndrome. What does weight have to do with it? *Ann Am Thorac Soc.* 2014;11:945-950.
*17. Piper A. **Obesity hypoventilation syndrome weighing in on therapy options. *Chest.* 2016;149:856-868.**

18. Bassi M, Furuya WI, Zoccal DB, et al. Facilitation of breathing by leptin effects in the central nervous system. *J Physiol.* 2016;594:1617-1625.

19. Leverton H, England C, Baxandall A. Carotid body activity – are we eating our way into the ventilatory pathway? *J Physiol.* 2018;596:2963-2964.

20. Caballero-Eraso C, Shin M-K, Pho H, et al. Leptin acts in the carotid bodies to increase minute ventilation during wakefulness and sleep and augment the hypoxic ventilatory response. *J Physiol.* 2019;597:151-172.

21. Ribeiro MJ, Sacramento JF, Gallego-Martin T, et al. High fat diet blunts the effects of leptin on ventilation and on carotid body activity. *J Physiol.* 2018;596:3187-3199.

22. Rozance PJ, Wright CJ. Preparing for the first breath: in the developing lung, maternal overnutrition takes centre stage. *J Physiol.* 2017;595:6595-6596.

23. Gnanalingham MG, Mostyn A, Gardner DS, et al. Developmental regulation of the lung in preparation for life after birth: hormonal and nutritional manipulation of local glucocorticoid action and uncoupling protein-2. *J Endocrinol.* 2006;188:375-386.

24. Tsuchiya T, Shimizu H, Horie T, et al. Expression of leptin receptor in lung: leptin as a growth factor. *Eur J Pharmacol.* 1999;365:273-279.

25. Thompson BR. Dysanapsis - once believed to be a physiological curiosity - is now clinically important. *Am J Respir Crit Care Med.* 2017;195:277-278.

*26. **Forno E, Weiner DJ, Mullen J, et al. Obesity and airway dysanapsis in children with and without asthma. *Am J Respir Crit Care Med.* 2017;195:314-323.**

27. Pianosi PT. Flow limitation and dysanapsis in children and adolescents with exertional dyspnea. *Resp Physiol Neurobiol.* 2018;252-253:58-63.

*28. **Umetsu DT. Mechanisms by which obesity impacts upon asthma. *Thorax.* 2017;72:174-177.**

29. Ferreira PG, Freitas PD, Silva AG, et al. Dynamic hyperinflation and exercise limitations in obese asthmatic women. *J Appl Physiol.* 2017;123:585-593.

30. Bel EH. Another piece to the puzzle of the "obese female asthma" phenotype. *Am J Respir Crit Care Med.* 2013;188:263-270.

31. Pakhale S, Baron J, Dent R, et al. Effects of weight loss on airway responsiveness in obese adults with asthma. Does weight loss lead to reversibility of asthma? *Chest.* 2015;147:1582-1590.

32. van Huisstede A, Rudolphus A, Cabezas MC, et al. Effect of bariatric surgery on asthma control, lung function and bronchial and systemic inflammation in morbidly obese subjects with asthma. *Thorax.* 2015;70:659-667.

33. Franssen FME, O'Donnell DE, Goossens GH, et al. Obesity and the lung: 5. Obesity and COPD. *Thorax.* 2008;63:1110-1117.

34. Peres A, Dorneles GP, Dias AS, et al. T-cell profile and systemic cytokine levels in overweight-obese patients with moderate to very-severe COPD. *Resp Physiol Neurobiol.* 2018;247:74-79.

35. Wouters EFM. Adiponectin: a novel link between adipose tissue and chronic obstructive pulmonary disease. *Am J Respir Crit Care Med.* 2013;188:522-523.

36. van den Borst B, Gosker HR, Schols AMWJ. Central fat and peripheral muscle. Partners in crime in chronic obstructive pulmonary disease. *Am J Respir Crit Care Med.* 2013;187:8-13.

37. Johnson BD, Babb TG. Is obesity deflating? *J Appl Physiol.* 2011;111:2-4.

38. Shapiro ML, Komisarow J. The obesity paradox and effects of early nutrition: is there a paradox, or is there not? *Crit Care Med.* 2017;45:918-919.

39. Ora J, Laveneziana P, Wadell K, et al. Effect of obesity on respiratory mechanics during rest and exercise in COPD. *J Appl Physiol.* 2011;111:10-19.

40. Crummy F, Piper AJ, Naughton MT. Obesity and the lung: 2. Obesity and sleep disordered breathing. *Thorax.* 2008;63:738-746.

16

High Altitude and Flying

KEY POINTS

- Low inspired oxygen partial pressure at altitude causes immediate hyperventilation, which increases further with acclimatization to produce hypocapnia and improve oxygen levels.
- The rate of ascent and altitude achieved are determinants of altitude-related illnesses, which vary from mild acute mountain sickness to potentially lethal high-altitude pulmonary oedema.

- High-altitude populations have adaptations to their environment such as lesser degrees of hyperventilation compensated for by a greater lung surface area for gas exchange.
- Commercial aircraft cabins are pressurized to an equivalent altitude of less than 2400 m (8000 ft), representing a level of hypoxia similar to breathing 15% oxygen at sea level.

With increasing altitude the barometric pressure falls, but the fractional concentration of oxygen in the air (0.21) and the saturated vapour pressure of water at body temperature (6.3 kPa or 47 mmHg) remain constant. The Po_2 of the inspired air is related to the barometric pressure as follows:

Inspired gas Po_2
$$= 0.21 \times (\text{Barometric pressure} - 6.3) \text{ kPa}$$

or

Inspired gas Po_2
$$= 0.21 \times (\text{Barometric pressure} - 47) \text{ mmHg}$$

The influence of the saturated vapour pressure of water becomes relatively more important until, at an altitude of approximately 19 000 m or 63 000 ft, the barometric pressure equals the water vapour pressure, and alveolar Po_2 and Pco_2 become zero.

Table 16.1 is based on the standard table relating altitude and barometric pressure. However, there are important deviations from the predicted barometric pressure under certain circumstances, particularly at low latitudes.[1] At the summit of Everest, the actual barometric pressure was found to be 2.4 kPa (18 mmHg) greater than predicted, and this was crucial to reaching the summit without oxygen. The uppermost curve in Figure 16.1 shows the expected Po_2 of air as a function of altitude, whereas the crosses indicate observed values in the Himalayas that are consistently higher than expected.

Equivalent Oxygen Concentration

The acute effect of altitude on inspired Po_2 may be simulated by reduction of the oxygen concentration of gas inspired at sea level (Table 16.1). This technique is extensively used for studies of hypoxia and for clinical assessment of patients before flying (see later), but there are theoretical reasons why the same inspired Po_2 at normal and low barometric pressure may have different physiological effects. These include the density of the gas being breathed and different PN_2 values in the tissues.[3]

Up to 10 000 m (33 000 ft), it is possible to restore the inspired Po_2 to the sea-level value by an appropriate increase in the oxygen concentration of the inspired gas (also shown in Table 16.1). Lower inspired Po_2 values may be obtained between 10 000 and 19 000 m, above which body fluids boil.

Respiratory System Responses to Altitude

Ascent to altitude presents three main challenges to the respiratory system, resulting from progressively reduced inspired Po_2, low relative humidity and, in outdoor environments, extreme cold. Hypoxia is by far the most important of these and requires significant physiological changes to allow continuation of normal activities at altitude. The efficiency of these changes depends on many factors such as the normal altitude at which the subject lives, the rate of ascent, the altitude attained and the health of the subject.

TABLE 16.1	Barometric Pressure Relative to Altitude						
Altitude		Barometric Pressure		Inspired Gas P_{O_2}		Equivalent Oxygen % at Sea Level	Percentage Oxygen Required to Give Sea-Level Value of Inspired Gas P_{O_2}
(ft)	(m)	(kPa)	(mmHg)	(kPa)	(mmHg)		
0	0	101	760	19.9	149	20.9	20.9
2000	610	94.3	707	18.4	138	19.4	22.6
4000	1220	87.8	659	16.9	127	17.8	24.5
6000	1830	81.2	609	15.7	118	16.6	26.5
8000	2440	75.2	564	14.4	108	15.1	28.8
10000	3050	69.7	523	13.3	100	14.0	31.3
12000	3660	64.4	483	12.1	91	12.8	34.2
14000	4270	59.5	446	11.1	83	11.6	37.3
16000	4880	54.9	412	10.1	76	10.7	40.8
18000	5490	50.5	379	9.2	69	9.7	44.8
20000	6100	46.5	349	8.4	63	8.8	49.3
22000	6710	42.8	321	7.6	57	8.0	54.3
24000	7320	39.2	294	6.9	52	7.3	60.3
26000	7930	36.0	270	6.3	47	6.6	66.8
28000	8540	32.9	247	5.6	42	5.9	74.5
30000	9150	30.1	226	4.9	37	5.2	83.2
35000	10700	23.7	178	3.7	27	3.8	–
40000	12200	18.8	141	2.7	20	2.8	–
45000	13700	14.8	111	1.8	13	1.9	–
50000	15300	11.6	87	1.1	8	1.1	–
63000	19200	6.3	47	0	0	0	–

Note: 100% oxygen restores sea-level inspired P_{O_2} at 10000 m (33000 ft).

Physiological Effects of Exposure to Altitude

Transport technology now permits altitude to be attained quickly and without the exertion of climbing. Within a few hours, rail, air, cable car or motor transport may take a passenger from near sea level to as high as 4000 m (13100 ft).

Ventilatory Changes

At high altitude the decrease in inspired gas P_{O_2} reduces alveolar, and therefore arterial, P_{O_2}. The actual decrease in alveolar P_{O_2} is mitigated by hyperventilation caused by the hypoxic drive to ventilation. However, on acute exposure to altitude, the ventilatory response to hypoxia is very short-lived because of a combination of the resultant hypocapnia and hypoxic ventilatory decline (page 52 and Fig. 4.7). During the first few days at altitude, this disadvantageous negative feedback is reversed by acclimatization (see later).

Signs and Symptoms

Visual impairment is the earliest sign of altitude hypoxia, and at 2400 m (8000 ft) under mesopic (twilight) light conditions there is impairment of both contrast acuity and chromatic sensitivity.[4] Under scotopic conditions (night vision) impairment may occur at altitudes of only 1200 m (4000 ft) because of the greater sensitivity to hypoxia of rods compared with cones in the retina.[5] However, the most serious aspect of exposure to altitude is impairment of mental performance, which is of particular relevance to aviation personnel. Although difficult to study, there is evidence of impaired memory, cognitive flexibility and reaction times at altitude, but fortunately these tend to occur at higher levels than the cabin altitude (page 214) of commercial aircraft.[5–7] Impaired cognitive function as a result of hypoxia is because of both a direct effect of hypoxia on

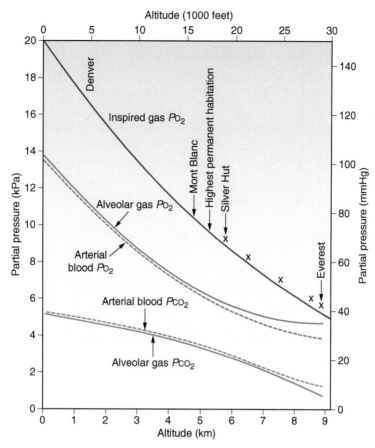

• **Fig. 16.1** Inspired, alveolar and arterial gas partial pressures at rest, as a function of altitude. The curve for inspired Po_2 (red) is taken from standard data in Table 16.1, but the crosses show actual measurements in the Himalayas. The alveolar gas data are from West JB, Hackett PH, Maret KH, et al. Pulmonary gas exchange on the summit of Mount Everest. *J Appl Physiol.* 1983;55:678-687, and agree remarkably well with the arterial blood data from the simulated ascent of Everest.[2]

brain tissue and cerebral vasoconstriction from the resulting hypocapnia.[8]

Acute exposure to high altitude ultimately leads to loss of consciousness, which usually occurs at altitudes in excess of 6000 m (about 20 000 ft). The time to loss of consciousness varies with altitude, and is of great practical importance to pilots in the event of loss of pressurization (Fig. 16.2). The shortest possible time to loss of consciousness (about 15 seconds) applies at greater than 16 000 m (52 000 ft), and is governed by lung-to-brain circulation time and the capacity of high energy phosphate stores in the brain (page 273).

Acclimatization to Altitude

Acclimatization refers to the processes by which tolerance and performance are improved over a period of hours to weeks after an individual who normally lives at relatively low altitude ascends to a higher area. Acclimatization never returns blood gases or performance back to sea-level values but can achieve impressive physiological results. For example, Everest has been climbed without oxygen by well-acclimatized lowlanders, although the barometric pressure on the summit would cause rapid loss of consciousness without acclimatization (Fig. 16.2). Adaptation to altitude (described later) refers to physiological differences in

permanent residents at high altitude and is quite different from acclimatization.

Earlier studies of acclimatization took place in the attractive, although somewhat hostile, environment of high-altitude expeditions in many mountain ranges. Technical limitations in these conditions led to two experiments, named Operation Everest II and III, in which volunteers lived in a decompression chamber in which an ascent to the summit of Everest was simulated.[9] These conditions permitted extensive physiological research to be undertaken at rest and during exercise.

Ventilatory Control

Prolonged hypoxia results in several complex changes in ventilation and arterial blood gases which are shown in Figure 16.3. The initial hypoxic drive to ventilation on acute exposure is short-lived, and after about 30 mintues ventilation returns to only slightly above normoxic levels, with Pco_2 just below control levels (Fig. 16.3). This poor ventilatory response causes significant arterial hypoxaemia and results in many of the symptoms seen during the first few hours and days at altitude. Over the next few days, ventilation slowly increases, with an accompanying reduction of Pco_2 and matching increase in arterial Po_2. This

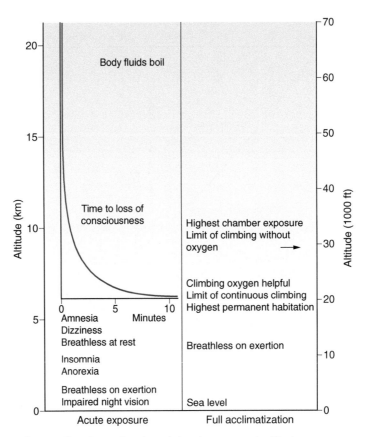

• **Fig. 16.2** Symptoms of acute and chronic exposure to altitude.

increase in Po_2 is of relatively small magnitude and can never correct Po_2 to normal (sea-level) values, but it does seem to be enough to ameliorate most of the symptoms of exposure to acute altitude.

There are significant differences between species in the rate at which acclimatization takes place, being just a few hours in most animals, and several days or weeks in humans.[3] Both the rate of ascent and the altitude attained influence the speed at which ventilatory acclimatization occurs, but in humans most subjects are fully acclimatized within 1 week.

There are many possible mechanisms to explain the ventilatory changes seen with acclimatization. In spite of the low blood Pco_2, stimulation of the central chemoreceptors almost certainly plays a part in the hyperventilation that occurs with acclimatization. It was first suggested, in 1963, that the restoration of cerebrospinal fluid (CSF) pH, by means of bicarbonate transport, might explain this acclimatization of ventilation to altitude. However, the time course of changes in CSF pH does not match changes in ventilation, and most studies showed a persistent increase in CSF pH at altitude. CSF pH therefore is unlikely to represent an important mechanism of acclimatization. Other studies, mainly in animals, indicate that acclimatization represents an increase in the responsiveness of the respiratory centre to hypoxia from both direct effects of prolonged hypoxia on the central nervous system and prolonged maximal afferent input from the peripheral chemoreceptors. This increased responsiveness may be mediated by alterations in the sensitivity to neurotransmitters involved in respiratory control (see Fig. 4.4). For example, increased sensitivity to glutamate will directly increase ventilation, or decreasing γ–aminobutyric acid (GABA) sensitivity will effectively reduce hypoxic ventilatory decline (page 52).

In addition to changes affecting the central chemoreceptors, there is evidence that peripheral chemoreceptor sensitivity is increased during prolonged hypoxia, contributing to the progressive hyperventilation seen with acclimatization. In humans, the acute hypoxic ventilatory response is increased during the first few days at altitude and for several days after return to sea level. The mechanism of this increased sensitivity to hypoxia is not known, but is independent of changes in Pco_2, and may reside either with increased sensitivity of the carotid bodies or with the increased responsiveness of the respiratory centre described in the previous paragraph.

Respiratory alkalosis at altitude is counteracted, over the course of a few days, by renal excretion of bicarbonate, resulting in a degree of metabolic acidosis that will tend to increase respiratory drive (see Fig. 4.6). This was formerly thought to be the main factor in the ventilatory adaptation to altitude, but it now appears to be of minor importance compared with the changes in the central and peripheral chemoreceptors.

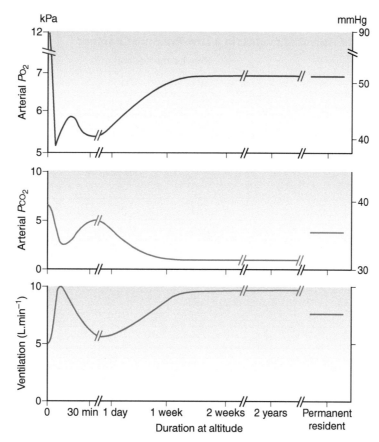

• **Fig. 16.3** Effects of prolonged hypoxia (equivalent to 4300 m, 14 100 ft) on ventilation and blood gases. The first section of the graph shows the acute hypoxic response and hypoxic ventilatory decline described in Chapter 4. Acclimatization then takes place, partially restoring P_{O_2} by means of long-term hyperventilation and hypocapnia, a situation that is maintained indefinitely while remaining at altitude. Individuals who reside throughout life at this altitude maintain similar P_{O_2} values with lesser degrees of hyperventilation, but still have a minute ventilation greater than sea level normal.

Blood Gases

Figure 16.3 shows the time course of blood gas changes during acclimatization, and Figure 16.1 shows changes in alveolar gas partial pressures with altitude in fully acclimatized mountaineers. Alveolar P_{O_2} is unexpectedly well preserved at extreme altitude, and at greater than 8000 m (26 000 ft) tends to remain close to 4.8 kPa (36 mmHg). Operations Everest II and III found arterial P_{O_2} values of 3.6 and 4.1 kPa (27 and 31 mmHg) at a pressure equivalent to the summit of Everest (Table 16.2), with an alveolar/arterial P_{O_2} difference of less than 0.3 kPa (2 mmHg) at rest.[10] The Caudwell Extreme Everest expedition in 2007 obtained arterial blood samples at 8400 m (27 559 ft) with an average P_{O_2} of 3.3 kPa (25 mmHg). There was also a significant alveolar to arterial P_{O_2} difference of 0.7 kPa (5 mmHg), which the authors suggested may have resulted from a diffusion barrier to oxygen at such low levels, possibly as a result of subclinical pulmonary oedema.[11]

Haemoglobin Concentration and Oxygen Affinity

An increase in haemoglobin concentration was the earliest adaptation to altitude to be demonstrated. Initially caused by a reduction in plasma volume, erythropoietin levels are raised within a few hours at altitude, and haemoglobin mass begins to increase within a few days, reaching a plateau after about three weeks.[1,12] Data from subjects at 8400 m (27 559 ft) reported an increase from 148 to 193 g.L^{-1}, which, at the resting value of 54% saturation, maintained an arterial oxygen content of almost 15 mL.dL^{-1}.[11]

The haemoglobin dissociation curve at altitude is affected by changes in both pH and 2,3-diphosphoglycerate (DPG) concentration (page 146). DPG concentrations are generally increased at high altitude,[2] displacing the curve to the right, whereas pH is invariably high because of hyperventilation, displacing the curve to the left. Conflicting reports of the P$_{50}$ (page 146) at altitude therefore exist, with differences resulting from the population studied (high-altitude natives or lowlanders), the degree of acclimatization, altitude of the study, and so on.[1] However, it is generally thought that the pH effect predominates, and that altitude causes a left shift of the curve; and in vivo data at 3600 m (12 000 ft) support this,[13] indicating that oxygen loading in the lung takes priority over maintaining P_{O_2} at the point of release.

TABLE 16.2	Cardiorespiratory Data Obtained at Rest and During Exercise at Extreme Reduction of Ambient Pressure During the Simulated Ascent of Everest in a Low-Pressure Chamber[10]				
		Sea-Level Equivalent		**Extreme Altitude Equivalent**	
Ambient pressure (kPa)		101		33.7	
(mmHg)		760		253	
Haemoglobin concentration (g.L^{-1})		135		170	
$\dot{V}_{O_2peak}$ (mL.min^{-1}, STPD)		3980		1170	
State		**Rest**	**Exercise**	**Rest**	**Exercise**
Exercise intensity (watts)		0	281	0	90
Ventilation (L.min^{-1}, BTPS)		11	107	42.3	157.5
$\dot{V}_{O_2peak}$ (mL.min^{-1}, STPD)		350	3380	386	1002
Ventilation equivalent		31	32	110	157
Arterial P_{O_2} (kPa)		13.2	12.0	4.0	3.7
(mmHg)		99.3	90.0	30.3	27.7
Arterial P_{CO_2} (kPa)		4.5	4.7	1.5	1.3
(mmHg)		33.9	35.0	11.2	10.1
Arterial/venous O_2 content difference (mL.dL^{-1})		5.7	15.0	4.6	6.7
Mixed venous P_{O_2} (kPa)		4.7	2.6	2.9	1.9
(mmHg)		35.1	19.7	22.1	14.3
Cardiac output (L.min^{-1})		6.7	27.2	8.4	15.7
Pulmonary arterial pressure (mean, mmHg)		15	33	33	48

Actual ambient pressure at simulated high altitude was 32 kPa (240 mmHg), but leakage of oxygen from masks worn by investigators had caused the oxygen concentration in the chamber to rise to 22%, the equivalent of 33.7 kPa at 21%, which is equivalent to the summit of Everest.
BTPS, body temperature and pressure, saturated STPD, standard temperature, pressure and dry.

Adaptation to Altitude[14]

Adaptation refers to physiological, epigenetic and genetic changes that occur over a period of years to generations in those who have taken up permanent residence at high altitude. There are qualitative as well as quantitative differences between acclimatization and adaptation, but each is remarkably effective. High-altitude residents have an impressive ability to exercise under grossly hypoxic conditions, but their adaptations show many striking differences from those in acclimatized lowlanders. Residents in different high-altitude areas of the world have differing adaptations.

Data regarding the mortality of climbers attempting to reach the summit of Mount Everest illustrate how effective adaptations to altitude are compared with acclimatization in lowlanders. Sherpa residents had a mortality of only 0.4%, compared with 2.7% amongst climbers.[15]

Physiological Adaptations

Long-term residence at altitude leads to a reduced ventilatory response to hypoxia,[1] which results in a reduction of ventilation compared with an acclimatized lowlander and a rise in P_{CO_2}, although neither of these returns to sea-level values (Fig. 16.3). High-altitude residents maintain similar arterial P_{O_2} values to those of acclimatized lowlanders

despite the reduced ventilation and therefore lower alveolar P_{O_2}. Pulmonary diffusing capacity must therefore be increased and depends on anatomical pulmonary adaptations increasing the area available for diffusion by the generation of greater numbers of alveoli and associated capillaries. This is an example of developmental plasticity occurring in infants who spend their formative years at altitude. In humans, the development of alveoli by septation of saccules formed in utero occurs mostly after birth (page 176), and it is this process that is stimulated by hypoxia, although the mechanism of this stimulation remains unknown.[16] An adult moving permanently to high altitude will therefore never achieve the same degree of adaptation as a native of the area, explaining the ability of high-altitude residents to exercise to a much greater degree than their nonresident visitors. Unfortunately, the enhanced growth of alveolar tissue is not matched by similar airway growth, and dysanapsis (page 202) occurs,[17] potentially rendering the individual susceptible to airway flow limitation.

Another major adaptation to altitude by long-term residents appears to be increased vascularity of heart and striated muscles, a change that is also important for the trained athlete. For the high-altitude resident, increased perfusion, probably mediated by higher levels of circulating nitric oxide products,[18] appears to compensate effectively for the reduced oxygen content of the arterial blood.

Epigenetic Adaptations

This term describes non–sequence-based changes to the genome,[14] and in hypoxic situations involves methylation of DNA, modifying the numerous transcriptional responses to hypoxia mediated by hypoxia-inducible factor (HIF, see Table 23.1). The methylation selectively silences genes responsible for HIF stabilization. Epigenetic changes are seen in adults, but animal studies suggest they also occur in utero or in infancy in response to intermittent hypoxia, and although the mechanisms are poorly understood, the changes can become inheritable and be passed on to subsequent generations.

Genetic Adaptations

Residents of high-altitude areas of the Andes hyperventilate less than residents at equivalent altitude in Tibet.[19] This higher ventilation in Tibetans may explain their reduced susceptibility, in comparison with populations in the Andes, to chronic mountain sickness (see next section) and some complications of pregnancy that are normally associated with high-altitude life. Human occupation of Tibet is believed to have begun earlier than in other high-altitude areas of the world, and these differences in Tibetan physiology could represent a more advanced genetic adaptation to the physiologically hostile environment.[20]

Polycythaemia is normal in high-altitude residents, and is influenced by altitude, population, sex and occupation.[19] Differences in haemoglobin levels between different high-altitude populations are described, with Tibetan populations generally being less polycythaemic than Andean people. Originally thought to represent genetic variation, further studies suggested that the difference may relate to occupational lung disease, for example from mining activities in Andean high-altitude areas, and that healthy individuals in both areas might have haemoglobin levels equivalent to those of acclimatized lowlanders.[19] Exercise at altitude is affected by haemoglobin concentration, with lower levels being associated with greater exercise capacity. This is believed to result from lower blood viscosity improving tissue blood flow and so oxygen delivery and suggests that polycythaemia may actually be a maladaptive response.[21]

Chronic Mountain Sickness (Monge Disease)[1]

A small minority of those who dwell permanently at very high altitude develop this dangerous illness. It is characterized by an exceptionally poor ventilatory response to hypoxia, resulting in low arterial P_{O_2} and high P_{CO_2}. There is cyanosis, high haematocrit, finger clubbing, pulmonary hypertension, right heart failure, dyspnoea and lethargy.

Exercise at High Altitude[22]

The summit of Everest was attained without the use of oxygen in 1978 by Messner and Habeler, and by many other climbers since then. Studies of exercise have been made at various altitudes up to and including the summit, and on the simulated ascents in Operations Everest II and III. Of necessity, these observations are largely confined to very fit subjects.

Capacity for Work Performed

There is a progressive decline in the external work that can be performed as altitude increases. On Operation Everest II,[2] 300 to 360 W was attained at sea level, 240 to 270 W at 59 kPa pressure (equivalent to 4300 m, 14000 ft) and 120 W at 37 kPa (7600 m, 25000 ft). Oxygen uptake during peak exercise ($\dot{V}_{O_{2peak}}$) also declines in accord with altitude to 1177 mL.min^{-1} at 32 kPa pressure. Resting cardiac output is unchanged at moderate altitude and only slightly increased at extreme altitude. During exercise, for a given power expenditure, the increase in cardiac output at altitude is the same as at sea level.[2]

Ventilation Equivalent of Oxygen Consumption

Figure 13.5 shows that ventilation as a function of oxygen consumption ($\dot{V}_{O_2}$) is comparatively constant. The length of the line increases with training, but the slope of the linear portion remains the same. With increasing altitude, the slope and intercept are both dramatically increased up to four times the sea-level value,[2] with maximal ventilation approaching 200 L.min^{-1} (Fig. 16.4). This is because ventilation is reported at body temperature and pressure satu-

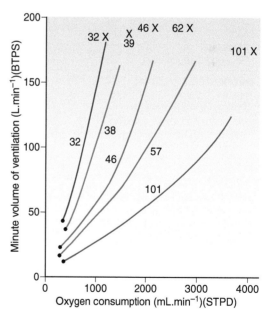

• **Fig. 16.4** The relationship between minute volume of ventilation and oxygen consumption at rest and during exercise at altitude. The relationship is radically changed at altitude, primarily because ventilation is reported at body temperature and pressure saturated *(BTPS)*, whereas oxygen consumption is reported at standard temperature and pressure dry *(STPD)*. Numbers in the figure indicate barometric pressure in kPa. •, resting points; ×, values at oxygen uptake during peak exercise ($\dot{V}_{O_{2peak}}$) from reference 10. (Data from reference 2.)

rated and oxygen consumption at standard temperature and pressure dry (see Appendix C).

Fortunately, the density of air is reduced in proportion to the barometric pressure at altitude. Resistance to turbulent flow is decreased, and therefore the work of breathing at a particular minute volume of respiration is less. Even with this mitigation, the extra ventilation needed to deliver the oxygen requirement at altitude means that the energy expenditure upon breathing for a given intensity of exercise is considerably higher than at sea level.

$P\text{co}_2$ and $P\text{o}_2$

During exercise at altitude, alveolar $P\text{co}_2$ falls, and alveolar $P\text{o}_2$ rises.[2] Arterial $P\text{co}_2$ falls with alveolar $P\text{co}_2$, but the alveolar/arterial $P\text{o}_2$ difference increases more than the alveolar $P\text{o}_2$ rises, and there is a consistent decrease in arterial $P\text{o}_2$ during exercise at altitude, leading to very low values for $P\text{o}_2$. The lower alveolar to pulmonary capillary $P\text{o}_2$ gradient, along with a faster pulmonary capillary transit time during exercise, causes diffusion limitation of oxygen uptake, and this may be improved by pulmonary vasodilation.[23] Elite athletes at altitude have worse exercise-induced hypoxaemia than less fit individuals because of their higher muscle oxygen-extracting capacity.[24]

Altitude Illness[25,26]

Acute Mountain Sickness

Acute mountain sickness (AMS) is characterized by a headache and at least one of the following: nausea, fatigue, dizziness and difficulty in sleeping (see later). Most research regarding AMS uses the Lake Louise questionnaire to quantify the occurrence and severity of the illness (Table 16.3).[25] Symptoms normally begin to occur at greater than 2000 m (6600 ft), with an abrupt increase in the incidence above 4500 m (14760 ft), affecting about one-half of trekkers at this altitude. The unacclimatized subject also has extreme dyspnoea on exertion at this level, and may have dyspnoea at rest. Severity varies greatly from a mild inconvenient headache to a severe life-threatening illness involving cerebral and pulmonary oedema.

The likelihood of developing AMS relates to altitude (particularly sleeping altitude), the rate of ascent and the degree of exertion. The mountaineer is therefore affected by altitude in a manner that differs from that of the aviator, because his physical exertion is much greater and the time course of exposure is different. Rate of ascent seldom exceeds 2000 m (6500 ft) per day from sea level, decreasing to only 300 m (1000 ft) per day at very high altitude. Smokers

TABLE 16.3	The Lake Louise Questionnaire for Acute Mountain Sickness[25]			
Symptom	**Score**	**Clinical Assessment**	**Score**	
Headache:		Change in mental status:	0	
None	0	No change	1	
Mild	1	Lethargy/lassitude	2	
Moderate	2	Disoriented/confused	3	
Severe, incapacitating	3	Stupor/semiconsciousness		
Gastrointestinal symptoms:		Ataxia (heel to toe walking):		
None	0	No ataxia	0	
Poor appetite or nausea	1	Manoeuvres to maintain balance	1	
Moderate nausea or vomiting	2	Steps off line	2	
Severe nausea or vomiting, incapacitating	3	Falls down	3	
			4	
Fatigue/weakness:		Can't stand		
Not tired or weak	0	Peripheral oedema:	0	
Mild fatigue/weakness	1	None	1	
Moderate fatigue/weakness	2	One location	2	
Severe fatigue/weakness, incapacitating	3	Two or more locations		
Dizzy/lightheadedness:				
Not dizzy	0			
Mild dizziness	1			
Moderate dizziness	2			
Severe, incapacitating	3			
Difficulty sleeping:				
Slept well as usual	0			
Did not sleep as well as usual	1			
Woke many times, poor night's sleep	2			
Could not sleep at all	3			

A subject who has recently arrived at a higher altitude, has a headache and has a score of >3 has acute mountain sickness.

have a lower incidence of AMS in the first few days after arriving at altitude, but smoking also impairs their long-term acclimatization.[27]

High-Altitude Pulmonary Oedema[28]

A small amount of subclinical pulmonary oedema probably occurs in all subjects at high altitude, but in a few percent the oedema becomes progressive and life-threatening.[1] As for AMS, the proportion of subjects who develop high-altitude pulmonary oedema (HAPE) depends on the altitude, the speed of ascent, the amount of strenuous exercise performed and individual susceptibility to the condition. It is most commonly seen in the unacclimatized and overambitious climber. Clinical features include cough, dyspnoea and hypoxia, with clinical and radiological signs of pulmonary oedema. Untreated, HAPE has a mortality rate of almost 50%, but with appropriate treatment this is normally less than 3%.

The pathophysiology of HAPE is complex.[29] Subjects with HAPE have significant pulmonary hypertension secondary to hypoxia, and low pulmonary capillary wedge pressures indicating normal left ventricular function. Subjects who are susceptible to HAPE seem to have an excessive hypoxic pulmonary vasoconstriction (HPV) response to hypoxia, and this may in part be as a result of impaired release of endothelial relaxing factors such as nitric oxide (page 80). Compared with subjects who are not susceptible to HAPE, susceptible subjects exhaled lower concentrations of nitric oxide during a high-altitude trip.[30] Pulmonary vasoconstrictors such as endothelin-1 are found in higher concentrations in HAPE-susceptible subjects, who also have greater sympathetic responses to hypoxia. On chest x-rays of subjects with HAPE, pulmonary shadows are typically patchy, indicating that some areas of lung have little blood flow, whereas others have greatly increased blood flow. Magnetic resonance imaging of the lung during hypoxia has shown that HPV is patchy in all subjects (page 81 and Fig. 6.9), but the uneven vasoconstriction is more pronounced in HAPE-susceptible subjects.[31] High capillary flow in some lung regions is believed to lead to 'stress failure' of capillaries, which in animals leads to haemorrhagic alveolar oedema. The same mechanism contributes to exercise-induced pulmonary haemorrhage in horses at sea level (page 313). Capillary stress failure also explains the association between exercise and HAPE, with increased cardiac output causing huge blood flows through less vasoconstricted regions of lung. Although inflammation is not believed to be a primary event in the pathogenesis of HAPE, it does occur in severe cases, and explains why coincidental lung inflammation from, for example, lower respiratory tract infections may exacerbate or even cause HAPE.

Other Medical Problems at Altitude

Cerebral oedema is also potentially lethal, is manifest in the early stages by ataxia, impaired mental capacity and decreased conscious level and if untreated may progress to coma and death.[25] Pulmonary and cerebral forms of severe AMS may both be present in the same patient, but a common aetiology has not been found. Mild, or localized, brain swelling is thought to occur in all people ascending to high altitudes, but it is unclear whether this always represents cerebral oedema.

Cough is another problem at altitude. Almost half of the trekkers in Nepal complain of a cough which may be severe. Coughing normally develops after a few days at altitude, and airway sensitivity to irritants is increased as a result of hyperventilation with low-humidity cold air. Development of a cough may, however, be the first manifestation of HAPE.

Sleep disturbance occurs at altitude.[32] Periodic breathing (page 54) occurs in most individuals at greater than 4000 m (13 000 ft) and does not reduce with acclimatization. There are cyclical changes in tidal volume, often associated with central (rather than obstructive) apnoeas, with or without arousal from sleep (see Fig. 14.2). Severe apnoeas can result in considerable additional hypoxaemia at high altitude, but in most cases mean Sa_{O_2} is maintained.[32] Periodic breathing is believed to result from the increased ventilatory responses to hypoxia and hypercapnia that occur at altitude, and is seldom seen in high-altitude residents, who have an attenuated hypoxic drive. Cerebral blood flow, and specifically the responsiveness of the cerebral circulation to carbon dioxide, seems to also play a role in attenuating the development of periodic breathing.[33]

Therapy for Altitude-Induced Illness[25]

For any severe forms of AMS, particularly if HAPE or cerebral oedema is suspected, administration of oxygen and descent to a lower altitude are the first essentials. First aid for life-threatening conditions also involves using a portable hyperbaric chamber which can be inflated using a foot pump to pressures that easily simulate 2000 m (6500 ft) of descent.[1]

People with mild AMS (Lake Louise score ≤ 4) do not need to be removed from high altitude, and with rest, hydration and symptomatic treatment most symptoms of AMS will resolve as acclimatization takes place. For moderate or severe AMS (Lake Louise score ≥ 5) drug treatment may be required, and a variety of options exist.

Acetazolamide is recommended as a prophylactic treatment to reduce AMS symptoms and may be used to treat established AMS. Inhibition of carbonic anhydrase (CA) by the drug (page 124) may reduce AMS by multiple mechanisms,[34] the most important of which is CA inhibition in the renal tubules causing a bicarbonate diuresis, inducing a metabolic acidosis which stimulates ventilation. Additional mechanisms include reducing transport of carbon dioxide out of cells which causes an intracellular acidosis, including in the cells of the medullary chemoreceptors, so driving respiration. Finally, CA inhibition in the choroid plexus reduces CSF formation, reducing intracranial pressure, and low-dose acetazolamide reduces cerebral oxygen requirements.[35] All these actions in effect accelerate acclimatization.

Dexamethasone, a glucocorticoid, is also beneficial for prevention and treatment of AMS, and increases exercise capacity at altitude. The mechanisms of this effect are mostly unknown, but may include sympatholysis, anti-inflammatory effects, reduced production of reactive oxygen species and attenuation of HPV.[36] The greater incidence of side effects with this drug limits its widespread use.

Nifedipine, a calcium channel blocker, is an established treatment for HAPE, and when used prophylactically prevents HAPE developing in susceptible individuals. It is an effective drug for treating pulmonary hypertension, and the convenience of administration by oral or sublingual route makes it a popular choice for mountaineers.

Sildenafil and tadalafil are pulmonary vasodilators acting via inhibition of phosphodiesterase 5 (page 84) and may be taken orally. Sildenafil has been shown to be effective at reducing the hypoxia-induced rise in pulmonary arterial pressure at altitude, and therefore has potential as a useful treatment for HAPE.[37]

Flying

Only a very small number of people will ever visit places of high enough altitude to induce any of the respiratory changes described in this chapter so far. However, worldwide, almost 2 billion people per year fly in commercial aircraft, so it is useful to consider the respiratory effects of aviation.

Altitude Exposure

For reasons of fuel economy and avoidance of weather systems, commercial aircraft operate at between 9000 and 12 000 m (30 000–40 000 ft). The passenger cabin must therefore be pressurized, and a typical design aims for a cabin pressure equivalent to less than 2400 m (8000 ft), referred to as the 'cabin altitude'. This cabin pressure is not obligatory, but is regarded as 'best practice' by the industry, and represents a compromise between an acceptable level of hypoxia for passengers, fuel costs and the effects of the inside-to-outside pressure difference on the structure of the aircraft.[38] In one study average peak cabin altitude on 207 commercial flights in the United States was approximately 1900 m (6300 ft), but in 10% of flights this exceeded 2400 m (8000 ft) at some point.[39] More recently designed aircraft with a fuselage composed of carbon fibre are more able to resist the stresses caused by a higher cabin pressure, and so aim for maximum cabin altitudes of 1800 m (6000 ft).

Military aircraft fly prolonged reconnaissance missions at altitudes around 22 400 m (73 500 ft), with the cockpit pressurized to an equivalent altitude of 9000 m (30 000 ft). Pilots must therefore breathe 100% oxygen by mask to maintain an inspired Po_2 close to sea level to facilitate the required mental performance. Hypergravity caused by

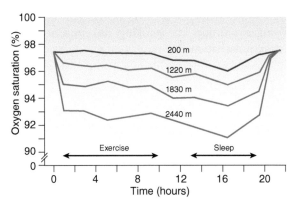

inertial forces in the head-to-foot direction along with hyperoxia (page 251) may lead to lung atelectasis in pilots.[40] At this altitude, military pilots are also at risk of altitude decompression sickness, which is discussed on page 224.

In theory, cabin altitudes of less than 2400 m (8000 ft) should represent a minimal physiological challenge to healthy individuals, resulting in a drop of only a few percent in Sa_{O_2}. In practice, a study of healthy cabin crews during normal flight patterns showed that over half had Sa_{O_2} drops to less than 90%.[41] The effects of this degree of hypoxia on performance are controversial, although impaired night vision or colour recognition may occur at this altitude (page 206). For passengers, average Sa_{O_2} values during a flight are approximately 92%, although this may be worse during exercise and sleep (Fig. 16.5).[42] Of more concern than lowered Sa_{O_2} is the effect of mild hypoxia on the pulmonary vasculature, with evidence from actual[43] and simulated[44] flights that HPV is active in healthy passengers. The rise in pulmonary vascular resistance (Fig. 16.6) takes about an hour to develop, suggesting that the second phase of HPV (page 81) is responsible, and is more pronounced in older subjects.

Depressurization

Loss of cabin pressure at altitude either through equipment failure or accident is extremely rare. In the case of slow loss of cabin pressure, oxygen is provided for passengers as an interim measure until the aircraft can descend: 100% oxygen provides adequate protection from loss of consciousness up to an altitude of about 12 000 m (40 000 ft), where the atmospheric pressure is roughly equal to the sea-level atmospheric Po_2.

There are sporadic reports of stowaway passengers undertaking long-haul flights in the wheel well of modern aircraft.[45] This environment affords little protection against the cold and severe hypoxia of altitude levels well above that

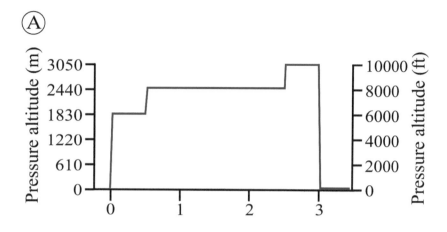

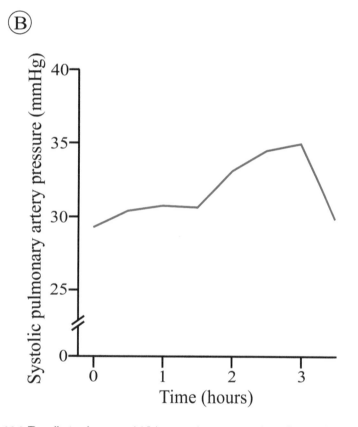

• **Fig. 16.6** The effects of commercial flying on pulmonary vascular resistance, based on healthy subjects on a simulated flight of 3 hours' duration in a hypobaric chamber. **(A)** The cabin pressure profile of the study. **(B)** Pulmonary vascular resistance, showing an increase only after about one hour of hypoxia. (From reference 44 with permission of the Aerospace Medical Association.)

of Everest. That half of these stowaways die is not surprising, but it is remarkable that half of them survive. Severe hypothermia is believed to protect them against the effects of hypoxia.

Air Travel in Patients with Respiratory Disease[46]

To patients with respiratory disease flying may present a significant challenge, particularly if arterial hypoxaemia already exists at sea level, and careful preflight assessment is required. A variety of preflight clinical evaluations and investigations have been recommended to determine the risk of flying for an individual patient with respiratory disease. A summary of the British Thoracic Society guidelines is shown in Table 16.4. In some patients a hypoxic challenge test is recommended to determine whether in-flight oxygen is required. This test involves measurement of arterial Po_2 while simulating flying conditions by using a hypoxic gas mixture, usually 15% oxygen. This inspired Po_2 equates to

TABLE 16.4	British Thoracic Society Recommendations on Assessing the Safety of Patients with Respiratory Disease Wishing to Fly, and Their Requirement for In-Flight Supplemental Oxygen[46]

Indicators that Further Clinical Assessment is Required:

- Previous air travel intolerance with significant respiratory symptoms (dyspnoea, chest pain, confusion or syncope)
- Severe COPD (FEV_1 <30% predicted) or asthma
- Bullous lung disease
- Severe (vital capacity <1 L) restrictive disease (including chest wall and respiratory muscle disease), especially with hypoxaemia and/or hypercapnia
- Cystic fibrosis
- Comorbidity with conditions worsened by hypoxaemia (cerebrovascular disease, cardiac disease or pulmonary hypertension)
- Pulmonary tuberculosis
- Within 6 weeks of hospital discharge for acute respiratory illness
- Recent pneumothorax
- Risk of or previous venous thromboembolism
- Preexisting requirement for oxygen, CPAP or ventilator support

Contraindications to Commercial Air Travel:

- Ongoing pneumothorax with persistent air leak
- Major haemoptysis
- Usual oxygen requirement at sea level at a flow rate exceeding 4 L.min^{-1}

Hypoxic Challenge Test:

PaO_2 ≥6.6 kPa (≥50 mmHg)	Oxygen not required
PaO_2 <6.6 kPa (<50 mmHg)	In-flight oxygen required at 2 L.min^{-1} via nasal cannulae

Hypoxic challenge test is arterial oxygen partial pressure after breathing 15% oxygen for 20 minutes.
COPD, Chronic obstructive pulmonary disease; *CPAP*, continuous positive airway pressure; FEV_1, Forced Expiratory Volume in 1 s.

a cabin altitude of 2400 m (8000 ft), and represents the lowest oxygen partial pressure that should be experienced during a commercial flight (Table 16.1).

Cabin Air Quality

Aircraft ventilation systems deliver 4 to 8 L.s^{-1} of air per passenger during flight. However, compression and temperature regulation of fresh air from outside are expensive in energy terms, and most current designs of aircraft incorporate cabin air recirculation systems.[47] Total air delivered remains unchanged, but up to 50% may be recirculated rather than fresh. This recirculation of cabin air has caused concerns about the potential transmission of airborne pathogens between passengers. These fears seem to be unfounded: recirculated air passes through a high-efficiency particulate air filter before reentering the cabin, and studies comparing passengers travelling on aircraft with recirculated compared with 100% fresh air ventilation systems found no difference in the likelihood of developing a common cold after the flight.[47]

Carbon dioxide concentration in aircraft often exceeds the generally accepted 'comfort' level of 1000 parts per million (ppm) and would be expected to be higher in aircraft with greater amounts of recirculated air. Concentrations observed in aircraft vary between around 700 and 1700 ppm,[48] and are highest when the aircraft is occupied but on the ground, and lowest whilst flying at cruise altitude. Carbon dioxide itself does not cause respiratory problems at

these levels but is used more as a marker of the adequacy of ventilation.

Humidity is invariably low in aircraft, with most studies finding relative humidity to be an average 14% to 19% during flight, compared with in excess of 50% in most sea-level environments. Like carbon dioxide, cabin humidity is maximal when on the ground and minimal at cruise altitude.[48] The low humidity occurring in aircraft is responsible for many minor symptoms such as irritation of the eyes and upper airway, although these symptoms are unusual with less than 3 to 4 hours of exposure.

With the exception of low humidity, there is therefore little evidence that the cabin air of aircraft poses any threat to healthy passengers. The numerous symptoms reported following air travel almost certainly have their origins in other activities associated with air travel, in particular the consumption of alcohol and adapting to differing time zones.

References

*1. West JB, Schoene RB, Luks AM, et al. *High Altitude Medicine and Physiology*. London: CRC Press; 2012.
2. Sutton JT, Reeves JT, Wagner PD, et al. Operation Everest II: oxygen transport during exercise at extreme simulated altitude. *J Appl Physiol*. 1988;64:1309-1321.
3. Conkin J, Wessell JH. Critique of the equivalent air altitude model. *Aviat Space Environ Med*. 2008;79:975-982.

4. Connolly DM. Oxygenation state and twilight vision at 2438 m. *Aviat Space Environ Med.* 2011;82:2-8.
5. Petrassi FA, Hodkinson PD, Walters PL, et al. Hypoxic hypoxia at moderate altitudes: review of the state of the science. *Aviat Space Environ Med.* 2012;83:975-984.
6. Asmaro D, Mayall J, Ferguson S. Cognition at altitude: impairment in executive and memory processes under hypoxic conditions. *Aviat Space Environ Med.* 2013;84:1159-1165.
7. Steinman Y, van den Oord MHAH, Frings-Dresen MHW, et al. Flight performance during exposure to acute hypobaric hypoxia. *Aerosp Med Hum Perform.* 2017;88:760-767.
8. van Dorpe E, Los M, Dirven P, et al. Inspired carbon dioxide during hypoxia: effects on task performance and cerebral oxygen saturation. *Aviat Space Environ Med.* 2007;78:666-672.
9. Richalet JP, Robach P, Jarrot S, et al. Operation Everest III (COMEX '97): effects of prolonged and progressive hypoxia on humans during a simulated ascent to 8848 m in a hypobaric chamber. *Adv Exp Med Biol.* 1999;474:297-317.
10. Wagner PD, Sutton JT, Reeves JT, et al. Operation Everest II: pulmonary gas exchange during a simulated ascent of Mt. Everest. *J Appl Physiol.* 1987;63:2348-2359.
11. Grocott MPW, Martin DS, Levett DZH, et al. Arterial blood gases and oxygen content in climbers on mount Everest. *N Engl J Med.* 2009;360:140-149.
12. Siebenmann C, Cathomen A, Hug M, et al. Hemoglobin mass and intravascular volume kinetics during and after exposure to 3,454 m altitude. *J Appl Physiol.* 2015;119:1194-1201.
13. Balaban DY, Duffin J, Preiss D, et al. The in-vivo oxyhaemoglobin dissociation curve at sea level and high altitude. *Respir Physiol Neurobiol.* 2013;186:45-52.
14. Julian CG. Epigenomics and human adaptation to high altitude. *J Appl Physiol.* 2017;123:1362-1370.
15. Firth PG, Zheng H, Windsor JS, et al. Mortality on Mount Everest, 1921–2006: descriptive study. *BMJ.* 2008;337:a2654.
16. Massaro D, Massaro GD. Pulmonary alveoli: formation, the 'call for oxygen', and other regulators. *Am J Physiol Lung Cell Mol Physiol.* 2002;282:L345-L348.
17. Llapur CJ, Martínez MR, Grassino PT, et al. Chronic hypoxia accentuates dysanaptic lung growth. *Am J Respir Crit Care Med.* 2016;194:327-332.
18. Erzurum SC, Ghosh S, Janocha AJ, et al. Higher blood flow and circulating NO products offset high-altitude hypoxia among Tibetans. *Proc Natl Acad Sci USA.* 2007;104:17593-17598.
19. Moore LG. Measuring high-altitude adaptation. *J Appl Physiol.* 2017;123:1371-1385.
*20. **Petousi N, Robbins PA. Human adaptation to the hypoxia of high altitude: the Tibetan paradigm from the pregenomic to the postgenomic era. *J Appl Physiol.* 2014;116:875-884.**
21. Simonson TS, Wei G, Wagner HE, et al. Low haemoglobin concentration in Tibetan males is associated with greater high-altitude exercise capacity. *J Physiol.* 2015;593:3207-3218.
22. Schoene RB. Limits of respiration at high altitude. *Clin Chest Med.* 2005;26:405-414.
23. de Bisschop C, Martinot J, Leurquin-Sterk G, et al. Improvement in lung diffusion by endothelin A receptor blockade at high altitude. *J Appl Physiol.* 2012;112:20-25.
24. Van Thienen R, Hespel P. Enhanced muscular oxygen extraction in athletes exaggerates hypoxemia during exercise in hypoxia. *J Appl Physiol.* 2016;120:351-361.
25. Imray C, Booth A, Wright A, et al. Acute altitude illnesses. *BMJ.* 2011;343:d4943.
*26. **Luks AM. Physiology in medicine: a physiologic approach to prevention and treatment of acute high-altitude illnesses. *J Appl Physiol.* 2015;118:509-519.**
27. Wu T-Y, Ding S-Q, Liu J-L, et al. Smoking, acute mountain sickness and altitude acclimatisation: a cohort study. *Thorax.* 2012;67:914-919.
28. Korzeniewski K, Nitsch-Osuch A, Guzekc A, et al. High altitude pulmonary edema in mountain climbers. *Respir Physiol Neurobiol.* 2015;209:33-38.
29. Hopkins SR. Stress failure and high-altitude pulmonary oedema: mechanistic insights from physiology. *Eur Respir J.* 2010;35:470-472.
30. Duplain H, Sartori C, Lepori M, et al. Exhaled nitric oxide in high-altitude pulmonary edema. Role in the regulation of pulmonary vascular tone and evidence for a role against inflammation. *Am J Respir Crit Care Med.* 2000;162:221-224.
31. Dehnert C, Risse F, Ley S, et al. Magnetic resonance imaging of uneven pulmonary perfusion in hypoxia in humans. *Am J Respir Crit Care Med.* 2006;174:1132-1138.
32. Ainslie PN, Lucas SJ, Burgess KR. Breathing and sleep at high altitude. *Respir Physiol Neurobiol.* 2013;188:233-256.
33. Burgess KR, Lucas SJ, Shepherd K, et al. Worsening of central sleep apnea at high altitude—a role for cerebrovascular function. *J Appl Physiol.* 2013;114:1021-1028.
34. Leaf DE, Goldfarb DS. Mechanisms of action of acetazolamide in the prophylaxis and treatment of acute mountain sickness. *J Appl Physiol.* 2007;102:1313-1322.
35. Wang K, Smith ZM, Buxton RB, et al. Acetazolamide during acute hypoxia improves tissue oxygenation in the human brain. *J Appl Physiol.* 2015;119:1494-1500.
36. Swenson ER. Pharmacology of acute mountain sickness: old drugs and newer thinking. *J Appl Physiol.* 2016;120:204-215.
37. Richalet J-P, Gratadour P, Robach P, et al. Sildenafil inhibits altitude-induced hypoxemia and pulmonary hypertension. *Am J Respir Crit Care Med.* 2005;171:275-281.
38. Aerospace Medical Association, Aviation Safety Committee, Civil Aviation Subcommittee. Cabin cruising altitudes for regular transport aircraft. *Aviat Space Environ Med.* 2008;79:433-439.
39. Hampson NB, Kregenow DA, Mahoney AM, et al. Altitude exposures during commercial flight: a reappraisal. *Aviat Space Environ Med.* 2013;84:27-31.
40. Dussault C, Gontier E, Verret C, et al. Hyperoxia and hypergravity are independent risk factors of atelectasis in healthy sitting humans: a pulmonary ultrasound and SPECT/CT study. *J Appl Physiol.* 2016;121:66-77.
41. Cottrell JJ, Lebovitz BL, Fennell RG, et al. Inflight arterial saturation: continuous monitoring by pulse oximetry. *Aviat Space Environ Med.* 1995;66:126-130.
42. Muhm JM, Rock PB, McMullin DL, et al. Effect of aircraft-cabin altitude on passenger discomfort. *N Engl J Med.* 2007;357:18-27.
43. Smith TG, Talbot NP, Chang RW, et al. Pulmonary artery pressure increases during commercial air travel in healthy passengers. *Aviat Space Environ Med.* 2012;83:673-676.
44. Turner BE, Hodkinson PD, Timperley AC, et al. Pulmonary artery pressure response to simulated air travel in a hypobaric chamber. *Aerosp Med Hum Perform.* 2015;86:529-534.
45. Veronneau SJH, Mohler SR, Pennybaker AL, et al. Survival at high altitudes: Wheel-well passengers. *Aviat Space Environ Med.* 1996;67:784-786.
46. Ahmedzai S, Balfour-Lynn IM, Bewick T, et al. On behalf of the British Thoracic Society Standards of Care Committee. Managing passengers with stable respiratory disease planning air travel: British Thoracic Society recommendations. *Thorax.* 2011;66:i1-i30.
47. Zitter JN, Mazonson PD, Miller DP, et al. Aircraft cabin air recirculation and symptoms of the common cold. *JAMA.* 2002;288:483-486.
48. Lindgren T, Norback D. Cabin air quality: indoor pollutants and climate during intercontinental flights with and without tobacco smoking. *Indoor Air.* 2002;12:263-272.

17

High Pressure and Diving

KEY POINTS

- When diving in water the increased density of inhaled gases and immersion in water cause an increase in the work of breathing, which can impair gas exchange during exercise.
- At greater than about 4 atmospheres absolute pressure nitrogen has anaesthetic effects, and divers must breathe helium, which also overcomes the problem of increased gas density.
- On ascent from a dive expansion of gases in closed body spaces and bubble formation in the tissues and blood can cause pulmonary barotrauma and decompression sickness.

Humans have sojourned temporarily in high-pressure environments since the introduction of the diving bell. The origin of this development is lost in antiquity, but Alexander the Great was said to have been lowered to the seabed in a diving bell.

The environment of the diver is often, but not invariably, aqueous. Saturation divers spend most of their time in a gaseous environment in chambers that are held at a pressure close to that of the depth of water at which they will be working. Tunnel and caisson workers may also be at high pressure in a gaseous environment. Those in an aqueous environment also have the additional effect of different gravitational forces applied to their trunks, which influence the mechanics of breathing and other systems of the body. Workers in both environments share the physiological problems associated with increased ambient pressures and partial pressures of respired gases.

In this field, as in others, we cannot escape from the multiplicity of units, and some of these are set out in Table 17.1. Note particularly that 'atmosphere gauge' is relative to ambient pressure. Thus 2 atm absolute (ATA) equals 1 atm gauge relative to sea level. Throughout this chapter atmospheres of pressure refer to absolute and not gauge.

Exchange of Oxygen and Carbon Dioxide

Effect of Pressure on Alveolar P_{CO_2} and P_{O_2}

Pressure has complicated and important effects on P_{CO_2} and P_{O_2}. The alveolar concentration of CO_2 equals its rate of production divided by the alveolar ventilation (page 107). However, both gas volumes must be measured under the same conditions of temperature and pressure. Alveolar CO_2 concentration at 10 ATA will be about one-tenth of sea-level values, that is, 0.56% compared with 5.3% at sea level. When these concentrations are multiplied by pressure to give P_{CO_2}, values are similar at sea level and 10 atm. Thus as a rough approximation, alveolar CO_2 concentration decreases inversely to the environmental pressure, but the P_{CO_2} remains near its sea-level value.

Effects on the P_{O_2} are slightly more complicated. The difference between the inspired and alveolar oxygen concentrations equals the ratio of oxygen uptake to inspired alveolar ventilation. This fraction, like the alveolar CO_2 concentration, decreases inversely with the increased pressure. However, the corresponding partial pressure will remain close to the sea-level value, as does the alveolar P_{CO_2}. Therefore the difference between the inspired and alveolar P_{O_2} will remain roughly constant, and the alveolar P_{O_2}, to a first approximation, increases by the same amount as the inspired P_{O_2} (Fig. 17.1). However, these considerations only take into account the direct effect of pressure on gas partial pressures. There are other, more subtle, effects on respiratory mechanics and gas exchange which must now be considered.

Effect on Mechanics of Breathing[1-3]

Two main factors must be considered. First, there is the increased density of gases at pressure, although this can be reduced by changing the composition of the inspired gas. The second factor is the pressure of water on the body, which alters the gravitational effects to which the respiratory system is normally exposed.

Gas density is increased in direct proportion to pressure. Thus air at 10 atm has 10 times the density of air at sea

TABLE 17.1 **Pressures and Po_2 Values at Various Depths of Seawater**

Depth of Seawater		Pressure (Absolute)		Po_2 Breathing Air					Percentage Oxygen to Give Sea-Level Inspired Po_2
				Inspired		Alveolar			
(m)	(ft)	(atm)	(kPa)	(kPa)	(mmHg)	(kPa)	(mmHg)		
0	0	1	101	19.9	149	13.9	104		20.9
10	32.8	2	203	41.2	309	35.2	264		10.1
20	65.6	3	304	62.3	467	56.3	422		6.69
50	164	6	608	126	945	120	900		3.31
Usual Limit for Breathing Air									
100	328	11	1,110						1.80
200	656	21	2,130						0.94
Usual Limit for Saturation Dives									
Threshold for High-Pressure Nervous Syndrome									
500	1640	51	5,170						0.39
1000	3280	101	10,200						0.20
Depth Reached by Sperm Whale									
2000	6560	201	20,400						0.098
2500	8200	251	25,400						0.078

Pressure reached by nonaquatic mammals with pharmacological amelioration of high-pressure nervous syndrome

Note: 10 m seawater = 1 atm (gauge). Alveolar Po_2 is assumed to be 6 kPa (45 mmHg) less than inspired Po_2.

level, which increases the resistance to turbulent gas flow (page 28). As a result airway resistance is increased, both at rest and, to a greater extent, during exercise,[3] and there are limits to the maximal breathing capacity (MBC) that can be achieved. In fact, it is usual to breathe a helium/oxygen mixture at pressures in excess of about 6 atm because of nitrogen narcosis (see later). Helium has only one-seventh the density of air, and so is easier to breathe. Furthermore, lower inspired oxygen concentrations are both permissible and indeed desirable as the pressure increases (Table 17.1). Therefore, at 15 atm it would be reasonable to breathe a mixture of 98% helium and 2% oxygen. This would more than double the MBC that the diver could attain while breathing air at that pressure. Hydrogen has even lower density than helium and has been used in gas mixtures for dives to more than 500 m deep.

The effect of immersion is additional to any change in the density of the respired gases. In open-tube snorkel breathing, the alveolar gas is close to normal atmospheric pressure, but the trunk is exposed to a pressure depending on the depth of the subject, which is limited by the length of the snorkel tube. This is equivalent to a standing subatmospheric pressure applied to the mouth, and it is difficult to inhale against a 'negative' pressure loading of more than 5 kPa (50 cmH$_2$O). This corresponds to a mean depth of immersion of only 50 cm, and it is therefore virtually impossible to

use a snorkel tube at a depth of 1 m. However, the normal length of a snorkel tube assures that the swimmer is barely more than awash, so these problems should not arise.

Negative pressure loading is prevented by supplying gas to the diver's airway at a pressure close to the hydrostatic pressure surrounding the diver. This may be achieved by providing an excess flow of gas with a pressure-relief valve controlled by the surrounding water pressure. Such an arrangement was used for the traditional helmeted diver supplied by an air pump on the surface. Free-swimming divers carrying their own compressed gas supply rely on inspiratory demand valves, which are also balanced by the surrounding water pressure.

These arrangements supply gas close to the hydrostatic pressure surrounding the trunk. However, the precise 'static lung loading' depends on the location of the pressure-controlling device in relation to the geometry of the chest. Minor differences result from the various postures that the diver may assume. Thus if he or she is 'head up' when using a valve at mouthpiece level, the pressure surrounding the trunk is higher than the airway pressure by a mean value of about 3 kPa (30 cmH$_2$O). If he or she is 'head down', airway pressure is greater than the pressure to which the trunk is exposed. The head-down position thus corresponds to positive pressure breathing, and the head-up position to negative pressure breathing. The latter causes a reduction of

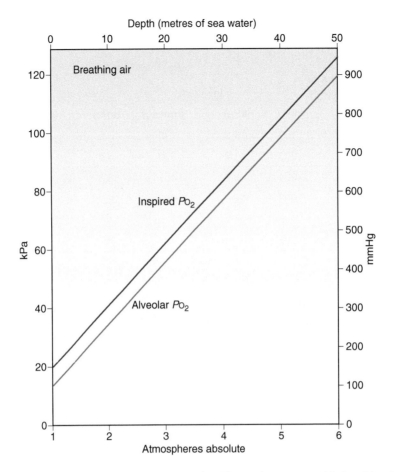

• **Fig. 17.1** Inspired and alveolar P_{O_2} values as a function of increasing pressure while breathing air at rest.

functional residual capacity of about 20% to 30%, but breathing is considered to be easier head up than head down.

Apart from these considerations, immersion has relatively little effect on respiratory function, and the additional respiratory work of moving extracorporeal water does not seem to add appreciably to the work of breathing.

Effect on Gas Exchange[1,2,4]

The best measure of the efficiency of oxygenation of the arterial blood is the alveolar/arterial P_{O_2} gradient. Measurement of arterial blood gas partial pressures presents formidable technical difficulties at high pressures. However, studies at 2.8, 47 and 66 ATA have reported only small increases in alveolar/arterial P_{O_2} gradient. Because it is customary to supply deep divers with an inspired oxygen partial pressure of at least 0.5 ATA, arterial hypoxaemia is unlikely to occur either from hypoventilation or from maldistribution of pulmonary ventilation and perfusion in healthy subjects.

The position for arterial P_{CO_2} is less clear. Hypercapnia is a well-recognized complication of diving, and divers may have a blunted P_{CO_2}/ventilation response of unknown cause. Hypercapnia in divers at rest is uncommon, but during exercise elevated end-tidal and arterial P_{CO_2} levels are

described, reaching levels in the range of 6.2 to 8.3 kPa (47–62 mmHg) during exercise at 66 ATA.[4] This is potentially hazardous, because 9 kPa is approaching the level at which there may be some clouding of consciousness, which is potentially dangerous at depth. High gas density at depth causing increased work of breathing is believed to be responsible for the inadequate ventilation during exercise.

Oxygen Consumption

The relationship between power output and oxygen consumption at pressures up to 66 ATA, whether under water or dry, is not significantly different from the relationship at normal pressure[4] shown in Figure 13.1. Oxygen consumption is expressed under standard conditions of temperature and pressure, dry (STPD; see Appendix C) and therefore represents an absolute quantity of oxygen. However, this volume, when expressed at the diver's environmental pressure, is inversely related to the pressure. Thus an oxygen consumption of 1 L.min^{-1} (STPD) at a pressure of 10 atm would be only 100 mL.min^{-1} when expressed at the pressure to which the diver is exposed. Similar considerations apply to CO_2 output.

The ventilatory requirement for a given oxygen consumption at increased pressure is also not greatly different from the normal relationship shown in Figure 13.5, provided that the oxygen consumption is expressed at STPD, and minute volume is expressed at body temperature, saturated with water vapour and at the pressure to which the diver is exposed (see Appendix C). Considerable confusion is possible as a result of the different methods of expressing gas volumes, and although the differences are trivial at sea level they become very important at high presures.

Exercise

Oxygen consumption may reach very high values during free swimming (see Fig. 13.1) of around 2 to 3 $L.min^{-1}$ (STPD) for a swimming speed of only 2 $km.h^{-1}$. Peak oxygen consumption during exercise is improved slightly at modest high pressures (<20 ATA), an observation that results from hyperoxia (0.3 ATA oxygen) normally used at this depth. With deeper dives, there is a progressive reduction in exercise capacity, irrespective of the oxygen pressure, as a result of respiratory limitation secondary to higher gas density.

Effects Attributable to the Composition of the Inspired Gas

Air

Oxygen

When breathing air at a pressure of 6 ATA, the inspired P_{O_2} will be about 126 kPa (945 mmHg), and the alveolar P_{O_2} about 120 kPa (900 mmHg). This is below the threshold for oxygen convulsions of about 2 ATA, but above the threshold for pulmonary oxygen toxicity if exposure is continued for more than a few hours (see Chapter 25).

Nitrogen

It is actually nitrogen that limits the depth to which air may be breathed. It has three separate undesirable effects.

First, nitrogen is an anaesthetic and, in accord with its lipid solubility, can cause full surgical anaesthesia at a partial pressure of about 30 ATA. The narcotic effect of nitrogen is first detectable when breathing air at about 4 ATA, and there is usually serious impairment of performance at 10 ATA. This effect is known as nitrogen narcosis or 'the rapture of the deep'. It is a general rule that nitrogen narcosis precludes the use of air at depths greater than 100 m of seawater (11 ATA pressure) and, in fact, air is not used at pressures greater than 6 ATA. Helium is the preferred substitute at higher pressures and has no detectable narcotic properties up to at least 100 ATA.

The second problem attributable to nitrogen at high pressures is its density, which causes greatly increased hindrance to breathing at high pressure (see earlier description). Helium has only one-seventh of the density of nitrogen, which is the second reason for its choice.

The third problem with nitrogen is its solubility in body tissues, with the resultant formation of bubbles on decompression. This is discussed in more detail in a later section.

Other inert gases, particularly helium, are less soluble in body tissues, which is the third reason to use helium at high pressures.

Helium/Oxygen Mixtures

For the reasons outlined in the previous section, helium is the preferred diluent inert gas at pressures greater than 6 ATA. The concentration of oxygen required to give the same inspired gas P_{O_2} as at sea level is shown in Table 17.1. In fact, it is usual practice to provide an inspired P_{O_2} of about 0.5 ATA (50 kPa or 375 mmHg) to give a safety margin in the event of error in gas mixing and to provide protection against hypoventilation or defective gas exchange. This level of P_{O_2} appears to be below the threshold for pulmonary oxygen toxicity, even during prolonged saturation dives.

A special problem with helium is its very high thermal conductivity, which tends to cause hypothermia unless the diver's environment is heated. Heat loss from radiation and evaporation remain generally unchanged, but convective heat loss from the respiratory tract and skin is greatly increased. It is usual for chambers to be maintained at temperatures as high as 30°C to 32°C during saturation dives on helium/oxygen mixtures.

Helium/Oxygen/Nitrogen Mixtures

The pressure that can be attained while breathing helium/oxygen mixtures is currently limited by high-pressure nervous syndrome (HPNS).[5] This is a hyperexcitable state of the central nervous system which appears to be because of hydrostatic pressure per se and not to any changes in gas partial pressures. It becomes a serious problem for divers at pressures in excess of 50 ATA, but is first apparent at about 20 ATA.

Various treatments can mitigate this effect and so increase the depth at which a diver can operate safely. The most practicable is the addition of 5% to 10% nitrogen to the helium/oxygen mixture. This in effect reverses HPNS with partial nitrogen narcosis, whilst the HPNS reverses the narcosis that would be caused by the nitrogen. Trimix containing 5% nitrogen allows divers to function normally at depths of over 600 m.

Types of Diving Activity and Their Respiratory Effects

Snorkelling is the simplest form of human diving, but, as described earlier, respiratory effects limit the diver to the top 50 cm of water. Many other forms of diving have therefore evolved.

Breath-Hold Diving[6]

The simplest method of diving is by breath holding, and this is still used for recreation and for collecting items from the seabed. After breathing air, breath-holding time is normally limited to 60 to 75 seconds, and the changes in alveolar gas partial pressures are shown in Figure 4.10. Astonishingly, the depth record is currently 214 m.[7] Many remarkable mechanisms interact to make this possible.

Lung Volume

As pressure increases, lung volume decreases by Boyle's law (page 415). Thus at 10 ATA, an initial lung volume of 6 L would be reduced to about 600 mL, well below residual volume (RV), and with the loss of 5.4 kg of buoyancy. During descent a point is reached when the body attains neutral buoyancy, and the body will sink below that depth. To increase lung volume before diving, breath-hold divers have developed a technique called glossopharyngeal insufflation, in which air is taken into the oropharynx and compressed before being forced into the already fully inflated lung. Lung volumes are increased above normal total lung capacity by 2 L or more. Pulmonary pressure is increased above atmospheric, which adversely affects venous return, cardiac filling and pulmonary blood flow,[8,9] and potentially causes barotrauma.[10] The same technique has also been used by patients with severe respiratory disease to improve expiratory air flow and so improve speech volume.[11] A similar procedure, glossopharyngeal exsufflation, allows the divers to practice reducing their lung volumes below RV. For dives to 200-m depth the lungs must be almost totally collapsed, and must be reinflated on the return ascent, and the ability of a human to perform this manoeuvre contradicts much of what we currently understand about lung mechanics.[7]

Alveolar P_{O_2}

This increases with greater depth as the alveolar gas is compressed, providing a doubling of P_{O_2} at about 8 m deep. More of the alveolar oxygen is therefore available at depth. Conversely, during ascent, alveolar P_{O_2} decreases caused partly by oxygen consumption, but mainly to decreasing pressure. There is thus danger of hypoxia before reaching the surface. However, when the alveolar P_{O_2} falls below the mixed venous P_{O_2}, there is a paradoxical transfer of oxygen from mixed venous blood to alveolar gas, and the arterial P_{O_2} is maintained above the very low partial pressure that would otherwise occur in the alveoli. This may be an important factor in preventing loss of consciousness in the final stages of ascent.

Alveolar P_{CO_2}

By a similar mechanism, alveolar P_{CO_2} is greater during a breath-hold dive than during a simple breath hold at sea level. At an environmental pressure of only 12 kPa (90 mmHg) gauge, the alveolar P_{CO_2} will be increased above the mixed venous P_{CO_2}, and there will be a paradoxical transfer of CO_2 from alveolus to arterial blood. Fortunately there is a limited quantity of CO_2 in the alveolar gas, and the process is reversed during late descent and ascent.

Limited Duration Dives

Most dives are of relatively brief duration and involve a rapid descent to operating depth and a period spent at depth, followed by an ascent, the rate of which is governed by the requirement to avoid release of inert gas dissolved in the tissues. The profile and the duration of the ascent are governed by the depth attained, the time spent at depth and the nature of the diluent inert gas.

The diving bell. The simplest and oldest technique was the diving bell. Air was trapped under the bell on the surface, but the internal water level rose as the air was compressed at depth. Useful time at depth was generally no more than 20 to 30 minutes. More recently, additional air was introduced into the bell under pressure from the surface.

The helmeted diver. From about 1820 until recently, the standard method of diving down to 100 m has been by a helmeted diver supplied with air pumped from the surface into the helmet and escaping from a relief valve controlled by the water pressure. This gave much greater mobility than the old diving bell and permitted the execution of complex tasks.

Self-contained underwater breathing apparatus (SCUBA) diving. There was for some years a desire to move towards free-swimming divers carrying their own gas supply, first achieved in 1943. This system is based on a demand valve controlled by both the ambient pressure and the inspiration of the diver. Air-breathing SCUBA dives are usually restricted to depths of 30 m. Greater depths are possible, but special precautions must then be taken to avoid decompression sickness. SCUBA divers are far more mobile than helmeted divers and can work in almost any body position.

Caisson and tunnel working. Since 1839, tunnel and bridge foundations have been constructed by pressurizing the work environment to exclude water. The work environment is maintained at pressure, normally of less than 4 ATA, with staff entering and leaving by airlocks. Entry is rapid, but exit requires adherence to the appropriate decompression schedule if the working pressure is in excess of 2 ATA.

Free submarine escape. It is possible to escape from a submarine by free ascent from depths down to about 100 m. The submariner first enters an escape chamber, which is then pressurized to equal the external water pressure. He then opens a hatch communicating with the exterior and leaves the chamber. During the ascent, the gas in his lungs expands according to Boyle's law. It is therefore imperative that he keeps his glottis and mouth open, allowing gas to escape in a continuous stream. If gas is not allowed to escape, barotrauma is almost certain to occur (see later). In an uneventful escape, the time spent at pressure is too short for there to be any danger of decompression sickness.

Saturation Dives

When prolonged and repeated work is required at great depths, it is more convenient to hold the divers in a dry living chamber kept on board a ship or oil rig and held at a pressure close to the pressure of their intended working depth. Divers transfer to a smaller chamber at the same pressure that is lowered to depth as and when required. The divers then leave the chamber for work, without any major change in pressure, but remain linked to the chamber by an umbilical cord. On return to the chamber, they can be raised to the surface where they wait, still at pressure, until they are next required. A normal tour of duty is about 3 weeks, the whole of which is spent at operating pressure, currently up to about 20 ATA, breathing helium/oxygen mixtures. During the long period at pressure, tissues are fully saturated with inert gas at the chamber pressure, and prolonged decompression is then required, which may last for several days.

Respiratory Aspects of Decompression Illness[12,13]

Returning to the surface after a dive is a hazardous procedure and can give rise to a variety of complications variously known as 'bends', 'chokes' or caisson disease. In its mildest form, subjects have short-lived joint pain, but more serious presentations include pulmonary barotrauma or neurological deficit that can result in permanent disability. In the late 19th century, before decompression illness was understood, the effects on caisson workers were severe. For example, of the 600 men involved in building the underwater foundations of the St Louis Bridge in the United States, 119 had serious decompression illness and 14 died. Today some form of decompression illness is thought to affect 1 in 5000 to 10 000 recreational dives, and 1 in 1000 commercial dives.[13] There are two main ways in which illness arises.

Barotrauma

Barotrauma as a result of change in pressure will affect any closed body space containing gas and tends to occur during ascent when the gas expands. The middle and inner ear, sinuses and teeth are the most commonly affected areas,[14] but pulmonary barotrauma, although rare, is much more dangerous. Pulmonary barotrauma may occur during rapid ascent in untrained subjects, for example during submarine escape training (see previous discussion) when the subject forgets to exhale during ascent. Barotrauma results in disruption of the airway or alveolar wall, and air may enter either the pulmonary vessels or interstitial tissue, from where it spreads along tissue planes to the pleura, mediastinum or subcutaneous tissues. Mediastinal or pleural air pockets continue to expand during ascent, until chest pain or breathing difficulties occur within a few minutes of surfacing.

Some divers develop barotrauma during relatively shallow dives, and efforts have been made to identify which divers are at risk.[15] In this case, barotrauma is believed to result from expansion of air trapped in the periphery of the lung by small airway closure. Subjects with reduced expiratory flow rates at low lung volume, including some patients with asthma, are therefore at a theoretically greater risk.[15]

Decompression Sickness

Tissue bubble formation occurs when tissues become 'supersaturated' with gases such that the sum of dissolved gas partial pressures (e.g., nitrogen, oxygen, helium and CO_2) exceeds the local absolute pressure.[13] For example, after SCUBA diving while breathing nitrogen and oxygen, when decompression occurs tissue partial pressure of nitrogen (P_{N_2}) becomes greater than the ambient pressure, and bubbles form, exactly as occurs in the bottle when opening a carbonated drink. Even in supersaturated tissues, bubble formation requires a 'micronucleus' around which the bubble can form, currently believed to be tissue microbubbles (<10 μm in diameter) of uncertain origin.[16] The increase in tissue P_{N_2} during descent and the decrease in P_{N_2} on ascent are both exponential curves. Tissues poorly perfused with blood have the slowest half-time for both uptake and elimination, hence, on decompression, tissue P_{N_2} decreases most slowly in poorly perfused tissues such as cartilage, giving rise to the bends. How these bubbles lead to decompression sickness is poorly understood. Most divers have microparticles (cell-derived membrane vesicles <1 μm in diameter) in their blood following a dive, and neutrophil activation is also common, but how these changes relate to symptomatic illness is unclear.[17]

Arterial gas embolism is another type of decompression sickness. Venous bubbles occur commonly during decompression, and the filtration provided by the lung is extremely effective. Overload of the filtration system or passage through pulmonary arteriovenous anastomoses (page 12) may result in arterial gas embolism, but this is only believed to be the case in severe decompression sickness. There is an increasing body of evidence that arterial gas embolism follows shunting of blood containing air bubbles from the right to left sides of the heart through an otherwise asymptomatic atrial septal defect (page 164). Whatever the origins, arterial gas embolism is believed to be the major factor causing the neurologic deficits of decompression sickness, and may contribute to long-term neurologic damage in professional divers.[18]

Treatment of decompression sickness is best achieved by avoidance. Detailed tables indicate the safe rate of decompression depending on the pressure and time of exposure. Administration of oxygen will reduce the blood P_{N_2}, and so accelerate the resorption of bubbles in both blood and tissue. In severe cases, including all divers with neurologic deficits, urgent recompression in a chamber is required, followed by slow decompression with oxygen and other therapeutic interventions.[13]

Altitude Decompression Sickness[19,20]

Flying at high altitude in military aircraft exposes pilots to significant degrees of decompression; a cabin altitude of 9000 m (30 000 ft) is equivalent to approximately 0.3 ATA. During actual flights, symptoms of decompression sickness tend to be underreported because these elite pilots may fear restrictions on their flying activities. However, during their careers, three-quarters of pilots experience problems, and almost 40% of trainee pilots develop symptoms during hypobaric chamber testing to normal cabin altitudes.[19] Joint pain is predictably the most common symptom, whereas the 'chokes' (substernal pain, cough and dyspnoea) occur in 1% to 3% of cases. Breathing 100% oxygen for 60 minutes before altitude exposure significantly attenuates the symptoms seen, and is required by the US Air Force before flying.

Flying in the partially pressurized cabin (page 214) of commercial aircraft shortly after underwater diving increases the risk of decompression sickness. The likelihood of developing symptoms is increased by both greater depth of the last dive and shorter duration of time between the dive and flying. Dives to less than 18.5 m deep and leaving over 24 hours between diving and flying, are generally accepted as resulting in a minimal, but not zero, risk of decompression sickness.[21]

References

1. Mummery HJ, Stolp BW, deL Dear G, et al. Effects of age and exercise on physiological dead space during simulated dives at 2.8ATA. *J Appl Physiol.* 2003;94:507-517.
2. Moon RE, Cherry AD, Stolp BW, et al. Pulmonary gas exchange in diving. *J Appl Physiol.* 2009;106:668-677.
3. Held HE, Pendergast DR. Relative effects of submersion and increased pressure on respiratory mechanics, work, and energy cost of breathing. *J Appl Physiol.* 2013;114:578-591.
4. Salzano JV, Camporesi EM, Stolp BW, et al. Physiological responses to exercise at 47 and 66 ATA. *J Appl Physiol.* 1984;57:1055-1068.
5. Halsey MJ. The effects of high pressure on the central nervous system. *Physiol Rev.* 1982;62:1341-1377.
*6. **Lindholm P, Lundgren CE. The physiology and pathophysiology of human breath-hold diving. *J Appl Physiol.* 2009;106:284-292.**
7. Fahlman A. The pressure to understand the mechanism of lung compression and its effect on lung function. *J Appl Physiol.* 2008;104:907-908.
8. Mijacika T, Frestad D, Kyhl K, et al. Blood pooling in extrathoracic veins after glossopharyngeal insufflation. *Eur J Appl Physiol.* 2017;117:641-649.
9. Mijacika T, Kyhl K, Frestad D, et al. Effect of pulmonary hyperinflation on central blood volume: An MRI study. *Respir Physiol Neurobiol.* 2017;243:92-96.
10. Linér MH, Andersson JPA. Suspected arterial gas embolism after glossopharyngeal insufflation in a breath-hold diver. *Aviat Space Environ Med.* 2010;81:74-76.
11. Maltais F. Glossopharyngeal breathing. *Am J Respir Crit Care Med.* 2011;184:381.
*12. **Bove AA. Diving medicine. *Am J Respir Crit Care Med.* 2014;189:1479-1486.**
13. Vann RD, Butler FK, Mitchell SJ, et al. Decompression illness. *Lancet.* 2010;377:153-164.
14. Nakdimon I, Zadik Y. Barodontalgia among aircrew and divers. *Aerosp Med Hum Perform.* 2019;90:128-131.
15. Bove AA. Pulmonary barotrauma in divers: can prospective pulmonary function testing identify those at risk? *Chest.* 1997;112:576-578.
16. Mahon RT. Tiny bubbles. *J Appl Physiol.* 2010;108:238-239.
17. Thom SR, Bennett M, Banham ND, et al. Association of microparticles and neutrophil activation with decompression sickness. *J Appl Physiol.* 2015;119:427-434.
18. Wilmshurst P. Brain damage in divers. *BMJ.* 1997;314:689-690.
19. Balldin UI, Pilmanis AA, Webb JT. Pulmonary decompression sickness at altitude: early symptoms and circulating gas emboli. *Aviat Space Environ Med.* 2002;73:996-999.
20. Jersey SL, Hundemer GL, Stuart RP, et al. Neurological altitude decompression sickness among U-2 pilots: 2002–2009. *Aviat Space Environ Med.* 2011;82:673-682.
21. Freiberger JJ, Denoble PJ, Pieper CF, et al. The relative risk of decompression sickness during and after air travel following diving. *Aviat Space Environ Med.* 2002;73:980-984.

18

Respiration in Closed Environments and Space

KEY POINTS

- Environments in which a closed atmosphere suitable for breathing is maintained include closed-circuit anaesthesia, submarines and space vehicles.
- Problems of maintaining acceptably low carbon dioxide concentrations and low levels of inhaled contaminants are common to all these environments.

- In the microgravity of space static lung volumes are reduced, ventilation and perfusion are better matched, and airway obstruction during sleep is uncommon.
- For atmospheric regeneration in long-term space missions of the future, a combination of physicochemical and biological systems is likely to be needed.

The fascination of the human race with exploration has taken humans well beyond the high altitude and underwater environments described in Chapters 16 and 17. Our ability to maintain life in space, the most hostile of environments yet explored, was developed as a result of techniques used to sustain breathing in other seemingly unrelated environments on Earth. All these environments share problems common to maintaining respiration while separated from the Earth's atmosphere.

Closed-System Anaesthesia

This may not represent the most dramatic example of closed-environment breathing but it is the most common. Careful control of the composition of respired gas is the hallmark of inhalational anaesthesia. The anaesthetist must maintain safe concentrations of oxygen and CO_2 in the patient's lungs while controlling with great precision the dose of inhaled anaesthetic. It was recognized over 100 years ago that anaesthesia could be prolonged by allowing patients to rebreathe some of their expired gas, including the anaesthetic vapour. Provided oxygen is added and CO_2 removed, other gases can be circulated round a breathing system many times, providing beneficial effects such as warm and humid inspired gas. Rebreathing systems are also useful as a method for reducing both the amount of anaesthetic used and the pollution of the operating theatre environment.

A totally closed system during anaesthesia means that all expired gases are recirculated to the patient, with oxygen added only to replace that consumed and anaesthetic agent added to replace that absorbed by the patient. In practice,

low-flow anaesthesia, in which over half of the patient's expired gases are recirculated, is much more commonly used. In each case, CO_2 is absorbed by chemical reaction with combinations of calcium, sodium, potassium or barium hydroxides, resulting in the formation of the respective carbonate and water. The reaction cannot be reversed, and the absorbent must be discarded after use.

Widespread use of closed-system anaesthesia is limited by perceived difficulties with maintaining adequate concentrations of gases that the patient is consuming, such as oxygen and anaesthetic agent. However, gas-monitoring systems are now universally used with low-flow anaesthesia, allowing accurate control of breathing system gas composition.

Accumulation of Other Gases in Closed Circuits

Closed breathing systems with a constant inflow and consumption of oxygen will allow retention of other gases entering the system either with the fresh gas or from the patient. This affects the patient in two quite distinct ways. First, inert gases such as nitrogen and argon may accumulate to such an extent that they dilute the oxygen in the system. Second, small concentrations of more toxic gases may develop within the breathing system.

Nitrogen enters the system from the patient at the start of anaesthesia. Body stores of dissolved nitrogen are small, but air present in the lungs may contain 2 to 3 L of nitrogen, which will be transferred to the system in the first few minutes. If nitrogen is not intended to be part of the closed-system gas mixture, the patient must 'denitrogenate' by breathing high concentrations of oxygen before being anaesthetized, or higher fresh gas flow rates must be used initially to flush the nitrogen from the closed system.

Argon is normally present in air at a concentration of 0.93%. Oxygen concentrators effectively remove nitrogen from air, concentrating argon in similar proportions to oxygen, resulting in argon concentrations of around 5%. In a study of closed-system breathing in volunteers using oxygen from an oxygen concentrator, argon levels in the breathing system reached 40% after only 80 minutes.[1] Cylinders of medical-grade oxygen and hospital supplies from liquid oxygen evaporators contain negligible argon, so the risk of accumulation is low.

Methane is produced in the distal colon by anaerobic bacterial fermentation and is mostly excreted directly from the alimentary tract. Some methane is, however, absorbed into the blood, where it has low solubility and is rapidly excreted by the lung, following which it will accumulate in the closed system. There is a large variation between subjects in methane production, and, therefore, the concentrations seen during closed-system anaesthesia. Mean levels in a circle system in healthy patients reached over 900 parts per million (ppm), well below levels regarded as unacceptable in other closed environments, but sufficient to cause interference with some anaesthetic gas analysers.[2]

Acetone, ethanol and carbon monoxide all have high blood solubility, so concentrations in the breathing system remain low, but rebreathing causes accumulation in the blood. Levels achieved are generally low,[2] but acetone accumulation may be associated with postoperative nausea. Closed-system anaesthesia is not recommended in patients with increased excretion of acetone or alcohol, such as in uncontrolled diabetes mellitus, after recent alcohol ingestion or during prolonged starvation.

Submarines

Submersible ships have been used for almost 100 years, almost exclusively for military purposes until the last few decades when they have become more widespread for undersea exploration and industrial use. Atmospheric pressure in the submarine remains approximately the same as at surface level during a dive, the duration of which is limited by the maintenance of adequate oxygen and CO_2 levels for the crew in the ship.

Diesel-Powered

Submarines were used extensively during both world wars and were powered by diesel engines like surface-based warships. Clearly, the oxygen requirement of the engines precluded them from use during dives, and battery-powered engines were used, thus limiting the duration of dives to just a few hours. A more significant limitation to dive duration was atmospheric regulation. No attempt was made to control the internal atmosphere, and, after ventilation at the surface, the submarine dived with only the air contained within. After approximately 12 hours the atmosphere contained 15% oxygen, 5% CO_2 and a multitude of odours and contaminants. The need to return to the surface was apparent when the

submariners became short of breath and were unable to light their cigarettes because of low levels of oxygen.

Nuclear-Powered

Short dive duration severely limited the use of diesel-powered submarines. The development of nuclear power allowed submarines to generate an ample supply of heat and electricity completely independent of oxygen supply, allowing prolonged activity underwater. Atmospheric regeneration was therefore needed, and current nuclear-powered submarines routinely remain submerged for weeks.

Atmosphere Regeneration

The plentiful supply of seawater and electricity make hydrolysis of water the obvious method for oxygen generation. Seawater must first have all electrolytes removed by a combination of evaporation and deionization. Theoretically, 1 L of water can yield 620 L of oxygen, so, even with less than 100% efficient electrolysis, large volumes of oxygen are easily produced. Submarine atmosphere oxygen concentration is maintained at 21% ± 2%.

Atmospheric CO_2 in submarines is absorbed by passage through monoethanolamine, which chemically combines with CO_2 to produce carbonates. When fully saturated, the absorber can either be replaced or be regenerated by heating with steam, when the CO_2 is released and can be vented into the sea. This method maintains the CO_2 concentration in submarines at 0.5% to 1.5%, and although further reduction is possible, the energy cost of doing so is prohibitive.

Atmospheric contamination during prolonged submarine patrols is well recognized, with many hundreds of substances entering the atmosphere, originating from both machinery and crew. These substances include volatile hydrocarbons such as benzene, oil droplets, carbon monoxide, cadmium and microbial organisms, with varying concentrations in different parts of the submarine. Continuous monitoring of many compounds is now performed, and maximum allowable levels during prolonged patrols are defined.[3] Submarine air-conditioning units include catalytic burners that oxidize carbon monoxide, hydrogen and other hydrocarbons to CO_2 and water, and charcoal absorbers to absorb any remaining contaminants. The health risks from submarine occupation are therefore believed to be extremely small.[3]

Physiological Effects of Prolonged Hypercapnia[4]

Definition of a 'safe' level of atmospheric CO_2 over long periods has concerned submarine designers for some years. Symptoms caused by elevated inhaled CO_2 are common, and include respiratory symptoms, flushing, sweating, dizziness and feeling faint,[5] but the levels normally seen in submarines are not associated with impaired cognition.[6] The respiratory response to inhalation of low concentrations of CO_2 (<3%) is similar to that at higher levels (page 48), but compensatory acid-base changes seem to be quite different.

Respiratory Changes[7]

Atmospheric CO_2 levels of 1% cause an elevation of inspired P_{CO_2} of 1 kPa (7.5 mmHg), which results in an average increase in minute ventilation of 2 to 3 $L.min^{-1}$. However, the degree of hyperventilation is highly variable between subjects, and presumably relates to their central chemoreceptor sensitivity to CO_2 (page 49). Measurements of arterial blood gases in submariners show that the elevated minute volume limits the increase in arterial P_{CO_2} to an average of only 0.14 kPa (1 mmHg). After a few days, the increase in ventilation declines, and minute volume returns towards normal, allowing arterial P_{CO_2} to increase further to reflect the inspired P_{CO_2}. The time course of the decline in ventilation is too short to result from blood acid-base compensation (see later) and is believed to reflect a small attenuation of the central chemoreceptor response.

Calcium Metabolism[8]

Elevation of arterial P_{CO_2} causes a respiratory acidosis, which is normally, over the course of 1 or 2 days, compensated for by the retention of bicarbonate by the kidney (page 271). The changes in pH seen when breathing less than 3% CO_2 appear to be too small to stimulate measurable renal compensation, and pH remains slightly lowered for some time. During this period, CO_2 is deposited in bone as calcium carbonate, and urinary and faecal calcium excretion is drastically reduced to facilitate this. Serum calcium levels also decrease, suggesting a shift of extracellular calcium to the intracellular space. After about 3 weeks, when bone stores of CO_2 are saturated, renal excretion of calcium and hydrogen ions begins to increase, and pH tends to return to normal. Abnormalities of calcium metabolism have been demonstrated with inspired CO_2 concentrations as low as 0.5%.

Some other effects of low levels of atmospheric CO_2 during space travel are described next (page 228).

Space[9]

Space represents the most hostile environment into which humans have sojourned. At 80 km (50 miles) above Earth there is insufficient air to allow aerodynamic control of a vehicle, and at 200 km (125 miles) there is an almost total vacuum. True space begins above 700 km (435 miles), where particles become so scarce that the likelihood of a collision between two atoms becomes negligible. Even under these conditions there are estimated to be 10^8 particles (mainly hydrogen) per cubic metre compared with 10^{25} on the Earth's surface. Maintenance of a respirable atmosphere in these circumstances is challenging, and both American and Soviet space pioneers lost their lives during the development of suitable technology. Current experience is based on expeditions in close proximity to Earth, involving Earth orbit or travel to the moon. This means that the raw materials for atmosphere regeneration can be repeatedly supplied from Earth.

Atmosphere Composition

A summary of manned space missions and the atmospheres used is shown in Table 18.1. Spacecraft have an almost

TABLE 18.1   Summary of Manned Space Missions and Their Respiratory Environments

Missions	Period of Use	Number of Crew	Habitable Volume (m³)	Cabin Pressure (kPa)	Cabin Pressure (mmHg)	Oxygen Conc. (%)	Atmosphere Regeneration Methods O₂ Supply	Atmosphere Regeneration Methods CO₂ Removal
Vostok	1961–1965	1	2.5	100	760	100	KO₂	KO₂
Mercury	1961–1963	1	1.6	34	258	100	Pressurized O₂	LiOH
Gemini	1965–1966	2	2.3	34	258	100	Liquid O₂	LiOH
Soyuz	1967–present	2/3	—	100	760	22	KO₂	KO₂/LiOH
Apollo	1968–1972	3	5.9	34	258	100[a]	Liquid O₂	LiOH
Salyut	1971–1986	5	100	100	760	21	KO₂	KO₂/LiOH
Skylab	1973–1974	3	361	34	258	72	Liquid O₂	Molecular sieve
Shuttle	1981–2011	7	74	100	760	21	Liquid O₂	LiOH
Mir	1986–2001	6	150	100	760	23	Electrolysis/ chemical	Molecular sieve
International Space Station	2001–present	6	388	100	760	21	Electrolysis/ chemical	Molecular sieve

[a]Oxygen concentration reduced to 60% during launch to reduce fire risk.

totally closed system of atmospheric control, and early Soviet space vehicles aimed to be completely sealed environments. Their designers had such confidence in the structure that emergency stores of oxygen were considered unnecessary until Soyuz 11 depressurized on reentry in 1971, tragically killing all three cosmonauts. American Apollo missions leaked approximately 1 kg of gas per day in space, even with a lower atmospheric pressure (Table 18.1).

The use of a total pressure of 34.5 kPa (259 mmHg) in early US space vehicles required a high atmospheric oxygen concentration to provide an adequate inspired Po_2 (Table 18.1). Because of the fatal fire on the launch pad in 1967, the composition of the atmosphere during launch was changed from 100% oxygen to 64% oxygen in 36% nitrogen at the same pressure, which still gave an inspired Po_2 in excess of the normal sea-level value. Previous Soviet designs were all based on maintaining normal atmospheric pressure, and space vehicles in current use continue to do so with inspired oxygen concentrations of nearly 21%. Extravehicular activity in space presents a particular problem. To maintain a functionally acceptable flexibility of the space suit in the vacuum of space, the internal pressure is only 28 kPa (212 mmHg). This entails the use of 100% oxygen after careful decompression and denitrogenation of the astronaut.

Oxygen Supply

Storage of oxygen and other gases in space presents significant problems. The weight of the containers used is critical during launch, and storage of significant quantities of oxygen requires high pressures and therefore strong heavy tanks.

Chemical generation of oxygen was used mainly by Soviet space missions. Potassium superoxide releases oxygen on exposure to moisture, a reaction that generates potassium hydroxide as an intermediate and so also absorbs CO_2:

$$4KO_2 + 3H_2O + 2CO_2 \rightarrow 2K_2CO_3 + 3H_2O + 3O_2$$

One kilogram of KO_2 can release over 200 L of oxygen, but the reaction is irreversible, and the used canisters must be discarded. Sodium chlorate candles, which release oxygen when simply ignited, were used for emergency oxygen generation in Soviet space missions and are still used for atmospheric regeneration in disabled submarines.

Electrolysis of water is an efficient way to produce oxygen in space, where solar panels provide the electricity. In contrast to submarines, water is scarce in space vehicles, again because of weight considerations at launch. In the International Space Station (ISS) oxygen is generated by electrolysis using wastewater from the occupants, although this alone does not produce sufficient oxygen for a reasonably active astronaut.

Carbon Dioxide Removal

Chemical absorption by lithium hydroxide was the mainstay of US space vehicles, whereas the Soviet program used KO_2, as previously described. Reversible chemical reactions such as those used in submarines have been adapted for space use and can be regenerated by exposure to the vacuum of space.

Molecular sieves allow CO_2 to be adsorbed into a chemical matrix without undergoing any chemical reaction. When saturated with CO_2, exposure to the space vacuum causes release of the adsorbed gas. Use of two- or four-bed molecular sieves allows continuous CO_2 removal by half the processors while the others are regenerated.

Maintenance of low levels of CO_2 on prolonged future space missions is likely to have unacceptable costs in terms of energy and consumables. This fact led to three space agencies worldwide undertaking a joint research programme to study the effects of 1.2% and 0.7% atmospheric CO_2 on a wide range of physiological systems. The study involved normal volunteers spending 22 days in a closed mock 'space station' on the ground. Some of the results have already been described (page 226).[7,8] Effects at 0.7% atmospheric CO_2 were generally concluded to be minimal.[10] At 1.2%, however, changes in respiration and calcium metabolism were significant and, more important, mental performance was impaired, with a loss of alertness and visuomotor performance.[11] Inspired Pco_2 on the ISS is maintained between 0.5 and 0.8 kPa (3.8–6.0 mmHg) or 0.5% to 0.8%.[4]

Atmospheric Contamination

Chemical contamination within space vehicles is mainly from within the habitable area of the vehicle, with external contamination from propellants, and so on, being very rare. The greatest contribution to atmospheric contamination is the astronauts themselves, but the compounds released such as carbon monoxide, ammonia, methane and indole are easily dealt with by standard methods. More complex chemicals may be released into the atmosphere by a process called off-gassing. Almost all nonmetallic substances, but particularly plastics, release small quantities of volatile chemicals for many months and years after manufacture. This is more likely to occur at low atmospheric pressure as on the earlier space missions, but remains a current problem on the ISS from the repeated deliveries of supplies.[12] Within a closed environment, these chemicals may accumulate to toxic levels, and complex air-conditioning units are required.

Long-Term Space Travel

Manned space travel to planets more distant than the moon requires expeditions of years' duration with no access to supplies from Earth. For example, the journey time to Mars is around 6 months, so the minimum realistic mission duration would be 2 years. The estimated mass of provisions required to sustain six crew members for this duration would be over 45 tons, which far exceeds the capacity of current space vehicles.[13] Regenerative life-support systems have, therefore, been studied extensively in recent years, and aim to reverse the effects of animal metabolism on a closed atmosphere. Biological solutions are believed by many to be the only feasible option, and biospheres are discussed in later sections. Physicochemical methods, however, are now realistic options, and are likely to act as valuable backup systems.

CO_2 reduction reactions convert CO_2 back into oxygen, and two main methods are described. The Sabatier reaction requires hydrogen to produce methane and water:

$$CO_2 + 4H_2 \rightarrow CH_4 + 2H_2O.$$

Methane can then be converted to solid carbon and hydrogen gas, which reenters the Sabatier reactor. The Bosch reaction produces solid carbon in one stage:

$$CO_2 + 2H_2 \rightarrow 2H_2 + \text{solid C}.$$

Electrolysis of water generates oxygen and hydrogen gas; the latter enters the Bosch or Sabatier reactions, and the water produced is recycled. Both reactions ultimately generate solid carbon which must be removed from the reactors periodically: current hardware can convert CO_2 into oxygen for 60 person-days before the carbon deposits must be emptied.

In situ resource utilization on Mars.[14] The atmosphere of Mars is composed of 95.3% CO_2, 2.7% N_2, 1.6% Ar, 0.13% O_2 and 0.07% CO. For any mission to Mars, these gases could be used for atmospheric regeneration, as shown in Figure 18.1. Separation of the gases in the atmosphere will produce a small amount of oxygen and larger volumes of nitrogen and argon, which may be used as buffer gas in the atmosphere. On prolonged missions, loss of buffer gas from the vehicle by leakage and from activation of airlocks is a substantial problem. The abundant CO_2 on Mars could enter a Sabatier reactor, and the methane produced may then be used as a propellant for the mission, the water used either by the crew or to provide oxygen for the life-support systems, and the hydrogen can reenter the Sabatier reactor.

Microgravity[15]

All bodies with mass exert gravitational forces on each other, so zero gravity is theoretically impossible. Once in space, away from the large mass of Earth or other planets, gravitational forces become negligible, and are referred to as microgravity. Space vehicles in orbit around Earth are still subject to its considerable gravitational forces, but these are matched exactly by the centrifugal force from the high tangential velocity of the space vehicle.[9] Occupants of orbiting space vehicles are normally subject to a gravitational force of approximately 10^{-6} times that on Earth's surface.

Chapter 7 contains numerous references to the effect of gravity on the topography of the lung and the distribution of perfusion and ventilation. Microgravity may therefore be predicted to have significant effects on respiratory function.

Early studies of short-term microgravity used a jet flying in a series of parabolic arcs, which gave around 25 seconds of weightlessness. This technique remains less expensive and complex than travel to space, and is still used for many physiological studies of microgravity.[16] Unfortunately, between each period of microgravity the subject is exposed to a similar duration of increased gravitational forces (2 G) as the jet pulls out of the parabolic arc portion of the flight, and this may influence the results of physiological studies. Sustained microgravity has been studied in space. In 1991 an extended series of investigations on seven subjects was undertaken in Spacelab SLS-1, which was carried into orbit by the space shuttle for a 9-day mission, and studies of prolonged microgravity on the ISS continue.[17]

Lung Volumes

Chest radiography in the sitting position during short-term microgravity showed the diaphragm to be slightly higher in some of the subjects at functional residual capacity (FRC). This accords with a 413 mL reduction in FRC also measured in parabolic arc studies on seated subjects.[18] Abdominal contribution to tidal excursion was increased at microgravity in the seated position, probably because of loss of postural tone in the abdominal muscles,[18] an observation now confirmed in space studies.[19]

During sustained microgravity, subdivisions of lung volume were again found to be intermediate between the sitting and supine volumes at 1 G, except for residual volume which was reduced below that seen in any position at 1 G (Fig. 18.2).[20] The FRC was reduced by 750 mL compared

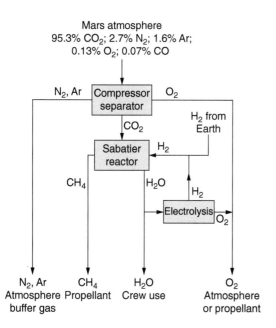

Mars atmosphere
95.3% CO_2; 2.7% N_2; 1.6% Ar;
0.13% O_2; 0.07% CO

• **Fig. 18.1** In situ resource utilization on Mars. Using a series of simple physicochemical processes, the atmosphere of Mars, supplemented by hydrogen transported from Earth, may be used to provide buffer gas and oxygen for the space-vehicle atmosphere, methane as propellant for the vehicle and water for use by the crew or for generation of oxygen. (From reference 14.)

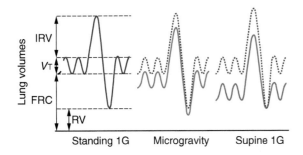

• **Fig. 18.2** Static lung volumes during sustained microgravity after 9 days in Earth orbit. The dotted line shows the normal standing values on Earth for comparison. Volumes at microgravity are generally intermediate between standing and supine values at 1 G, except residual volume, which is further reduced. *FRC*, Functional residual capacity; *IRV*, inspiratory reserve volume; *RV*, residual volume; *V*T, tidal volume.

with preflight standing values. These changes in lung volume are ascribed to altered respiratory mechanics and increased thoracic blood volume.

Topographic Inequality of Ventilation and Perfusion

Early results in the Lear jet, using single-breath nitrogen wash-out (page 92), indicated a substantial reduction in topographic inequality of ventilation and perfusion during weightlessness, as expected. However, more detailed studies in Spacelab showed that a surprising degree of residual inequality of blood flow and ventilation persisted despite the major improvement at zero gravity. Ventilatory inequality with microgravity is believed to result from continued airway closure at low lung volume, airway closure possibly occurring in a patchy fashion.[21] The most likely explanation for the continued perfusion inequality is the central to peripheral 'radial' gradient within each horizontal slice of lung (page 94), which is mostly overshadowed at 1 G by the large vertical perfusion gradient.

Other Changes to Respiratory Physiology in Microgravity

Snoring and airway obstruction during sleep are common, and a contributory factor is reduced activity of pharyngeal dilator muscles allowing gravity on Earth to initiate obstruction (page 192). This role of gravity in sleep-disordered breathing was confirmed by a study of astronauts sleeping in the orbiting space shuttle, where there were dramatic reductions in their apnoea/hypopnoea index (page 193), and snoring was virtually eliminated.[22] Exercise capacity (based on peak O_2 consumption) in microgravity is reduced in most astronauts, with contributions from reduced blood volume decreasing muscle oxygen supply,[23] impaired diffusion of oxygen within muscle[24] and muscle detraining effects.[25] Finally, the behaviour of inhaled particles (page 166) is altered in space, with sedimentation impossible in microgravity as the particles are weightless. Although this reduces the proportion of inhaled particles retained in the lung, it also causes small particles (1 μm) to be deposited in the lung periphery rather than the airways.[26]

Biospheres[9]

A biosphere is defined as 'a closed space of two or more connected ecosystems in equilibrium with their environment'. Only energy enters and leaves a biosphere. Earth is the largest and most successful known biosphere, although the equilibrium between its ecosystems is almost certainly changing (Chapter 34). Attempts to create smaller biospheres have mostly been driven by the prospect of long-term space travel. Physicochemical methods of sustaining life, as described earlier, have many limitations, whereas a biological system has numerous advantages. Plants perform the complex CO_2-reduction chemistry using chlorophyll, and at the same time, rather than generating carbon, they produce varying amounts of food. Plants also act as efficient water-purification systems via transpiration.

Small-Scale Biological Atmospheric Regeneration

The first report of prolonged biological atmosphere regeneration was described in 1961, when a single mouse was maintained in a closed chamber for 66 days.[27] Air from the chamber was circulated through a second chamber containing 4 L of *Chlorella* alga solution illuminated with artificial light. Over the course of the experiment, the oxygen concentration in the chamber increased from 21% to 53%, and the CO_2 concentration remained less than 0.2%. Subsequent experiments by both American and Soviet researchers demonstrated the feasibility of human life support by *Chlorella*, culminating in a 30-day closure of a single researcher in a 4.5-m^3 room, maintained by just 30 L of alga solution. Algae alone are unsuitable for long-term life support.[9] Their excellent atmospheric regeneration properties result from a very fast rate of growth, but *Chlorella* is generally regarded as inedible, presenting a significant disposal problem in a totally closed system. In addition, if the algal solution becomes acidic for any reason, such as bacterial contamination, algae produce carbon monoxide in unacceptable quantities.

Unknown to the scientific community at large, starting in 1963 the Soviet Union ran a 'Bios' research centre at the Institute of Biophysics in Krasnoyarsk, Siberia.[9,28] In 1983, two researchers successfully spent 5 months in a biosphere (Bios 3), which provided all their atmospheric regeneration needs and over three-quarters of their food.[28] In these studies, plants were grown hydroponically, that is, without soil with their roots bathed in a carefully controlled nutrient solution. Light was provided with continuous xenon lighting to maximize growth to such an extent that, under these conditions, wheat can be harvested six times per year. An estimated 13 m^2 of planted area will then produce enough oxygen for one human, although over 30 m^2 is probably required to produce almost enough food as well.

American research of controlled ecological life-support systems (CELSS) began in 1977, and has focused on basic plant physiology.[9] Atmospheric regeneration is usually the easiest problem to overcome, whereas the plant species used has important implications for the dietary intake and psychological well-being of the CELSS inhabitants.[28] In contrast to this American project, the European Space Agency is developing a life-support system for long-term space travel centred around microorganisms, which are more versatile biochemically.[29] For example, bacteria may be used to compost crew waste and inedible plant components into nitrogenous compounds to enhance the plant growth.

Biosphere 2[9]

Small-scale biosphere experiments never attained a totally closed system, particularly with respect to food supplies and waste disposal, and always struggled with the accumulation of toxic atmospheric compounds. With these problems in mind, an ambitious series of biosphere experiments were established in Arizona, culminating in the Biosphere 2 project in 1991.

A totally sealed complex, covering 3.15 acres (1.3 hectares) was purpose-built with a stainless-steel underground lining and principally a glass cover. Two flexible walls, or 'lungs', were included to minimize pressure changes within the complex with expansion and contraction of the atmosphere. A 2-year closure was planned, with the complex containing a wide range of flora and fauna, including eight humans. Soil was chosen as the growing medium for all plants in preference to the hydroponic techniques used previously. This was to facilitate air purification by soil bed reactors, in which atmospheric air is pumped through the soil where bacterial action provides an adaptable and efficient purification system. A CO_2 'scrubber' system was included in Biosphere 2 to control atmospheric CO_2 levels, particularly during winter when shorter days reduce photosynthetic activity. Also, the amount of O_2-consuming biomass relative to atmosphere volume was known to be high, therefore small increases in CO_2 levels were anticipated.

Biosphere 2 aimed, wherever possible, to use ecological engineering. By the inclusion of large numbers of species (3800 in total), it was hoped that there would be sufficient flexibility between systems to respond to changes in the environment. In particular, microbial diversity is believed to be extremely important in maintaining Biosphere 1 (Earth), and multiple habitats were established to facilitate this type of diversity in Biosphere 2.

Outcome from the 2-Year Closure

Concentrations of oxygen and CO_2 in Biosphere 2 were very unstable (Fig. 18.3), and after 16 months, oxygen concentration had fallen to only 14%. Extensive symptoms were reported by the human inhabitants, including significantly reduced work capacity, and external oxygen had to be added to the atmosphere. CO_2 levels did increase slightly during winter months (Fig. 18.3) when the CO_2 was removed by the scrubber system.

It was never expected that all species introduced into Biosphere 2 would survive, and extinction of some species

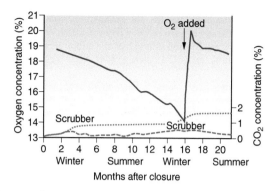

• **Fig. 18.3** Changes in atmospheric concentrations of oxygen (solid red line) and carbon dioxide (dashed orange line) during the 2-year closure of Biosphere 2. Less daylight during winter months reduces photosynthesis causing increased levels of carbon dioxide *(CO₂)*. CO_2 was therefore removed using a CO_2 scrubber system during the periods shown. Even when CO_2 absorption by the scrubbers is taken into account (blue dotted line), it can clearly be seen that the reduction in O_2 concentration exceeds the increase in CO_2 concentration; after 16 months, O_2 had to be added to the biosphere. See text for details. (From references 9 and 30.)

was seen as a natural response to stabilization of the ecosystem. However, after 21 months, extinct species were numerous, including 19 of 25 vertebrates and most insects, including all pollinators.[30] In contrast, ants and cockroaches thrived.

The success of Biosphere 2 as a closed ecosystem was therefore limited, and, in contrast to the smaller biospheres previously used, basic atmospheric regeneration was a significant problem. Any increase in CO_2 concentration should be matched by an equivalent decrease in O_2 concentration, as biological reactions between CO_2 and O_2 are generally equimolar. Even when the CO_2 removed by the recycling system is taken into account, it can clearly be seen from Figure 18.3 that oxygen losses were much greater. The explanation for this is believed to be twofold. First, oxygen depletion occurred because of respiration in the biosphere proceeding faster than photosynthesis, most likely as a result of excessive microbial activity in the soil. Second, much of the CO_2 produced by this respiration was lost from the atmosphere by chemical reaction with the concrete from which the biosphere complex was built.

We remain some way away from being able to establish a long-term habitable atmosphere away from Earth.

References

1. Parker CJR, Snowdon SL. Predicted and measured oxygen concentrations in the circle system using low fresh gas flows with oxygen supplied by an oxygen concentrator. *Br J Anaesth*. 1988;61: 397-402.

2. Versichelen L, Rolly G, Vermeulen H. Accumulation of foreign gases during closed-system anaesthesia. *Br J Anaesth*. 1996;76: 668-672.

3. Dean MR. Benzene exposure in Royal Naval submarines. *J R Soc Med*. 1996;89:286P-288P.

*4. Zouboules SM, Day TA. The exhausting work of acclimating to chronically elevated CO_2. *J Physiol*. 2019;597:61421-1423.

5. Law J, Young M, Alexander D, et al. Carbon dioxide physiological training at NASA. *Aerosp Med Hum Perform*. 2017;88: 897-902.

*6. Rodeheffer CD, Chabal S, Clarke JM, et al. Acute exposure to low-to-moderate carbon dioxide levels and submariner decision making. *Aerosp Med Hum Perform*. 2018;89:520-525.

7. Elliott AR, Prisk GK, Schöllmann C, et al. Hypercapnic ventilatory response in humans before, during, and after 23 days of low level CO_2 exposure. *Aviat Space Environ Med*. 1998;69:391-396.

8. Drummer C, Friedel V, Börger A, et al. Effects of elevated carbon dioxide environment on calcium metabolism in humans. *Aviat Space Environ Med*. 1998;69:291-298.

9. Churchill SE. *Fundamentals of Space Life Sciences*. Malabar, Florida: Krieger Publishing; 1997.

10. Frey MAB, Sulzman FM, Oser H, et al. The effects of moderately elevated ambient carbon dioxide levels on human physiology and performance: a joint NASA-ESA-DARA study—overview. *Aviat Space Environ Med*. 1998;69:282-284.

11. Manzey D, Lorenz B. Effects of chronically elevated CO_2 on mental performance during 26 days of confinement. *Aviat Space Environ Med*. 1998;69:506-514.

12. Romoser AA, Scully RR, Limero TF, et al. Predicting air quality at first ingress into vehicles visiting the International Space Station. *Aerosp Med Hum Perform*. 2017;88:104-113.

13. Grigoriev AI, Kozlovskaya IB, Potapov AN. Goals of biomedical support of a mission to Mars and possible approaches to achieving them. *Aviat Space Environ Med*. 2002;73:379-384.

14. Sridhar KR, Finn JE, Kliss MH. In-situ resource utilisation technologies for Mars life support systems. *Adv Space Res*. 2000;25:249-255.

*15. Prisk GK. The lung in space. *Clin Chest Med*. 2005;26:415-438.

16. Shelhamer M. Parabolic flight as a spaceflight analog. *J Appl Physiol*. 2016;120:1442-1448.

17. Prisk GK, Fine JM, Cooper TK, et al. Vital capacity, respiratory muscle strength, and pulmonary gas exchange during long-duration exposure to microgravity. *J Appl Physiol*. 2006;101:439-447.

18. Paiva M, Estenne M, Engel LA. Lung volumes, chest wall configuration, and pattern of breathing in microgravity. *J Appl Physiol*. 1989;67:1542-1550.

19. Wantier M, Estenne M, Verbanck S, et al. Chest wall mechanics in sustained microgravity. *J Appl Physiol*. 1998;84:2060-2065.

20. Elliott AR, Prisk GK, Guy HJB, et al. Lung volumes during sustained microgravity on Spacelab SLS-1. *J Appl Physiol*. 1994;77:2005-2014.

21. Dutrieue B, Verbanck S, Darquenne C, et al. Airway closure in microgravity. *Respir Physiol Neurobiol*. 2005;148:97-111.

22. Elliott AR, Shea SA, Dijk D-J, et al. Microgravity reduces sleep-disordered breathing in humans. *Am J Respir Crit Care Med*. 2001;164:478-485.

23. Moore AD, Downs ME, Lee SMC, et al. Peak exercise oxygen uptake during and following long-duration spaceflight. *J Appl Physiol*. 2014;117:231-238.

24. Ade CJ, Broxterman RM, Moore AD, et al. Decreases in maximal oxygen uptake following long-duration spaceflight: role of convective and diffusive O_2 transport mechanisms. *J Appl Physiol*. 2017;122:968-975.

25. Hoffmann U, Moore Jr AD, Koschate J, et al. $\dot{V}O_2$ and HR kinetics before and after International Space Station missions. *Eur J Appl Physiol*. 2016;116:503-511.

26. Darquenne C, Prisk GK. Particulate deposition in the human lung under lunar habitat conditions. *Aviat Space Environ Med*. 2013;84:190-195.

27. Bowman RO, Thomae FW. Long-term nontoxic support of animal life with algae. *Science*. 1961;134:55-56.

28. Ivanov B, Zubareva O. To mars and back again on board Bios. *Soviet Life*. 1985;4:22-25.

29. Hendrickx L, De Wever H, Hermans V, et al. Microbial ecology of the closed artificial ecosystem MELiSSA (Micro-Ecological Life Support System Alternative): reinventing and compartmentalising the Earth's food and oxygen regeneration system for long-haul space exploration missions. *Res Microbiol*. 2006;157:77-86.

30. Cohen JE, Tilman D. Biosphere 2 and biodiversity: the lessons so far. *Science*. 1996;274:1150-1151.

19

Drowning

KEY POINTS

- Immersion in thermoneutral water activates protective airway reflexes, and aspiration does not occur until lung oxygen stores have been used up and hypoxia causes the airway to open.

- In cold water, the cold shock reflex causes gasping and hyperventilation under water, with inhalation of large quantities of water and rapid severe hypoxia.

It is estimated that there are more than 360 000 victims of drowning worldwide each year.[1] In most countries drowning is a major cause of accidental death, particularly amongst children. Drowning is more common in low- or middle-income countries than in high-income countries, is more common for men than for women and is frequently associated with alcohol ingestion. For each victim of death by drowning, there are estimated to be several cases of 'near-drowning' that are severe enough to require hospital admission, and probably hundreds of other less severe incidents. Death from pulmonary complications ('secondary drowning') may occur a considerable time after the accident in patients who were initially normal.

The essential feature of drowning is asphyxia, but many of the physiological responses depend on how much aspiration of water occurs and upon the substances that are dissolved or suspended in the water. The temperature of the water is crucially important, and hypothermia after near-drowning in very cold water is a major factor influencing survival.

Physiology of Immersion[2]

The hydrostatic pressure exerted on the body during immersion can be substantial. As a result there is a huge increase in venous return, causing increased pulmonary blood volume, cardiac output and, soon afterwards, a significant diuresis. Cephalad displacement of the diaphragm from raised abdominal pressure coupled with direct chest compression increases the work of breathing by about 65%. Three reflexes affect the respiratory system and come into play in drowning:

1. *Airway irritant reflexes.* Aspiration of water into the mouth initially stimulates swallowing followed by coughing, glottic closure and laryngospasm. If water penetrates deeper into the respiratory tract, below the vocal folds, bronchospasm results.

2. *Cold shock.* This describes a combination of several cardiovascular and respiratory reflexes that occur in response to sudden total-body immersion in cold water.[3,4] Sudden immersion in water below 25°C is a potent stimulus to respiration, and causes an initial large gasp followed by substantial hyperventilation. The stimulus is increased with colder temperatures, reaching a maximum at 10°C. Functional residual capacity is acutely increased, and individuals may find themselves breathing almost at total lung capacity, giving a sensation of dyspnoea. Breath-hold time is severely reduced, often to less than 10 seconds, which impairs the ability of victims to escape from a confined space underwater or to orientate themselves before seeking safety.

3. *Diving reflex.* In response to cold water stimulation of the face and eyes, the diving reflex produces bradycardia, peripheral vasoconstriction and apnoea in most mammals. It is particularly well-developed in diving mammals (page 311) to reduce oxygen consumption and facilitate long-duration dives. The reflex is present in humans, and is more active in infants than adults. In healthy adults sudden immersion of the head in cold water initially causes a cold shock response with hyperventilation, but within 1 minute respiratory rate decreases in keeping with a diving reflex.[4]

Physiological Mechanisms of Drowning

Glottic closure from inhaled water, pulmonary aspiration, cold shock and the diving response all influence the course of events following submersion in water; the relative importance of each depends, amongst many other factors, on the age of the victim and the temperature of the water.

Conflicting influences on the heart from activation of both the parasympathetic (diving reflex) and sympathetic (cold shock) systems are believed to contribute to death from cardiac dysrhythmia in some victims.[3]

Drowning Without Aspiration of Water

This occurs in fewer than 10% of drowning victims. In thermoneutral water, when cold-stimulated reflexes will be minimal, the larynx is firmly closed during submersion, and some victims will lose consciousness before water is aspirated. The rate of decrease of alveolar, and therefore arterial, Po_2 depends on the lung volume and the oxygen consumption. Oxygen stored in the alveolar gas after a maximal inspiration is unlikely to exceed 1 L, and an oxygen consumption of 3 L.min^{-1} would not be unusual in a subject either swimming or struggling. Loss of consciousness from decreased alveolar Po_2 usually occurs very suddenly and without warning.

In cold water, hypoxia secondary to glottic closure may still occur. In addition, the cold shock and diving reflexes both leave the victim vulnerable to cardiovascular complications such as arrhythmias and sudden circulatory failure, leading to death before aspiration can occur. This is likely to be more common in elderly individuals.

Drowning with Aspiration of Water

Almost 90% of drowning victims have aspirated significant volumes of water. Following sudden immersion in cold water the cold shock response is believed to be more common than the diving reflex, and hyperventilation rapidly leads to aspiration. In thermoneutral water, glottic closure may either be overcome by the conscious victim or eventually subside because of hypoxia; in both circumstances aspiration is likely to continue. Once aspiration occurs, reflex bronchospasm quickly follows, further worsening respiratory function.

Freshwater

Aspiration of freshwater further down the bronchial tree causes rapid and profound changes to the alveolar surfactant, leading to loss of the normal elastic properties of the alveoli and disturbed ventilation/perfusion ratios. In freshwater drowning, alveolar water is quickly absorbed, resulting in alveolar collapse and a pulmonary shunt, in addition to the changes resulting from dilution of surfactant. A significant shunt is therefore quickly established, with resulting hypoxia. Some studies indicate that neurogenic pulmonary oedema because of cerebral hypoxia might coexist with alveolar flooding from aspirated water.[5] The pulmonary changes caused by immersion appear to be quickly reversible,[5] with good prospects of return to normal pulmonary function in those who survive immersion.

A substantial volume of water may be absorbed from the lungs, and profound hyponatraemia, leading to fits, has been described in infants drowned in freshwater.[6] However,

most human victims absorb only small quantities of water, and redistribution rapidly corrects the blood volume. Hypovolaemia is the more common problem after near-drowning.[6]

Seawater

Seawater is hypertonic, with more than three times the osmolarity of blood. Consequently, seawater in the lungs is not initially absorbed, and instead draws fluid from the circulation into the alveoli. Animal studies found that, after aspiration of seawater, it is possible to recover from the lungs 50% more than the original volume inhaled. This clearly maintains the proportion of flooded alveoli, and results in a persistent shunt with reduction in arterial Po_2.

The Role of Hypothermia[2]

Some degree of hypothermia is usual in near-drowned victims, and body temperature is usually in the range of 33°C to 36°C. Hypothermia-induced reduction in cerebral metabolism is protective during hypoxia, and is believed to contribute to the numerous reports of survival after prolonged immersion in cold water, particularly in children. There have been reports of survival of near-drowned children and adults trapped for periods as long as 80 minutes beneath ice.[6] However, for the reasons outlined earlier, arterial hypoxaemia is believed to develop very quickly, and there is controversy surrounding how body temperature can decrease quickly enough to provide any degree of cerebral protection. Surface cooling is not believed to allow a rapid enough fall in temperature, as normal physiological responses to cold such as peripheral vasoconstriction and shivering limit the decline in temperature. Even so, the greater body surface area of children relative to their body size will theoretically result in more rapid cooling by heat conduction from the body surface.[2]

Absorption of cold water either from the lungs or stomach will contribute to hypothermia during prolonged immersion, but quantitatively the volumes required are unlikely to be absorbed, particularly in seawater. Heat loss from the flushing of cold water in and out of the respiratory tract, without absorption occurring, is another possible explanation. Animal studies have shown that airway flushing with cold water reduces carotid artery blood temperature by several degrees within a few minutes, which is sufficient to produce a useful reduction in cerebral oxygen requirement. Finally, repeated aspiration of cold water may directly cool deep areas of the brain through conductive heat loss to the nasopharynx.[2,7]

Despite these potential benefits, hypothermia in most drowning victims probably does more harm than good. Consciousness is lost at around 32°C, making further aspiration almost inevitable, and ventricular fibrillation or asystole commonly occur at temperatures below 28°C. Once rescued, near-drowned patients often cool further before arrival at hospital.

Principles of Therapy for Near-Drowning

There is a high measure of agreement on general principles of treatment.[6,8]

Immediate Treatment

In-water resuscitation may be used by highly trained rescuers, and involves artificial ventilation before removing the victim from the water; cardiac compressions are not possible until on land, but early ventilation may improve survival.[8] Circulatory failure and loss of consciousness may occur when a patient is lifted from the water in a vertical position, for example by a helicopter winch. This is probably because of the loss of water pressure resulting in relative redistribution of blood volume into the legs. It is now recommended that victims are removed from the water in the prone position wherever possible.

At the scene of the drowning, it can be very difficult to determine whether there has been cardiac or even respiratory arrest. However, there are many records of apparently dead victims who have recovered without evidence of brain damage after long periods of total immersion. It is therefore essential that cardiopulmonary resuscitation (CPR) be undertaken in all victims until fully assessed in hospital, no matter how hopeless the outlook may appear at the scene.

Early treatment of near-drowning is crucial, and this requires efficient instruction in CPR for those who may be available in locations where drowning is likely to occur. CPR should follow standard algorithms, except that it is recommended to give five initial rescue breaths rather than the standard two before commencing chest compressions to try and clear water from the lungs.[8] Out of hospital, mouth-to-mouth ventilation is the method of choice, but high inflation pressures are usually required when there has been flooding of the lungs. Attempts to drain water from the lungs by postural drainage or an abdominal thrust (the Heimlich manoeuvre) are to be avoided because these are likely to cause regurgitation of stomach contents with possible aspiration, and will delay the institution of artificial ventilation. Tracheal intubation should be performed as soon as possible to protect the airway from aspiration. Most survivors will breathe spontaneously within 1 to 5 minutes after removal from the water. The decision to discontinue resuscitation should not be taken until assessment in hospital, particularly if the state of consciousness is confused by hypothermia.

Hospital Treatment

On arrival at hospital, patients should be triaged into these categories:
1. Awake
2. Impaired consciousness (but responsive)
3. Comatose

There should be better than 90% survival in the first two categories, but patients should still be admitted for observation and followed up after discharge. Late deterioration of pulmonary function may occur, and is known as 'secondary drowning', which is a form of acute lung injury (see Chapter 31). This can develop in any patient who has aspirated water, and the onset is usually within 4 hours of the aspiration.[2] Patients who are comatose or hypoxic will require admission to a critical care unit. Treatment follows the general principles for hypoxic cerebral damage and aspiration lung injury. If spontaneous breathing does not result in satisfactory levels of arterial Po_2 and Pco_2, continuous positive airway pressure may be tried, and is frequently useful. If this is unsuccessful, or if the patient has neurological impairment, artificial ventilation is required.

References

*1. Anon. Drowning: a silent killer. *The Lancet.* 2017;389:1859.
2. Giesbrecht GG. Cold stress, near drowning and accidental hypothermia: a review. *Aviat Space Environ Med.* 2000;71:733-752.
3. Datta A, Tipton M. Respiratory responses to cold water immersion: neural pathways, interactions, and clinical consequences awake and asleep. *J Appl Physiol.* 2006;100:2057-2064.
4. Gagnon DD, Pretorius T, McDonald G, et al. Cardiovascular and ventilatory responses to dorsal, facial, and whole-head water immersion in eupnea. *Aviat Space Environ Med.* 2013;84: 573-583.
5. Rumbak MJ. The etiology of pulmonary edema in fresh water near drowning. *Am J Emerg Med.* 1996;14:176-179.
6. Harries M. Near drowning. *BMJ.* 2003;327:1336-1338.
7. Takeda Y, Hashimoto H, Fumoto K, et al. Effects of pharyngeal cooling on brain temperature in primates and humans. A study for proof of principle. *Anesthesiology.* 2012;117:117-125.
8. Szpilman D, Bierens JJLM, Handley AJ, et al. Drowning. *N Engl J Med.* 2012;366:2102-2110.

20

Smoking and Air Pollution

KEY POINTS

- Although becoming less popular, one-fifth of the UK population still smokes tobacco, and worldwide, the number of smokers is increasing.
- Smoking involves the regular inhalation of a variety of toxic compounds that stimulate airway irritant receptors and activate inflammatory pathways in the lung.

- The effects of passive smoking begin in utero, when lung development is impaired, leaving the infant susceptible to lower respiratory tract illness for the first few years of life.
- Air pollution with carbon monoxide, ozone, nitrogen dioxide and particulate matter can occur either indoors or outside, and is associated with a variety of respiratory diseases and symptoms.

The air we breathe is rarely a simple mixture of oxygen, nitrogen and water vapour. For much of the world's population, air also contains a variety of other, more noxious, gases and particles. In addition, a substantial proportion of people choose to further contaminate the air that they, and others, breathe with tobacco smoke.

Tobacco Smoke

In the Americas tobacco was used for medicinal purposes for many centuries before being introduced from the New World into Europe in the 16th century. Through his acquaintance with Queen Elizabeth I, Sir Walter Raleigh made smoking tobacco an essential fashionable activity of every gentleman. Thereafter the practice steadily increased in popularity until the explosive growth of the habit after the First World War (1914–1918).

There have always been those opposed to smoking, and King James I (1603–1625) described it as 'a custom loathsome to the eye, hateful to the nose, harmful to the brain and dangerous to the lungs'. However, firm evidence to support his last conclusion was delayed by some 350 years. Only relatively recently did it become clear that smokers had a higher mortality, and that the causes of the excess mortality included many respiratory diseases.[1] There are currently over a billion smokers worldwide. In high-income countries, the proportion of the population that smokes has generally declined since evidence of serious health consequences emerged; in the UK and the US this is now around 20%. Globally, however, the number of smokers is increasing. The health costs of tobacco smoking are enormous: over 80% of smokers are in low- and middle-income countries,[2] where the smoking prevalence amongst males may exceed 70%. Worldwide, one-third of people who smoke will die as a result of their habit, and it is estimated that during this century smoking will cause 1000 million premature deaths.[3]

Constituents of Tobacco Smoke

More than 2000 potentially noxious constituents have been identified in tobacco smoke, some in the gaseous phase and others in the particulate or tar phase. The particulate phase is defined as the fraction eliminated by passing smoke through a filter of pore size 0.1 μm. This is not to be confused with the 'filter tip', which allows passage of considerable quantities of particulate matter.

There is great variation in the yields of the different constituents between different brands and different types of cigarettes. This is achieved by using leaves of different species of plants, by varying the conditions of curing and cultivation and by using filter tips. Ventilated filters have a ring of small holes in the paper between the filter tip and the tobacco. These holes admit air during a puff, and dilute all constituents of the smoke.

Gaseous Phase

Carbon monoxide (CO) is present in cigarette smoke at a concentration issuing from the butt of the cigarette during a puff of around 1% to 5%, which is far into the toxic range. A better indication of the extent of CO exposure is the percentage of carboxyhaemoglobin in blood. For nonsmokers, the value is normally less than 1.5%, but is influenced by exposure to air pollution and other people's cigarette smoke (see later). Typical values for smokers range from 2% to 12%. The value is influenced by the number of cigarettes smoked, the type of cigarette and the pattern of inhalation of smoke.

Tobacco smoke also contains very high concentrations (about 400 parts per million [ppm]) of nitric oxide (NO) and trace concentrations of nitrogen dioxide, the former being slowly oxidized to the latter in the presence of oxygen. The toxicity of these compounds is well known. Nitrogen dioxide hydrates in alveolar lining fluid to form a mixture of nitrous and nitric acids. In addition, the nitrite ion converts haemoglobin to methaemoglobin.

Other constituents of the gaseous phase include hydrocyanic acid, cyanogen, aldehydes, ketones, nitrosamines and volatile polynuclear aromatic hydrocarbons (PAHs).

Particulate Phase

The material removed by a Cambridge filter is known as the 'total particulate matter', with an aerosol particle size in the range of 0.2 to 1 μm. The particulate phase comprises water, nicotine and 'tar'. Nicotine ranges from 0.05 to 2.5 mg per cigarette, and 'tar' from 0.5 to 35 mg per cigarette.

Individual Smoke Exposure

Individual smoke exposure is a complex function of the quantity of cigarettes that are smoked and the pattern of inhalation.

Quantifying Cigarettes Smoked

Exposure is usually quantified in 'pack-years'. This equals the product of the number of packs (20 cigarettes) smoked per day, multiplied by the number of years that that pattern was maintained. The totals for each period are then summated for the lifetime of the subject.

Pattern of Inhalation

There are very wide variations in patterns of smoking. Air is normally drawn through the cigarette in a series of 'puffs' with a volume of about 25 to 50 mL per puff. The puff may be simply drawn into the mouth and rapidly expelled without appreciable inhalation. However, the habituated smoker will either inhale the puff directly into the lungs or, more commonly, pass the puff from the mouth to the lungs by inhaling air either through the mouth or else through the nose while passing the smoke from the mouth into the pharynx by apposing the tongue against the palate, obliterating the gas space in the mouth. The inspiration is often especially deep, to flush into the lung any smoke remaining in the dead space.

The quantity of nicotine, tar and CO obtainable from a single cigarette is therefore variable, and the number and type of cigarettes smoked are not the sole determinants of effective exposure. Habituated smokers adjust their smoking pattern to maintain a particular blood level of nicotine.

For example, after changing to a brand with a lower nicotine yield, it is common practice to modify the pattern of inhalation to maximize nicotine absorption.

Respiratory Effects of Smoking

Cigarette smoking has extensive effects on respiratory function, and is clearly implicated in the aetiology of a number of respiratory diseases, particularly chronic obstructive pulmonary disease (COPD) and bronchial carcinoma, which are discussed in Chapters 28 and 30, respectively. Why only around one-fifth of smokers go on to develop COPD remains uncertain, but is likely to relate to a genetic susceptibility to the effect of tobacco smoke (page 331). Studies of the modification of the expression of several genes in smokers via methylation of DNA have identified associations with this and a decline in lung function, the development of COPD and lung cancer.[4] Pulmonary endothelial cell injury because of cigarette smoke includes barrier dysfunction, endothelial inflammation, apoptosis and altered vasoactive mediator production. These processes are implicated in the development of conditions including acute respiratory distress syndrome (ARDS), emphysema and vascular remodeling in COPD.[5]

Airway Mucosa

There are conflicting laboratory reports regarding the sensitivity of airway reflexes in smokers, with increased sensitivity demonstrated in response to inhalation of small concentrations of ammonia vapour and decreased sensitivity in response to capsaicin. There are also variable effects of smoking cessation on the cough reflex. There is, however, general agreement that smokers have hyperresponsive airway reflexes secondary to airway inflammation, probably caused by increased excitability of vagal sensory nerves in response to inflammatory mediators.[6]

Ciliary movement is inhibited by both particulate and gas phase compounds in vitro, but in vivo studies have shown contradictory results, with some studies showing increased ciliary activity in response to cigarette smoke. Ciliary structure may be abnormal, with some work showing smoking reduces the length of cilia by reducing expression of the intraflagellar transport gene responsible for normal ciliary production.[7] A small reduction in ciliary length may significantly impair its mucus-clearing function (page 166).

There is agreement that mucus production is increased in long-term smokers, who have hyperplasia of submucosal glands and increased numbers of goblet cells even when asymptomatic. Mucus clearance is universally found to be impaired in smokers, which, coupled with increased mucus production and airway sensitivity, gives rise to the normally productive smoker's cough. Three months after smoking cessation, many of these changes are reversed, except in those patients who have developed airway damage from long-term airway inflammation.

Airway Diameter

Airway diameter is reduced acutely with smoking as a result of reflex bronchoconstriction in response to inhaled particles

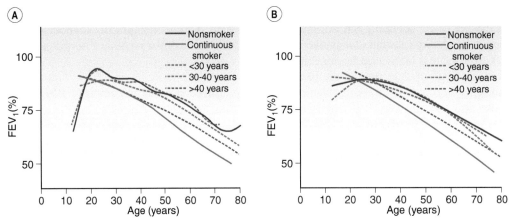

• **Fig. 20.1** Schematic diagram showing the effects of smoking on lifelong changes in the forced expiratory volume in one second *(FEV₁)*. **(A)** Male subjects; **(B)** female subjects. Red lines show lifelong nonsmokers. Males take longer than females to reach their early adult peak in lung volumes. The increase in very elderly males is caused either by health survivor bias or the diminishing sample size. In lifelong smokers (blue lines) the decline in lung function begins immediately and proceeds at a faster rate than in nonsmokers. The effect of stopping smoking depends on the age at which the subject permanently quits *(dashed lines)*, with little adverse effect on FEV₁ if this occurs before the age of 30 years. FEV₁ is expressed as a percentage of the volume at age 25. (Data from reference 8.)

and the increased mucus production already described. Long-term small airway inflammation causes chronic airway narrowing that has a multitude of effects on lung function. Airway narrowing promotes premature airway closure during expiration, which results in an increase in closing volume and disturbed ventilation/perfusion relationships. Distribution of inspired gas as indicated by the single-breath nitrogen test (page 92) is therefore often abnormal in smokers. Small airway narrowing over many years gives rise to a progressive reduction in the forced expiratory volume in one second (FEV_1), described later. Many of these changes are at an advanced stage before smokers develop respiratory symptoms.

Ventilatory Capacity

Although males take longer than females for their FEV_1 to reach its peak in early adulthood, in both sexes the value remains high until around 40 years of age, before declining steadily as the subject grows older (Fig. 20.1). Longitudinal studies of FEV_1 reveal that, for smokers, the decline in FEV_1 begins in early adulthood and proceeds at a faster rate than in nonsmokers, as illustrated in Figure 20.1.[8] Eventually, this decline in lung function results in lung pathology.

Passive Smoking

A nonsmoker is exposed to all the constituents of tobacco smoke while indoors in the presence of smokers. Exposure varies with many factors, including size and ventilation of the room, number of people smoking and absorption of smoke constituents on soft furnishings and clothing. CO concentrations of 20 ppm have been reported, which is above the recommended environmental concentration (see later discussion). 'Side-stream' smoke from a smouldering cigarette stub produces greater quantities of potentially noxious substances than 'main-stream' smoke produced when a cigarette burns in a stream of air drawn through it during a puff. On average, side-stream smoke is generated during 58 seconds in each minute of cigarette smoking, and this is not included in the measured yield of a cigarette.

Evidence for adverse health effects of passive smoking is now convincing: passive smoking by adults has been linked to lung cancer, cardiovascular disease, asthma and COPD.

Maternal Smoking

Infants whose mothers smoke during pregnancy have low birthweight, are more likely to be born prematurely and are at greater risk of sudden infant death syndrome (page 181). Up to 2 years of age, infants with parents who smoke are more prone to lower respiratory tract illnesses and episodes of wheezing, and when older they have reduced lung volumes and higher carboxyhaemoglobin levels and are more likely to have asthma even at 14 years of age. It remains unclear whether this results from passive smoking in utero or from postnatal exposure to tobacco smoke in the home,[9] but evidence for an in utero contribution is mounting, mediated by reduced innate immunity in the child born to a mother who smokes.[10] The increased risk of lower respiratory tract illness in passive-smoking infants is believed to result from smaller airway calibre at birth causing a greater propensity to airway closure with the normal infective or allergic challenges of infancy. After a few years of normal growth, airway size increases sufficiently to reduce symptoms, and these children 'grow out' of their susceptibility to respiratory illness, although their lung function remains poorer than that of children who did not have lower airways disease in early life.

Smoking and Perioperative Complications

The increased sensitivity of the airway to inhaled irritants seen in smokers causes a greater incidence of adverse events such as cough, breath hold or laryngospasm on induction of general anaesthesia, even in passive smokers.[11]

There is ample evidence that smokers have an increased incidence of perioperative complications, including death and postoperative pulmonary complications (page 263).

Smoking Cessation

Smoking cessation helps to reverse and limit pathological changes in the airways, as well as reduce longer term risks associated with smoking, for example, the development of lung cancer. Use of a combination of interventions, including behavioural support and pharmacotherapy such as nicotine replacement therapy, produce the best 'quit rates'.[12]

E-Cigarettes

There are now 2 million e-cigarette users in the UK,[13] but the rising popularity of electronic nicotine delivery systems has caused controversy. E-cigarettes produce an aerosol by heating a liquid that contains a solvent and nicotine.[14] They are an effective form of nicotine replacement therapy, and improve smoking cessation rates.[13,15] Passive inhalation of nicotine is known to occur, but because the vapour is only released when the user 'puffs' on the device, a smaller amount of toxic substance is released into the environment when compared with a burning cigarette. Although using e-cigarettes is likely to be less harmful than smoking tobacco, decades of exposure may be required to establish long-term health effects. Substituting e-cigarettes for tobacco smoking still involves delivery of nicotine into the lungs and may still cause harm. In recent studies, e-cigarettes have been found to affect markers of tissue injury and inflammation.[16,17] Mice exposed to e-cigarette solution for 4 months demonstrated changes associated with the development of COPD, including cytokine expression, airway hyperreactivity and lung tissue destruction.[18] Increased rates of chronic bronchitis symptoms were found in adolescent e-cigarette users, even after adjustment for cigarette and second-hand smoke exposure.[19] There are concerns that the perception of e-cigarettes as 'safe' nicotine may be attracting children into a nicotine addiction that will lead to smoking, and although guidelines to regulate the manufacturing, marketing and consumption of e-cigarettes in public spaces are being developed, these are new and incomplete.[20]

Mechanisms of Smoking-Related Lung Damage

Many of the compounds present in cigarette smoke have direct irritant and toxic effects on the lungs. In the longer term these effects are likely to be mediated by changes in gene expression by the airway, and even quite low-level smoke exposure, as seen with passive smoking, causes changes in the expression of 128 different genes with a host of physiological roles.[21] There are three major mechanisms by which lung damage occurs.

Oxidative Injury

Oxidative injury, including peroxidation of membrane lipids, is an important component of the pulmonary damage caused by cigarette smoke. These effects are likely to be mediated by upregulation of the genes for phospholipase A_2 and various peroxidase enzymes.[21]

Direct Oxidative Damage

The tar phase contains reactive oxygen species such as quinone and hydroquinone, and the gas phase contains NO. These compounds can reduce oxygen in the body, to yield the superoxide anion and thence the highly damaging hydroxyl radical (see Fig. 25.3).

Cell-Mediated Oxidative Damage

This results from smoking-induced activation of, or enhancement of, neutrophil and macrophage activity in the respiratory tract.[6] Bronchoalveolar lavage in humans has shown that smokers have larger numbers of intraalveolar macrophages, and also significant numbers of neutrophils that are not normally present in nonsmokers. It is the particulate component of smoke that is responsible for the recruitment and activation of neutrophils in the alveoli. This suggests that the interaction of particulate matter and alveolar macrophages releases a neutrophil chemoattractant, and that neutrophils are subsequently activated to release either proteases or reactive oxygen species. This activation may be a direct response to cigarette smoke, or may represent excessive reactive oxygen species production in response to minor infective challenge in smokers.

Evidence of in vivo oxidative stress in smokers is based mainly on measures of antioxidant activity in both the lungs and blood. Compared with nonsmokers, human smokers have reduced levels of vitamin E in alveolar fluid, reduced plasma concentrations of vitamin C and greatly increased superoxide dismutase and catalase activity in alveolar macrophages.

Carcinogenesis

Smoking contributes to the development of cancer in many organs, but the respiratory tract clearly receives the greatest exposure to tobacco smoke carcinogens. There are two groups of compounds with carcinogenic activity, found mostly in the tar of the particulate phase. Some hydrocarbons, in particular PAHs, are carcinogenic, whereas others such as aromatic phenols (phenol, indole and catechol) are cocarcinogens and tumour promoters, without which the carcinogenic compounds are relatively innocuous. Tobacco-related nitrosamines and nicotine derivatives are also carcinogenic, and, because of their ease of absorption into the blood, are responsible for cancer formation not only in the respiratory tract and oesophagus but also in more distant organs such as the pancreas. Knowledge about these carcinogens has led to many attempts to reduce their concentration in smoke by modifying the cigarette, and tar levels in cigarettes have declined almost 3-fold since 1955. However, these changes have had little impact on the incidence of lung cancer (page 357), and smoking cessation remains the best way to avoid all smoking-related cancers.

Immunological Activation

Smokers have elevated serum immunoglobin (Ig)E levels compared with nonsmokers, the cause of which is uncertain but may be 2-fold. Direct toxicity and oxidative cell damage result in greater airway mucosal cell permeability, allowing better access for allergens to underlying immunologically active cells. Smoking also increases the activity of some T-lymphocyte subsets that are responsible for producing interleukin-4, a cytokine well known for stimulating IgE production, and is known to produce a long-term systemic inflammatory response.

Air Pollution[22]

Pollution is the world's largest environmental cause of disease and premature death and is responsible for an estimated 9 million deaths annually. Air pollution carries a significant burden of morbidity, including respiratory, cardiovascular and neurological impairment, and possibly pregnancy complications and low birthweight.[23] Most adversely affected are the world's poorest and most vulnerable, with almost 92% of pollution-related deaths occurring in low- and middle-income countries. Children, the elderly and those with cardiopulmonary disease are also more susceptible. It has been estimated that in Europe up to 21% of the urban population are exposed to levels of pollutants in excess of European Union regulations.[24] Fuel combustion (either fossil fuels or the burning of biomass) accounts for 85% of airborne particulate pollution. Worldwide, household air pollution is slowly declining, but ambient air pollution continues to worsen. As a recognized global problem, the World Health Organization (WHO) Air Quality Guidelines[25] set standards for maximum acceptable levels of common pollutants, and the State of Global Air report produced annually since 2017 brings together information on air quality and health.[26] WHO recommendations on the reduction of the short-lived climate pollutants black carbon, ozone (O_3) and methane (which persist for days to decades, rather than greenhouse gases which persist for hundreds to thousands of years) could lead to a reduction in 3.5 million deaths per year by 2030 and a slowing of global warming within 10 years.[27]

Air pollution is associated with a greater prevalence of cardiac disease,[28] a greater incidence of lung cancer[29] and an increased rate of natural-cause mortality,[30] although a link with nonmalignant respiratory mortality remains unproven.[31] Despite this last observation, there is some evidence that traffic-related air pollution increases the prevalence of both COPD and asthma, and wider agreement that, in patients with these diseases, pollution exacerbates their condition. Epidemiological research has also found effects of air pollution on lung function in children, showing that the closer children live to busy roads the slower is the rate at which their FEV_1 increases as they grow,[32] and the more likely they are to develop respiratory disease, including infections[33] and asthma. Similar observations have been made relating lung function in adults with proximity to road traffic.[34] In children, early-life exposure to traffic-related air pollution appears to lead to an increased risk of wheeze, but long-term exposure throughout childhood is needed to increase the risk of developing asthma.[35] Fine particulate matter[36] and nitrogen dioxide[37] (see later) seem to be the main pollutants responsible for increased mortality.

Sources of Pollutants

Primary Pollutants

These are substances released into the atmosphere directly from the polluting source and are mostly derived from the combustion of fossil fuels. Petrol engines that ignite the fuel in an oxygen-restricted environment produce varying quantities of CO, nitrogen oxides and hydrocarbons such as benzene and polycyclic aromatic compounds. All of these pollutants are reduced by the use of a catalytic converter. In contrast, diesel engines burn fuel with an excess of oxygen, producing little CO but more nitrogen oxides and particulate matter. Burning of coal, oil and biomass is now restricted almost entirely to power generation, and the pollutants produced depend on the type of fuel used and the amount of effort expended on 'cleaning' the emissions. However, particulates and nitrogen oxides are invariably produced, and this remains a source of sulphur dioxide.

Secondary Pollutants

These are formed in the atmosphere from chemical changes to primary pollutants. NO produced from vehicle engines is quickly converted to nitrogen dioxide (NO_2), and during this process may react with O_3, reducing the atmospheric concentration of the latter. Alternatively, when exposed to sunlight in the lower atmosphere, both NO and NO_2 react with oxygen to produce O_3.

Meteorological Conditions

Meteorological conditions influence air pollution. In conditions of strong wind, pollutants are quickly dispersed; in cloudy weather the development of secondary pollutants is unlikely. Ground-level pollution in urban areas is exacerbated by clear, calm weather when 'temperature inversion' can occur. On a clear night, heat is lost from the ground to the atmosphere by radiation, and the ground level air cools dramatically (Fig. 20.2, *A*). At dawn the ground is quickly heated by the sun's radiation and warms the air, which lifts a blanket of cool air to approximately 50 to 100 m high.

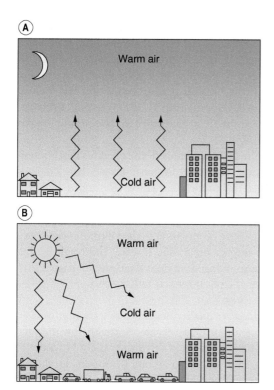

• **Fig. 20.2** Temperature inversion producing pollution in the morning rush hour. **(A)** At night, the ground loses heat to the atmosphere by radiation, and ground level air cools. **(B)** In the morning, with strong sun and still conditions, the ground heats up quickly and displaces the blanket of cold air upwards, so preventing effective air mixing and trapping vehicular pollution at ground level.

Because in still conditions mixing of air masses is slow to occur, the relatively cold air sits on top of the warm air below. In the meantime, the morning rush hour produces large amounts of pollutants that are unable to disperse and become trapped near the ground (Fig. 20.2, *B*).

Respiratory Effects of Pollutants

Recommended maximum levels of common pollutants are shown in Table 20.1. The extent to which these levels are achieved varies greatly between different countries and from year to year.

CO is found in the blood of patients, in trace concentrations, as a result of its production in the body, but mainly as a result of smoking and air pollution. The amount of carboxyhaemoglobin formed when breathing air polluted with CO will depend on the subject's minute volume. One study reported carboxyhaemoglobin levels of 0.4% to 9.7% in London taxi drivers, but the highest level in a nonsmoking driver was 3%.[38] Recommended levels shown in Table 20.1 are calculated to result in a carboxyhaemoglobin concentration of less than 2.5% even during moderate exercise. CO levels similar to those seen in smokers are only likely to occur during severe outdoor pollution episodes, although indoor pollution with CO may be more common (see later).

Nitrogen dioxide is mainly a primary pollutant, but a small amount is produced from NO. In the UK, about half

TABLE 20.1 World Health Organization Air Quality Guidelines[25]

Pollutant	Short (≤1 h)	Moderate (8–24 h)	Annual
		Duration of Exposure	
Ozone		$100\ \mu g.m^{-3}$	
Particulate PM$_{10}$	$50\ \mu g.m^{-3}$		$20\ \mu g.m^{-3}$
Particulate PM$_{2.5}$	$25\ \mu g.m^{-3}$		$10\ \mu g.m^{-3}$
Sulphur dioxide	$500\ \mu g.m^{-3}$	$20\ \mu g.m^{-3}$	
Nitrogen dioxide	$200\ \mu g.m^{-3}$		$40\ \mu g.m^{-3}$
Carbon monoxide	25–87 ppm	10 ppm	

ppm, Parts per million; PM, particulate matter.

of atmospheric NO$_2$ is derived from vehicles. Indoor levels of NO$_2$ commonly exceed outdoor levels, and the respiratory effects of NO$_2$ are therefore described in the next section.

O$_3$ is a secondary pollutant formed by the action of sunlight on nitrogen oxides, and therefore the highest levels tend to occur in rural areas downwind from cities and roads. In all areas, the dependence on sunlight means that O$_3$ levels slowly increase throughout the day, reaching peak levels shortly after the evening rush hour. The oxidative stress brought about by exposure to O$_3$ causes lipid oxidation and airway inflammation. The toxic effects on the respiratory tract are dependent on both concentration and duration of exposure. Exposure to concentrations of $200\ \mu g.m^{-3}$ for just a few hours commonly causes throat irritation, chest discomfort and cough, resulting from both direct stimulation of irritant receptors in the airway and activation of inflammatory pathways. Bronchoconstriction may occur, accompanied by a decrease in FEV$_1$, and exercise capacity is limited. There is a large variability between individuals in their spirometric response to O$_3$, with approximately 10% of subjects having a severe response. This variability in response is partly a result of differing genetic susceptibility.[39] It is interesting that laboratory studies have failed to demonstrate that asthmatic subjects are more susceptible to O$_3$-induced pulmonary symptoms. Even so, there is good evidence that high O$_3$ concentrations are associated with increased hospital attendance and respiratory problems, particularly in children. In adults, it has been calculated that for every 5 parts per billion (ppb) increment in long-term ambient O$_3$ exposure, the risk of mortality from a chronic lower respiratory disease increases by 5%.[40]

Declining use of coal has substantially reduced the production of sulphur dioxide in recent years, and two-thirds of production in the UK now originates from oil-burning power stations. Normal atmospheric levels have no short-term effect on healthy subjects, but asthmatic patients may develop bronchoconstriction at between 100 and 250 ppb.

Particulate matter consists of a mixture of soot, liquid droplets, recondensed metallic vapours and organic debris. The disparate nature of particulate pollution reflects its extremely varied origins, but in the urban environment, diesel engines are a major source. Only particles of less than 10 μm diameter are considered to be 'inhalable' into the lung (page 166), so particulate pollution is measured as the concentration of particles smaller than this diameter, known as PM_{10}. Particulate matter is further subdivided into the following:

- Coarse particles, between 2.5 and 10 μm diameter, make up a smaller proportion of PM_{10} than the other particles and are less well studied, but are still believed to contribute significantly to the adverse health effects of particulate pollution.[41]
- Fine particles, or $PM_{2.5}$, are less than 2.5 μm in diameter, are the most numerous particle present in air pollution and are responsible for most of the adverse effects. It has been estimated through large-scale epidemiological research that, for every 10 μg m^{-3} increase in the concentration of $PM_{2.5}$, all-cause mortality increases by 7.3%.[42] The mechanism appears to relate to an imbalance between oxidants and antioxidants. Assays are being developed for use as a research tool to characterize the oxidative potential of $PM_{2.5}$ particles, that is, their ability to generate reactive oxygen species.[43]
- Ultrafine particles are carbon particles less than 0.1 μm in size. Their small size means they should be breathed in and out without being trapped by the airway lining fluid (page 166). However, some particles are retained in the lung, where they remain in the long term, probably contained within macrophages, and without any evidence of systemic absorption. Their contribution to the health effects of particulate pollution is uncertain.

Acute effects of particles on lung function again include airway irritation and small reductions in lung volumes such as FEV_1 and forced vital capacity. It is, however, associations between $PM_{2.5}$ levels and overall mortality that have been the focus of most research.[36] Particulate pollution has widespread proinflammatory effects on lung epithelial cells and alveolar macrophages, causing inflammatory responses both locally, in the lung, and in distant sites where activation of clotting pathways may explain PM-induced increases in death from cardiovascular disease.

Indoor Air Pollution[44]

Worldwide, the most common source of household air pollution (HAP) is smoke produced by open fires used for cooking, leading to calls for improved cook stoves to reduce the use of indoor open fires.[45] The combustion of biomass fuels produces large amounts of particulate matter, and is associated with the development of respiratory morbidity, including respiratory infections in children.[46] Studies investigating whether cleaner-burning biomass stoves affect the incidence of childhood pneumonia are inconclusive, and reducing emissions from cooking

sources alone is unlikely to have major beneficial health effects unless as part of a more comprehensive clean air strategy.[47,48] In addition, the extent of HAP reduction required to produce a health benefit is unknown. Although the biological plausibility of a link between HAP and the development of COPD is strong, this also remains unproven, with large studies to date producing conflicting results.[49,50]

In the developed world, the effective heating systems and extensive insulation in most homes has led to dramatic changes in indoor air quality, relating to higher temperatures, higher humidity levels and reduced ventilation. It is estimated that most people spend in excess of 80% of their time indoors, so any indoor air pollution may have a considerable impact on public health. The respiratory effects of passive smoking were described earlier (page 238), and the impact of environmental radon exposure on lung cancer is discussed on page 356.

Indoor air quality generally reflects that of the outdoor air, except that O_3 levels are invariably low indoors because of the rapid reaction of O_3 with household synthetic materials. In addition to pollutants from outside, there are three specific indoor pollutants.

Allergens

Warm moist air, poor ventilation and extensive floor coverings provide ideal conditions for house dust mite infestation and the retention of numerous other allergens. This is believed to contribute to the recent upsurge in the prevalence of atopic diseases such as asthma, and is discussed in Chapter 28.

Carbon Monoxide

Malfunctions of heating equipment in the home may release CO into the indoor environment. Acute CO poisoning from this cause is common, and the occurrence of prolonged low-level exposure to indoor CO may be underestimated. Headache, malaise and flu-like symptoms are all features of long-term CO poisoning, although these symptoms are believed to be completely reversible once the exposure to CO is stopped. Smokers, who have permanently elevated carboxyhaemoglobin levels, appear to be resistant to these symptoms.

Nitrogen Dioxide

Gas-fired cookers, stoves and boilers all produce NO_2, the amount being dependent on the arrangements for waste gas exclusion. In this respect, gas cookers are the worst culprits, as they are rarely associated with chimneys and flues, and normally discharge their waste gases directly into the kitchen atmosphere. During cooking, NO_2 levels may reach over 750 μg.m^{-3}, which is well in excess of outdoor pollution targets (Table 20.1). Mild airway irritant effects are seen at levels of around 550 μg.m^{-3} in asthmatic subjects, or at 1800 μg.m^{-3} in nonasthmatic subjects. Clinically significant effects of long-term exposure include the worsening of asthma symptoms in children.[51]

References

1. Doll R, Hill AB. Smoking and carcinoma of the lung. *BMJ.* 1950;2:739-748.

2. Zwar NA, Mendelsohn CP, Richmond RL. Supporting smoking cessation. *BMJ.* 2014;348:f7535.

*3. **Frieden TR, Bloomberg MR. How to prevent 100 million deaths from tobacco. *Lancet.* 2007;369:1758-1761.**

4. DeMeo D. The recursive trek of epigenetics from the bench to the bedside. *Am J Respir Crit Care Med.* 2018;198:145-155.

5. Lu Q, Gottlieb E, Rounds S. Effects of cigarette smoke on epithelial cells. *Am J Physiol Lung Cell Mol Physiol.* 2018;314: L743-L756.

6. Kou YR, Kwong K, Lee L-Y. Airway inflammation and hypersensitivity induced by chronic smoking. *Respir Physiol Neurobiol.* 2011;178:395-405.

7. Hessel J, Heldrich J, Fuller J, et al. Intraflagellar transport gene expression associated with short cilia in smoking and COPD. *PLoS ONE.* 2014;9:e85453.

8. Kohansal R, Martinez-Camblor P, Agustí A, et al. The natural history of chronic airflow obstruction revisited. An analysis of the Framingham offspring cohort. *Am J Respir Crit Care Med.* 2009; 180:3-10.

9. Johnson CC, Wegienka GR. Cigarette exposure in very early life leads to persistent respiratory effects. *Am J Respir Crit Care Med.* 2014;189:380-381.

10. Le Souef PN. Adverse effects of maternal smoking during pregnancy on innate immunity in infants. *Eur Respir J.* 2006;28:675-677.

11. Schwilk B, Bothner U, Schraag S, et al. Perioperative respiratory events in smokers and nonsmokers undergoing general anaesthesia. *Acta Anaesthesiol Scand.* 1997;41:348-355.

12. Carrick M, Robson J, Thomas C. Smoking and anaesthesia. *Br J Anaesth Educ.* 2019;19:1-6.

13. Britton J. Electronic cigarettes and smoking cessation in England. *BMJ.* 2016;354:i4819.

14. Dinakar C, O'Connor G. The health effects of electronic cigarettes. *N Engl J Med.* 2016;375:1372-1381.

15. Hajek P, Phillips-Waller A, Przulj D, et al. A randomized trial of e-cigarettes versus nicotine-replacement therapy. *N Engl J Med.* 2019;380:629-637.

16. Chun L, Moazed F, Calfee C, et al. Pulmonary toxicity of e-cigarettes. *Am J Physiol Lung Cell Mol Physiol.* 2017;313:L193-L206.

17. Scott A, Lugg ST, Aldridge K, et al. Pro-inflammatory effects of e-cigarette vapour condensate on human alveolar macrophages. *Thorax.* 2018;73:1161-1169.

18. Garcia-Arcos I, Geraghty P, Baumlin N, et al. Chronic electronic cigarette exposure in mice induces features of COPD in a nicotine-dependent manner. *Thorax.* 2016;71:1119-1129.

19. McConnell R, Barrington-Trimis J, Wang K, et al. Electronic cigarette use and respiratory symptoms in adolescents. *Am J Respir Crit Care Med.* 2017;195:1043-1049.

20. Evans C, Dickey B, Schwartz D. E-cigarettes: mucus measurements make marks. *Am J Respir Crit Care Med.* 2018;197:420-421.

21. Strulovici-Barel Y, Omberg L, O'Mahony M, et al. Threshold of biologic responses of the small airway epithelium to low levels of tobacco smoke. *Am J Respir Crit Care Med.* 2010;182:1524-1532.

22. Landrigan P, Fuller R, Acosta N. The Lancet Commission on pollution and health. *Lancet.* 2018;391:462-512.

23. Stock S, Clemens T. Traffic pollution is linked to poor pregnancy outcomes. *BMJ.* 2017;359:j5511.

24. Paulin L, Hansel N. Physical activity and air pollution. *Am J Respir Crit Care Med.* 2016;194:786-787.

*25. **World Health Organization. *WHO Air quality guidelines for particulate matter, ozone, nitrogen dioxide and sulfur dioxide. Global update 2005. Summary of risk assessment.* Geneva: WHO; 2006.**

26. Health Effects Institute. *State of Global Air 2019. Special Report.* Boston MA: Health Effects Institute; 2019.

27. Anonymous. Short-lived climate pollutants: a focus for hot air? *Lancet.* 2015;386:1707.

28. Brauer M, Mancini GBJ. Where there's smoke . . . Poor air quality is an important contributor to cardiovascular risk. *BMJ.* 2014;348:g40.

29. Bhaskaran K, Armstrong B, Wilkinson P, et al. Air pollution as a carcinogen further strengthens the rationale for accelerating progress towards a low carbon economy. *BMJ.* 2013;347:f7607.

30. Beelen R, Raaschou-Nielsen O, Stafoggia M, et al. Effects of long-term exposure to air pollution on natural-cause mortality: an analysis of 22 European cohorts within the multicentre ESCAPE project. *Lancet.* 2014;383:785-795.

31. Dimakopoulou K, Samoli E, Beelen R, et al. Air pollution and nonmalignant respiratory mortality in 16 cohorts within the ESCAPE project. *Am J Respir Crit Care Med.* 2014;189:684-696.

32. Grigg J. Traffic-derived air pollution and lung function growth. *Am J Respir Crit Care Med.* 2012;186:1208-1209.

33. Grigg J. Air pollution and respiratory infection: an emerging and troubling association. *Am J Respir Crit Care Med.* 2018;198: 700-701.

34. Adam M, Schikowski T, Carsin A, et al. Adult lung function and long term air exposure. ESCAPE; a multicentre cohort study and meta-analysis. *Eur Respir J.* 2015;45:38-50.

35. Brunst K, Ryan P, Brokamp C, et al. Timing and duration of traffic-related air pollution exposure and the risk for childhood wheeze and asthma. *Am J Respir Crit Care Med.* 2015;192: 421-427.

36. Atkinson RW, Kang S, Anderson HR, et al. Epidemiological time series studies of PM2.5 and daily mortality and hospital admissions: a systematic review and meta-analysis. *Thorax.* 2014;69: 660-665.

37. Faustini A, Rapp R, Forastiere F. Nitrogen dioxide and mortality: review and meta-analysis of long-term studies. *Eur Respir J.* 2014; 44:744-753.

38. Jones RD, Commins BT, Cernik AA. Blood lead and carboxyhaemoglobin levels in London taxi drivers. *Lancet.* 1972;2:302-303.

39. Brunekreef B, Holgate ST. Air pollution and health. *Lancet.* 2002;360:1233-1242.

40. Hao Y, Balluz L, Strosnider H, et al. Ozone, fine particulate matter and chronic lower respiratory disease mortality in the United States. *Am J Respir Crit Care Med.* 2015;192:337-341.

41. Strickland M. Taking another look at ambient coarse particles. *Am J Respir Crit Care Med.* 2018;197:697-698.

42. Berger R, Ramaswami R, Solomon C, et al. Air pollution still kills. *N Engl J Med.* 2017;376:2591-2592.

43. Weichenthal S, Lavigne E, Evans, G et al. Fine particulate matter and emergency room visits for respiratory illness; effect modification by oxidative potential. *Am J Respir Crit Care Med.* 2016; 194:577-586.

44. Samet JM, Spengler JD. Indoor environments and health: moving into the 21st century. *Am J Public Health.* 2003;93:1489-1493.

45. Naeher LP. Biomass-fueled intervention stoves in the developing world. Potential and challenges. *Am J Respir Crit Care Med.* 2009; 180:586-587.

46. Emmelin A, Wall S. Indoor air pollution. A poverty-related cause of mortality among the children of the world. *Chest.* 2007; 132:1615-1623.

47. Gordon S, Mortimer K, Grigg J, et al. In control of ambient and household air pollution – how low should we go? *Lancet Respir Med.* 2017;5:918-919.

48. Sood A, Assad NA, Barnes PJ, et al. ERS/ATS workshop report on respiratory health effects of household air pollution. *Eur Respir J.* 2018;51:1700698.

49. Balmes J, Eisen E. Household air pollution and chronic obstructive airway disease. *Am J Respir Crit Care Med.* 2018;197:547-549.

50. van Zyl-Smit RN, Balmes JR. Seeing the wood for the trees: household air pollution and lung disease. *Am J Respir Crit Care Med.* 2019;199:264-265.

51. Belanger K, Gent JF, Triche EW, et al. Association of indoor nitrogen dioxide exposure with respiratory symptoms in children with asthma. *Am J Respir Crit Care Med.* 2006;173:297-303.

21

Anaesthesia

KEY POINTS

- All anaesthetic drugs reduce ventilation and impair the ventilatory response to both hypercapnia and hypoxia.
- Upper airway muscle function is inhibited by anaesthesia, leading to airway obstruction, usually at the level of the soft palate.
- Functional residual capacity is reduced within a few minutes of induction of anaesthesia as a result of altered respiratory muscle activity causing changes to the shape and volume of the thoracic cavity.

- Most patients develop small areas of atelectasis during anaesthesia, reexpansion of which requires high lung inflation pressures.
- Oxygenation is impaired by these changes, with wider scatter of ventilation/perfusion ($\dot{V}/\dot{Q}$) ratios along with increased alveolar dead space and pulmonary shunt.

Only 12 years after the first successful public demonstration of general anaesthesia in 1846, John Snow reported the pronounced changes that occur in respiration during the inhalation of chloroform.[1] Subsequent observations have confirmed that anaesthesia has profound effects on the respiratory system. However, these effects are diverse and highly specific; some aspects of respiratory function are profoundly modified, whereas others are scarcely affected at all.

Control of Breathing

Unstimulated Ventilation

It is well known that anaesthesia diminishes pulmonary ventilation, and hypercapnia is common if spontaneous breathing is preserved. Reduced minute volume is due partly to a reduction in metabolic demand, but mainly to interference with the chemical control of breathing, in particular a reduced sensitivity to carbon dioxide, as described later. In an uncomplicated anaesthetic there should not be sufficient resistance to breathing to affect the minute volume. However, the minute volume may be greatly decreased if there is respiratory obstruction.

At lower concentrations of inhaled anaesthetics, minute volume may remain unchanged, but smaller tidal volumes with higher respiratory frequency often occur resulting in reduced alveolar ventilation and an increase in $P\text{CO}_2$. With higher concentrations of anaesthetic, breathing becomes slower, and spontaneous minute volume may decrease to very low levels, particularly in the absence of surgical stimulation, and this will inevitably result in hypercapnia. Clearly

there is no limit to the rise that may occur if the anaesthetist is prepared to tolerate gross hypoventilation.

There are anaesthetists in many parts of the world who do not believe that temporary hypercapnia during anaesthesia is harmful to a healthy patient. Many hundreds of millions of patients must have been subjected to this transient physiological trespass since 1846, and there seems to be no convincing evidence of harm resulting from it—except perhaps increased surgical bleeding. In other parts of the world the departure from physiological normality is regarded with concern, and it is usual either to assist spontaneous respiration by manual compression of the reservoir bag or, more commonly, to paralyse and ventilate artificially as a routine.

Quite different conditions apply during anaesthesia with artificial ventilation. The minute volume can then be set at any level deemed appropriate by the anaesthetist, and in the past there was a tendency to hyperventilate patients, resulting in hypocapnia. Now that monitoring of end-expiratory $P\text{CO}_2$ is routine, artificial ventilation can be adjusted to maintain the preselected target $P\text{CO}_2$.

Effect on $P\text{CO}_2$/Ventilation Response Curve

Progressive increases in the alveolar concentration of all inhalational anaesthetic agents decrease the slope of the $P\text{CO}_2$/ventilation response curve, and, at deep levels of anaesthesia, there may be no response at all to $P\text{CO}_2$. Furthermore, the anaesthetized patient, as opposed to the awake subject, always becomes apnoeic if $P\text{CO}_2$ is reduced below the apnoeic threshold $P\text{CO}_2$ (page 50). In Figure 21.1, the purple flat curve rising to the left represents the starting points for various $P\text{CO}_2$/ventilation response curves. Without added

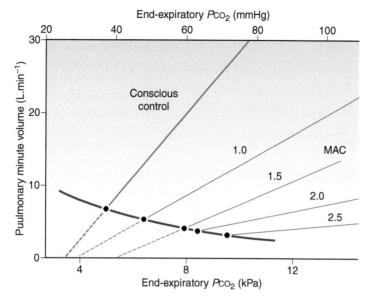

• **Fig. 21.1** Displacement of the P_{CO_2}/ventilation response curve with different end-expiratory concentrations of halothane. The purple curve sloping down to the right indicates the pathway of P_{CO_2} and ventilation change resulting from depression without the challenge of exogenous carbon dioxide. The broken lines indicate extrapolation to apnoeic threshold P_{CO_2}. MAC; Minimum alveolar concentration.

carbon dioxide in the inspired gas, deepening anaesthesia is associated with decreasing ventilation and a rising P_{CO_2}, and points moving progressively down and to the right. At intervals along this curve are shown P_{CO_2}/ventilation response curves resulting from adding carbon dioxide to the inspired gas.

At an equivalent depth of anaesthesia, currently available inhaled anaesthetics depress the ventilatory response to P_{CO_2} by a similar amount. This is conveniently shown by plotting the slope of the P_{CO_2}/ventilation response curve against equianaesthetic concentrations of different anaesthetics (Fig. 21.2), shown as multiples of minimum alveolar concentration (MAC), although the validity of using MAC multiples in this way has been questioned. With low doses of inhaled anaesthetics (0.2 MAC), there is almost no

depression of the hypercapnic ventilatory response,[2] in contrast to the response to hypoxia described later.

Surgical stimulation antagonizes the effect of anaesthesia on the P_{CO_2}/ventilation response curve. It may easily be observed that, in a spontaneously breathing patient, a surgical incision increases the ventilation, whatever the depth of anaesthesia. During prolonged anaesthesia without surgical stimulation, there is no progressive change in the response curve up to 3 hours. With the exception of ketamine, intravenous anaesthetics have a similar effect on ventilation as inhalational anaesthetics.

Effect on P_{O_2}/Ventilation Response Curve[3,4]

The normal relationship between P_{O_2} and ventilation was described on pages 50 et seq. It was long believed that this reflex was the ultimum moriens and, unlike the P_{CO_2}/ventilation response curve, unaffected by anaesthesia. This doctrine was a source of comfort to many generations of anaesthetists until the 1970s, when halothane anaesthesia was shown to reduce the acute hypoxic ventilatory response (AHVR) in humans. It was soon shown that not only was the hypoxic response affected by inhalational anaesthetics it was also, in fact, exquisitely sensitive (Fig. 21.3).[5] Hypoxic drive was markedly attenuated at 0.1 MAC, a level of anaesthesia that would not be reached for a considerable time during recovery from anaesthesia. Similar effects were found with all the currently used inhalational agents and propofol.[3]

These findings were widely accepted for some years, until a study by Temp et al.[6] in 1992 showed that AHVR was only diminished in hypercapnic conditions. This study initiated a

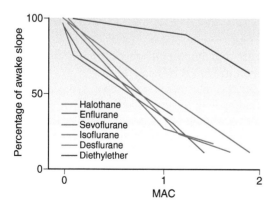

• **Fig. 21.2** Relative depression of the ventilatory response to CO_2 by different inhalational anaesthetics as a function of minimum alveolar concentration (MAC).

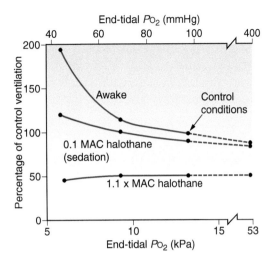

• **Fig. 21.3** Effect of halothane anaesthesia on the ventilatory response to hypoxia. The data shown in this figure have now been challenged; see text for details. *MAC*, Minimum alveolar concentration. (From reference 12.)

great deal of further research. A summary of the findings of these and many other studies are shown in Figure 21.4. The most notable feature of these results is their diversity, with, for example, different studies of similar concentrations of isoflurane, particularly at sedative levels, resulting in completely opposite results. However, for the other agents there does seem to be a generally dose-dependent depression of the hypoxic ventilatory response, although at 0.1 MAC considerable variation remains. There are many possible explanations for these results, mostly relating to methodological differences between studies:

Anaesthetic agent. Differences between anaesthetic agents in their effects on AHVR are not obvious from Figure 21.4. However, a quantitative review of 37 studies did find differences, with the least depression of the response by low-dose sevoflurane, progressively increasing depression

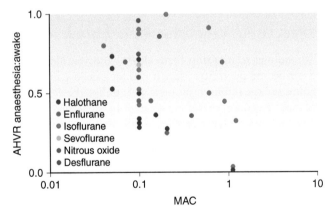

• **Fig. 21.4** Summary of studies of the acute hypoxic ventilatory response and inhalational anaesthesia or sedation. The ordinate is the ratio of the increase in minute volume with hypoxia during anaesthesia or sedation and the awake (control) response. Thus a ratio of unity represents no depression of the response, and zero represents a completely abolished response. All studies were performed under isocapnic conditions, except the two green circles which used poikilocapnia with isoflurane. See text for details. *AHVR*, Acute hypoxic ventilatory response; *MAC*, minimum alveolar concentration.

by isoflurane and enflurane, with halothane having the greatest effect.[3]

Subject stimulation. The degree of arousal of subjects is known to affect the AHVR. Studies of hypoxic response at 'sedative' levels of anaesthesia ($\leq$0.2 MAC) differed in the amount of stimulation provided, with some forcing the subjects to remain awake and others leaving subjects undisturbed. Although not a significant factor in determining the overall degree of depression of AHVR by inhaled anaesthetics, subject stimulation may be a factor for some anaesthetic agents at low concentrations.

Hypoxic challenge. The rate of onset, degree and duration of hypoxia can all affect the ventilatory response, which is normally biphasic, with hypoxic ventilatory decline (HVD) occurring a few minutes after the onset of hypoxia (see Fig. 4.7). Some studies of AHVR used rapid 'step' changes into hypoxic conditions, whereas others used a 'ramp' onset of hypoxia over several minutes, such that the response under the latter conditions will be a combination of AHVR and HVD. However, the hypoxic stimulus used does not seem to be a major influence on the response, and HVD seems to be uninfluenced by anaesthesia.

Carbon dioxide concentration. This may be maintained at normal, prehypoxic, levels (isocapnia) or allowed to find its own level (poikilocapnia). This has a large effect in the awake subject, with the hypoxic response greatly attenuated during poikilocapnia (see Fig. 4.7). During anaesthesia with up to 0.85 MAC isoflurane, the hypoxic ventilatory response during poikilocapnia is essentially maintained; that is, the increase in ventilation with hypoxic challenge is the same when asleep as when awake. This has led to the suggestion that anaesthesia has less effect on the hypoxic ventilatory response itself, but may reduce the normally additive interaction between the ventilatory responses to hypoxia and hypercapnia (see Fig. 4.8).[7]

It is generally agreed that the effect of anaesthetics on AHVR is on the peripheral chemoreceptors, possibly exclusively so at sedative levels.[8]

Implications of the Depression of Acute Hypoxic Ventilatory Response by Anaesthetic Agents

There are four important practical implications of the attenuation of AHVR by anaesthesia:

1. Patients cannot act as their own hypoxia alarm by responding with hyperventilation.
2. Patients who already have a reduced sensitivity to $P\text{CO}_2$ (e.g., some patients with chronic respiratory failure) may stop breathing after induction of anaesthesia has abolished their hypoxic drive.
3. Anaesthesia may be dangerous at very high altitude or in other situations where survival depends on hyperventilation in response to hypoxia (Chapter 16).
4. Because hypoxic drive is obtunded at subanaesthetic concentrations, this effect will persist into the early

postoperative period after patients have regained consciousness and are apparently able to fend for themselves.

This uncertainty about the effect of subanaesthetic concentrations on AHVR casts doubt on the validity of extrapolating the results of earlier studies to patients recovering from anaesthesia. The degree of stimulation of patients is likely to affect their AHVR, which will therefore be affected by many factors such as pain control and the amount of activity in their surroundings. A patient should behave like a poikilocapnic subject, and so depression of AHVR will be minimal.[3,7] Finally, patients recovering from an anaesthetic will frequently be hypercapnic secondary to opioid administration, sometimes compounded by airway obstruction. Under these circumstances the ventilatory response to the combination of hypoxia and hypercapnia is almost certainly reduced to less than that seen when awake. Although doubt has been cast on the relevance of the earlier studies of Knill and Gelb[5] (Fig. 21.3), there remains ample evidence that a sleeping patient in the recovery room is at risk of failing to mount a suitable ventilatory response to hypoxia.

Pattern of Contraction of Respiratory Muscles

One of the most remarkable examples of the specificity of anaesthetic actions is on the muscles associated with respiration. Many of these effects could hardly have been predicted, but, nevertheless, have great clinical importance, and underlie many of the secondary effects described later in this chapter.

Pharynx

Anaesthesia usually causes obstruction of the pharyngeal airway unless measures are taken for its protection. Figure 21.5 shows changes in the sagittal geometry of the pharynx immediately after induction of anaesthesia with thiopentone in the supine position. The soft palate falls against the posterior pharyngeal wall, occluding the nasopharynx in almost every patient, presumably due to interference with the action of some or all of the pharyngeal muscles (page 59). Similar findings are also reported using magnetic resonance imaging, when the mean anteroposterior diameter of the pharynx at the level of the soft palate decreased from 6.6 mm when awake to 2.7 mm during propofol anaesthesia.[9] Radiographic studies have shown considerable posterior movement of tongue and epiglottis, but usually not sufficient to occlude the oral or hypopharyngeal airway (Fig. 21.5).

Secondary changes occur when the patient attempts to breathe. Upstream obstruction then often causes major passive downstream collapse of the entire pharynx (Fig. 21.6), a mechanism with features in common with the sleep apnoea/hypopnoea syndrome (page 193). This secondary collapse of the pharynx is due to interference with the normal action of pharyngeal dilator muscles, particularly the

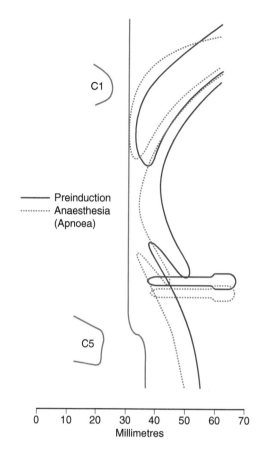

- **Fig. 21.5** Median sagittal section of the pharynx to show changes between the conscious state (*continuous red lines*) and following induction of anaesthesia (*broken blue lines*). The most consistent change was occlusion of the nasopharynx. (From Nandi PR, Charlesworth CH, Taylor SJ, et al. Effect of general anaesthesia on the pharynx. *Br J Anaesth*. 1991;66:157-162. With permission of the Editor of the *British Journal of Anaesthesia* and Oxford University Press.)

genioglossus. The epiglottis may be involved in hypopharyngeal obstruction during anaesthesia, and posterior movement is clearly seen in Figures 21.5 and 21.6.

Maintenance of Pharyngeal Airway Patency

Extension of the neck moves the origin of the genioglossus anteriorly by 1 to 2 cm, and usually clears the hypopharyngeal airway. Protrusion of the mandible moves the origin of genioglossus still further forward. The use of a pharyngeal airway, such as that of Guedel, is frequently helpful, but the tip may become lodged in the vallecula, or the tongue may be pushed downwards and backwards to obstruct the tip of the airway. In current practice for most unintubated patients the laryngeal mask airway (LMA) is used, and provides an airtight seal around the laryngeal perimeter, allowing spontaneous ventilation. None of these methods provide protection from regurgitated gastric contents, in which case a tracheal tube is required.

Inspiratory Muscles

John Snow's early observations of respiration during anaesthesia describe that a decrease in thoracic respiratory excursion

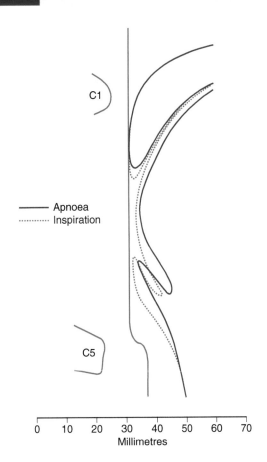

C1

——— Apnoea
.... Inspiration

C5

| 0 | 10 | 20 | 30 | 40 | 50 | 60 | 70 |

Millimetres

• **Fig. 21.6** Median sagittal section of the pharynx during anaesthesia to show changes between the apnoeic state (*continuous red lines*, corresponding to the broken blue lines in Fig. 21.5) and following attempted inspiration (*broken blue lines*). Upstream obstruction in the nasopharynx results in downstream collapse of the oropharynx and hypopharynx. (From Nandi PR, Charlesworth CH, Taylor SJ, et al. Effect of general anaesthesia on the pharynx. *Br J Anaesth.* 1991;66:157-162. With permission of the Editor of the *British Journal of Anaesthesia* and Oxford University Press.)

may be used as a sign of deepening anaesthesia, and selective depression of some inspiratory rib cage muscles does indeed occur. Electromyography (EMG) of the parasternal intercostal muscles in humans shows their activity to be consistently abolished by 1 MAC of anaesthesia and absent in some subjects at just 0.2 MAC.[10] Thiopentone decreases the EMG activity of the sternothyroid, sternohyoid and scalene muscles, whereas diaphragmatic function seems to be well-preserved during anaesthesia, particularly phasic EMG activity during inspiration. This combination of changes in muscle activity commonly gives rise to paradoxical inspiratory movements in which diaphragmatic contraction causes expansion of the lower rib cage and abdomen while the upper rib cage is drawn in due to the negative intrathoracic pressure and a lack of support from upper rib cage respiratory muscles. This pattern of breathing is seen commonly in children, who have a more compliant chest wall than adults, and in adults when respiratory resistance is increased causing a greater fall in intrathoracic pressure. Some studies have, however, found no

reduction in rib cage movement with, for example, isoflurane at 1 MAC,[11] and it is possible that changes in spinal curvature during anaesthesia caused earlier studies of rib cage movement to overestimate the changes.[12] Thus earlier descriptions of selective depression of rib cage movement should not be regarded as an invariable feature of anaesthesia with spontaneous ventilation, particularly at the depth of anaesthesia used clinically and with a low-resistance, unobstructed airway.

The resting position and dimensions of the rib cage and diaphragm during anaesthesia are described next.

Expiratory Muscles[13]

General anaesthesia causes expiratory phasic activity of the abdominal muscles, which are normally silent in the conscious supine subject. Anaesthetic agents, opioids[14] and hypercapnia are all involved in stimulating the expiratory muscle activity. This activity begins in some subjects at only 0.2 MAC of halothane,[10] and is very difficult to abolish as long as spontaneous breathing continues. Activation of expiratory muscles seems to serve no useful purpose and does not appear to have any significant effect on the change in functional residual capacity (FRC).

Respiratory muscle coordination often becomes disturbed during anaesthesia with spontaneous ventilation.[11,15] Paradoxical movements between the upper and lower chest wall, and the chest and abdominal muscles, are accompanied by changes in respiratory timing between inspiratory and expiratory muscle groups. These are believed to originate in selective effects of anaesthesia on different respiratory neuronal groups in the central pattern generator, and are more marked when airway resistance is higher.[15] The most usual pattern seen is a phase delay between abdominal and rib cage movement, as illustrated in Figure 21.7.

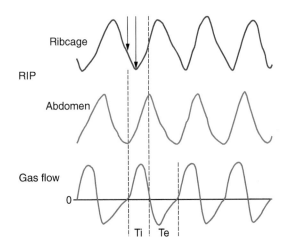

Ribcage

RIP

Abdomen

Gas flow

0

Ti   Te

• **Fig. 21.7** Respiratory inductance plethysmography (RIP) tracings of rib cage and abdominal movements during 1.5 minimum alveolar concentration halothane anaesthesia in children, and the accompanying respiratory gas flows. Note the phase delay between abdominal and rib cage movements, indicated by solid arrows, which in the example shown is approximately 30% of the inspiratory time. Ti, Inspiratory time; Te, expiratory time. (From reference 31, with permission of the authors and the publishers of *Anesthesiology*.)

Change in Functional Residual Capacity

In 1963 Bergman was the first to report a decrease of FRC during anaesthesia.[16] The reduction in FRC is now known to have the following characteristics:

- FRC is reduced during anaesthesia with all anaesthetic drugs that have been investigated, by a mean value of about 15% to 20% of the awake FRC in the supine position, although there is considerable individual variation.
- FRC is reduced immediately on induction of anaesthesia, reaches its final value within the first few minutes and does not seem to fall progressively throughout anaesthesia. It does not return to normal until some hours after the end of anaesthesia.
- FRC is reduced to the same extent during anaesthesia whether the patient is paralysed or not.
- The reduction in FRC has a weak but significant correlation with the age of the patient.
- The reduction in FRC is greater in obese patients.[17]

Cause of the Reduction in FRC[18]

There is general agreement that three factors may contribute to the reduced FRC, as follows.

Chest shape. Computed tomography (CT) scanners first demonstrated that, during anaesthesia, there is a reduction in the cross-sectional area of the rib cage corresponding to a decrease in lung volume of about 200 mL.[19] Improved CT scanning technology subsequently allowed scans of half the chest to be obtained in just 0.3 seconds, followed by three-dimensional (3D) reconstruction and analysis of the volume of chest structures.[10] These studies confirmed that changes in chest-wall shape account for a reduction in FRC of about 200 mL. There is less agreement about why the chest wall changes shape; possible explanations include the changes in respiratory muscle activity already described, diaphragmatic position and activity or spinal curvature.

Diaphragm position. In the conscious subject in the supine position there is residual end-expiratory tone in the diaphragm, which prevents the weight of the abdominal viscera pushing the diaphragm too far into the chest in the supine position. In the early 1970s Froese and Bryan demonstrated that, under anaesthesia, the dependent part of the diaphragm is displaced cephalad,[20] whereas little or no movement of the nondependent regions occurs.[19] Studies using 3D reconstructions of CT scans confirmed that diaphragm shape rather than position alters during anaesthesia.[18,21] The change in FRC that can be ascribed to changes in diaphragm shape is on average less than 30 mL.[10] A summary of the changes in chest wall and diaphragm positions during anaesthesia is shown in Figure 21.8.

Thoracic blood volume. A shift of blood from the peripheral circulation into the chest during anaesthesia has been postulated as a cause of reduced FRC,[22] although this

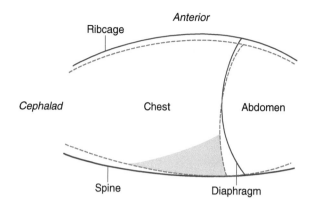

• **Fig. 21.8** Schematic diagram showing a midsagittal section of the chest wall and diaphragm awake (*solid red line*) and during anaesthesia (*dashed blue line*). Note the reduction in rib cage volume, the increased spinal curvature and the change in diaphragmatic position. The shaded area shows where atelectasis usually occurs during anaesthesia.

observation has not been confirmed[10] and is currently regarded as an unlikely contributory factor.

Atelectasis During Anaesthesia[18]

'Miliary atelectasis' during anaesthesia was first proposed by Bendixen et al. in 1963 as an explanation of the increased alveolar/arterial Po_2 difference during anaesthesia.[23] Conventional radiography, however, failed to show any appreciable areas of collapse, presumably because of most atelectasis being behind the diaphragm on anteroposterior radiographs (see next). Hedenstierna's group in Sweden was the first to demonstrate pulmonary opacities on CT scans of subjects during anaesthesia. These opacities usually occurred in the dependent areas of lung just above the diaphragm, and were termed 'compression atelectasis'. Their extent correlated very strongly with the calculated intrapulmonary shunt, and animal studies showed that the areas of opacity had a typical histological appearance of collapsed lung.[24] More recently, lung ultrasonography has been used to demonstrate areas of atelectasis in the basal and dependent areas of the lung which correlated moderately to hypoxia, as calculated by a $Pa_{O_2}/F_{I_{O_2}}$ ratio of less than 300.[25]

Atelectasis occurs in between 75% and 90% of healthy individuals having general anaesthesia with muscle paralysis (Fig. 21.9), and persists into the postoperative period in a similar percentage.[26] It is unrelated to patient age. Atelectasis is most easily quantified from a single CT scan slice, taken immediately above the dome of the right diaphragm, and is expressed as the percentage of the cross-sectional area containing atelectasis. The percentage of atelectasis during anaesthesia recorded in this way seems small, usually around 3%, but the atelectatic areas contain many more alveoli per unit volume than aerated lung, and this 3% of cross-sectional area equates to around 10% of lung tissue.[27]

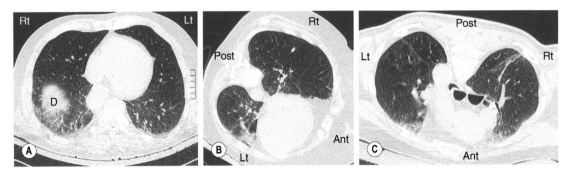

• **Fig. 21.9** Computed tomography (CT) of transverse sections of the thoracic cage in three patients in different positions during general anaesthesia. **(A)** Supine position. **(B)** Semilateral position. **(C)** Prone position. Increased lung density because of atelectasis is seen in the dependent regions of the lungs, irrespective of the patient's position. Note that in CT scans of the chest the patient is being viewed from the feet. *Rt*, Right; *Lt*, left; *Post*, posterior; *Ant*, anterior; *D*, diaphragm.

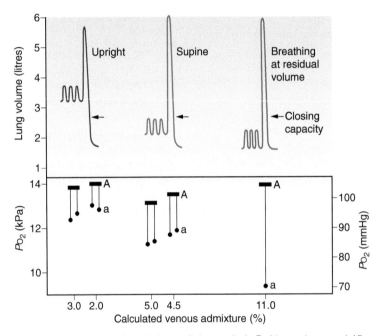

• **Fig. 21.10** Changes in tidal excursion relative to vital capacity in Dr Nunn when aged 45 years; arrows indicate the closing capacity. Ideal alveolar *(A)* P_{O_2} is shown by the horizontal bar, and arterial *(a)* P_{O_2} by the black circles. Venous admixture was calculated on the assumption of an arterial/mixed venous oxygen content difference of 5 mL.dL^{-1}. (From Nunn JF. Measurement of closing volume. *Acta Anaesthiol Scand Suppl.* 1978;70:154-160. With permission of the editors of *Acta Anaesthesiologica Scandinavica*.)

Causes of Atelectasis

There are three mechanisms involved, all closely interrelated, and it is likely that all three are involved in the formation of atelectasis in vivo.

Airway closure as a result of the reduced FRC may lead to atelectasis. In the supine position, the expiratory reserve volume has a mean value of approximately 1 L in males and 600 mL in females. Therefore the reduction in FRC following the induction of anaesthesia will bring the lung volume close to residual volume. This will tend to reduce the end-expiratory lung volume below the closing capacity (CC), particularly in older patients (see Fig. 2.11), resulting in airway closure and collapse of lung. Pulmonary atelectasis can easily be demonstrated in conscious

subjects who voluntarily breathe oxygen close to residual volume, and Figure 21.10 shows the effect on arterial P_{O_2} of simulating the reduction in FRC that occurs during anaesthesia. Even if lung collapse does not occur, the airway narrowing caused by reduced lung volume creates areas with low $\dot{V}/\dot{Q}$ ratios that contribute to impaired gas exchange.[28]

An important aspect of this problem is any change to CC during anaesthesia. Early studies suggested that CC remained constant, but subsequent work concluded that FRC and CC are both reduced in parallel following the induction of anaesthesia.[29] It is possible that bronchodilation caused by the anaesthetic (see later) counteracts the reduction in airway calibre that would be expected to result from the reduction in FRC.

Compression atelectasis may occur because of changes in chest wall and diaphragm position, which lead to the transmission of high intraabdominal pressure to the chest and compression of areas of lung. As shown in Figure 21.9 the predominantly dependent distribution of atelectasis also points to a role for changes in the position of the dependent regions of the diaphragm.

Absorption atelectasis develops when an airway becomes partially or totally closed and the gas contained within the pulmonary units distal to the airway is absorbed into the blood. Absorption of gas does not cause atelectasis, but in effect accelerates collapse should airway narrowing or closure occur from either of the preceding mechanisms. The rapid uptake of oxygen into the blood makes an important contribution to the development of absorption atelectasis (see the following section).

Prevention of Atelectasis[30]

Recognition of atelectasis during anaesthesia has led to great interest in ways to prevent its occurrence. Several interesting findings have emerged.

Inspired Oxygen Concentration

Administration of high concentrations of oxygen during anaesthesia would be expected to promote atelectasis, and there is evidence for this at a variety of stages during a general anaesthetic.

- *Preoxygenation.* An F_{IO_2} of 1.0 immediately before induction of anaesthesia leads to significantly more atelectasis than in patients with an F_{IO_2} of 0.3 or 0.21 during induction.[31] The crucial F_{IO_2} for worsening atelectasis seems to be greater than 0.6, as a study comparing an F_{IO_2} of 1.0, 0.8 or 0.6 found cross-sectional areas of atelectasis on CT scans following induction of 5.6%, 1.3% and 0.2%, respectively.[32]
- *Maintenance.* Following reexpansion of atelectasis during anaesthesia (see later), a high F_{IO_2} causes a more rapid recurrence of atelectasis.[33] However, it remains unclear whether a high F_{IO_2} during anaesthesia causes postoperative respiratory problems. Two studies have compared maintenance of anaesthesia with a F_{IO_2} of 0.3 or greater than or equal to 0.8, and found no differences in postoperative oxygenation in the first 24 hours.[34,35]
- *Before extubation.* Use of a F_{IO_2} of 1.0 before removal of the tracheal tube at the completion of surgery is associated with more CT-demonstrated atelectasis in the immediate postoperative period.[36]

Using 100% inspired oxygen before, during and at the conclusion of a general anaesthetic therefore seems to be associated with more pulmonary atelectasis. These observations have led to the suggestion that it is time to challenge the routine use of 100% oxygen during anaesthesia.[37] Anaesthetists use 100% oxygen before induction and extubation to provide a longer time period before hypoxia occurs, should there be difficulty in maintaining a patent airway. However, this safety period will be shortened only slightly by preoxygenating with an F_{IO_2} of 0.8, the use of which may significantly reduce the amount of atelectasis that occurs.[32]

Nitrous Oxide

Mathematical modelling of the rate at which absorption atelectasis occurs suggests that using N_2O rather than N_2 with oxygen is unimportant.[38] Looking at diffusion of gases into and out of a closed lung unit, this model finds that the diffusion of N_2O into the lung unit from the mixed venous blood is faster than the diffusion of N_2 out of the lung unit, so its volume is maintained and collapse prevented. The in vivo situation is clearly more complex. Partial pressures of N_2O in lung units and blood are rarely in a steady state, and the time at which lung units become closed will vary, causing unpredictable effects of N_2O on atelectasis (page 350).

Positive Airway Pressures

Application of a tight-fitting face mask to the patient before induction allows the use of continuous positive airway pressure (CPAP) before the patient is asleep, and positive end-expiratory pressure (PEEP) after induction. Using low levels of CPAP (6 cmH2O) before induction has been shown to abolish the formation of atelectasis,[39] and also to prolong the time taken for oxygen saturation to fall to 90% during the apnoea that normally follows induction of anaesthesia.[40]

During maintenance of anaesthesia, moderate levels of PEEP (10 cmH2O) prevent the occurrence of atelectasis following a reexpansion manoeuvre (see later). Use of PEEP (7–9 cmH2O) alone has been shown to reduce atelectasis occurrence in healthy subjects undergoing nonabdominal surgery,[41] although much higher levels are needed to reexpand existing atelectasis.

At emergence from anaesthesia it seems to be more difficult to prevent the development of impaired oxygenation in the postanaesthesia care unit, which is normally presumed to be because of atelectasis. The amount of coughing on the tracheal tube before extubation does not influence early postoperative oxygenation,[42] and use of CPAP before extubation is also ineffective.[43] A study in patients with lung disease found that use of a F_{IO_2} of 1.0 rather than 0.3 before extubation was associated with worse gas exchange at 60 minutes postoperatively, but this was felt by the authors to have resulted from changes to pulmonary blood flow and not atelectasis.[44]

Reexpansion of Atelectasis

Two methods have been described to reexpand collapsed areas of lung, and these recruitment manoeuvres (RMs) are shown in Figure 21.11.

Continuous Positive Airway Pressure Manoeuvres

The first RM reported to reexpand atelectasis consisted of a series of hyperinflation manoeuvres using three breaths to an airway pressure of 30 cmH2O followed by a final breath to

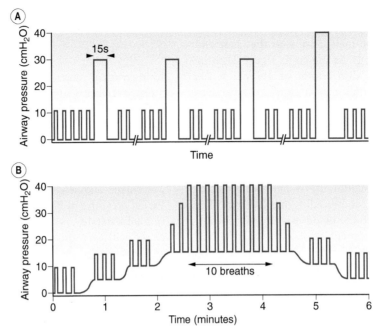

• **Fig. 21.11** Schematic representation of manoeuvres to reexpand atelectasis during anaesthesia. **(A)** Vital capacity manoeuvre involving three large breaths sufficient to achieve airway pressures of 30 cmH$_2$O followed by a single breath to 40 cmH$_2$O, each sustained for 15 s. The breaks on the abscissa represent 3 to 5 minutes of intermittent positive pressure ventilation with normal tidal volume. **(B)** Positive end-expiratory pressure (PEEP) and large tidal volumes showing progressive application of PEEP up to 15 cmH$_2$O, followed by increased tidal volume until a peak airway pressure of 40 cmH$_2$O or tidal volume of 18 mL.kg^{-1} is achieved, which is then maintained for 10 breaths. (From Rothen HU, Sporre B, Engberg G, et al. Reexpansion of atelectasis during general anaesthesia: a computed tomography study. *Br J Anaesth.* 1993;71:788-795 and Tusman G, Böhm SH, Vazquez de Anda GF, et al. 'Alveolar recruitment strategy' improves arterial oxygenation during general anaesthesia. *Br J Anaesth.* 1999;82:8-13. With permission of the authors and Oxford University Press.)

40 cmH$_2$O, each sustained for 15 seconds (Fig. 21.11, *A*). Between these large breaths normal intermittent positive pressure ventilation was continued for 3 to 5 minutes. CT scanning during this manoeuvre shows that the first hyperinflation of 30 cmH$_2$O reduces the area of atelectasis by half, and the subsequent inflations to 30 cmH$_2$O have little additional effect, but the final breath to 40 cmH$_2$O completely reexpands the atelectasis. Subsequent work by the same group showed that the inflation pressure of 40 cmH$_2$O did not need to be sustained for 15 seconds, with half of the atelectasis reexpanded after only 2 seconds, and all the atelectasis reexpanded after 7 to 8 seconds in three-quarters of patients.[45]

Positive End-Expiratory Pressure

High levels of PEEP are required to reexpand atelectasis. Also, resolution of atelectasis is not complete, and collapse recurs within minutes when PEEP is discontinued.[46] In addition, high levels of PEEP cause significant changes to $\dot{V}/\dot{Q}$ relationships within the lung and may not improve oxygenation. Increasing levels of PEEP are more useful if used in conjunction with large tidal volumes. One widely accepted technique involves stepwise increases in PEEP levels to 15 cmH$_2$O or 20 cmH$_2$O, and then tidal volume is increased until peak airway pressures of 40 cmH$_2$O are achieved (Fig. 21.11, *B*).

In both these techniques for reexpansion of atelectasis, airway pressures reach 40 cmH$_2$O. An airway pressure this high is not without risk, including the possibility of pulmonary barotrauma (Chapter 32) or cardiovascular disturbance. It is therefore good practice to interrupt the RM if mean blood pressure or heart rate change by more than 20% during the procedure. Similarly to PEEP, these RMs reduce intrapulmonary shunt, but increase $\dot{V}/\dot{Q}$ mismatch, such that there is often only a small improvement in oxygenation (see later).

Respiratory Mechanics[47]

Calibre of the lower airways

Effect of Reduced Functional Residual Capacity

Figures 3.5 and 21.12 both show the hyperbolic relationship between lung volume and airway resistance. Figure 21.12 clearly shows that the curve is steep in the region of FRC in the supine position; therefore the reduction in FRC that occurs during anaesthesia might be expected to result in a marked increase in airway resistance. However, most anaesthetics may have some bronchodilator effect, as outlined in the following paragraph, and this effect almost exactly offsets the effect of reduction in lung volume. Thus

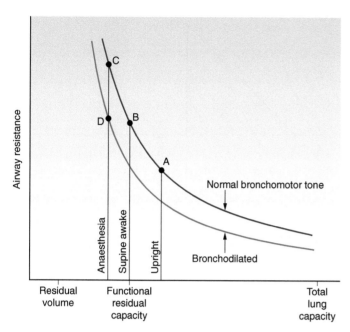

• **Fig. 21.12** Airway resistance as a function of lung volume with normal bronchomotor tone and when bronchodilated. *A,* Upright and awake; *B,* supine and awake; *C,* supine and anaesthetized without bronchodilation; *D,* supine, anaesthetized and with the degree of bronchodilatation that normally occurs during anaesthesia. Note that the airway resistance is similar at *B* and *D,* bronchodilation approximately compensating for the decrease in functional residual capacity.

total respiratory system resistance during anaesthesia is only slightly greater than in the awake supine subject, most of the change occurring in the lung/airway components rather than the chest wall (Table 21.1).

Inhalational Anaesthetics

All inhalational anaesthetics may act as bronchodilators by direct relaxation of airway smooth muscle,[48] suppression of airway vagal reflexes or inhibition of the release of

bronchoconstrictor mediators. In healthy patients, results from studies of modern inhalational anaesthetics are variable, with some demonstrating reduced resistance at 1 MAC[49] and others finding no effect.[50] Desflurane may even increase airway resistance, particularly at high MAC values, and probably because of increased gas density.[50] Therefore it appears that inhaled anaesthetic agents at clinically used concentrations have little effect as bronchodilators acting directly on the airway, and that when used clinically to overcome increased airway resistance from asthma, smoking, and soon, they are more likely to be working simply by suppression of airway reflexes.

Intravenous anaesthetics have effects similar to inhalational anaesthetics. Their direct effects on smooth muscle are mostly weak in comparison with inhaled agents, and in clinical practice their ability to attenuate neural reflex bronchoconstriction predominates.

Other Sites of Increased Airway Resistance

Breathing systems. Excessive resistance or obstruction may arise in apparatus such as breathing systems, valves, connectors and tracheal tubes. The tubes may be kinked, the lumen may be blocked or the cuff may herniate and obstruct the lower end, which may also abut against the carina or the side wall of the trachea. A reduction in diameter of a tracheal tube greatly increases its resistance; the pattern of flow is intermediate between laminar and turbulent for the conditions shown in Figure 21.13. With artificial ventilation this high resistance increases gas velocity, which affects the distribution of inspired gas within the lung, depending on the position and direction of the tracheal tube in the airway (Fig. 21.14).[51] Resistance imposed by an LMA is less than that of a corresponding size of tracheal tube.[52]

Pharynx and larynx. The pharynx is commonly obstructed during anaesthesia by the mechanisms described earlier in this

TABLE 21.1 Respiratory Mechanics During Anaesthesia

Compliance (Static)	Anaesthetized		Awake Normal Range	
	L.kPa⁻¹	mL.cmH₂O⁻¹	L.kPa⁻¹	mL.cmH₂O⁻¹
Respiratory system	0.81	81	0.5–1.9	47–190
Lungs	1.5	150	0.9–4.0	90–400
Chest wall	2.0	203	1.0–3.5	100–350
Resistance	kPa.L⁻¹.s	cmH₂O.L⁻¹.s	kPa.L⁻¹.s	cmH₂O.L⁻¹.s
Respiratory system	0.48	4.8	0.12–0.44	1.2–4.4
Lung tissue/airway	0.35	3.5	0.07–0.24	0.7–2.4
Chest wall	0.13	1.3	0.05–0.20	0.5–2.0

(Data during anaesthesia are in the supine position from Pelosi P, Croci M, Calappi E, et al. The prone position during general anesthesia minimally affects respiratory mechanics while improving functional residual capacity and increasing oxygen tension. *Anesth Analg.* 1995;80:955-960.)

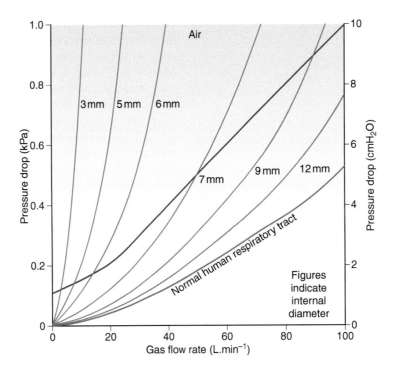

• **Fig. 21.13** Flow rate/pressure drop plots of a range of tracheal tubes, with their connectors and catheter mounts. The heavy purple line is the author's suggested upper limit of acceptable resistance for an adult. Pressure drop does not quite increase according to the fourth power of the radius because the catheter mount offers the same resistance throughout the range of tubes. With 70% N_2O/30% O_2, the pressure drop is about 40% greater for the same gas flow rate when flow is turbulent but is little different when the flow is chiefly laminar.

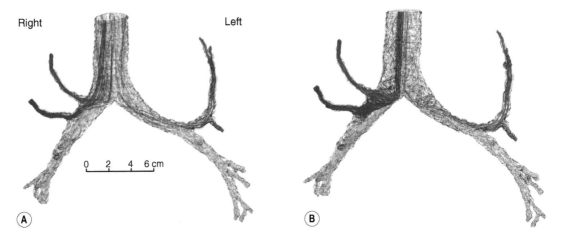

• **Fig. 21.14** Computational fluid dynamic modelling of gas flow in the airway using a three-dimensional mathematical model of a human airway derived from computed tomography scans. **(A)** No tracheal tube in place; **(B)** an 8-mm internal diameter tracheal tube centrally placed in the trachea 4 cm proximal to the carina. The coloured lines are streamlines of gas flow, each colour corresponding to the lung lobe which the gas finally enters. Note that the gas exiting the tracheal tube forms a high velocity jet, resulting in turbulence in the airway. Gas flow rate for both drawings is a constant 30 L.min⁻¹, corresponding to normal peak inspiratory flow. (**(B)** From reference 90, with permission of the publishers of *Anaesthesia*.)

chapter, unless active steps are taken to preserve patency. Reflex laryngospasm is still possible at depths of anaesthesia that suppress other airway protective reflexes. In most cases the spasm eventually resolves spontaneously, but it may be improved by application of CPAP or terminated by deepening anaesthesia or neuromuscular blockade.

Compliance

Total respiratory system compliance is reduced during anaesthesia to a figure approaching the lower end of the normal range (Table 21.1). Both static and dynamic measurements (page 24) are reduced compared with the awake

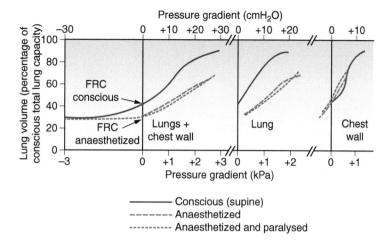

• **Fig. 21.15** Pressure/volume relationships before and after the induction of anaesthesia and paralysis. The first section shows the relationship for the respiratory system (lungs and chest wall). The second and third sections represent the lungs and the chest wall, respectively. There are only insignificant differences between observations during anaesthesia with and without paralysis. There are, however, major differences in pressure/volume relationships of the lung and total respiratory system following the induction of anaesthesia. Arrows indicate the functional residual capacity, which, during anaesthesia, is only slightly greater than the residual volume. *FRC*, Functional residual capacity. (From Westbrook PR, Stubbs SE, Sessler AD, et al. Effects of anesthesia and muscle paralysis on respiratory mechanics in normal man. *J Appl Physiol.* 1973;34:81-86.)

state. Compliance seems to be reduced very early in anaesthesia, and the change is not progressive.

Figure 21.15 summarizes the effect of anaesthesia on the pressure/volume relationships of the lung and chest wall. The diagram shows the major differences between the conscious state and anaesthesia. There are only minor differences between anaesthesia with and without paralysis. The left-hand section shows the relationship for the whole respiratory system comprising lungs plus chest wall. The curves obtained during anaesthesia clearly show the reduction in FRC (lung volume with zero-pressure gradient from alveoli to ambient). Application of a positive pressure as high as 30 cmH$_2$O (3 kPa) to the airways expands the lungs to barely 70% of the preoperative total lung capacity, which implies a reduced overall compliance. Table 21.1 and the two sections on the right of Figure 21.15 show that the major changes are in the lung rather than the chest wall.

The cause of this observed reduction in lung compliance has been difficult to explain. There is no convincing evidence that anaesthesia affects pulmonary surfactant in humans at clinically used concentrations. A more likely explanation is that the reduced lung compliance is simply the consequence of breathing at reduced lung volume.

Gas Exchange

Every factor influencing gas exchange may be altered during anaesthesia, and many of the changes must be considered as normal features of the anaesthetized state. These 'normal' changes usually pose no threat to the patient, because their effects can easily be overcome by simply increasing F_{IO_2} and the minute volume. The 'normal' changes may be contrasted

with a range of pathological alterations in gas exchange that may arise during anaesthesia from such circumstances as airway obstruction, apnoea, bronchospasm or pneumothorax. These may be life threatening and require urgent action for their correction.

The major changes that adversely affect gas exchange during anaesthesia are reduced minute volume of ventilation (described earlier), increased dead space and shunt (considered in terms of the three-compartment model described on page 96 and in Fig. 7.10) and altered distribution of ventilation and perfusion in relation to $\dot{V}/\dot{Q}$ ratios.

Dead Space

With allowance for the apparatus dead space of the tracheal tube and its connections, the dead space/tidal volume ratio from carina downwards averages 32% during anaesthesia with either spontaneous or artificial ventilation. This is approximately equal to the ratio for the normal conscious subject including trachea, pharynx and mouth (approximately 70 mL). Physiological dead space equals the sum of its anatomical and alveolar components, and the subcarinal anatomical dead space is not normally increased. Therefore the increase in subcarinal physiological dead space during anaesthesia must be in the alveolar component.

In the study shown in Figure 21.16, subcarinal anatomical dead space was always significantly less than physiological, reaching a maximum of about 70 mL at tidal volumes greater than 350 mL. This roughly accords with the expected geometric dimensions of the lower respiratory tract. At smaller tidal volumes, the anatomical dead space was less than the expected geometric volume. Values of less than

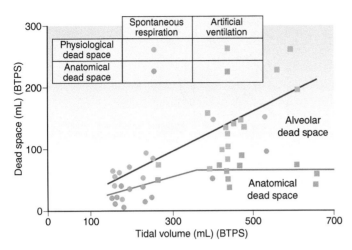

• **Fig. 21.16** Data and regression lines for physiological and anatomical dead space (the difference indicating alveolar dead space) as a function of tidal volume. There were no significant differences between anaesthesia with and without paralysis. Note the range over which physiological dead space appeared to be a constant fraction of tidal volume. Anatomical dead space was constant at a tidal volume greater than 350 mL, resulting in increased alveolar dead space. *BTPS,* Body temperature and pressure saturated (From Nunn JF, Hill DW. Respiratory dead space and arterial to end-tidal CO_2 tension difference in anesthetized man. *J Appl Physiol.* 1960;15:383-389. With permission of the editor and publishers of the *Journal of Applied Physiology.*)

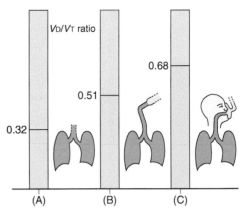

• **Fig. 21.17** Physiological plus apparatus dead space (where applicable) as a fraction of tidal volume in anaesthetized patients from carina downwards **(A)**; including tracheal tube or laryngeal mask airway and connector **(B)**; and including upper airway, facemask and connector **(C)**.

30 mL were recorded in some patients with tidal volumes of less than 250 mL. This is attributed to axial streaming and the mixing effect of the heartbeat and is clearly an important and beneficial factor in patients with depressed breathing.

Alveolar dead space increases with tidal volume, so that the sum of anatomical and alveolar (= physiological) dead space remains about 32% of tidal volume (Fig. 21.16). The cause of the increase in alveolar dead space during uncomplicated general anaesthesia is not immediately obvious. There is no evidence that it is the result of pulmonary hypotension causing development of a zone 1 (page 78), and the reduced vertical height of the lung in the supine position would mitigate against this. The alternative explanation is maldistribution with overventilation of *relatively* underperfused alveoli. Studies of $\dot{V}/\dot{Q}$ relationships outlined next give some support to this view, but such patterns of maldistribution have not invariably been observed during anaesthesia.

Use of a tracheal tube or LMA will bypass much of the normal anatomical dead space arising in the mouth and pharynx. However, for practical purposes the apparatus dead space of the tracheal tube or LMA[53] and their connections must be included for the purpose of calculating alveolar ventilation during anaesthesia. The total dead space then increases to about 50% of tidal volume (Fig. 21.17). When using a facemask, it is necessary to add the volume of the mask and its connections to the physiological dead space, which now also includes the trachea, pharynx and mouth. The total dead space then amounts to about two-thirds of the tidal volume. Thus a seemingly adequate minute volume

of 6 $L.min^{-1}$ may be expected to result in an alveolar ventilation of only 2 $L.min^{-1}$, which would almost inevitably result in hypercapnia.

Compensation for increased dead space may be made by increasing the minute volume to maintain the alveolar ventilation. In artificially ventilated anaesthetized patients the problem hardly exists. The patient may have a large dead space, but the high minute volumes that are usually selected provide more than adequate compensation. Thus the alveolar ventilation is almost always greater than necessary for carbon dioxide homeostasis. With monitoring of end-expiratory P_{CO_2}, there is seldom any difficulty in maintaining a normal value. However, the existence of an alveolar dead space means that the arterial P_{CO_2} during anaesthesia is usually 0.3 to 0.5 kPa (2.5–3.7 mmHg) greater than the end-expiratory P_{CO_2}.[54]

In the case of the hypoventilating patient who is allowed to breathe spontaneously during anaesthesia, the reduction in dead space at smaller tidal volumes shown in Figure 21.16 prevents some of the alveolar hypoventilation that would be expected if the volume of the dead space remained constant. This, together with the reduced metabolic rate, results in the hypercapnia being much less than the values for minute volume sometimes observed during anaesthesia. No doubt, over the years, many patients have owed their lives to these factors.

Shunt

Magnitude of the Change During Anaesthesia

In the conscious healthy subject, the shunt or venous admixture amounts to only 1% to 2% of cardiac output (page 101). This results in an alveolar/arterial P_{O_2} gradient of less than 1 kPa (7.5 mmHg) in the young healthy subject breathing air, but the gradient increases with age and lung disease. During anaesthesia, the alveolar/arterial P_{O_2} difference is usually increased to a value that corresponds to an average shunt of about 10%. Measurements of pulmonary venous admixture, taking into account the mixed venous oxygen content, have also been made, and these concur with shunts of the order of 10%. This provides an acceptable basis for predicting arterial Po_2 during an uncomplicated anaesthetic, and it also permits calculation of the concentration of oxygen in the inspired gas that will provide an acceptable arterial Po_2. About 30% to 40% inspired oxygen is usually adequate in an uncomplicated anaesthetic.

Cause of Venous Admixture During Anaesthesia

About half of the observed venous admixture is true shunt through the areas of atelectasis described earlier. There is a very strong correlation between the shunt (measured as perfusion of alveoli with a $\dot{V}/\dot{Q}$ ratio <0.005) and the area or volume of atelectasis seen on CT scans.[19] Studies using isotope techniques have demonstrated intrapulmonary shunting in the same areas of lung where atelectasis is seen on CT scans.[55] However, the venous admixture during anaesthesia also contains components because of dispersion of the $\dot{V}/\dot{Q}$ distribution and to perfusion of alveoli with low $\dot{V}/\dot{Q}$ ratios.

Ventilation/Perfusion Relationships

The three-compartment model of the lung (page 96) provides a definition of lung function in terms of dead space and shunt, parameters that are easily measured, reproducible and provide a basis for corrective therapy. Nevertheless, it does not pretend to provide a true picture of what is going on in the lung. A far more sophisticated approach is provided by the analysis of the distribution of pulmonary ventilation and perfusion in terms of $\dot{V}/\dot{Q}$ ratios, determined either by the multiple inert gas elimination (page 107) or radioisotopic scanning techniques.

During general anaesthesia both ventilation and perfusion are found to be distributed to a wider range of $\dot{V}/\dot{Q}$ ratios than when awake (Fig. 21.18), irrespective of whether the patient is paralysed and ventilated[19] or breathing spontaneously.[56] Other studies of $\dot{V}/\dot{Q}$ mismatch during anaesthesia with paralysis and artificial ventilation have consistently found ventilation to be preferentially distributed to

ventral lung areas (see Fig. 32.7), irrespective of body position, whereas perfusion remains partly gravity-dependent (page 93).[57] As a result, $\dot{V}/\dot{Q}$ ratios are more evenly matched when prone. The ventral redistribution of ventilation is a result of positive pressure ventilation rather than anaesthesia, because it is not seen in spontaneously breathing anaesthetized subjects.[58]

Effect of Age on $\dot{V}/\dot{Q}$ Ratios During Anaesthesia

In awake subjects, increasing age causes a widening of the distribution of $\dot{V}/\dot{Q}$ ratios, and the distribution widens still further with anaesthesia.[19] It would thus be expected that intrapulmonary shunt during anaesthesia would also increase with age, but studies of this effect have produced variable results, probably because of differences in measurement techniques and degrees of lung pathology in older patients. The most thorough study, which only included 45 patients, ranging in age from 23 to 69 years, concluded that atelectasis (as seen with CT) and true intrapulmonary shunt (determined by multiple inert gas elimination technique as alveoli with $\dot{V}/\dot{Q}$ <0.005) did not relate to age.[19] However, both were substantially increased during anaesthesia and correlated with each other, and this study confirmed the enhanced decline in arterial Po_2 with increasing age during anaesthesia. Venous admixture (calculated as for the three-compartment model) was increased significantly from a mean value of 5.5% of cardiac output before anaesthesia to 9.2% during anaesthesia. Venous admixture increased steeply with age (0.17% per year), and this was attributed to an age-dependent increase in the spread of $\dot{V}/\dot{Q}$ ratios (Fig. 21.19) and to greater perfusion of alveoli with low $\dot{V}/\dot{Q}$ ratios (0.005–0.1).

Effect of Positive End-Expiratory Pressure

It has long been known that, in contrast to the situation in intensive care, PEEP often does little to improve the arterial Po_2 during anaesthesia.[59] There are two reasons why PEEP is not associated with improved oxygenation. First, the decrease in cardiac output associated with PEEP reduces the oxygen saturation of the blood traversing the remaining shunt, and so reduces arterial Po_2. Second, in the supine position PEEP

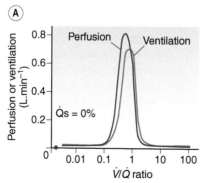
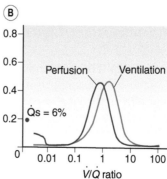

• **Fig. 21.18** Distribution of ventilation and perfusion as a function of ventilation/perfusion ratios in an awake **(A)** and anaesthetized paralysed **(B)** subject. (Data from reference 41.)

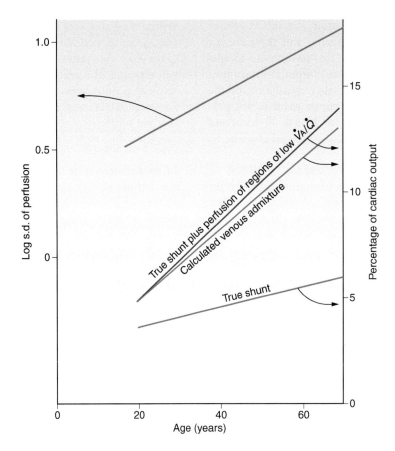

• **Fig. 21.19** Age dependence of various factors influencing alveolar/arterial P_{O_2} difference during anaesthesia.[41] The logarithm of standard deviation of distribution of perfusion (*orange line*) is significantly greater during anaesthesia (shown) than when awake (not shown) and has a significant regression against age under both circumstances. True shunt (*green line*) is significantly increased almost 10-fold compared with before anaesthesia, but the correlation with age is not significant. Perfusion of areas of poorly ventilated regions ($0.005 <$ ventilation/prefusion ($\dot{V}/\dot{Q}$) < 0.1) was significantly increased compared with before anaesthesia and correlated with age in both circumstances. Venous admixture (*blue line*) here refers to the value obtained from the shunt equation (page 101) and agrees well with the sum of shunt and perfusion of regions of low $\dot{V}/\dot{Q}$ (*purple line*).

increases ventilation in dependent areas, but causes similar changes in perfusion such that regional $\dot{V}/\dot{Q}$ ratios are virtually unchanged (Fig. 21.20). The essential difference from the patient undergoing critical care is probably the lack of protection of intrathoracic blood vessels from raised airway pressure that is afforded by stiff lungs in most patients requiring critical care.

Other Factors Affecting Ventilation/Perfusion Relationships During Anaesthesia

Hypoxic pulmonary vasoconstriction (HPV) contributes to maintaining a normal $\dot{V}/\dot{Q}$ ratio by reducing perfusion to underventilated alveoli (pages 80). Inhalational anaesthetics inhibit HPV (page 260), and so in theory may worsen $\dot{V}/\dot{Q}$ mismatch during anaesthesia. There is some evidence from animal studies that this is the case, and one human study of anaesthesia with intravenous barbiturates, which are believed to have less effect on HPV, demonstrated only a small amount of intrapulmonary shunting.[60] High concentrations of inspired oxygen will inhibit HPV by maintaining alveolar P_{O_2} at a high level even in poorly ventilated alveoli. Some

work has shown that lower inspired oxygen concentrations during anaesthesia (30%) are associated with less $\dot{V}/\dot{Q}$ scatter than when breathing 100% oxygen.[31]

Summary

These studies of $\dot{V}/\dot{Q}$ relationships during anaesthesia complement one another and give greatly increased insight into the effect of anaesthesia on gas exchange. The effect of anaesthesia on gas exchange is summarized as follows:

- Uniformity of distribution of ventilation and perfusion is decreased by anaesthesia. The magnitude of the change is age-related and may be affected by the inspired oxygen concentration and anaesthetic agents used.
- The increase in alveolar dead space appears to be because of increased distribution of ventilation to areas of high (but not usually infinite) $\dot{V}/\dot{Q}$.
- Venous admixture is increased in anaesthesia to around 5% to 10%, but the change is markedly affected by age and is minimal in the young.

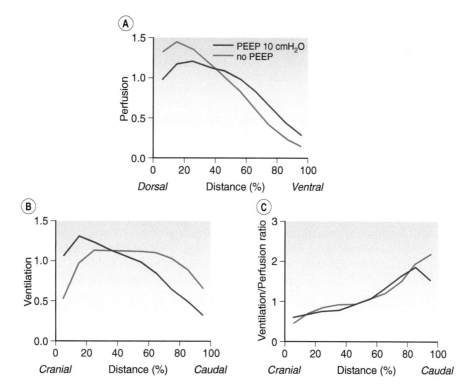

• **Fig. 21.20** Effect of positive end-expiratory pressure *(PEEP)* on perfusion **(A)**, ventilation **(B)** and ventilation/prefusion *(V̇/Q̇)* ratios **(C)** during anaesthesia with paralysis and ventilation in supine healthy subjects. Data obtained using a dual isotope SPECT method (page 106). Ventilation and perfusion shown are the values for that lung region relative to the means for all regions. Note how the application of PEEP changes both regional ventilation and perfusion in a similar manner, so having little effect on *V̇/Q̇* ratios. (From Petersson J, Ax M, Frey J, et al. Positive end-expiratory pressure redistributes regional blood flow and ventilation differently in supine and prone humans. *Anesthesiology.* 2010;113:1361-1369. With permission of the publishers of *Anesthesiology.*)

• The increased venous admixture during anaesthesia is due partly to an increase in true intrapulmonary shunt (because of atelectasis) and partly to increased distribution of perfusion to areas of low (but not zero) *V̇/Q̇* ratios.

• The major differences are between the awake and the anaesthetized states. Paralysis and artificial ventilation do not greatly alter the parameters of gas exchange in spite of the different spatial distribution of ventilation.

• Both PEEP and lung hyperinflation manoeuvres reduce the shunt, but the beneficial effect on arterial Po_2 is offset by greater *V̇/Q̇* mismatch and a decrease in cardiac output which reduces the mixed venous oxygen content. Typical values for the various factors discussed are shown in Table 21.2.

TABLE 21.2	Changes in Factors Influencing Gas Exchange After Induction of Anaesthesia			
		Anaesthetized		
	Awake	SPONTANEOUS VENTILATION	IPPV	IPPV + PEEP
F_{IO_2}	0.21	0.4	0.4	0.4
$\dot{Q}s/\dot{Q}_t$ (%)	1.6	6.2	8.6	4.1
V_D/V_T	30	35	38	44
Cardiac output (L.min⁻¹)	6.1	5.0	4.5	3.7
Pa_{O_2} (kPa)	10.5	17.6	18.8	20.5
Pa_{O_2} (mmHg)	79	132	141	153
$\dot{V}$—mean ($\dot{V}/\dot{Q}$)	0.81	1.3	2.20	3.03
$\dot{Q}$—mean ($\dot{V}/\dot{Q}$)	0.47	0.51	0.83	0.55

IPPV, Intermittent positive pressure ventilator; *PEEP*, positive end-expiratory pressure.
(From Nunn JF. Oxygen—friend and foe. *J R Soc Med.* 1985;78:618-622.)

Other Effects of General Anaesthesia on the Respiratory System

Response to Added Resistance

The preceding sections would lead one to expect that anaesthesia would cause grave impairment of the ability of patients to increase their work of breathing in the face of added resistance. Surprisingly, this is not the case, and anaesthetized patients preserve a remarkable ability to overcome added resistance. The anaesthetized patient responds to inspiratory loading in two phases. First, there is an instant augmentation of the force of contraction of the inspiratory muscles, mainly the diaphragm, during the first loaded breath. Detection of the inspiratory resistance may be mediated by either airway or lung receptors, and is only slightly inhibited by anaesthesia.[61] The second response is much slower, and overshoots when the loading is removed, and the time course suggests that this is mediated by an increase in Pco_2. In combination, these two mechanisms enable the anaesthetized patient to achieve good compensation with inspiratory loading up to about 0.8 kPa (8 cmH$_2$O). Even more remarkable is the preservation of the elaborate response to expiratory resistance (see Fig. 3.11), with a large increase in minute volume occurring with expiratory resistive loading during inhalational anaesthesia.

Hypoxic Pulmonary Vasoconstriction[62]

The contribution to $\dot{V}/\dot{Q}$ mismatch of disturbed HPV during anaesthesia has already been described, but the effects of anaesthesia on HPV merit further discussion. Early animal studies using isolated lungs found that several inhalational anaesthetics inhibit HPV, but no such effect was found with intravenous anaesthetics. Although in vitro studies gave clear evidence that inhalational anaesthetics depressed HPV, in vivo studies were inconsistent. One cause of this inconsistency was the concomitant depression of cardiac output by inhalational anaesthetics. In Chapter 6 it was explained how hypoxia influences pulmonary vascular resistance not only by the alveolar Po_2 but also, in part, by the mixed venous Po_2. A reduction in cardiac output must decrease the mixed venous Po_2 if oxygen consumption remains unchanged, and this would intensify pulmonary vasoconstriction. Thus an inhalational anaesthetic will inhibit HPV by direct action, whereas it may intensify HPV by reducing mixed venous Po_2 as a result of decreasing cardiac output. Most investigators' results are consistent with the view that inhalational anaesthetics depress HPV, provided that allowance is made for the effect of concomitant changes of cardiac output. An example of when HPV may be relevant in clinical anaesthesia is during one-lung ventilation, which is described on page 403.

Anaesthesia in Specific Patient Groups

Paediatrics[63]

Perioperative respiratory adverse events are a major cause of morbidity and mortality in the paediatric population. Children under the age of 2 years are at greatest risk of developing respiratory failure during anaesthesia, attributed to factors such as immaturity of respiratory control (page 179) and reflexes leading to a blunted response to inadequate gas exchange, and the small size and greater collapsibility of both upper and lower airways. Lower efficiency of respiratory muscles and a reduced surface area for gas exchange are also important. Although healthy term neonates exhibit an exaggerated ventilatory response to hypercapnia, the response of preterm infants is attenuated. In addition, following AHVR, the subsequent HVD is especially marked in preterm infants, in whom respiratory rates decrease to below baseline after only 1 to 2 minutes of hypoxia. Neonates (especially up to the age of 2 months) are predisposed to dynamic upper airway obstruction because of muscular hypotonia and neuronal immaturity. Anything affecting neuronal function, such as anaesthesia, increases the likelihood of upper airway collapse. The FRC of children undergoing anaesthesia, as in the adult population, is reduced. In children under 11 years of age the decrease is even more marked, and is as great as 44% of awake FRC. In addition to the causes of reduced FRC in adults, children demonstrate less elastic recoil of the supporting lung parenchyma, and this leads to reduced support for the small airways. Atelectasis occurs more commonly in children because of their compliant chest wall,[64] and as in adults may be exacerbated by using a high concentration of oxygen.[65] Compared with adults the reduction in lung compliance observed during anaesthesia is greater in neonates and infants; if spontaneously breathing, the increased work of breathing can lead to fatigue.

Obesity[66]

The effects of obesity on respiratory function are described in Chapter 15. Obese patients already have a small FRC when supine, and the further reduction with anaesthesia results in an exponential decrease in FRC during anaesthesia with increasing body mass index. Similarly, with increasing obesity there is a greater fall in lung compliance and increase in lung resistance under anaesthesia. Obese patients develop more atelectasis during anaesthesia, the development of which may be attenuated by noninvasive ventilation before induction of anaesthesia.[67] Atelectasis also persists longer into the postoperative period. Performance of a RM as described earlier is particularly effective in obese patients, and leads to reexpansion of atelectasis and improved oxygenation, although higher airway pressures of 50 to 55 cmH$_2$O may be required.[68] Analysis of clinical data from obese patients indicates that high tidal volume and low PEEP ventilation are often used without performing RMs.[69] Cardiovascular effects of a RM are less pronounced in fluid-loaded obese patients,[70] but the beneficial effects of an intraoperative RM do not seem to continue into the postoperative period.[71] The uncertain role of PEEP during anaesthesia in nonobese subjects is similar for those with obesity. In morbidly obese patients (BMI = 40 kg.m^{-2}), modest levels of PEEP (10 cmH$_2$O) improve FRC and elastance but have variable effects on oxygenation.[72]

When selecting tidal volume settings for ventilation of morbidly obese patients during anaesthesia, it is particularly important to base these on ideal rather than actual body weight; 8 mL.kg^{-1} in a patient weighing 150 kg (331 lb) will quickly result in high airway pressures, overdistension of lung tissue and potential barotrauma.

Special Circumstances Relevant During Anaesthesia

Patient position

Lateral

In Chapter 7 it was explained that in an awake patient in the lateral position there is preferential distribution of inspired gas to the lower lung (see Table 7.1), and this accords approximately with the distribution of pulmonary blood flow. This favourable distribution of inspired gas is disturbed by anaesthesia whether respiration is spontaneous or artificial in the anaesthetized patient, with preferential ventilation of the nondependent (upper) lung and continued preferential perfusion of the dependent lung. This predictably leads to a greater spread of $\dot{V}/\dot{Q}$ ratios and a further fall in P_{O_2} compared with the supine position. Atelectasis seen on CT scanning forms only in the dependent lung, but the overall amount of atelectasis and the intrapulmonary shunt are similar to that seen when anaesthetized and paralysed when supine (page 404 and Fig. 21.9).

Prone

A patient anaesthetized in the prone position should have the upper chest and pelvis supported, to allow free movement of the abdomen and lower chest. In subjects anaesthetized and paralysed in this position, respiratory mechanics are only minimally affected, and both FRC and arterial P_{O_2} are greater than when supine. Compared with a supine subject, artificial ventilation in the prone position increases regional ventilation to ventral, now dependent, areas. Perfusion remains largely gravity-dependent, with a similar increase in perfusion to ventral-dependent areas, thus establishing better $\dot{V}/\dot{Q}$ matching than when supine. Use of 10 cmH$_2$O of PEEP in the prone position redistributes both ventilation and perfusion and may worsen gas exchange.[73]

Laparoscopic Surgery

Compared with open surgery, the benefits of many laparoscopic procedures are now well-established and have led to an expansion in the number of surgical procedures performed via laparoscopy. As confidence in, and understanding of, the technique improves, procedures become more complex and more prolonged, and are attempted in less fit patients.

Absorption of gas from the peritoneal cavity depends on the partial pressure of gas present and its solubility in peritoneal tissue. Gas mixtures are rarely used, so the partial pressure is normally equal to the insufflation pressure. Insoluble gases such as helium or nitrogen would be absorbed to a much smaller extent, but would also be more disastrous during the rare complication of gas embolus. Air, oxygen and nitrous oxide all support combustion, preventing the use of diathermy, which is fundamental to laparoscopic surgery. Thus carbon dioxide remains the usual gas used for the erroneously named 'pneumoperitoneum'. Laparoscopic operations involve the insufflation of carbon dioxide into the peritoneum to a pressure of 10 to 15 mmHg, and normally also involve positioning the patient head up (for upper abdominal surgery) or head down (for lower abdominal and pelvic procedures). These procedures have two adverse effects on respiration.

Respiratory Mechanics

In addition to the changes already described for general anaesthesia, the increased intraabdominal pressure during laparoscopy causes further restriction of the diaphragm and lower chest wall. Respiratory system compliance is significantly reduced,[74] sometimes accompanied by increased airway resistance, particularly in obese patients. An increase in airway pressures invariably occurs. The head-up position may attenuate some of these changes, but patients in the head-down position during laparoscopy have a further cause for substantially reduced compliance. In healthy patients, these significant changes in respiratory system mechanics have only a small effect on $\dot{V}/\dot{Q}$ distribution. An animal study showed that perfusion of poorly ventilated dependent lung regions was reduced by establishing a pneumoperitoneum, possibly because of enhanced HPV from the hypercapnia (page 83).[75] A study of nine healthy patients using the multiple inert gas elimination technique to characterize $\dot{V}/\dot{Q}$ ratios found only a transient reduction in pulmonary shunt and no significant changes in alveolar dead space or in areas of abnormally high or low $\dot{V}/\dot{Q}$ ratios.[76] Successful artificial ventilation during laparoscopy faces all the same challenges as described below, exacerbated by obesity and the head-down position. Once again, the combination of RMs and modest PEEP (10 cmH$_2$O) seems to be the most effective strategy.

Carbon Dioxide Absorption[77]

Transperitoneal absorption of carbon dioxide into the blood begins within a few minutes of commencing a laparoscopic procedure, and is estimated to be 30 to 50 mL.min^{-1}. If ventilation remains unchanged, this will quickly increase arterial P_{CO_2}, and carbon dioxide will begin diffusing into the medium and slow compartments of the body's huge carbon dioxide stores (see page 131 and Fig. 9.10). After a prolonged procedure, with elevated arterial P_{CO_2}, hypercapnia may be present for many hours postoperatively as the carbon dioxide stores empty. Unfortunately, this is a period when the patient is no longer receiving artificial ventilation and is recovering from a general anaesthetic, and so may struggle to meet the increased ventilatory requirement. Increasing the minute volume during surgery should allow the maintenance of a normal arterial P_{CO_2} to prevent this scenario from developing. In patients who are obese or have respiratory disease, the changes in compliance described previously will further impair the excretion of carbon dioxide and require an even larger minute volume. End-tidal carbon dioxide monitoring may be used to estimate the required ventilation, but in some patients $\dot{V}/\dot{Q}$ disturbances mean that there may be an unpredictable end-tidal to arterial P_{CO_2} gradient.

Regional Anaesthesia

Epidural or spinal anaesthesia may be expected to influence the respiratory system, either by a central effect of drugs absorbed from the spinal canal or by affecting the pattern or strength of contraction of respiratory muscle groups.[78] These effects are generally small, but of great importance in view of the tendency to use regional anaesthetic techniques in patients with respiratory disease or in obstetric practice when respiratory function is already abnormal.

Control of Breathing

Thoracic epidural anaesthesia may cause a small reduction in resting tidal volume as a result of reduced rib cage movement, and predictably this does not occur following lumbar epidural anaesthesia. Studies of hypercapnic and hypoxic ventilatory responses during epidural anaesthesia have produced conflicting results. Thoracic anaesthesia may reduce the ventilatory response to hypercapnia by inhibition of intercostal muscle activity. Lumbar epidurals have been reported to increase the response to hypercapnia, which is believed to be stimulated by anxiety (the study was performed immediately before surgery) or because of a direct stimulant effect of lignocaine on the respiratory centre.[79] The AHVR is unaffected by thoracic epidural anaesthesia, but lumbar epidurals may increase ventilation in response to hypoxia by a poorly understood mechanism.

Respiratory muscle function has been extensively studied using EMGs and CT scans during high lumbar (block up to T1 dermatome) epidural anaesthesia,[80] which confirmed the reduced contribution of the rib cage to resting ventilation. FRC was increased by 300 mL as a result of both caudad movement of the diaphragm and reduced thoracic blood volume. In spite of these changes, most respiratory function measurements remain essentially unchanged during epidural anaesthesia, with only small changes in forced vital capacity and peak expiratory flow rate (PEFR). The situation is quite different in late pregnancy, when regional anaesthesia is commonly used. Significant reductions in forced vital capacity, PEFR and peak expiratory pressure, a measure of abdominal muscle activity, have all been reported after regional anaesthesia.

Oxygenation during epidural anaesthesia is largely unaffected. In a study by Hedenstierna's group, lumbar epidural anaesthesia produced no changes in $\dot{V}/\dot{Q}$ relationships or pulmonary shunt, and no CT evidence of atelectasis, except in one subject with a higher than normal body mass index in the lithotomy position.[81]

Respiratory Function in the Postoperative Period

Reversal of Intraoperative Physiological Changes

In the first few minutes of recovery, alveolar P_{O_2} may be reduced by elimination of nitrous oxide, which dilutes alveolar oxygen (diffusion hypoxia) and carbon dioxide, but this effect is usually transient. Both the reduced FRC and the increased alveolar/arterial P_{O_2} gradient observed during anaesthesia usually return to normal during the first few hours after minor operations. Following major surgery, the restoration of a normal alveolar/arterial P_{O_2} gradient may take many days, and episodes of hypoxia are common. There are several contributory factors.

Reduced lung volume and atelectasis contribute to postoperative changes, and there is a continued reduction in FRC, usually reaching its lowest value 1 to 2 days after surgery before slowly returning to normal values within a week. Reduction of the FRC is greatest in patients having surgery close to the diaphragm, that is, those with upper abdominal or thoracic incisions. The effect is less pronounced following laparoscopic surgery in the upper abdomen. Atelectasis seen on CT imaging during anaesthesia persists for at least 24 hours in patients having major surgery. The effects of these changes on $\dot{V}/\dot{Q}$ relationships and oxygenation are similar to those seen during anaesthesia, but the provision of adequate inspired oxygen concentration in the postoperative period is less reliable. Blinded postoperative continuous oxygen saturation monitoring for 48 hours postoperatively has shown that hypoxaemia occurs frequently, and may be severe: 21% of patients spent 10 or more minutes with oxygen saturations below 90%, and 5% spent 5 or more minutes with saturations less than 85%.[82]

Normal activity of almost all respiratory muscles may be impaired following major surgery, including the airway muscles, abdominal muscles and diaphragm.[83,84] Factors giving rise to this situation include anaesthetic agents and neuromuscular blocking agents (NMBAs), postoperative analgesic drugs (especially opioids), pain, disturbed sleep patterns and the inflammatory response to surgery. Abnormal respiratory muscle activity arises not only from muscle weakness, but also from impaired coordination between the different muscle groups and failure of the normal physiological reflexes and control mechanisms on which their activity depends.[84]

Effort-dependent lung function tests such as forced vital capacity, forced expiratory volume in one second and PEFR are all reduced significantly following surgery, particularly if pain control is inadequate. Laparoscopic surgery is again associated with lesser, but still significant reductions in lung function, and the degree of change is again related to the site of surgery. Respiratory control may be abnormal for several weeks following anaesthesia and surgery,[85] with reduced responses to hypercapnia and hypoxia. This has major implications for overcoming airway obstruction when asleep. The responses are still slightly impaired 6 weeks after surgery, even in the absence of inflammation, pain and analgesic use, suggesting plasticity in the respiratory control mechanisms at the time of surgery that takes some time to return to normal.[85]

Postoperative Pulmonary Complications

Postoperative pulmonary complication (PPC) is a term widely used to describe a large collection of complications including, among others, pneumonia, atelectasis, pulmonary aspiration and acute respiratory distress syndrome (ARDS).[86] Intraoperative reduced FRC, increased $\dot{V}/\dot{Q}$ mismatch and atelectasis are believed to contribute to the aetiology of PPCs. Patients who develop a PPC have increased morbidity and mortality, a higher risk of unplanned intensive care unit admission and an increased length of hospital stay.[87]

Preoperative Interventions to Avoid Postoperative Pulmonary Complications

Numerous attempts have been made to predict those at risk of developing a PPC, and both modifiable and nonmodifiable factors identified.[87–89] The elective preoperative period allows modifiable risk factors to potentially be corrected; these include anaemia, recent respiratory infection and low preoperative oxygen saturation ([Sao_2] <96%). Some evidence exists that preoperative physiotherapy interventions and education on postoperative breathing exercises can reduce the incidence of PPCs in patients undergoing major open upper abdominal surgery.[90] Optimizing respiratory function in those with chronic lung disease such as asthma and COPD should be undertaken if possible, particularly if they have a history of a recent infection.

Postoperative pulmonary complications are known to be several times more common in smokers, depending on the definitions used. This is attributable to increased secretions, impaired mucus clearance and small airway narrowing. Most studies of the perioperative effects of smoking have been carried out on patients undergoing major surgery, usually cardiothoracic or upper abdominal surgery. The high incidence of respiratory complications in this group makes them an ideal study population, but there is relatively less known about the respiratory effects of perioperative smoking after more minor surgery.

A key strategy to reduce the risk of a PPC is therefore preoperative smoking cessation (page 239). The duration of smoking abstinence required to significantly reduce the incidence of PPCs is controversial.[91,92] Nicotine, which is responsible for many untoward cardiovascular changes, has a half-life of only 30 minutes, whereas carboxyhaemoglobin has a half-life of 4 hours when breathing air. A smoking fast of just a few hours will therefore effectively remove the risks associated with carbon monoxide and nicotine. Some older studies in patients undergoing cardiac surgery found a greater incidence of PPCs in patients who stopped smoking for less than 8 weeks before surgery compared with those who continued smoking until the day before surgery. Other studies have failed to demonstrate this effect, and there are concerns that the original investigations had insufficient statistical power to draw this conclusion.[91] Current advice is therefore that smokers should always strive to stop smoking preoperatively, and that the longer the period of cessation the greater will be the likelihood of avoiding a PPC.[93] Patients presenting for emergency surgery clearly do not allow for preoperative optimization, and other nonmodifiable factors such as increased age and comorbidities all put patients into a high risk group for PPCs. Attempts to reduce the risk of developing a PPC in these patients can only be carried out in the intra- and postoperative period.

Intraoperative Considerations

Intraoperative approaches to reduce the risk of a PPC are based on lung protective ventilation strategies.[94,95] Until recently, ventilation strategies in anaesthetized patients received little attention compared with patients with injured lungs (Chapter 31). It was believed that the relatively short duration of ventilation and the usually healthy lungs of patients during anaesthesia meant they were at minimal risk of ventilator-induced lung injury (VILI, page 392). Increasing evidence to the contrary is emerging. For example, after only 3 hours of general anaesthesia there is reduced lung-diffusing capacity, not explained solely by lung volume loss, and biomarker evidence of alveolar damage.[96] The pathophysiological mechanisms that lead to VILI in critically ill patients (page 392) occur in some patients during anaesthesia, and include atelectasis, opening and closing of airways with each breath (atelectrauma), overdistension of alveoli and a significant systemic inflammatory response. These changes are more likely to occur in some patient groups, such as those having cardiac, thoracic or open abdominal surgery, in whom the respiratory effects of anaesthesia and surgery continue into the early postoperative period.[95] These factors have led to calls for ventilation during anaesthesia to follow similar protocols as in lung-injured patients (page 371), the so-called 'protective ventilation'.[97] Conventional ventilation during anaesthesia aimed to reduce pulmonary collapse by using large V_T (10–15 mL.kg^{-1}), usually with no PEEP. This regimen probably developed simply because, in the past, the basic mechanical ventilators used in theatre were unable to deliver anything else. Features of protective ventilation comprise a smaller V_T, some PEEP and regular RMs (page 251). A number of randomized controlled trials[98,99] and meta-analyses[100,101] have shown better clinical outcomes with protective ventilation. There is now general agreement that a V_T of 6 to 8 mL.kg^{-1} of ideal body weight is optimal, but the use of RMs intraoperatively and the best level of PEEP remain unclear.[102] Optimal PEEP can be considered as the end-expiratory pressure that prevents atelectrauma while avoiding overdistension of ventilated alveoli, and this pressure varies from patient to patient. Various approaches to determining this level have been described. One method is to use invasive techniques such as oesophageal manometry to assess transpulmonary pressure (page 17). Less invasive methods include using electrical impedance tomography to map ventilation distribution in real-time,[103,104] or by subtracting inspiratory and expiratory V_T following a change in PEEP.[105] This allows the change in end-expiratory lung volume to be determined and V_T to be adjusted accordingly. Small V_T and low PEEP (<5 cmH$_2$O) may be associated with increased perioperative mortality,[106] and 5 cmH$_2$O PEEP has been found insufficient to prevent atelectrauma.[107] Conversely, animal studies show that high PEEP (10 cmH$_2$O) increases lung inflammatory markers,[108] and in humans using a high PEEP level (12 vs 2 cmH$_2$O) was associated with a similar incidence of PPCs and a greater incidence of cardiovascular problems.[109]

Lung strain is a concept defined in an attempt to understand mechanisms whereby artificial ventilation leads to lung injury. The V_T delivered (i.e., the change in lung volume) and the FRC to which it is delivered define the degree of strain. Driving pressure (ΔP) is the difference between plateau pressure and PEEP, and represents V_T normalized to respiratory system compliance.[110] Higher ΔP has been shown to be associated with poorer outcomes in ARDS (see Chapter 31). A meta-analysis of 2250 patients undergoing anaesthesia and artificial ventilation also found a higher ΔP to be associated with the development of PPCs,[111] with a predictive value greater than that of V_T. Defining useful bedside measures which accurately reflect physiological variables that can predict clinical outcomes is the subject of ongoing research.

There is considerable variation in protocols, patient groups studied and outcome measures across trials designed to investigate the effects of intraoperative ventilation on PPCs. For example, studies already using a basic lung protective strategy in the control group have not demonstrated improved outcomes in the intervention groups receiving more individualized ventilation settings.[112] Standardizing perioperative outcome measures may help to address this problem,[113] but further research is required to find the optimal ventilation strategy in different patient groups during anaesthesia. In patients with COPD, use of neuraxial block techniques has shown a reduced rate of PPCs when compared with those undergoing general anaesthesia, and where possible, the avoidance of artificial ventilation altogether in these patients may be beneficial.[114]

Postoperative Considerations

Airway obstruction, often associated with residual muscle paralysis, is a common potential cause of hypoxia shortly after anaesthesia. This may be compounded by the residual effects of anaesthetic agents on ventilatory control that have been described previously. Another significant risk to adequate respiratory function in the early postoperative period and the development of a PPC is the use of NMBAs and their reversal with neostigmine. Careful management when reversing NMBAs can help to reduce the risk of postoperative neuromuscular block,[115] but where residual NMBA activity persists, defined as a train-of-four ratio less than 0.9, significantly lower values for forced vital capacity and PEFR are demonstrated.[116] Even when seemingly adequately reversed, use of NMBAs is still associated with an increased incidence of PPCs, potentially caused by residual respiratory muscle weakness despite reversal, or by an effect of neostigmine on respiratory muscle or airway function.[117] Many intraoperative factors such as choice of induction and maintenance agents, as well as use of opioid analgesia, also contribute to the function of postoperative airway reflexes and respiratory muscles.[118] The speed of return of protective airway reflexes postoperatively has been shown to vary with choice of volatile for the maintenance of anaesthesia intraoperatively; desflurane promotes a faster return of airway reflexes when compared with sevoflurane, even when NMBA usage and reversal are standardized.[119]

Sputum retention occurs in many patients following surgery. General anaesthesia, particularly with a tracheal tube, causes impairment of mucociliary transport in the airways, an effect that may persist into the postoperative period. This, coupled with reduced FRC, residual atelectasis and an ineffective cough, contributes to the development of PPCs. Multidisciplinary approaches in the postoperative period can reduce the incidence of PPCs, with an emphasis on incentive spirometry, coughing and deep breathing, good oral care, early mobilization and patient education.[120]

References

1. Snow J. *On Chloroform and Other Anaesthetics: Their Action and Administration*. London: Churchill; 1858.
2. Pandit JJ. Effect of low dose inhaled anaesthetic agents on the ventilatory response to carbon dioxide in humans: a quantitative review. *Anaesthesia*. 2005;60:461-469.
3. Pandit JJ. The variable effect of low-dose volatile anaesthetics on the acute ventilatory response to hypoxia in humans: a quantitative review. *Anaesthesia*. 2002;57:632-643.
4. Dahan A, Teppema LJ. Influence of anaesthesia and analgesia on the control of breathing. *Br J Anaesth*. 2003;91:40-49.
5. Knill RL, Gelb AW. Ventilatory responses to hypoxia and hypercapnia during halothane sedation and anesthesia in man. *Anesthesiology*. 1978;49:244-251.

6. Temp JA, Henson LC, Ward DS. Does a subanaesthetic concentration of isoflurane blunt the ventilatory response to hypoxia. *Anesthesiology*. 1992;77:1116-1124.

7. Sjögren D, Sollevi A, Ebberyd A, et al. Isoflurane anesthesia (0.6 MAC) and hypoxic ventilatory response in humans. *Acta Anaesthesiol Scand*. 1995;39:17-22.

8. van den Elsen M, Sarton E, Teppema L, et al. Influence of 0.1 minimum alveolar concentration of sevoflurane, desflurane and isoflurane on dynamic ventilatory response to hypercapnia in humans. *Br J Anaesth*. 1998;80:174-182.

9. Mathru M, Esch O, Lang J, et al. Magnetic resonance imaging of the upper airway. Effects of propofol anesthesia and nasal continuous positive airway pressure in humans. *Anesthesiology*. 1996;84:273-279.

10. Warner DO, Warner MA, Ritman EL. Human chest wall function while awake and during halothane anesthesia: I Quiet breathing. *Anesthesiology*. 1995;82:6-19.

11. Lumb AB, Petros AJ, Nunn JF. Rib cage contribution to resting and carbon dioxide stimulated ventilation during 1 MAC isoflurane anaesthesia. *Br J Anaesth*. 1991;67:712-721.

12. Morton CPJ, Drummond GB. Change in chest wall dimensions on induction of anaesthesia: a reappraisal. *Br J Anaesth*. 1994;73:135-139.

13. Drummond GB. The abdominal muscles in anaesthesia and after surgery. *Br J Anaesth*. 2003;91:73-80.

14. Drummond GB, Dhonneur G, Kirov K, et al. Effects of an opioid on respiratory movements and expiratory activity in humans during isoflurane anaesthesia. *Respir Physiol Neurobiol*. 2013;185:425-434.

15. Reigner J, Ameur MB, Ecoffey C. Spontaneous ventilation with halothane in children: a comparative study between endotracheal tube and laryngeal mask airway. *Anesthesiology*. 1995;83:674-678.

16. Bergman NA. Distribution of inspired gas during anesthesia and artificial ventilation. *J Appl Physiol*. 1963;18:1085-1089.

17. Futier E, Constantin J-M, Petit A, et al. Positive end-expiratory pressure improves end-expiratory lung volume but not oxygenation after induction of anaesthesia. *Eur J Anaesthesiol*. 2010;27:508-513.

18. Duggan M, Kavanagh BP. Pulmonary atelectasis. A pathogenic perioperative entity. *Anesthesiology*. 2005;102:838-854.

19. Gunnarsson L, Tokics L, Gustavsson H, et al. Influence of age on atelectasis formation and gas exchange impairment during general anaesthesia. *Br J Anaesth*. 1991;66:423-432.

20. Froese A, Bryan C. Effects of anaesthesia and paralysis on diaphragmatic mechanics in man. *Anesthesiol*. 1974;41:242-255.

21. Reber A, Nylund U, Hedenstierna G. Position and shape of the diaphragm: implications for atelectasis formation. *Anaesthesia*. 1998;53:1054-1061.

22. Krayer S, Rehder K, Beck KC, et al. Quantification of thoracic volumes by three-dimensional imaging. *J Appl Physiol*. 1987;62:591-598.

23. Bendixen HH, Hedley-Whyte J, Laver MB. Impaired oxygenation in surgical patients during general anesthesia with controlled ventilation. *N Engl J Med*. 1963;269:991-996.

24. Hedenstierna G, Tokics L, Strandberg A, et al. Correlation of gas exchange impairment to development of atelectasis during anaesthesia and muscle paralysis. *Acta Anaesthesiol Scand*. 1986;30:183-191.

25. Monastesse A, Girard F, Massicotte N, et al. Lung ultrasonography for the assessment of perioperative atelectasis: a pilot feasibility study. *Anesth Analg*. 2017;124:494-504.

26. Mavros MN, Velmahos GC, Falagas ME. Atelectasis as a cause of postoperative fever. Where is the clinical evidence? *Chest*. 2011;140:418-424.

27. Hedenstierna G. Invited editorial on "Kinetics of absorption atelectasis during anaesthesia: a mathematical model". *J Appl Physiol*. 1999(suppl 6):1114-1115.

28. Rothen HU, Sporre B, Engberg G, et al. Airway closure, atelectasis and gas exchange during general anaesthesia. *Br J Anaesth*. 1998;81:681-686.

29. Bergman NA, Tien YK. Contribution of the closure of pulmonary units to impaired oxygenation during anesthesia. *Anesthesiology*. 1983;59:395-401.

30. Magnusson L, Spahn DR. New concepts of atelectasis during general anaesthesia. *Br J Anaesth*. 2003;91:61-72.

31. Rothen HU, Sporre B, Engberg G, et al. Prevention of atelectasis during general anaesthesia. *Lancet*. 1996;345:1387-1391.

32. Edmark L, Kostova-Aherdan K, Enlund M, et al. Optimal oxygen concentration during induction of general anesthesia. *Anesthesiology*. 2003;98:28-33.

33. Rothen HU, Sporre B, Engberg G, et al. Influence of gas composition on recurrence of atelectasis after a reexpansion maneuver during general anesthesia. *Anesthesiology*. 1995;82:832-842.

34. Akça O, Podolsky A, Eisenhuber E, et al. Comparable postoperative pulmonary atelectasis in patients given 30% or 80% oxygen during and 2 hours after colon resection. *Anesthesiology*. 1999;91:991-998.

35. Mackintosh N, Gertsch MC, Hopf HW, et al. High intraoperative inspired oxygen does not increase postoperative supplemental oxygen requirements. *Anesthesiology*. 2012;117:271-279.

36. Benoit Z, Wicky S, Fischer JF, et al. The effect of increased F_{IO_2} before tracheal extubation on postoperative atelectasis. *Anesth Analg*. 2002;95:1777-1781.

37. Lumb AB. Just a little oxygen to breathe as you go off to sleep ... is it always a good idea? *Br J Anaesth*. 2007;99:769-771.

38. Joyce CJ, Williams AB. Kinetics of absorption atelectasis during anaesthesia: a mathematical model. *J Appl Physiol*. 1999;86:1116-1125.

39. Rusca M, Proietti S, Schnyder P, et al. Prevention of atelectasis formation during induction of general anesthesia. *Anesth Analg*. 2003;97:1835-1839.

40. Herriger A, Frascarolo P, Spahn DR, et al. The effect of positive airway pressure during pre-oxygenation and induction of anaesthesia upon duration of non-hypoxic apnoea. *Anaesthesia*. 2004;59:243-247.

41. Östberg E, Thorisson A, Enlund M, et al. Positive end-expiratory pressure alone minimizes atelectasis formation in nonabdominal surgery: a randomized controlled trial. *Anaesthesiol*. 2018;128:1117-1124.

42. Lumb AB, Bradshaw K, Gamlin FMC, et al. The effect of coughing at extubation on oxygenation in the post-anaesthesia care unit. *Anaesthesia*. 2015;70:416-420.

43. Lumb AB, Greenhill SJ, Simpson MP, et al. Lung recruitment and positive airway pressure before extubation does not improve oxygenation in the post-anaesthesia care unit: a randomized clinical trial. *Br J Anaesth*. 2010;104:643-648.

44. Kleinsasser AT, Pircher I, Truebsbach S, et al. Pulmonary function after emergence on 100% oxygen in patients with chronic obstructive pulmonary disease. A Randomized, Controlled trial. *Anesthesiology*. 2014;120:1146-1151.

45. Rothen HU, Neumann P, Berglund JE, et al. Dynamics of reexpansion of atelectasis during general anaesthesia. *Br J Anaesth*. 1999;82:551-556.

46. Hedenstierna G, Tokics L, Lundquist H, et al. Phrenic nerve stimulation during halothane anaesthesia. Effects on atelectasis. *Anesthesiology*. 1994;80:751-760.

47. Milic-Emili J, Robatto FM, Bates JHT. Respiratory mechanics in anaesthesia. *Br J Anaesth*. 1990;65:4-12.

48. Yamakage M. Effects of anaesthetic agents on airway smooth muscle. *Br J Anaesth*. 2002;88:624-627.

49. Dikmen Y, Eminoglu E, Salihoglu Z, et al. Pulmonary mechanics during isoflurane, sevoflurane and desflurane anaesthesia. *Anaesthesia*. 2003;58:745-748.

50. Nyktari V, Papaioannou A, Volakakis N, et al. Respiratory resistance during anaesthesia with isoflurane, sevoflurane, and

desflurane: a randomized clinical trial. *Br J Anaesth.* 2011;107:454-461.

51. Lumb AB, Burns AD, Figueroa Rosette JA, et al. Computational fluid dynamic modelling of the effect of ventilation mode and tracheal tube position on air flow in the large airways. *Anaesthesia.* 2015;70:577-584.

52. Bhatt SB, Kendall AP, Lin ES, et al. Resistance and additional inspiratory work imposed by the laryngeal mask airway: a comparison with tracheal tubes. *Anaesthesia.* 1992;47:343-347.

53. Casati A, Fanelli G, Torri G. Physiological dead space/tidal volume ratio during face mask, laryngeal mask, and cuffed oropharyngeal airway spontaneous ventilation. *J Clin Anesth.* 1998;10:652-655.

54. Yamauchi H, Ito S, Sasano H, et al. Dependence of the gradient between arterial and end-tidal Pco_2 on the fraction of inspired oxygen. *Br J Anaesth.* 2011;107:631-635.

55. Tokics L, Hedenstierna G, Svensson L, et al. $\dot{V}/\dot{Q}$ distribution and correlation to atelectasis in anesthetized paralyzed humans. *J Appl Physiol.* 1996;81:1822-1833.

56. Nyrén S, Radell P, Mure M, et al. Inhalation anesthesia increases $\dot{V}/\dot{Q}$ regional heterogeneity during spontaneous breathing in healthy subjects. *Anesthesiology.* 2010;113:1370-1375.

57. Nyrén S, Radell P, Lindahl SGE, et al. Lung ventilation and perfusion in prone and supine postures with reference to anesthetized and mechanically ventilated healthy volunteers. *Anesthesiology.* 2010;112:682-687.

58. Radke OC, Schneider T, Heller AR, et al. Spontaneous breathing during general anesthesia prevents the ventral redistribution of ventilation as detected by electrical impedance tomography. A randomized trial. *Anesthesiology.* 2012;116:1227-1234.

59. Nunn JF, Bergman NA, Coleman AJ. Factors influencing the arterial oxygen tension during anaesthesia with artificial ventilation. *Br J Anaesth.* 1965;37:898-914.

60. Anjou-Lindskog E, Broman L, Broman M, et al. Effects of intravenous anesthesia on VA/Q distribution: a study performed during ventilation with air and with 50% oxygen, supine and in the lateral position. *Anesthesiology.* 1985;62:485-492.

61. Drummond GB, Cullen JP. Detection of inspiratory resistive loads after anaesthesia for minor surgery. *Br J Anaesth.* 1997;78:308-310.

62. Lumb AB, Slinger PS. Hypoxic pulmonary vasoconstriction: physiology and anesthetic implications. *Anesthesiology.* 2015;122:932-946.

63. Trachsel D, Svendsen J, Erb T. Effects of anaesthesia on paediatric lung function. *Br J Anaesth.* 2016;117:151-163.

64. Serafini G, Cornara G, Cavalloro F, et al. Pulmonary atelectasis during paediatric anaesthesia: CT evaluation and effect of positive end-expiratory pressure (PEEP). *Paediatr Anaesth.* 1999;9:225-228.

65. de la Grandville B, Petak F, Albu G, et al. High inspired oxygen fraction impairs lung volume and ventilation heterogeneity in healthy children: a double-blind randomised controlled trial. *Br J Anaesth.* 2019;122:682-691.

66. Pelosi P, Croci M, Ravagnan I, et al. The effects of body mass on lung volumes, respiratory mechanics, and gas exchange during anesthesia. *Anesth Analg.* 1998;87:654-660.

67. Futier E, Constantin J-M, Pelosi P, et al. Noninvasive ventilation and alveolar recruitment maneuvers improve respiratory function during and after intubation of morbidly obese patients. A randomized controlled study. *Anesthesiology.* 2011;114:1354-1363.

68. Reinius H, Jonsson L, Gustafsson S, et al. Prevention of atelectasis in morbidly obese patients during general anesthesia and paralysis. A computerized tomography study. *Anesthesiology.* 2009;111:979-987.

69. Ball L, Hemmes S, Neto A, et al. Intraoperative ventilation settings and their associations with postoperative pulmonary complications in obese patients. *Br J Anaesth.* 2018;121:899-908.

70. Bohm SH, Thamm OC, von Sanersleben A, et al. Alveolar recruitment strategy and high positive end-expiratory pressure levels do not affect hemodynamics in morbidly obese intravascular volume-loaded patients. *Anesth Analg.* 2009;109:160-163.

71. Defresne AA, Hans GA, Goffin PJ, et al. Recruitment of lung volume during surgery neither affects the postoperative spirometry nor the risk of hypoxaemia after laparoscopic gastric bypass in morbidly obese patients: a randomized controlled study. *Br J Anaesth.* 2014;113:501-507.

72. Yoshino J, Akata T, Takahashi S. Intraoperative changes in arterial oxygenation during volume- controlled mechanical ventilation in modestly obese patients undergoing laparotomies with general anesthesia. *Acta Anaesthesiol Scand.* 2003;47:742-750.

*73. Petersson J, Ax M, Frey J, et al. Positive end-expiratory pressure redistributes regional blood flow and ventilation differently in supine and prone humans. *Anesthesiology.* 2010;113:1361-1369.

74. Loring SH, Behazin N, Novero A, et al. Respiratory mechanical effects of surgical pneumoperitoneum in humans. *J Appl Physiol.* 2014;117:1074-1079.

75. Strang CM, Fredén F, Maripuu E, et al. Ventilation–perfusion distributions and gas exchange during carbon dioxide-pneumoperitoneum in a porcine model. *Br J Anaesth.* 2010;105:691-697.

76. Andersson L, Lagerstrand L, Thörne A, et al. Effect of CO_2 pneumoperitoneum on ventilation-perfusion relationships during laparoscopic cholecystectomy. *Acta Anaesthesiol Scand.* 2002;46:552-560.

77. Kazama T, Ikeda K, Kato T, et al. Carbon dioxide output in laparoscopic cholecystectomy. *Br J Anaesth.* 1996;76:530-535.

78. Veering BT, Cousins MJ. Cardiovascular and pulmonary effects of epidural anaesthesia. *Anesth Intensive Care.* 2000;28:620-635.

79. Labaille T, Clergue F, Samii K, et al. Ventilatory response to CO_2 following intravenous and epidural lidocaine. *Anesthesiology.* 1985;63:179-185.

80. Warner DO, Warner MA, Ritman EL. Human chest wall function during epidural anesthesia. *Anesthesiology.* 1996;85:761-773.

81. Reber A, Bein T, Högman M, et al. Lung aeration and pulmonary gas exchange during lumbar epidural anaesthesia and in the lithotomy position in elderly patients. *Anaesthesia.* 1998;53:854-861.

82. Sun Z, Sessler D, Dalton J, et al. Post-operative hypoxemia is common and persistent; a prospective, blinded observational study. *Anesth Analg.* 2015;121:709-715.

83. Drummond GB. Diaphragmatic dysfunction: an outmoded concept. *Br J Anaesth.* 1998;80:277-280.

84. Sasaki N, Meyer MJ, Eikermann M. Postoperative respiratory muscle dysfunction pathophysiology and preventive strategies. *Anesthesiology.* 2013;118:961-978.

85. Nieuwenhuijs D, Bruce J, Drummond GB, et al. Ventilatory responses after major surgery and high dependency care. *Br J Anaesth.* 2012;108:864-871.

86. Miskovic A, Lumb AB. Postoperative pulmonary complications. *Br J Anaesth.* 2017;118:317-334.

87. Fernandez-Bustamante A, Frendl G, Sprung J, et al. Postoperative pulmonary complications, early mortality, and hospital say following noncardiothoracic surgery. *JAMA Surg.* 2017;152:157-166.

88. Canet J, Gallart L, Gomar C, et al. Prediction of postoperative pulmonary complications in a population-based surgical cohort. *Anesthesiol.* 2010;113:1338-1350.

89. Neto A, da Costa G, Hemmes S, et al. The LAS VEGAS risk score for prediction of postoperative pulmonary complications: An observational study. *Eur J Anaesthesiol.* 2018;35:691-701.

90. Boden I, Skinner E, Browning L, et al. Pre-operative physiotherapy for the prevention of respiratory complications after upper abdominal surgery: pragmatic, double-blinded, multicenter randomized controlled trial. *BMJ.* 2017;360:1-15.

91. Warner DO. Perioperative abstinence from cigarettes. Physiologic and clinical consequences. *Anesthesiol.* 2006;104:356-367.

92. Tønnesen H, Nielsen PR, Lauritzen JB, et al. Smoking and alcohol intervention before surgery: evidence for best practice. *Br J Anaesth.* 2009;102:297-306.

93. Mills E, Eyawo O, Lockhart I, et al. Smoking cessation reduces postoperative complications: a systematic review and meta-analysis. *Am J Med.* 2011;124:144-154.

*94. **Vidal Melo MF, Eikermann M. Protect the lungs during abdominal surgery. It may change the postoperative outcome. *Anesthesiology.* 2013;118:1254-1257.**

95. Coppola S, Froio S, Chiumello D. Protective lung ventilation during general anesthesia: is there any evidence? *Crit Care.* 2014;18:210.

96. Di Marco F, Bonacina D, Vassena E, et al. The effects of anesthesia, muscle paralysis, and ventilation on the lung evaluated by lung diffusion for carbon monoxide and pulmonary surfactant protein B. *Anesth Analg.* 2015;120:373-380.

97. Pelosi P, Gama de Abreu M. Tidal volumes during general anesthesia. Size does matter! *Anesthesiology.* 2012;116:985-986.

98. Futier E, Constantin J-M, Paugam-Burtz C, et al. A trial of intraoperative low-tidal-volume ventilation in abdominal surgery. *N Engl J Med.* 2013;369:428-437.

99. Futier E, Constantin JM, Paugam-Burtz C, et al. A trial of intraoperative low-tidal-volume ventilation in abdominal surgery. *N Engl J Med.* 2013;369:428-437.

*100. **Neto AS, Cardoso SO, Manetta JA, et al. Association between use of lung-protective ventilation with lower tidal volumes and clinical outcomes among patients without acute respiratory distress syndrome. a meta-analysis. *JAMA.* 2012;308:1651-1659.**

101. Yang D, Grant M, Stone A, et al. A meta-analysis of intraoperative ventilation strategies to prevent pulmonary complications. Is low tidal volume alone sufficient to protect healthy lungs? *Ann Surg.* 2016;263:881-887.

102. Hedenstierna G, Edmark L. Protective ventilation during anaesthesia; is it meaningful? *Anaesthesiol.* 2016;125:1079-1082.

103. Nestler C, Simon P, Petroff D. Individualised end-expiratory pressure in obese patients during general anaesthesia: a randomized controlled clinical trial using electrical impedance tomography. *Br J Anaesth.* 2017;119:1194-1205.

104. Pereira SM, Tucci MR, Morais CCA, et al. Individual positive end-expiratory pressure settings optimize intraoperative mechanical ventilation and reduce postoperative atelectasis. *Anesthesiology.* 2018;129:1070-1081.

105. Shaefi S, Eikermann M. Analysing tidal volumes early after a positive end-expiratory pressure increase: a new way to determine optimal PEEP in the operating theatre? *Br J Anaesth.* 2018;120:626-628.

106. Levin MA, McCormick PJ, Lin HM, et al. Low intraoperative tidal volume ventilation with minimal PEEP is associated with increased mortality. *Br J Anaesth.* 2014;113:97-108.

107. Wirth S, Baur M, Spaeth J, et al. Intraoperative positive end-expiratory pressure evaluation using the intratidal compliance-volume profile. *Br J Anaesth.* 2015;114:483-490.

108. Hong CM, Xu D-Z, Lu Q, et al. Low tidal volume and high positive end-expiratory pressure mechanical ventilation results in increased inflammation and ventilator-associated lung injury in normal lungs. *Anesth Analg.* 2010;110:1652-1660.

109. The PROVE Network Investigators for the Clinical Trial Network of the European Society of Anaesthesiology. High versus low positive end-expiratory pressure during general anaesthesia for open abdominal surgery (PROVHILO trial): a multicentre randomised controlled trial. *Lancet.* 2014;384:495-503.

110. Fernandez-Bustamente A, Vidal Melo MF. Bedside assessment of lung aeration and stretch. *Br J Anaesth.* 2018;121:1001-1004.

111. Neto A, Hemmes S, Barbas C, et al. Association between driving pressure and development of postoperative pulmonary complications in patients undergoing mechanical ventilation for general anaesthesia: a meta-analysis of individual patient data. *Lancet Respir Med.* 2016;4:272-280.

112. Ferrando C, Soro M, Unzueta C, et al. Individualised perioperative open-lung approach versus standard protective ventilation in abdominal surgery (iPROVE): a randomized controlled trial. *Lancet Respir Med.* 2018;6:193-203.

113. Abbott T, Fowler A, Pelosi P. A systematic review and consensus definitions for standardised end-points in perioperative medicine: pulmonary complications. *Br J Anaesth.* 2018;120:1066-1079.

114. Hausman MS, Jewell ES, Engoren M. Regional versus general anesthesia in surgical patients with chronic obstructive pulmonary disease: does avoiding general anesthesia reduce the risk of postoperative complications? *Anesth Analg.* 2015;120:1405-1412.

115. Murphy G, Kopman A. Neostigmine as an antagonist of residual block: best practices do not guarantee predictable results. *Br J Anaesth.* 2018;121:225-227.

116. Kumar GV, Nair AM, Murthy HS, et al. Residual neuromuscular blockade affects postoperative pulmonary function. *Anesthesiology.* 2012;117:1234-1244.

117. Sasaki N, Meyer MJ, Malviya SA, et al. Effects of neostigmine reversal of nondepolarizing neuromuscular blocking agents on postoperative respiratory outcomes. A prospective study. *Anesthesiology.* 2014;121:959-968.

118. Kirmeier E, Eriksson L, Lewald H, et al. Post anaesthesia pulmonary complications after use of muscle relaxants (POPULAR); a prospective, observational multi-centre study. *Lancet Respir Med.* 2019;7:129-140.

119. McKay R, Hall K, Hills N. The effect of anaesthetic choice (sevoflurane versus desflurane) and neuromuscular management on speed of airway reflex recovery. *Anesth Analg.* 2016;122:393-401.

120. Cassidy MR, Rosenkranz P, McCabe K, et al. I COUGH: reducing postoperative pulmonary complications with a multidisciplinary patient care programme. *JAMA Surg.* 2013;148:740-746.

22

Changes in the Carbon Dioxide Partial Pressure

KEY POINTS

- Hypocapnia occurs when alveolar ventilation is excessive relative to carbon dioxide production, and usually results from hyperventilation because of hypoxia, acidosis or lung disease.
- Hypercapnia most commonly occurs because of inadequate alveolar ventilation from a multitude of causes, or more rarely from increased carbon dioxide production.

- Arterial P_{CO_2} affects the cerebral circulation—hypocapnia may cause potentially harmful vasoconstriction, whereas vasodilatation from hypercapnia may increase intracranial pressure.
- Hypercapnia, and the resulting acidosis, both have depressant effects on the cardiovascular system, but these are opposed by the stimulant effects of catecholamine release.

Routine monitoring of end-expiratory and arterial P_{CO_2} means it should now be possible to avoid both hypocapnia and hypercapnia under almost all clinical circumstances. However, interest in hypercapnia has continued over recent years for two reasons. First, changes in the approach to artificial ventilation in severe lung injury have led to the use of 'permissive hypercapnia' (page 370). Second, a massive expansion of laparoscopic surgical techniques using carbon dioxide for abdominal insufflation has led to the anaesthetist having to control arterial P_{CO_2} under conditions of significantly increased pulmonary carbon dioxide output (page 261).

Before describing the effects of carbon dioxide on various physiological systems, this chapter will briefly outline the causes of changes in arterial P_{CO_2}.

Causes of Hypocapnia[1]

Hypocapnia can result only from alveolar ventilation that is excessive in relation to carbon dioxide production. Low values of arterial P_{CO_2} are commonly found, resulting from artificial ventilation with an excessive minute volume or from voluntary hyperventilation because of psychological disturbances such as anxiety. A low arterial P_{CO_2} may also result simply from hyperventilation during arterial puncture. Persistently low values may be because of an excessive respiratory drive resulting from one or more of the following causes.

Hypoxaemia is a common cause of hypocapnia, occurring in congenital heart disease with right-to-left shunting, residence at high altitude, pulmonary pathology or any other condition that reduces the arterial P_{O_2} below about

8 kPa (60 mmHg). Hypocapnia secondary to hypoxaemia opposes the ventilatory response to the hypoxaemia (page 53).

Metabolic acidosis produces a compensatory hyperventilation ('air hunger'), which minimizes the fall in pH that would otherwise occur. This is a pronounced feature of diabetic ketoacidosis; arterial P_{CO_2} values less than 3 kPa (22.5 mmHg) are not uncommon in severe metabolic acidosis. This is a vital compensatory mechanism. Failure to maintain the required hyperventilation, either from fatigue or inadequate artificial ventilation, leads to a rapid life-threatening decrease in arterial pH.

Mechanical abnormalities of the lung may drive respiration through vagal reflexes, resulting in moderate reduction of the P_{CO_2}. Thus conditions such as pulmonary fibrosis, pulmonary oedema and asthma are usually associated with a low to normal P_{CO_2} until the patient passes into type 2 respiratory failure (page 316).

Neurological disorders may result in hyperventilation and hypocapnia. This is most commonly seen in those conditions that lead to the presence of blood in the cerebrospinal fluid, such as after a head injury or subarachnoid haemorrhage.

Causes of Hypercapnia

It is uncommon to encounter an arterial P_{CO_2} above the normal range in a healthy subject. Any value of more than 6.1 kPa (46 mmHg) should be considered abnormal, but values up to 6.7 kPa (50 mmHg) may be transiently attained by breath holding.

When a patient is hypercapnic, there are only four possible causes:

1. *Increased concentration of carbon dioxide in the inspired gas.* This normally iatrogenic cause of hypercapnia is uncommon, but it is dangerous and differs fundamentally from the other causes listed here. It should therefore be excluded at the outset in any patient unexpectedly found to be hypercapnic when breathing via any external equipment. The carbon dioxide may be endogenous from rebreathing or exogenous from carbon dioxide added to the inhaled gases. Hypercapnia from rebreathing is more common, but fortunately its severity is limited by the rate at which the P_{CO_2} can increase. If all the carbon dioxide produced by metabolism is retained and distributed in the body stores, arterial P_{CO_2} can increase no faster than about 0.4 to 0.8 $kPa.min^{-1}$ (3–6 $mmHg.min^{-1}$).

2. *Increased carbon dioxide production.* If the pulmonary minute volume is fixed by artificial ventilation and carbon dioxide production is increased by, for example, malignant hyperpyrexia, hypercapnia is inevitable. Like the previous category, this is a rare but dangerous cause of hypercapnia during anaesthesia. A less dramatic, but very common, reason for increased carbon dioxide production is sepsis leading to pyrexia, which often results in hypercapnia in artificially ventilated patients. Although not strictly an increase in production, absorption of carbon dioxide from the peritoneum during laparoscopic surgery or pleura during thoracic surgery have the same respiratory effects.

3. *Hypoventilation.* An inadequate pulmonary minute volume is by far the commonest cause of hypercapnia. Pathological causes of hypoventilation are numerous and considered in Chapter 27 and Figure 27.2. In respiratory medicine, the commonest cause of long-standing hypercapnia is chronic obstructive pulmonary disease (COPD).

4. *Increased dead space.* This cause of hypercapnia is usually diagnosed by a process of exclusion when a patient has a high P_{CO_2} despite a normal minute volume and no evidence of a hypermetabolic state or inhaled carbon dioxide. The cause may be incorrectly configured breathing apparatus or a large alveolar dead space (page 97) from a variety of pathological causes.

Effects of Carbon Dioxide on the Nervous System

A number of special difficulties hinder an understanding of the effects of changes in P_{CO_2} on any physiological system. First, there is the problem of species difference, which is a formidable obstacle to the interpretation of animal studies in this field. The second difficulty arises from the fact that carbon dioxide can exert its effect either directly or in consequence of (respiratory) acidosis. The third difficulty arises from the fact that carbon dioxide acts at many different sites in the body, sometimes

producing opposite effects on a particular function, such as blood pressure (see later discussion).

Carbon dioxide has at least five major effects on the brain:

1. It is a major factor governing cerebral blood flow (CBF).
2. It influences the intracerebral pressure through changes in CBF.
3. It is the main factor influencing the intracellular pH, which is known to have important effects on the metabolism, and therefore function, of the cell.
4. It may be presumed to exert the inert gas narcotic effect in accord with its physical properties, which are similar to those of nitrous oxide.
5. It influences the excitability of certain neurones, particularly relevant in the case of the reticular activating system.

The interplay of these effects is difficult to understand, although the gross changes produced are well established.

Effects on Consciousness

Carbon dioxide has long been known to cause unconsciousness in dogs entering the Grotto del Cane in Italy, where carbon dioxide issuing from a fumarole forms a layer near the ground. It has been widely used as an anaesthetic for short procedures in small laboratory animals. Inhalation of 30% carbon dioxide is sufficient to produce anaesthesia in humans but is complicated by the frequent occurrence of convulsions. In patients with ventilatory failure, carbon dioxide narcosis occurs when the P_{CO_2} rises above about 12 kPa (90–120 mmHg).

Narcosis by carbon dioxide is probably not caused primarily by its inert gas narcotic effects, because its oil solubility predicts a much weaker narcotic than it seems to be. It is likely that the major effect on the central nervous system is by alteration of the intracellular pH, with consequent derangements of metabolic processes. In animals the narcotic effect correlates better with cerebrospinal fluid pH than with arterial P_{CO_2}.

The effects of inhaling low concentrations of carbon dioxide for a prolonged period of time are described on page 226.

Cerebral Blood Flow[2]

CBF increases with arterial P_{CO_2} at a rate of about 7 to 15 $mL.100~g^{-1}.min^{-1}$ for each kPa increase in P_{CO_2} (1–2 $mL.100~g^{-1}.min^{-1}$ per mmHg) within the approximate range 3 to 10 kPa (20–80 mmHg). The full response curve is S-shaped (Fig. 22.1). The response at very low P_{CO_2} is probably limited by the vasodilator effect of tissue hypoxia, and the response above 16 kPa (120 mmHg) seems to represent maximal vasodilatation. P_{CO_2} also influences the autoregulation of CBF with both hypocapnia and hypercapnia, reducing the range of cerebral perfusion pressures between which CBF is maintained constant.[3] Finally, the relationship between CBF and P_{CO_2} has a circadian

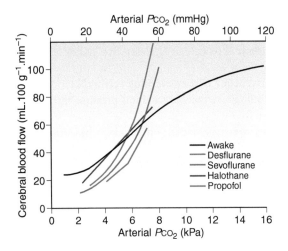

• **Fig. 22.1** Relationship of cerebral blood flow to arterial P_{CO_2} and the effect of general anaesthesia. The awake line can only be derived from animal experiments because of the extreme P_{CO_2} values used. The lines during anaesthesia are from various human studies, and all represent the effect at approximately one minimum alveolar concentration or equivalent. The changes shown represent the brain as a whole, and it is not possible to generalize about regional changes.

rhythm, being higher in the morning,[4] and is modified by sympathetic nervous system activity.[5]

Mechanisms

In the intact animal, CBF is increased in response to P_{CO_2} by a combination of vasodilatation of cerebral blood vessels and an increase in blood pressure (see later). Changes in P_{CO_2} lead to a complex series of events that bring about vasodilation of cerebral blood vessels.[2] In adults, the effect is initiated by changes in the extracellular pH in the region of the arterioles, which alters intracellular calcium levels both directly and indirectly via nitric oxide production and the formation of cyclic guanosine monophosphate. With prolonged hypocapnia, and to a lesser extent hypercapnia, changes in CBF return towards baseline after a few hours, an effect thought to result from changes in cerebrospinal fluid pH correcting the extracellular acidosis. Sensitivity of the cerebral circulation to carbon dioxide may be lost in a variety of pathological circumstances such as cerebral tumour, infarction or trauma. There is commonly a fixed vasodilatation in damaged areas of brain, which if widespread may cause dangerous increases in intracranial pressure (ICP).

Anaesthesia

Inhalational anaesthetics have a direct cerebral vasodilator effect and increase normocapnic CBF considerably.[6] They also accentuate the response to both hypocapnia and hypercapnia; that is, they increase the slope of the relationship between P_{CO_2} and CBF (Fig. 22.1). Despite the increased slope during hypocapnia, global CBF during anaesthesia with hyperventilation is normally still greater than when awake.[2] Intravenous anaesthetics such as thiopentone and propofol[7] reduce CBF at normal P_{CO_2} in accordance with the reduced cerebral oxygen consumption.

Vasoconstriction in response to hyperventilation continues to occur (Fig. 22.1), but at deeper levels of anaesthesia the response is reduced compared with when awake.[2]

ICP tends to rise with increasing P_{CO_2} as a result of cerebral vasodilatation. Hyperventilation was used for many years as a standard method of acutely reducing ICP after head injury, but the reduction in ICP may only be short lived, and the effects on CBF are variable. The possibility of *increased* CBF as a result of lowered ICP must be offset against reduced CBF from hypocapnic vasoconstriction. It is therefore preferable to monitor ICP, and if this is not possible hyperventilation should only be used to reduce ICP when other therapeutic approaches have failed.

Effects on the Autonomic and Endocrine Systems

Survival in severe hypercapnia is, to a large extent, dependent on the autonomic response. A great many of the effects of carbon dioxide on other systems are due wholly or in part to the autonomic response to carbon dioxide.

Animal studies have shown an increase in plasma levels of both adrenaline and noradrenaline in response to an elevation of P_{CO_2} during apnoeic mass-movement oxygenation. Similar, although variable, changes have been obtained over a lower range of P_{CO_2} in human volunteers inhaling carbon dioxide mixtures.[8] Animal studies indicate that the increase in catecholamine release is mediated by direct stimulation of ventrolateral medullary neurones, which respond to elevated P_{CO_2} by increasing sympathetic nerve discharge.[9]

The effect of an increased level of circulating catecholamines is, to a certain extent, offset by a decreased sensitivity of target organs when the pH is reduced. This is additional to the general depressant direct effect of carbon dioxide on target organs.

Effects on Other Body Systems

Respiratory System

Chapter 4 describes the role of carbon dioxide in the control of breathing, and this is not discussed further here. Animal studies suggest that hypercapnia has multiple adverse effects on lung tissue. Examples include impaired clearance of oedema fluid mediated by endocytosis, and so inactivation of the Na^+/K^+-ATPase (page 341) and inhibition of cytokines interleukin-6 and tumour necrosis factor, which are crucial components of innate immunity in the lung.[10]

Pulmonary Circulation

An elevated P_{CO_2} causes vasoconstriction in the pulmonary circulation (page 83), but the effect is less marked than that of hypoxia. Nevertheless, in healthy subjects an end-expiratory P_{CO_2} of 7 kPa (52 mmHg) increased pulmonary vascular resistance by 32%, which, along with elevated cardiac output, led to a 60% increase in mean pulmonary arterial pressure.[11] Although regional variations in blood flow have not been demonstrated, this effect is believed to act in a similar fashion to hypoxic pulmonary vasoconstriction (HPV) (page 80), diverting blood away from underventilated alveoli. Hypocapnia significantly attenuates HPV in animals, although this has not been described in humans. There is evidence that pH is responsible for CO_2-mediated changes in the pulmonary vasculature, rather than P_{CO_2} per se.[12]

Oxygenation of the Blood

Quite apart from its effect on ventilation, carbon dioxide exerts three other important effects that influence the oxygenation of the blood. First, if the concentration of nitrogen (or other 'inert' gas) remains constant, the concentration of carbon dioxide in the alveolar gas can increase only at the expense of oxygen, which must be displaced. Second, an increase in P_{CO_2} causes a displacement of the oxygen dissociation curve to the right (page 146). Finally, in animals, changes in P_{CO_2} are known to affect the distribution of ventilation/perfusion ratios as measured by the multiple inert gas elimination technique (page 107). This results from changes in pH influencing pulmonary vessels, as described in the previous paragraph, as well as causing changes in the size of small-diameter bronchi.

Cardiovascular System

The effects of carbon dioxide on the circulation are complicated by the alternative modes of action on different components of the system. In general, both hypercapnia and acidosis have direct depressant effects on cardiac myocytes and vascular smooth muscle cells, effects that are normally opposed by the increase in catecholamines caused by elevated P_{CO_2}. Under different circumstances these opposing effects make the overall effect of carbon dioxide on the cardiovascular system unpredictable. Despite this problem, moderate degrees of hypercapnia have been proposed to have therapeutic potential in treating septic shock when its effects can mimic inotropes such as dobutamine.[13]

Myocardial Contractility and Heart Rate

Both contractility and heart rate are diminished by elevated P_{CO_2} in the isolated preparation, probably as a result of change in pH. However, in the intact subject the direct depressant effect of carbon dioxide is overshadowed by the stimulant effect mediated through the sympathetic system. In artificially ventilated humans, increased P_{CO_2} raises cardiac output and slightly reduces total peripheral resistance,[8] therefore blood pressure tends to be increased. Awake healthy subjects studied with noninvasive Doppler echocardiography show similar changes.[11] With an end-expiratory P_{CO_2} of 7 kPa (52 mmHg) cardiac output was increased by about 1 L.min^{-1} as a result of increases in both heart rate and stroke volume, and accompanied by a small rise in blood pressure. Measurements of left ventricular systolic and diastolic function were unchanged, confirming the

dominance of catecholamine stimulation compared with direct depressant effects on the heart. The response of cardiac output to hypercapnia is diminished by most anaesthetics.[8]

Arrhythmias

Arrhythmias have been reported in awake humans during acute hypercapnia, but seldom seem to be of serious import. One study of normal subjects with modest degrees of hypercapnia did, however, demonstrate an increase in QT dispersion of the electrocardiogram during hypercapnia.[11] This finding reflects regional repolarization abnormalities of the ventricles, and under other circumstances, such as ischaemic heart disease, indicates a propensity to develop life-threatening arrhythmias.

Blood Pressure

As described earlier, an elevated P_{CO_2} usually causes a small increase in blood pressure, an effect seen in both conscious and anaesthetized patients. However, the response is variable, and certainly cannot be relied upon as an infallible diagnostic sign of hypercapnia. Hypotension accompanies an elevation of P_{CO_2} if there is blockade of the sympathetic system by, for example, spinal anaesthesia.

Effect on the Kidney

Renal blood flow and glomerular filtration rate are little influenced by minor changes of P_{CO_2}. However, at high levels of P_{CO_2} there is constriction of the glomerular afferent arterioles, leading to anuria. Long-term hypercapnia results in increased resorption of bicarbonate by the kidneys, further raising the plasma bicarbonate level and constituting a compensatory metabolic alkalosis. Long-term hypocapnia decreases renal bicarbonate resorption, resulting in a further fall of plasma bicarbonate and producing a compensatory metabolic acidosis. In each case the arterial pH returns towards the normal value, but the bicarbonate ion concentration departs even further from normality.

Effect on Blood Electrolyte Levels

The acidosis that accompanies hypercapnia causes leakage of potassium ions from the cells into the plasma. Because it takes an appreciable time for the potassium ions to be transported back into the intracellular compartment, repeated bouts of hypercapnia at short intervals result in a stepwise rise in plasma potassium.

A reduction in the ionized fraction of the total calcium has, in the past, been thought to be the cause of the tetany that accompanies severe hypocapnia. However, the changes that occur are too small to account for tetany, which occurs in parathyroid disease only when there has been a fairly gross reduction of ionized calcium. Hyperexcitability affects all nerves, and spontaneous activity ultimately occurs. The muscle spasms probably result from activity in proprioceptive fibres causing reflex muscle contraction.

Hypercapnia in Clinical Practice

Clinical Signs

Hyperventilation is the cardinal sign of hypercapnia because of an increased concentration of carbon dioxide in the inspired gas, whether it is endogenous or exogenous. However, this sign will be absent in patients in whom hypercapnia is the result of hypoventilation, and such patients, including those with COPD, constitute the great majority of occurrences of hypercapnia.

Dyspnoea may or may not be present. In patients with central failure of respiratory drive, dyspnoea may be entirely absent. On the other hand, when hypoventilation results from mechanical failure in the respiratory system (airway obstruction, pneumothorax, pulmonary fibrosis, etc.), dyspnoea is usually obvious.

In patients with COPD hypercapnia is usually associated with a flushed skin and a full and bounding pulse with occasional extrasystoles. The blood pressure is often raised, but this is not a reliable sign. Muscle twitching and a characteristic flap of the hands may be observed when coma is imminent. Convulsions may occur. The patient will become comatose when the $P\text{CO}_2$ is in the range 12 to 16 kPa (90–120 mmHg). Hypercapnia should always be considered in cases of unexplained coma.

Hypercapnia cannot be reliably diagnosed on clinical examination. This is particularly true when there is a neurological basis for hypoventilation. An arterial $P\text{CO}_2$ should be measured in all cases of doubt.

Severe Hypercapnia

Cases of severe hypercapnia without hypoxia are documented in sufficient numbers to indicate that complete recovery is possible and may even be the rule. One report from 1990[14] detailed five instances of hypercapnia without hypoxia in children with arterial $P\text{CO}_2$ values in the range of 21 to 36 kPa (155–269 mmHg). All were comatose or stuporous but recovered. A single case report of massive grain aspiration reported survival following a $P\text{CO}_2$ of 66.8 kPa (501 mmHg).[15] These cases indicate that, of the reported cases, full recovery seems to be the usual outcome. Hypoxia seems to be much more dangerous than hypercapnia.

References

1. Laffey JG, Kavanagh BP. Hypocapnia. *N Engl J Med.* 2002; 347:43-53.
2. Brian JE. Carbon dioxide and the cerebral circulation. *Anesthesiology.* 1998;88:1365-1386.
3. Meng L, Gelb AW. Regulation of cerebral autoregulation by carbon dioxide. *Anesthesiology.* 2015;122:196-205.
4. Strohm J, Duffin J, Fisher JA. Circadian cerebrovascular reactivity to CO_2. *Respir Physiol Neurobiol.* 2014;197:15-18.
5. Peebles KC, Ball OG, MacRae BA, et al. Sympathetic regulation of the human cerebrovascular response to carbon dioxide. *J Appl Physiol.* 2012;113:700-706.
6. Cho S, Kujigaki T, Uchiyama Y, et al. Effects of sevoflurane with and without nitrous oxide on human cerebral circulation. *Anesthesiology.* 1996;85:755-760.
7. Eng C, Lam AM, Mayberg TS, et al. The influence of propofol with and without nitrous oxide on cerebral blood flow velocity and CO_2 reactivity in humans. *Anesthesiology.* 1992;77:872-879.
8. Cullen DJ, Eger EI. Cardiovascular effects of carbon dioxide in man. *Anesthesiology.* 1974;41:345-349.
9. Toney GM. Sympathetic activation by the central chemoreceptor 'reflex': new evidence that RVLM vasomotor neurons are involved … but are they enough? *J Physiol.* 2006;577:3.
10. Shigemura M, Lecuona A, Sznajder JI. Effects of hypercapnia on the lung. *J Physiol.* 2017;595(8):2431-2437.
11. Kiely DG, Cargill RI, Lipworth BJ. Effects of hypercapnia on hemodynamic, inotropic, lusitropic, and electrophysiological indices in humans. *Chest.* 1996;109:1215-1221.
12. Loeppky JA, Scotto P, Riedel CE, et al. Effects of acid-base status on acute hypoxic pulmonary vasoconstriction and gas exchange. *J Appl Physiol.* 1992;72:1787-1797.
*13. **Wang Z, Su F, Bruhn A, et al. Acute hypercapnia improves indices of tissue oxygenation more than dobutamine in septic shock. *Am J Respir Crit Care Med.* 2008;177:178-183.**
14. Goldstein B, Shannon DC, Todres ID. Supercarbia in children: clinical course and outcome. *Crit Care Med.* 1990;18:166-168.
15. Slinger P, Blundell PE, Metcalf IR. Management of massive grain aspiration. *Anesthesiology.* 1997;87:993-995.

23

Hypoxia

KEY POINTS

- Intracellular acidosis from anaerobic metabolism occurs soon after the onset of cellular hypoxia and is worse when there is a plentiful supply of blood and glucose to the cell.
- Lack of high-energy substrates such as adenosine triphosphate (ATP) and direct effects of hypoxia both inhibit the activity of ion channels, decreasing the transmembrane potential of the cell, leading to increased intracellular calcium levels.
- In nervous tissue the uncontrolled release of excitatory amino acids exacerbates the hypoxic damage.
- Hypoxia causes the activation of a transcription protein hypoxia-inducible factor 1 (HIF-1), which induces the production of numerous proteins with diverse biological functions.

All but the simplest forms of life have evolved to exploit the immense advantages of oxidative metabolism. The price they have paid is to become dependent on oxygen for their survival. The essential feature of hypoxia is the cessation of oxidative phosphorylation (page 152) when the mitochondrial Po_2 falls below a critical level. Anaerobic pathways, in particular the glycolytic pathway (see Fig. 10.12), then come into play. These trigger a complex series of cellular changes leading first to reduced cellular function and ultimately to cell death. This chapter describes changes that occur with acute hypoxia—physiological effects of long-term hypoxia are described on page 207.

Biochemical Changes in Hypoxia

Depletion of High-Energy Compounds

Anaerobic metabolism produces only one-nineteenth of the yield of the high-energy phosphate molecule adenosine triphosphate (ATP) per mole of glucose, compared with aerobic metabolism (page 153). In organs with a high metabolic rate such as the brain, it is impossible to increase glucose transport sufficiently to maintain the normal level of ATP production. Therefore, during hypoxia, the ATP/adenosine diphosphate (ADP) ratio falls, and there is a rapid decline in the level of all high-energy compounds (Fig. 23.1). Similar changes occur in response to arterial hypotension. These changes will rapidly block cerebral function, but organs with a lower energy requirement will continue to function for a longer time and are thus more resistant to hypoxia (see later).

Under hypoxic conditions, there are two ways in which reductions in ATP levels may be minimized, both of which are effective for only a short time. First, the high-energy phosphate bond in phosphocreatine may be used to create ATP,[1] and initially this slows the rate of reduction of ATP (Fig. 23.1). Second, two molecules of ADP may combine to form one of ATP and one of adenosine monophosphate (AMP; the adenylate kinase reaction). This reaction is driven forward by the removal of AMP, which is converted to adenosine (a potent vasodilator) and thence to inosine, hypoxanthine, xanthine and uric acid, with irreversible loss of adenine nucleotides. The implications for production of reactive oxygen species by this pathway are discussed on page 288.

End Products of Metabolism

The end products of aerobic metabolism are carbon dioxide and water, both of which are easily diffusible and lost from the body. The main anaerobic pathway produces hydrogen and lactate ions which, from most of the body, escape into the circulation, where they may be measured or quantified in terms of the base deficit. However, the blood–brain barrier is relatively impermeable to charged ions, therefore hydrogen and lactate ions are retained within the neurones of the hypoxic brain. Lactacidosis can only occur when circulation is maintained to provide the large quantities of glucose required for conversion to lactic acid.

In severe cerebral hypoxia, a major part of the dysfunction and damage is because of intracellular acidosis rather than simply depletion of high-energy compounds (see later). Gross hypoperfusion is more damaging than total ischaemia, because the latter limits glucose supply and therefore the formation of lactic acid. Similarly, patients who have an episode of cerebral ischaemia whilst hyperglycaemic (e.g., a stroke) have been found to have more severe brain injury

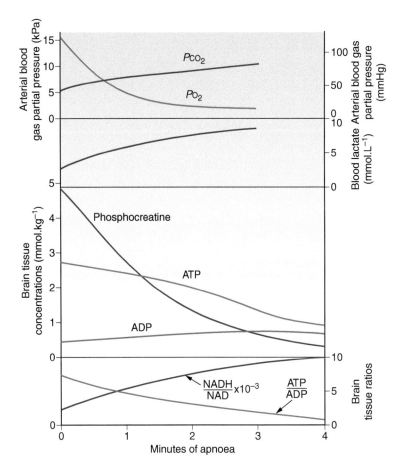

• **Fig. 23.1** Biochemical changes during 4 minutes of respiratory arrest in rats previously breathing 30% oxygen. Recovery of all values, except blood lactate, was complete within 5 minutes of restarting pulmonary ventilation. (Data from reference 1.) *ADP*, Adenosine diphosphate; *ATP*, adenosine triphosphate; *NAD*, nicotinamide adenine dinucleotide.

than those with normal or low blood glucose levels at the time of the hypoxic event.[2]

Initiation of Glycolysis

The enzyme 6-phosphofructokinase (PFK) is the rate-limiting element of the glycolytic pathway (see Fig. 10.12). Activity of PFK is enhanced by the presence of ADP, AMP and phosphate, which will rapidly accumulate during hypoxia, thus accelerating glycolysis. PFK is, however, inhibited by acidosis, which will quickly limit the formation of ATP from glucose. The intracellular production of phosphate from ATP breakdown also promotes the activity of glycogen phosphorylase, which cleaves glycogen molecules to produce fructose-1,6-diphosphate. This enters the glycolytic pathway below the rate-limiting PFK reaction, avoiding the expenditure of two molecules of ATP in its derivation from glucose. Therefore four molecules of ATP are produced from one of fructose-1,6-diphosphate in comparison with two from one molecule of glucose. There is no subsequent stage in the glycolytic pathway that is significantly rate limited by acidosis. Provided glycogen is available within the cell, this second pathway therefore provides a valuable reserve for the production of ATP.

Mechanisms of Hypoxic Cell Damage

Many mechanisms contribute to cell damage or death from hypoxia. The precise role of each is unclear, but there is general agreement that different tissues respond to hypoxia in quite varied ways. Also, the nature of the hypoxic insult has a large effect with differing speed of onset, degree of hypoxia, blood flow, blood glucose concentration and tissue metabolic activity all influencing the resulting tissue dysfunction.

Immediate Cellular Responses to Hypoxia[3]

Because of the dramatic clinical consequences of nervous system damage, neuronal cells are the most widely studied, and therefore form the basis for the mechanisms described in this section.[1] Changes in the transmembrane potential of a hypoxic neurone are shown in Figure 23.2, along with the major physiological changes that occur. At the onset of anoxia, central nervous system cells immediately become either slightly hyperpolarized (as shown in Fig. 23.2) or depolarized, depending on the cell type. This is followed by a gradual reduction in membrane potential until a 'threshold' value is reached, when a spontaneous rapid depolarization

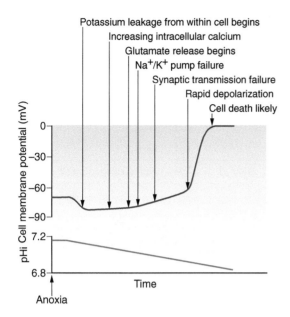

Potassium leakage from within cell begins
Increasing intracellular calcium
Glutamate release begins
Na^+/K^+ pump failure
Synaptic transmission failure
Rapid depolarization
Cell death likely

• **Fig. 23.2** Changes in transmembrane potential and intracellular pH (pHi) in a neuronal cell following the sudden onset of anoxia. Significant physiological events in the course of the hypoxic insult are shown. Once membrane potential reaches zero, cell death is almost inevitable (see text for details). The time between anoxia and rapid depolarization is highly variable, between about 4 minutes with complete ischaemia to almost 1 hour with hypoxia and preserved blood flow. (From reference 1.)

occurs. At this stage there are gross abnormalities in ion channel function, and the normal intracellular and extracellular ionic gradients are abolished, leading to cell death.

Potassium and Sodium Flux

Hypoxia has a direct effect on potassium channels (page 51), increasing transmembrane potassium conductance and causing the immediate hyperpolarization. Potassium begins to leak out from the cell, increasing the extracellular potassium concentration, thus tending to depolarize the cell membrane. Potassium leakage, along with sodium influx, is accelerated when falling ATP levels cause failure of the Na^+/K^+-ATPase pump. Following rapid depolarization, sodium and potassium channels probably simply remain open, allowing free passage of ions across the cell membrane and leading to cellular destruction.

Calcium

Intracellular calcium concentration increases shortly after the onset of hypoxia. Voltage-gated calcium channels open in response to the falling transmembrane potential, and the increasing intracellular sodium concentration causes the membrane-bound Na/Ca exchanger to reverse its activity. An altered transmembrane potential is detected within the cell by ryanodine receptors on intracellular organelles, leading to release of calcium from the endoplasmic reticulum and mitochondria. This increase in intracellular calcium is generally harmful, causing the activation of ATPase enzymes just when ATP may be critically low, the activation of proteases to damage sarcolemma and the cytoskeleton

and the uncontrolled release of neurotransmitters (see later). At this stage, the cell has probably not been irretrievably damaged by spontaneous depolarization, but derangement of calcium channel function effectively prevents normal synaptic transmission and therefore cellular function. Extracellular adenosine, formed from the degradation of AMP, is also believed to play a role in blocking calcium channels during anoxia.[1]

Glutamate Release

The excitatory amino acid glutamate, and to a lesser extent aspartate, is released from many neurones at concentrations of two to five times the normal concentration early in the course of a hypoxic insult, followed by further dramatic increases following rapid depolarization. Glutamate reuptake mechanisms also fail, and extracellular concentrations quickly reach neurotoxic levels, acting via the N-methyl-D-aspartate (NMDA) receptor. Cells with depleted energy stores are particularly susceptible, but the mechanism by which glutamate and aspartate bring about cell damage is unknown.

Nonglutamate Mechanisms

Other mechanisms of hypoxic cell damage include the effects of extracellular ATP. In a normally functioning cell, the intracellular concentration of ATP is approximately 10 mM, compared with 10 nM outside of the cell.[4] In a malfunctioning hypoxic cell ATP molecules may be transported out of the intracellular space via various ion channels. Once in the extracellular space ATP acts on the P2Y or P2X purinergic receptors, activation of which further increases membrane permeability, damages the cytoskeleton and leads to cytokine release.

Other nonglutamate mechanisms include the effects on potassium channels already described, and activation of transient receptor potential (TRP) channels, which are nonspecific cation channels. In the brain, TRPM7 contributes to calcium and magnesium homeostasis and influences cell growth, but in hypoxic conditions, in response to abnormal membrane potential and calcium levels, contributes to cell death.[5] Drugs affecting TRP function therefore have potential as neuroprotective agents.

Delayed Cellular Responses to Hypoxia

Following brain injury in humans, cerebral oedema often continues to develop for some hours after the initial insult. There are several possible explanations for this delayed neuronal damage, with activation of many different cellular systems implicated. However, it is a quite different clinical problem that has recently focussed attention on cellular adaptations to hypoxia. The core of many solid malignant tumours has a poor blood supply, caused by the failure of angiogenesis to keep up with the rapid tumour growth. Tumour hypoxia is associated with highly malignant, aggressive tumours, which often respond poorly to treatment. For this reason, much recent research has focussed on

TABLE 23.1	Genes Induced by Hypoxia and Their Effects		
Function	**Gene**		**Biological Action**
Oxygen transport	Erythropoietin		Stimulation of red cell production
	Transferrin		Iron transport
Increased blood flow	VEGF		Angiogenesis
	NO synthase		Vasodilatation
ATP production	Glucose transporter-1		Transfer of glucose into cell
	Hexokinase		
	Aldolase		Glycolysis (see Fig. 10.12)
	Lactate dehydrogenase		
	Pyruvate dehydrogenase kinase		Mitochondrial O_2 consumption
pH correction	Carbonic anhydrase		Buffering of metabolic acidosis
Inflammation	Interleukin-6, -8		Activation of inflammatory cells

ATP, Adenosine triphosphate; *NO*, nitric oxide; *VEGF*, vascular endothelial growth factor.

understanding the cellular effects of hypoxia, with a view to developing new therapeutic approaches.

Table 23.1 shows the numerous genes that may be induced by hypoxia. Most of the systems activated by hypoxia assist the cell in overcoming the hypoxic conditions, for example, erythropoietin to increase haemoglobin concentration, or glycolytic enzymes to increase anaerobic ATP formation. Some activated genes may accelerate cell proliferation and therefore increase tumour malignancy, whereas other genes are activated that encourage apoptosis and impair tumour growth.[6]

Hypoxia-Inducible Factor 1[7,8]

Many of these cellular adaptations to hypoxia are mediated by a transcription-regulating protein called hypoxia-inducible factor 1 (HIF-1). HIF-1 is a dimeric protein, with the HIF-1α subunit found in cytoplasm and the HIF-1β subunit constitutively expressed in the nucleus.[9,10] Under normal conditions cytoplasmic HIF-1α is ubiquitous, but a prolyl-hydroxylase protein (PHD-1) rapidly hydroxylates HIF-1α, rendering it inactive. Oxygen is required as a co-substrate for this reaction, such that, when cellular hypoxia occurs, hydroxylation by PHD-1 fails, and HIF-1α remains stable for long enough to enter the nucleus and combine with HIF-1β to initiate transcription of multiple hypoxia-induced genes, the best known of which are shown in Table 23.1. Other cofactors for the hydroxylation of HIF-1 include molecules from the citric acid cycle (see Fig. 10.13) such as succinate and fumarate, and iron. The last of these explains the influence of iron status on hypoxic responses in the pulmonary circulation (page 82). The HIF-1 system is implicated in many diseases, including intestinal inflammation, cancer, vascular disease and pulmonary hypertension, and so is now a major potential target for therapeutic agents.[9]

Ischaemic Preconditioning[11]

Prior exposure of a tissue to a series of short periods of hypoxia, interspersed with normal oxygen levels, has been found to influence the tissue's subsequent response to a prolonged ischaemic insult, a phenomenon known as ischaemic preconditioning. Although ischaemic preconditioning has been demonstrated in many tissues, the phenomenon has mostly been studied in heart muscle, and three forms are described.

Early Protection

Reduction in the damage occurring from an ischaemic period begins immediately after the preconditioning has occurred, and lasts for 2 to 3 hours. Activation of sarcolemmal and mitochondrial ATP-dependent K^+ channels (K_{ATP}) is believed to be the main mechanism by which protection from ischaemia occurs. After preconditioning, the enhanced activity of K_{ATP} channels helps to maintain the transmembrane potential nearer to normal values, slowing the rate of progression of the immediate cellular responses to hypoxia described earlier. During prolonged hypoxia, fluid and electrolyte imbalances also occur across the mitochondrial membrane, impairing the ability of the cell to make the best use of any oxygen remaining in the cell. Activated mitochondrial K_{ATP} channels will again reduce the rate at which these changes occur. Extracellular triggers that bring about preconditioning include adenosine, purines, bradykinin or catecholamines, all acting via G-proteins and protein kinase C to cause activation of the K_{ATP} channels.

Late Protection

This describes the protection from ischaemia seen about 12 hours after the preconditioning, and is less effective than early protection. It is again mediated by activation of K_{ATP} channels, this time brought about by transcription of genes encoding proteins such as inducible nitric oxide synthase, superoxide dismutase (page 290) or cyclooxygenase (page 170).

Remote Ischaemic Preconditioning[12,13]

This phenomenon offers the most potential for clinical use. The technique involves multiple (usually three to four) short periods of ischaemia induced in an arm or leg by inflating a blood pressure cuff above systolic blood pressure for 5 minutes. Damage caused by ischaemia in a remote organ, usually the heart during revascularization surgery, has then been demonstrated to be less in the 'preconditioned' patients. Unfortunately, improvements in biomarkers of injury have not translated into improved clinical outcomes, with two studies of remote ischaemic preconditioning in heart surgery finding no clinical benefit.[13] The reasons for this are multifactorial, and include effects of the anaesthetic agents used (see next section) or patient factors such as diabetes, which may render patients resistant to preconditioning.

Agents Used for Preconditioning

Several drugs, but particularly inhalational anaesthetics, can precondition cardiac muscle in a manner similar to brief ischaemic episodes.[11] The mechanism is also similar, with most of the effective drugs somehow enhancing K_{ATP} channel activity. Similar responses occur to the noble gases helium and xenon, possibly mediated by modulation of nitric oxide antagonism of the NMDA receptor[14] or activation of K_{ATP} channels.[15] Xenon may potentially be useful for neuroprotection against encephalopathy from cerebral ischaemia in neonates.[16]

Therefore, unfortunately, despite impressive laboratory results, ischaemic preconditioning has thus far failed to translate into a useful option in routine clinical practice, but it does show enormous potential for situations where ischaemia can be predicted in advance.

Po_2 Level at Which Hypoxia Occurs

'Critical Po_2' refers to the oxygen partial pressure below which oxidative cellular metabolism fails. For isolated mitochondria, this is known to be less than 0.13 kPa (1 mmHg), and possibly as low as 0.01 kPa (0.1 mmHg) in muscle cells, despite their large oxygen consumption. Venous Po_2 approximates to end-capillary Po_2 and, although highly variable, is usually in excess of 3 kPa (~20 mmHg), even in maximally working skeletal muscle. Thus when the minimal Po_2 in the nearby capillary is approximately 200 times greater than that required by the mitochondria, it is difficult to envisage how cellular hypoxia can occur in all but the most extreme situations. There are reasons why this is not the case in vivo.

Measurement of intracellular Po_2 is difficult. The most widely used technique is applicable only to muscle cells, and involves measurement of myoglobin saturation, from which Po_2 may be determined. These studies have indicated that intracellular Po_2 is in the range 0.5 to 2 kPa (3–15 mmHg), depending on cell activity. Diffusion of oxygen within cells is believed to be slow because of the proteinaceous nature of the cytoplasm, and therefore large variations in intracellular Po_2 are likely to exist. Thus, in intact cells, as opposed to isolated mitochondria, critical Po_2 is more likely to be of the order of 0.5 to 1.3 kPa (3–10 mmHg), which is much closer to the end-capillary value.

Critical Arterial Po_2 for Tissue Function

The minimal safe level of arterial Po_2 is that which will maintain a safe tissue Po_2. This will depend on many factors besides arterial Po_2, including haemoglobin concentration, tissue perfusion and tissue oxygen consumption. These factors are in accord with Barcroft's classification of 'anoxia' into anoxic, anaemic and stagnant (page 155).

This argument may be extended to consider in which circumstances the venous Po_2 (and by implication tissue Po_2) may fall below its critical level corresponding, in normal blood, to 32% saturation and oxygen content of 6.4 mL.dL^{-1}. If the brain has a mean oxygen consumption of 46 mL.min^{-1} and a blood flow of 620 mL.min^{-1}, the arterial/venous oxygen content difference will be 7.4 mL.dL^{-1}. Therefore, with normal cerebral perfusion, haemoglobin concentration, pH, and so on, this would correspond to a critical arterial oxygen content of 13.8 mL.dL^{-1}, saturation 68% and Po_2 4.8 kPa (36 mmHg). However, the other factors listed will probably not be normal. They may be unfavourable as a result of multiple pathologies in the patient (e.g., anaemia or a decreased cerebral blood flow). Alternatively, there may be favourable factors, such as polycythaemia in chronic hypoxaemia or reduced cerebral oxygen requirements during hypothermia or anaesthesia. The possible combinations of circumstances are so great that it is not feasible to consider every possible situation.

The most important message of this discussion is that there is no simple answer to the question: What is the safe lower limit of arterial Po_2? Acclimatized mountaineers have remained conscious at high altitude with arterial Po_2 values as low as 3.28 kPa (25 mmHg; Chapter 16). Patients presenting with severe respiratory disease tend to remain conscious down to similar levels of arterial Po_2. However, both acclimatized mountaineers and patients with chronic respiratory disease have compensatory polycythaemia and maximal cerebral vasodilatation. Uncompensated subjects who are acutely exposed to hypoxia are unlikely to remain conscious at such low values for arterial Po_2, but considerable individual variation must be expected.

Effects of Hypoxia

Hypoxia presents a serious threat to the body, and compensatory mechanisms usually take priority over other changes. Thus for example, in hypoxia with concomitant hypocapnia, hyperventilation and an increase in cerebral blood flow occur in spite of the decreased Pco_2. Certain compensatory mechanisms will come into play whatever the reason for the hypoxia, although their effectiveness will depend to a large extent on the cause.

For example, hyperventilation will be largely ineffective in stagnant or anaemic hypoxia because hyperventilation while breathing air can do little to increase the oxygen content of arterial blood, and usually nothing to increase perfusion.

Hyperventilation results from a decreased arterial Po_2, but the response is nonlinear (see Fig. 4.8). There is little effect until arterial Po_2 is reduced to about 7 kPa (52 mmHg): maximal response is at 4 kPa (30 mmHg). The interrelationship between hypoxia and other factors in the control of breathing is discussed in Chapter 4.

Pulmonary distribution of blood flow is improved by hypoxia as a result of hypoxic pulmonary vasoconstriction (page 80).

The sympathetic system is concerned in many of the responses to hypoxia, particularly the increase in organ perfusion. The immediate response is a reflex increase in sympathetic nerve discharge initiated by chemoreceptor stimulation, which occurs before any measurable increase in circulating catecholamines, although this does occur in due course. The increase in sympathetic nervous activity occurs even with intermittent hypoxia,[17] which has serious implications for patients with sleep-disordered breathing (page 193). Reduction of cerebral and probably myocardial vascular resistance is not dependent on the autonomic system but depends on local responses in the vicinity of the vessels themselves. With the exception of pulmonary vessels, hypoxia causes vasodilatation of blood vessels almost everywhere in the body. This results mainly from a direct effect of adenosine and other metabolites generated by hypoxia.

Cardiac output is increased by hypoxia, together with the regional blood flow to almost every major organ, particularly the brain.

Haemoglobin concentration is transiently increased with acute hypoxia in humans, particularly during apnoea, caused by splenic contraction.[18] The response is probably mediated by catecholamines, and although of minor importance for humans is a vital reflex for diving mammals (page 311). Haemoglobin is increased in chronic hypoxia because of residence at altitude or respiratory disease.

The oxyhaemoglobin dissociation curve is displaced to the right by an increase in 2,3-diphosphoglycerate and by acidosis, which may also be present. This tends to increase tissue Po_2 (see Fig. 10.10).

References

1. Martin RL, Lloyd HGE, Cowan AI. The early events of oxygen and glucose deprivation: setting the scene for neuronal death? *Trends Neurosci.* 1994;17:251-256.
2. Candelise L, Landi G, Orazio EN, et al. Prognostic significance of hyperglycaemia in acute stroke. *Arch Neurol.* 1985;42:661-663.
3. Ransom BR, Brown AM. Intracellular Ca^{2+} release and ischemic axon injury: the Trojan horse is back. *Neuron.* 2003;40:2-4.
4. Zhao H, Kilgas S, Alam A, et al. The role of extracellular adenosine triphosphate in ischemic organ injury. *Crit Care Med.* 2016;44:1000-1012.
5. Sun H-S. Role of TRPM7 in cerebral ischaemia and hypoxia. *J Physiol.* 2017;595(10):3077-3083.
6. Harris AL. Hypoxia—key regulatory factor in tumour growth. *Nat Rev Cancer.* 2002;2:38-46.
7. Berchner-Pfannschmidt U, Frede S, Wotzlaw C, et al. Imaging of the hypoxia-inducible factor pathway: insights into oxygen sensing. *Eur Respir J.* 2008;32:210-217.
8. Prabhakar NR, Semenza GL. Adaptive and maladaptive cardiorespiratory responses to continuous and intermittent hypoxia mediated by hypoxia-inducible factors 1 and 2. *Physiol Rev.* 2012;92:967-1003.
9. Kennel KB, Burmeister J, Schneider M, et al. The PHD1 oxygen sensor in health and disease. *J Physiol.* 2018;596:3899-3913.
*10. **West JB. Physiological effects of chronic hypoxia. *N Engl J Med.* 2017;376:1965-1971.**
11. Zaugg M, Lucchinetti E, Uecker M, et al. Anaesthetics and cardiac preconditioning. *Part I. Signalling and cytoprotective mechanisms. Br J Anaesth.* 2003;91:551-565.
*12. **Kharbanda RK, Nielsen TT, Redington AN. Translation of remote ischaemic preconditioning into clinical practice. *Lancet.* 2009;374:1557-1565.**
13. Mouton R, Soar J. Remote ischaemic preconditioning: an intervention for anaesthetists? *Br J Anaesth.* 2017;118:288-291.
14. Banks P, Franks NP, Dickinson R. Competitive inhibition at the glycine site of the N-methyl-D-aspartate receptor mediates xenon neuroprotection against hypoxia–ischemia. *Anesthesiology.* 2010;112:614-622.
15. Dickinson R, Franks NP. Bench-to-bedside review: molecular pharmacology and clinical use of inert gases in anesthesia and neuroprotection. *Crit Care.* 2010;14:229.
16. Smit E, Thoresen M. Xenon as a neuroprotective treatment in neonatal encephalopathy. *Infant.* 2014;10:1-4.
17. Mifflin S, Cunningham JT, Toney GM. Neurogenic mechanisms underlying the rapid onset of sympathetic responses to intermittent hypoxia. *J Appl Physiol.* 2015;119:1441-1448.
18. Lodin-Sundström A, Chagataye S. Spleen contraction during 20 min normobaric hypoxia and 2 min apnea in humans. *Aviat Space Environ Med.* 2010;81:545-549.

24

Anaemia

KEY POINTS

- Anaemia has little effect on pulmonary gas exchange but decreases oxygen carriage in the arterial blood in direct proportion to the reduction in haemoglobin concentration.
- Mechanisms that compensate for the reduced oxygen delivery include increased cardiac output, increased tissue oxygen extraction and a right shift of the oxyhaemoglobin dissociation curve.
- Older patients or those with poor cardiac reserve compensate less well when anaemic.

naemia is a widespread pathophysiological disorder that interferes with oxygen transport to the tissues. A quarter of the world's population is anaemic, with women and children being more affected, particularly in low-income countries.[1] In high-income countries it has a varied aetiology, including iron deficiency, chronic haemorrhage and end-stage renal failure. However, in low- and middle-income countries anaemia is endemic as a result of dietary deficiencies and infection with parasites such as hookworm and malaria.

Anaemia per se has no major direct effects on pulmonary function. Arterial Po_2 and saturation should remain within the normal range in uncomplicated anaemia, and the crucial effect is on the arterial oxygen content, and therefore oxygen delivery. Important compensatory changes are increased cardiac output, greater oxygen extraction from the arterial blood and, to a lesser extent, the small rightward displacement of the oxyhaemoglobin dissociation curve. However, there are limits to these adaptations, which define the minimal tolerable haemoglobin concentration, and also the exercise limits attainable with various degrees of severity of anaemia.

Physiological aspects of blood transfusion and blood substitutes are discussed on page 147.

Pulmonary Function

Gas Exchange

Alveolar Po_2 is determined by dry barometric pressure, inspired oxygen concentration and the ratio of oxygen consumption to alveolar ventilation (page 107). Assuming that the first two are unchanged, and with good evidence that the latter two factors are unaffected in the resting state by anaemia down to a haemoglobin concentration of at least 50 g.L^{-1} (see later), then there is no reason why alveolar Po_2 or Pco_2 should be affected by uncomplicated anaemia down to this level.

The increased cardiac output (see later discussion) will cause a small reduction in pulmonary capillary transit time, which, together with the reduced mass of haemoglobin in the pulmonary capillaries, causes a modest decrease in diffusing capacity (page 119). However, such is the reserve in the capacity of pulmonary capillary blood to reach equilibrium with the alveolar gas (see Fig. 8.2) that it is highly unlikely that this would have any measurable effect on the alveolar/end-pulmonary capillary Po_2 gradient, which in the normal subject is believed to be negligible. Thus pulmonary end-capillary Po_2 should also be normal in anaemia.

Continuing down the cascade of oxygen partial pressures from ambient air to the site of use in the tissues, the next step is the gradient in Po_2 between pulmonary end-capillary blood and mixed arterial blood. The Po_2 gradient at this stage is caused by shunting and the perfusion of relatively underventilated alveoli. There is no evidence that these factors are altered in anaemia, and arterial Po_2 should therefore be normal. Because the peripheral chemoreceptors are stimulated by reduction in arterial Po_2 and not arterial oxygen content (page 50), then there should be no stimulation of respiration, unless the degree of hypoxia is sufficient to cause anaerobic metabolism and lactacidosis.

Haemoglobin Dissociation Curve

It is well established that red blood cell 2,3-diphosphoglycerate levels are increased in anaemia (page 147), typical changes being from a normal value of 5 mmol.L^{-1} to around 7 mmol.L^{-1} at a haemoglobin concentration of 60 g.L^{-1}. This results in an increase in P_{50} from 3.6 to 4.0 kPa (27–30 mmHg). This rightward shift of the dissociation curve has a negligible effect on arterial saturation, but will increase the P_{O_2} at which oxygen is unloaded in the tissues, mitigating to a small extent the effects of reduction in oxygen delivery so far as tissue P_{O_2} is concerned.

Arterial Oxygen Content

Although the arterial oxygen saturation usually remains normal in anaemia, the oxygen content of the arterial blood will be reduced in approximate proportion to the decrease in haemoglobin concentration. Arterial oxygen content can be expressed as follows:

$$
\begin{array}{ccccccc}
Ca_{O_2} & = & ([Hb] & \times & Sa_{O_2} & \times & 1.39) & + & 0.3 \\
mL.dL^{-1} & & g.dL^{-1} & & \%/100 & & mL.g^{-1} & & mL.dL^{-1} \\
e.g., 20 & = & 14.7 & \times & 0.97 & \times & 1.39) & + & 0.3
\end{array}
$$

$$[\text{Eq. 24.1}]$$

where Ca_{O_2} is arterial oxygen content, [Hb] is haemoglobin concentration, Sa_{O_2} is arterial oxygen saturation, 1.39 is the combining power of haemoglobin with oxygen (page 144) and 0.3 is dissolved oxygen at normal arterial P_{O_2}.

Oxygen Delivery

The important concept of oxygen delivery $\dot{D}_{O_2}$ is considered in detail on page 154. It is defined as the product of cardiac output ($\dot{Q}$) and Ca_{O_2}.

$$
\begin{array}{ccccc}
\dot{D}_{O_2} & = & \dot{Q} & \times & Ca_{O_2} \\
mL.min^{-1} & & 1.min^{-1} & & mL.dL^{-1} \\
e.g., 1050 & = & 5.25 & \times & 20
\end{array}
$$

$$[\text{Eq. 24.2}]$$

(the right-hand side is multiplied by a scaling factor of 10 to account for the differing units of volume). Combining Equations 24.1 and 24.2:

$$
\begin{array}{ccccccccc}
\dot{D}_{O_2} & = & \dot{Q} & \times & \{([Hb] & \times & Sa_{O_2} & \times & 1.39) & + & 0.3\} \\
mL.min^{-1} & & 1.min^{-1} & & g.dL^{-1} & & \%/100 & & mL.g^{-1} & & mL.dL^{-1} \\
e.g., 1050 & = & 5.25 & \times & \{(14.7 & \times & 0.97 & \times & 1.39) & + & 0.3\}
\end{array}
$$

$$[\text{Eq. 24.3}]$$

(the right-hand side is again multiplied by a scaling factor of 10).

Normal values give an oxygen delivery of approximately 1000 mL.min^{-1}, which is about four times the normal resting oxygen consumption of 250 mL.min^{-1}. Extraction of oxygen from the arterial blood is thus 25%, and this accords with an arterial saturation of 97% and mixed venous saturation of 72%.

If the small quantity of dissolved oxygen (0.3 mL.dL^{-1}) is ignored, then oxygen delivery is seen to be proportional to the product of cardiac output, haemoglobin concentration and arterial oxygen saturation. There is, of course, negligible

scope for any compensatory increase in saturation in a patient with uncomplicated anaemia at sea level.

Effect of Anaemia on Cardiac Output

Equation 24.3 shows that, if other factors remain the same, a reduction in haemoglobin concentration will result in a proportionate reduction in oxygen delivery. Thus a haemoglobin concentration of 75 g.L^{-1}, with unchanged cardiac output, would halve delivery to give a resting value of 500 mL.min^{-1}, which would be approaching the likely critical value. However, patients with quite severe anaemia usually show little evidence of hypoxia at rest and, furthermore, achieve surprisingly good levels of exercise. Because arterial saturation cannot be increased, full compensation can be achieved only by a reciprocal relationship between cardiac output and haemoglobin concentration. Thus if haemoglobin concentration is halved, maintenance of normal delivery will require a doubling of cardiac output. Full compensation may not occur, but fortunately a reduction in haemoglobin concentration is usually accompanied by some increase in cardiac output.

Acute Anaemia

Early studies of cardiac output and anaemia involved measurement of cardiovascular parameters in patients before and after treatment for uncomplicated anaemia. Cardiac output was significantly greater before the patients' haemoglobin concentration increased. There was, however, a negative correlation between age and cardiac index in the anaemic state, reflecting the relative inability of the older patient to compensate. More recent studies have involved deliberately reducing the haemoglobin concentration isovolaemically in volunteers and patients.[2,3] One of these studies reduced the haemoglobin concentration from 131 to 50 g.L^{-1}, and the effects of this on the cardiovascular system are shown in Figure 24.1.[3] In these healthy volunteers the predictable linear relationship between cardiac index and haemoglobin concentration can easily be seen (Fig. 24.1, *B*).

The mechanism underlying the increase in cardiac output is not clear, but results from increases in both stroke volume and heart rate.[3] Likely explanations for these changes include reduced cardiac afterload because of lowered blood viscosity (Fig. 24.1, *A*) and increased preload because of greater venous return secondary to increased tone in capacitance vessels.

Chronic Anaemia

In one study of isovolaemic reduction of haemoglobin concentration, down to a mean value of 100 g.L^{-1}, the anaemia was then maintained at the same level for 14 days.[2] Immediately after induction of anaemia there was a marked increase in cardiac output (55%), but this decreased to only 17% above control levels after 14 days.

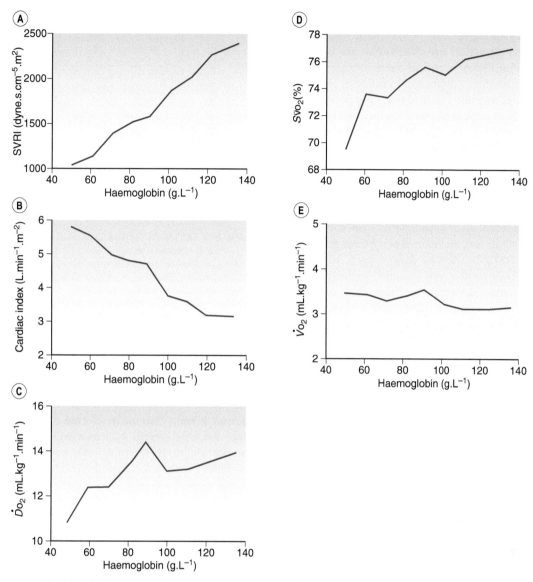

• **Fig. 24.1** Cardiovascular changes in response to acute isovolaemic reduction of mean haemoglobin concentration from 131 to 50 g.L^{-1} in healthy volunteers. **(A)** Systemic vascular resistance index (SVRI) falls in direct proportion to hemoglobin (Hb) concentration as blood viscosity decreases; **(B)** cardiac index doubles when Hb has fallen to 50 g.L^{-1}; **(C)** oxygen delivery ($\dot{D}o_2$) remains mostly unchanged until Hb is less than 80 g.L^{-1}; **(D)** mixed venous oxygen saturation ($S\bar{v}o_2$) is approximately maintained until Hb is less than 60 g.L^{-1}; **(E)** oxygen consumption ($\dot{V}o_2$) is maintained despite the fall in $\dot{D}o_2$ by increasing oxygen extraction, hence the fall in $S\bar{v}o_2$. (After reference 3.)

The Influence of Cardiac Output on Oxygen Delivery

After the acute reduction of haemoglobin concentration in healthy subjects,[2,3] cardiac output increases sufficiently to maintain near-normal oxygen delivery with moderate anaemia (Hb 100 g.L^{-1}),[2] but with more severe acute anaemia (Hb 50 g.L^{-1}) oxygen delivery may not be maintained (Fig. 24.1, C), and mixed venous oxygen saturation falls (Fig. 24.1, D).[3] However, in prolonged anaemia (2 weeks), the increase in cardiac output (only 17%) is insufficient to maintain oxygen delivery, which decreases to 27% below control values.[2]

Without an increase in cardiac output, it is likely that a haemoglobin concentration of 60 to 80 g.L^{-1} would be a significant physiological challenge. It is clear that the ability of the cardiovascular system to respond to anaemia with an increase in cardiac output is an essential aspect of accommodation to anaemia, and this is less effective in anaesthetized patients, the elderly or other subjects with reduced cardiac reserve.

Relationship Between Oxygen Delivery and Consumption

The relationship between oxygen delivery and consumption has been considered on page 155 et seq. When oxygen delivery is reduced, for whatever reason, oxygen consumption is at first maintained at its normal value, but with increasing oxygen extraction and therefore decreasing mixed venous saturation. Below a 'critical' value for oxygen delivery, oxygen consumption decreases as a function of delivery, and is usually accompanied by evidence of hypoxia, such as increased lactate in peripheral blood. Values for critical oxygen delivery depend on the pathophysiological state of the patient and vary from one condition to another.

It has not been clearly established what is the critical level of oxygen delivery in uncomplicated anaemia in humans. Studies of acutely induced anaemia have found no evidence of reduced oxygen consumption (Fig. 24.1, *E*) or tissue hypoxia even at a haemoglobin concentration of 50 g.L^{-1}.[3] In volunteers maintained at a haemoglobin concentration of 100 g.L^{-1} for 14 days, oxygen delivery decreased from about 1200 to 900 mL.min^{-1}, whereas oxygen consumption remained virtually unchanged.[2] Patients with long-term anaemia seem to remain above the critical value for oxygen delivery down to haemoglobin values of about 60 g.L^{-1}.

Anaemia and Exercise

Maintenance of constant oxygen consumption in the face of reduced delivery can only be achieved at the expense of a reduction in mixed venous saturation, as a result of increased extraction of oxygen from the arterial blood. This has been clearly demonstrated in both acute (Fig. 24.1, *D*) and sustained anaemia.[2] A reduction in the oxygen content of mixed venous blood curtails the ability of the anaemic patient to encroach on a useful reserve of oxygen, which is an important response to exercise. Reduction of haemoglobin to 100 g.L^{-1} resulted in a curtailment of oxygen consumption attained at maximal exercise from the control values of 3.0 L.min^{-1} (normalized to 70 kg body weight) down to 2.5 L.min^{-1} in the acute stage, and 2.1 L.min^{-1} after 14 days of sustained anaemia (Fig. 24.2).[2] The increase in cardiac output required for the same increase in oxygen consumption was greater in the anaemic state, and cardiac output at maximal oxygen consumption was slightly less than under control conditions. Maximal exercise in the anaemic state resulted in a reduction of mixed venous oxygen saturation to the exceptionally low value of 12%, compared with control values of 23% during maximal exercise with a normal haemoglobin concentration.

Brisk walking on level ground normally requires an oxygen consumption of about 1 L.min^{-1} and a cardiac output of about 10 L.min^{-1}. At a haemoglobin level of 50 g.L^{-1}, this would require a cardiac output of about 20 L.min^{-1} to permit an oxygen consumption of 1 L.min^{-1} with a satisfactory residual level of mixed venous oxygen saturation. It will be clear that, at this degree of anaemia, cardiac function is a critical factor determining the mobility of a patient.

Exercise tolerance may be limited by either respiratory or circulatory capacity. In uncomplicated anaemia, there is no reason to implicate respiratory limitation, and exercise

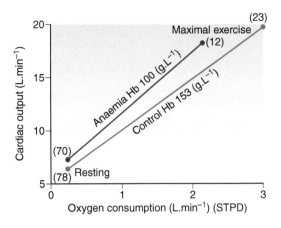

• **Fig. 24.2** Cardiac output as a function of oxygen consumption during rest and maximal exercise under control and isovolaemic anaemic conditions. Numbers in parentheses indicate mean mixed venous oxygen saturation. (Redrawn from reference 2 on the assumption that mean weight of the subjects was 70 kg, by permission of the author, as well as the editors and publishers of *Journal of Applied Physiology*.) *STPD,* Standard temperature and pressure, dry.

tolerance is, therefore, to a first approximation, governed by the remaining factors in the oxygen delivery Equation 24.3. On the assumption that the maximal sustainable cardiac output is only marginally affected by anaemia, it is to be expected that exercise tolerance will be reduced in direct proportion to the haemoglobin concentration. Available evidence supports this hypothesis (Fig. 24.3).

Using Haemoglobin to Enhance Athletic Performance

The corollary of the preceding description is the question of improving athletic performance by increasing haemoglobin concentration above the normal range. This used to be

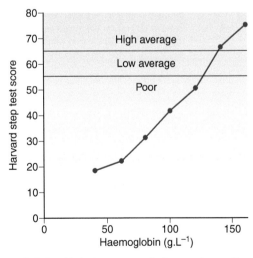

• **Fig. 24.3** Relationship between capacity for exercise and haemoglobin concentration. (After Viteri FE, Torun B. Anaemia and physical work capacity. *Clin Hematol.* 1974;3:609-626, by permission of the authors, as well as the editor and publishers of *Clinics in Haematology*.)

achieved by removal of blood for replacement of red cells after a few weeks when the subject's haemoglobin concentration had already been partially restored, a procedure known as blood doping. The same effect is now much more conveniently achieved by the administration of erythropoietin. Studies of trained athletes in this area are notoriously difficult, and it is easy to confuse the effects of changes in blood volume and haemoglobin concentration. However, the strategy is effective. For example, in a well-controlled study of highly trained runners,[4] in which a mean haemoglobin concentration of 167 g.L^{-1} was attained, there were significant increases in maximal oxygen uptake from 4.8 to 5.1 L.min^{-1}.

Anaemia in the Clinical Setting?[5]

Evolution has resulted in a haemoglobin concentration of 130 to 160 g.L^{-1} presumably for sound biological reasons, and this value must represent the best compromise between oxygen carriage, cardiac output and blood viscosity. For many years a haemoglobin concentration of over 100 g.L^{-1} was regarded as acceptable. At this level, cardiac output increases are modest, and although exercise tolerance may be reduced this is unlikely to trouble the patient. There is evidence that much lower values will be acceptable in some circumstances. Jehovah's Witnesses, whose religious beliefs prevent them from consenting to blood transfusion, frequently undergo major surgery, and survival is reported following haemoglobin values of less than 30 g.L^{-1}, albeit with substantial cardiovascular and respiratory support. There is also a suggestion that low haemoglobin values may actually be beneficial, with lowered blood viscosity improving blood flow through diseased vessels and so increasing tissue oxygenation, although the role of this effect in patients is unknown.

However, blood transfusion has always been, and currently remains, a hazardous and financially costly procedure, so in recent years there have been many studies addressing the haemoglobin level below which a blood transfusion should be used, the transfusion trigger (TT). Many studies in varied clinical situations compared restrictive TTs (70–90 g.L^{-1}) with liberal TTs (100–120 g.L^{-1}) and mostly found the restrictive strategies to be at least equivalent to, if not better than, liberal ones. TT values recommended by a variety of expert bodies worldwide are now all close to a threshold of 70 g.L^{-1}, although these are not applicable to patients with acute coronary syndrome or chronic cardiovascular disease in whom values should be maintained at greater than 80 g.L^{-1}.[6] There is also some evidence that perioperative TTs of 70 to 75 g.L^{-1} may be associated with higher mortality rates, and so a more liberal TT is advised.[7]

The organ that limits the acceptable degree of anaemia is inevitably the heart, where oxygen extraction is normally in excess of 50%. Increased oxygen extraction as a compensatory mechanism is therefore limited, and coronary blood flow must increase to facilitate the greater oxygen requirement of a raised cardiac output. Thus any patient with impaired coronary blood supply will be considerably less tolerant of anaemia than those with normal coronary arteries, as recognized in the previous recommendations.

This recent change in practice to deliberately allow patients to become severely anaemic has driven further basic science research into its effects on various body systems. Animal studies have demonstrated significant hypoxia-inducible factor 1 activation (page 276) in brain, kidney and liver at haemoglobin values of 50 g.L^{-1}, and this was also reported in the liver at 70 g.L^{-1},[8] a level often seen in patients. Secondary neurological injury occurs in animals at haemoglobin concentrations in the range 60 to 70 g.L^{-1}, close to that seen in patients. An important compensatory mechanism in the brain at this severity of anaemia is increased activity of all isoforms of nitric oxide synthase (page 80) leading to vasodilatation, and so improved oxygen delivery.[9]

Anaemia and Renal Failure

Chronic kidney disease leads to a lack of renal erythropoietin release, and severe symptomatic anaemia results, with patients commonly having haemoglobin levels of less than 80 g.L^{-1}. The availability of erythropoiesis-stimulating agents[10] has allowed partial correction of anaemia in many patients, leading to a substantial improvement in quality of life for most. There is, however, debate about the optimal target haemoglobin concentration.[11] There is good evidence that the chronic severe anaemia associated with renal disease commonly leads to cardiac complications. Unfortunately, there is also some evidence that correction of haemoglobin to normal values is associated with increased cardiac complications in these patients, and a value of around 115 g.L^{-1} seems to be the safest compromise.[10,11]

References

1. Balarajan Y, Ramakrishnan U, Özaltin E, et al. Anaemia in low-income and middle-income countries. *Lancet.* 2011;378:2123-2135.
2. Woodson RD, Wills RE, Lenfant C. Effect of acute and established anemia on O$_2$ transport at rest, submaximal and maximal work. *J Appl Physiol.* 1978;44:36-43.
3. Weiskopf RB, Viele MK, Feiner J, et al. Human cardiovascular and metabolic response to acute, severe isovolemic anemia. *JAMA.* 1998;279:217-221.
4. Buick FJ, Gledhill N, Froese AB, et al. Effect of induced erythrocythemia on aerobic work capacity. *J Appl Physiol.* 1980;48:636-642.
5. Goodnough LT, Levy JH, Murphy MF. Concepts of blood transfusion in adults. *Lancet.* 2013;381:1845-1854.
6. Docherty AB, O'Donnell R, Brunskill S, et al. Effect of restrictive versus liberal transfusion strategies on outcomes in patients with cardiovascular disease in a non-cardiac surgery setting: systematic review and meta-analysis. *BMJ.* 2016;352:i1351.
7. Chong MA, Krishnan R, Cheng D, et al. Should transfusion trigger thresholds differ for critical care versus perioperative patients? A meta-analysis of randomized trials. *Crit Care Med.* 2018;46:252-263.

8. Tsui AK, Marsden PA, Mazer CD, et al. Differential HIF and NOS responses to acute anemia: defining organspecific hemoglobin thresholds for tissue hypoxia. *Am J Physiol Regul Integr Comp Physiol*. 2014;307:R13-R25.

9. Hare GMT, Tsui AKY, McLaren AT, et al. Anemia and cerebral outcomes: many questions, fewer answers. *Anesth Analg*. 2008;107:1356-1370.

10. Drüeke TB. Anemia treatment in patients with chronic kidney disease. *N Engl J Med*. 2013;368:387-389.

11. Phrommintikul A, Haas SJ, Elsik M, et al. Mortality and target haemoglobin concentrations in anaemic patients with chronic kidney disease treated with erythropoietin: a meta-analysis. *Lancet*. 2007;369:381-388.

25

Oxygen Toxicity and Hyperoxia

KEY POINTS

- Breathing oxygen at increased atmospheric pressure achieves very high arterial Po_2 values, but venous Po_2, and therefore minimum tissue Po_2, only increases at 3 atm absolute pressure.
- Normal metabolic processes, particularly in the mitochondria, produce a range of powerful oxidizing derivatives of oxygen, some of which are referred to as reactive oxygen species.
- The harmful effects of reactive oxygen species are countered by a combination of ubiquitous enzymes that inactivate reactive oxygen species and endogenous antioxidant molecules.

- The lungs are susceptible to oxygen toxicity, the first measurable signs occurring in healthy subjects after breathing 100% oxygen for approximately 24 hours. The clinical effects of hyperoxia in the perioperative and critical care setting, as well as in acute medical conditions, are becoming better understood.
- Hyperbaric oxygen is used to treat a variety of conditions such as tissue infections, carbon monoxide poisoning and sports injuries, but its use remains controversial.

Chapter 23 described the disastrous consequences of lack of oxygen for life forms that depend on it, but for most organisms hypoxia is an infrequent event. However, oxygen itself also has toxic effects at the cellular level, which organisms have had to oppose by the development of complex antioxidant systems. The activity of toxic oxygen derivatives and antioxidant systems is perfectly balanced most of the time. Nevertheless, there is a strengthening opinion that over many years oxidative mechanisms predominate and may be responsible for the generalized deterioration in function associated with ageing.[1] In a variety of diseases, or when exposed to extra oxygen, the balance is radically disturbed, and unwanted physiological changes or direct tissue damage results.

Hyperoxia

Hyperventilation while breathing air can raise the arterial Po_2 to about 16 kPa (120 mmHg). Higher levels can be obtained only by oxygen enrichment of the inspired gas and/or by elevation of the ambient pressure. Although the arterial Po_2 can be raised to very high levels, the increase in arterial oxygen content is usually relatively small (Table 25.1). The arterial oxygen saturation is normally greater than 95% and, apart from raising saturation to 100%, additional oxygen can be carried only in physical solution. Provided that the arterial/mixed venous oxygen content difference remains

constant, it follows that venous oxygen content will rise by the same value as the arterial oxygen content. The consequences in terms of venous Po_2 (Table 25.1) are important, because minimum tissue Po_2 approximates more closely to venous than to arterial Po_2. The rise in venous Po_2 is trivial when breathing 100% oxygen at normal barometric pressure, and it is necessary to breathe oxygen at 3 atm absolute (ATA) pressure before there is a large increase in venous and therefore tissue Po_2. This is because most of the body requirement can then be met by dissolved oxygen, and the saturation of capillary and venous blood remains close to 100%.

It is convenient to consider two degrees of hyperoxia. The first applies to the inhalation of oxygen-enriched gas at normal atmospheric pressure, whereas the second involves inhaling oxygen at raised pressure and is termed *hyperbaric hyperoxia*. Firstly, however, it is necessary to understand the molecular basis by which oxygen causes damage to biological molecules.

Oxygen Toxicity

The Oxygen Molecule and Reactive Derivatives[2]

The dioxygen molecule (Fig. 25.1) is unusual because it has two unpaired electrons in the outer (2P) shell, but stability is conferred because the orbits of the two unpaired electrons

TABLE 25.1	Oxygen Levels Attained in the Normal Subject by Changes in the Oxygen Partial Pressure of Inspired Gas			
	At Normal Barometric Pressure		At 2 ATA	At 3 ATA
	Air	Oxygen	Oxygen	Oxygen
Inspired Gas P_{O_2} (Humidified)				
(kPa)	20	96	190	285
(mmHg)	150	713	1425	2138
Arterial P_{O_2}[a]				
(kPa)	13	80	175	270
(mmHg)	98	600	1313	2025
Arterial Oxygen Content[b]				
(mL.dL^{-1})	19.3	21.3	23.4	25.5
Arterial/Venous Oxygen Content Difference				
(mL.dL^{-1})	5.0	5.0	5.0	5.0
Venous Oxygen Content				
(mL.dL^{-1})	14.3	16.3	18.4	20.5
Venous P_{O_2}				
(kPa)	5.2	6.4	9.1	48.0
(mmHg)	39	48	68	360

Oxygen-induced vasoconstriction means tissue perfusion may be reduced by elevation of P_{O_2}. This tends to increase the arterial/venous oxygen content difference, which will limit the rise in venous P_{O_2}. The increases in venous P_{O_2} shown in this table are therefore likely to be greater than in vivo.
[a]Reasonable values have been assumed for P_{CO_2} and alveolar/arterial P_{O_2} difference.
[b]Normal values assumed for Hb, pH, and so on.

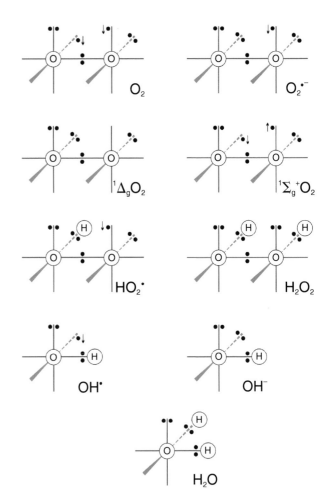

• **Fig. 25.1** Outer p-orbitals of electrons in (from the top left): ground state oxygen or dioxygen (O_2); superoxide anion ($O_2^{\bullet-}$); two forms of singlet oxygen ($1O_2$); hydroperoxyl radical ($HO_2^{\bullet}$); hydrogen peroxide (H_2O_2); hydroxyl radical ($OH^{\bullet}$); hydroxyl ion (OH^-); and water. The three lines represent the x, y and z axes of the orbitals, and arrows indicate the direction of rotation of unpaired electrons. See text for properties and interrelationships.

are parallel. The two unpaired electrons also confer the property of paramagnetism, which has been exploited as a method of gas analysis that is almost specific for oxygen (page 158).

Although ground state oxygen (dioxygen) is a powerful oxidizing agent, the molecule is stable and has an indefinite half-life. However, as discussed below, the oxygen molecule can be transformed into a range of reactive oxygen species (ROS) and other highly toxic substances, most of which are far more reactive than oxygen itself.

Singlet Oxygen

Internal rearrangements of the unpaired electrons of dioxygen result in the formation of two highly reactive species, both known as singlet oxygens ($1O_2$). In $1\Delta gO_2$ one unpaired electron is transferred to the orbit of the other (Fig. 25.1), imparting an energy level of 22.4 kcal.mol^{-1} above the ground state. With no remaining unpaired electron, $1\Delta gO_2$ is not a ROS. In $1\Sigma g^+$ the rotation of one unpaired electron is

reversed, which imparts an energy level of 37.5 kcal.mol^{-1} above the ground state, and this molecule is a ROS. $1\Sigma g^+$ is extremely reactive and rapidly decays to the $1\Delta gO_2$ form, which is particularly relevant in biological systems, and especially in lipid peroxidation.

Superoxide Anion

Under circumstances considered below, the oxygen molecule may be partially reduced by receiving a single electron, which pairs with one of the unpaired electrons, forming the superoxide anion ($O_2^{\bullet-}$ in Fig. 25.1), which is both an anion and a ROS. It is the first and crucial stage in the production of a series of toxic oxygen-derived ROS and other compounds. The superoxide anion is relatively stable in aqueous solution at body pH, but has a rapid biological decay because of the ubiquitous presence of superoxide dismutase (see later). Because it is charged, a superoxide anion does not readily cross cell membranes.

Hydroperoxyl Radical

The hydroperoxyl radical is a ROS. A superoxide anion may acquire a hydrogen ion to form the hydroperoxyl radical thus:

$$O^{\bullet-} + H^+ = HO_2^{\bullet}$$

The reaction is pH-dependent with a pK of 4.8, so the equilibrium is far to the left in biological systems.

Hydrogen Peroxide

Superoxide dismutase (SOD) catalyses the transfer of an electron from one molecule of the superoxide anion to another. The donor molecule becomes dioxygen, while the recipient rapidly combines with two hydrogen ions to form hydrogen peroxide (Fig. 25.1). Although hydrogen peroxide is not a ROS, it is a powerful and toxic oxidizing agent that plays an important role in oxygen toxicity. The overall reaction is as follows:

$$2O_2^{\bullet-} + 2H^+ \rightarrow H_2O_2 + O_2.$$

Hydrogen peroxide is continuously generated in the body. Two enzymes ensure its rapid removal. Catalase is a highly specific enzyme active against only hydrogen, methyl and ethyl peroxides. Hydrogen peroxide is reduced to water thus:

$$2H_2O_2 \rightarrow 2H_2O + O_2.$$

Glutathione peroxidase acts against a much wider range of peroxides (R–OOH), which react with glutathione (GSH) thus:

$$\begin{aligned} ROOH + 2G-SH \rightarrow \\ R-OH + G-S-S-G + H_2O. \end{aligned}$$

Catalase and glutathione peroxidase are discussed further in a later section.

Three-Stage Reduction of Oxygen

Figure 25.2 summarizes the three-stage reduction of oxygen to water, which is the fully reduced and stable state. This contrasts with the more familiar single-stage reduction of oxygen to water that occurs in the terminal cytochrome (page 153). Unlike the single-stage reduction of oxygen, the three-stage reaction shown in Figure 25.2 is not inhibited by cyanide.

Secondary Derivatives of the Products of Dioxygen Reduction

Although both the superoxide anion and hydrogen peroxide have direct toxic effects, they interact to produce even more dangerous species. On the right side of Figure 25.3 is the *Fenton or Haber–Weiss reaction*, which results in the formation of the harmless hydroxyl ion together with two extremely reactive species, the hydroxyl free radical (OH$^{\bullet}$) and singlet oxygen (1O$_2$)

$$O^{\bullet-} + H_2O_2 \rightarrow OH^- + OH^{\bullet} + 1O_2.$$

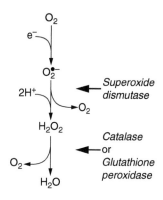

• **Fig. 25.2** Three-stage reduction of oxygen to water. The first reaction is a single electron reduction to form the superoxide anion reactive oxygen species. In the second stage the first products of the dismutation reaction are dioxygen and a short-lived intermediate, which then receives two protons to form hydrogen peroxide. The final stage forms water, the fully reduced form of oxygen.

The hydroxyl free radical is the most dangerous ROS derived from oxygen.

On the left side of Figure 25.3 is the reaction of hydrogen peroxide with a chloride ion to form hypochlorous acid. This occurs in the phagocytic vesicle of the neutrophil and plays a role in killing bacteria, facilitated by the enzyme myeloperoxidase. The myeloperoxidase reaction also occurs immediately after fertilization of the ovum, and hypochlorous acid thus formed causes polymerization of proteins to form the membrane that prevents further entry of spermatozoa.

The changes previously described have many features in common with those caused by ionizing radiation; the hydroxyl radical (OH$^{\bullet}$) is the most dangerous product in both cases. It is not, therefore, surprising that the effect of radiation is increased by high partial pressures of oxygen. As tissue Po$_2$ is reduced below about 2 kPa (15 mmHg), there is progressively increased resistance to radiation damage until, at zero Po$_2$, resistance is increased threefold. This unfortunate effect promotes

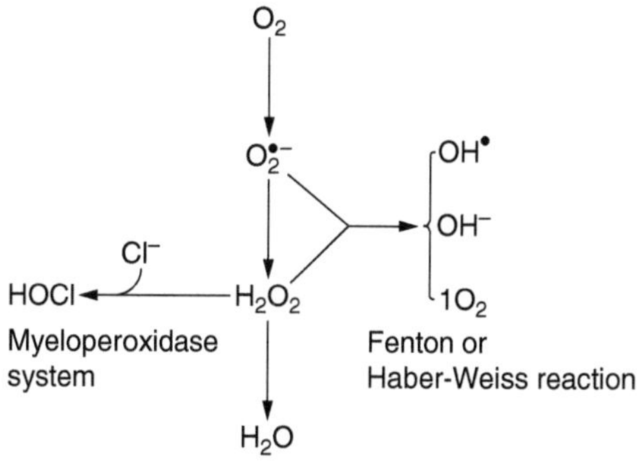

• **Fig. 25.3** Interaction of superoxide anion and hydrogen peroxide in the Fenton or Haber–Weiss reaction to form hydroxyl free radical, hydroxyl ion and singlet oxygen. Hypochlorous acid is formed from hydrogen peroxide by the myeloperoxidase system. (From Nunn JF. Oxygen—friend or foe. *J Roy Soc Med*. 1985;78:618-622, by courtesy of the editor of the *Journal of the Royal Society of Medicine*.)

resistance to radiotherapy of malignant cells in hypoxic areas of tumours (page 360).

Nitric oxide may behave as a ROS by reacting with the superoxide anion to produce peroxynitrite ($ONOO^-$). This molecule can either rearrange itself into relatively harmless nitrite or nitrate (page 148) or give rise to derivatives with similar biological activity to the hydroxyl radical. Conversely, nitric oxide may act as an antioxidant, binding to ferrous iron molecules and preventing them from contributing to the formation of a superoxide anion (see next) or the Fenton reaction. The in vivo role of nitric oxide as a ROS or antioxidant therefore remains unclear.[3]

Sources of Electrons for the Reduction of Oxygen to Superoxide Anion

Figure 25.3 shows the superoxide anion as the starting point for the production of many other ROS. The first stage reduction of dioxygen to the superoxide anion is therefore critically important in oxygen toxicity.

Mitochondrial Enzymes

Complex 1 (nicotinamide adenine dinucleotide + hydrogen oxidoreductase [NADH oxidoreductase]) and a variety of other mitochondrial enzymes may 'leak' electrons to molecular oxygen, producing superoxide anions during normal oxidative respiration.[4] Animal studies indicate that this may account for almost 2% of total mitochondrial oxygen consumption, indicating the importance of the highly efficient mitochondrial form of SOD (see later). The concentration of mitochondrial ROS molecules must be carefully controlled, a task undertaken by the mitochondrial permeability transition pore (mPTP) channels in the mitochondrial membrane. In response to an unfavourable redox state within the mitochondrion, the mPTP channels open very briefly to allow the ROS out into the cell for removal by cytoplasmic antioxidant systems. Excess ROS in the mitochondrion leads to more prolonged opening of mPTP channels, which can damage the mitochondrion and cell. Thus ROS are acting as a signalling pathway during normal circumstances to control their own levels, but can easily become a pathological cause of cell damage.[4]

NADPH Oxidase System

The NADPH oxidase system is the major electron donor in neutrophils and macrophages. The electron is donated from NADPH by the enzyme NADPH oxidase, which is located within the membrane of the phagocytic vesicle. This mechanism is activated during phagocytosis, and is accompanied by a transient increase in the oxygen consumption of the cells, a process known to be cyanide resistant. This is the so-called respiratory burst, and occurs in all phagocytic cells in response to a wide range of stimuli including bacterial endotoxin, immunoglobulins and interleukins. Superoxide anion is released into the phagocytic vesicle, where it is reduced to hydrogen peroxide, which then reacts with chloride ions to form hypochlorous acid in the myeloperoxidase

reaction (Fig. 25.3). For many years the release of ROS into the phagocyte was believed to be the main way in which bacteria were killed by phagocytes. Recent work on pulmonary neutrophils in mice with pneumococcal infection has refuted this claim, finding no evidence of bacterial killing by neutrophil-generated ROS, although ROS were involved in neutrophil regulation.[5] Powerful protease enzymes released into the phagosome by the neutrophil may be the most important bactericidal mechanism.

Although the NADPH oxidase system has extremely important biological functions, there seems little doubt that its inappropriate activation in marginated neutrophils can damage the endothelium of the lung, and it may well play a part in the production of acute lung injury (Chapter 31).

Xanthine Oxidoreductase and Reperfusion Injury[6]

The enzyme xanthine oxidoreductase (XOR) is responsible for the conversion of hypoxanthine and xanthine to uric acid (Fig. 25.4). XOR is a large (300 kDa) protein involving two separate substrate binding sites, one including flavine adenine dinucleotide cofactor and the other a

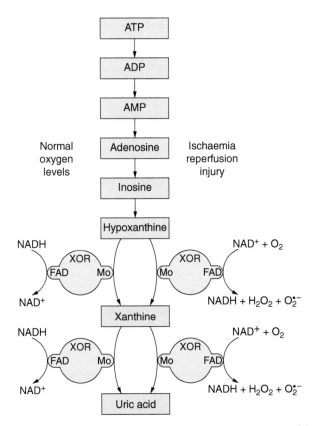

• **Fig. 25.4** Generation of superoxide anion from oxygen by the activity of xanthine oxidoreductase (XOR). With normal cellular oxygen levels (left side) nicotinamide adenine dinucleotide (NADH) is the cofactor, binding at the flavine adenine dinucleotide (FAD) site whilst the substrate reacts with the molybdenum binding site at the opposite side of the XOR molecule. Following a period of ischaemia (right side), reperfusion causes oxidized nicotinamide adenine dinucleotide and oxygen rather than NADH to react at the FAD binding site of XOR, resulting in the production of hydrogen peroxide or superoxide anion.

molybdenum molecule. In vivo, XOR exists in two interchangeable forms, with about 80% existing as xanthine dehydrogenase and the remainder as xanthine oxidase. In both forms XOR catalyses the conversion of both hypoxanthine to xanthine and of xanthine to uric acid, and under normal conditions uses NADH as a cofactor. In ischaemic or hypoxic tissue large quantities of hypoxanthine accumulate (page 273), the availability of NADH declines, and the ratio of the oxidase and dehydrogenase forms of XOR may be reversed. As a result of these changes, when oxygen is restored to the cell, the XOR catalysis of xanthine and hypoxanthine is altered, with NAD^+ and dioxygen now used as cofactors, resulting in the production of hydrogen peroxide and superoxide anions (Fig. 25.4). Thus during reperfusion there may be extensive production of ROS.

Ferrous Iron

Ferrous iron (Fe^{2+}) loses an electron during conversion to the ferric (Fe^{3+}) state. This is an important component of the toxicity of ferrous iron. A similar reaction also occurs during the spontaneous oxidation of haemoglobin to methaemoglobin (page 149). It is for this reason that large quantities of SOD, catalase and other protective agents are present in the young red blood cell. Their depletion may well determine the life span of the cell. Apart from ferrous iron acting as an electron donor, it is a catalyst in the Fenton reaction (see previous discussion).

High Po_2

Whatever other factors may apply, the production of ROS is increased at high levels of Po_2 by the law of mass action. It would seem that the normal tissue defences against ROS (discussed later) are usually effective only up to a tissue Po_2 of about 60 kPa (450 mmHg). This accords with the development of clinical oxygen toxicity, as discussed in a later section.

Exogenous Compounds

Various drugs and toxic substances can act as an analogue of NADPH oxidase and transfer an electron from NADPH to molecular oxygen. The best example of this is paraquat, which can, in effect, insert itself into an electron transport chain, alternating between its singly and doubly ionized forms. This process is accelerated at high levels of Po_2, and so there is a synergistic effect between paraquat and oxygen. Paraquat is concentrated in the alveolar epithelial type II cell where the Po_2 is as high as anywhere in the body. Because of the very short half-life of ROS, damage is confined to the lung. Bleomycin and some antibiotics (e.g., nitrofurantoin) can act in a similar manner (see next).

Biological Effects of Reactive Oxygen Species

Their use in the regulation of phagocytes, and possibly in the killing of microorganisms, is a beneficial role for ROS. Elsewhere within cells, the balance between the detrimental effects of ROS and the antioxidants that counter these (see later discussion) is described as the redox state of the cell. Cellular, and more specifically mitochondrial, redox state is believed to be part of an essential, yet poorly understood, cell signalling system,[4] involved, for example, in the sensing of oxygen levels in the carotid body. Otherwise, most effects of ROS on biological systems are harmful, and alterations in redox state are linked to a diverse range of diseases.

The three main biochemical targets for ROS damage are DNA, lipids and sulphydryl-containing proteins. All three are also sensitive to ionizing radiation. The mechanisms of both forms of damage have much in common and synergism occurs.

1. *DNA*. Breakage of chromosomes in cultures of animal lung fibroblasts by high concentrations of oxygen was first demonstrated in 1978.[7] Subsequent work has demonstrated that ROS are involved in damaging both nuclear and mitochondrial DNA, including repair errors, double-strand breaks and activation of transcription factors and signal proteins. These mechanisms are all believed to underpin the role of ROS in carcinogenesis.[8] In vivo studies of therapeutic hyperbaric oxygen in humans have also shown DNA damage. However, adverse clinical outcomes from hyperbaric oxygen have not been demonstrated, although susceptible subgroups that have less effective cellular antioxidant or DNA repair systems may exist.[9]

2. *Lipids*. There is little doubt that lipid peroxidation is a major mechanism of tissue damage by ROS. The interaction of a ROS with an unsaturated fatty acid not only disrupts that particular lipid molecule, but also generates another ROS, so that a chain reaction ensues until stopped by an antioxidant. Lipid peroxidation disrupts cell membranes and accounts for the loss of integrity of the alveolar/capillary barrier in pulmonary oxygen toxicity.

3. *Proteins*. Damage to sulphydryl-containing proteins results in formation of disulphide bridges, which inactivates a range of proteins.

Interference with these fundamental cellular molecules has widespread physiological implications. Superoxide anion and the peroxynitrite formed from nitric oxide initiate a wide range of pathological processes, including inactivation of neurotransmitters, inhibition of proteins, release of cytokines and exertion of direct cytotoxic effects (Fig. 25.5).[10] Inevitably, cell dysfunction will rapidly occur, followed in the longer term by the occurrence of inflammation, malignancy or cell death. Over an animal's lifetime, ROS-induced damage is now known to be closely linked to cardiovascular and neurologic disease, cancer and the degenerative changes of ageing.[1,8]

Defences Against Reactive Oxygen Species

Life in an oxidizing environment is possible only because of powerful antioxidant defences, which all aerobes have developed (Chapter 34).

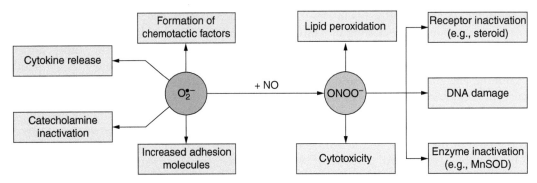

• **Fig. 25.5** Biochemical effects of superoxide anion and peroxynitrite. These potent cellular effects initiate numerous pathological processes, including inflammation, malignancy or cell death. *MnSOD*, Manganese superoxide dismutase. (From reference 10, with permission of the publishers of *Nature Reviews Drug Discovery*.)

Antioxidant Enzymes

These enzymes are widely distributed in different organs and different species, but are deficient in most obligatory anaerobic bacteria. Young animals normally have increased levels of SOD and catalase, which confer greater resistance to oxygen toxicity. The reactions catalysed by antioxidant enzymes were described earlier.

Superoxide Dismutase[11]

Three types of SOD exist, each derived from a separate gene: extracellular SOD, cytoplasmic SOD containing manganese (MnSOD) and mitochondrial SOD containing both copper and zinc (CuZnSOD). Extra production of SOD may be induced by several mechanisms, of which hyperoxia is the most notable, but inflammatory cytokines such as interferon, tumour necrosis factor, interleukins and lipopolysaccharide are important stimulants of SOD production in the intact animal.

Animal studies have consistently shown that induction of SOD confers some protection against the toxic effects of oxygen, and, by implication, enhanced SOD activity may be protective against the wide range of pathological processes already described. There are difficulties in the therapeutic use of SOD, because the most important forms are intracellular or mitochondrial enzymes, which have very short half-lives in plasma. Therefore there is little scope for their use by direct intravenous injection. It is possible for SOD to enter cells if it is administered in liposomes, and extracellular SOD has been used by direct instillation into the lungs. Recent attempts to enhance SOD activity for therapeutic purposes have switched to the development of SOD mimetics.[10] A number of small polycyclic compounds, mostly containing a central manganese molecule, have been found to catalyse the same reactions as SOD. SOD mimetics are being investigated in clinical trials, but results are still pending.

Catalase has a cellular and extracellular distribution similar to SOD, with which it is closely linked in disposing of the superoxide anion (Fig. 25.2). Although studied less extensively, catalase production is believed to be induced by the same factors as SOD. Similarly, trials of exogenous antioxidant enzymes have usually given better results when both SOD and catalase are administered.

The glutathione peroxidase system scavenges not only the ROS, but also reactive species formed during lipid peroxidation. Two molecules of the tripeptide (glycine-cysteine-glutamic acid) GSH are oxidized to one molecule of reduced glutathione (GSSG) by the formation of a disulphide bridge linking the cysteine residues. GSH is reformed from GSSG by the enzyme glutathione reductase, with protons supplied by NADPH.

Endogenous Antioxidants

Ascorbic acid is a small molecule with significant antioxidant properties which are particularly important for removal of the hydroxyl free radical. Apart from a direct chemical effect on the cell redox state, ascorbic acid also has effects on nitric oxide synthesis, and may influence cell biochemistry by this mechanism as well.[12] Humans, along with guinea pigs and bats, lack the enzyme required for the production of ascorbic acid, and must ingest sufficient vitamin C to compensate. In these mammals, SOD activity is markedly higher than in those able to produce endogenous ascorbic acid.

Vitamin E (α-tocopherol) is a highly fat-soluble compound, and is therefore found in high concentrations in cell membranes. Predictably, its main antioxidant role is in the prevention of lipid peroxidation chain reactions, as described earlier.

Glutathione is found in high concentrations in the airway lining fluid as part of the glutathione peroxidase system previously described. Widespread use of paracetamol, which at high doses can reduce glutathione levels in the lung, may attenuate the antioxidant activity provided by glutathione, increasing oxidative stress and possibly contributing to the increasing incidences of asthma and chronic obstructive pulmonary disease (COPD; Chapter 28).[13]

Surfactant may act as an antioxidant in the lung. Animal studies have shown that administration of exogenous surfactant prolongs the duration of oxygen exposure required to cause lung damage.[14]

Exogenous Antioxidants

Allopurinol. Because XOR plays a pivotal role in the reactions shown in Figure 25.4, it seemed logical to explore the use of allopurinol, which inhibits a range of enzymes including XOR. As expected, benefit was seen mainly following ischaemia–reperfusion injury, but under these conditions allopurinol has multiple effects on purine metabolism, and may not be acting as a XOR inhibitor at all.[6]

Iron-chelating agents. Because ferrous iron is both a potent source of electrons for conversion of oxygen to the superoxide anion and a catalyst in the Fenton reaction, the iron-chelating agent desferrioxamine has antioxidant properties in vitro.

Mitochondrial-targeted antioxidants. The development of diaphragm weakness in chronic heart failure has been linked to the presence of elevated oxidants, and this impairment of diaphragmatic function leads to an exacerbation of dyspnea. In animal studies, pharmacological targeting of mitochondrial ROS has been shown to counteract diaphragm weakness, and suggests a possible approach to managing this in clinical practice,[15] although this remains experimental.

These compounds, along with other in vitro antioxidants such as *n*-acetyl cysteine, β-carotene and dimethylsulphoxide, have generally failed to live up to their expectations in human disease. There are three possible explanations. First, studies of ROS production and antioxidants in human cells are relatively rare, and there is known to be considerable species variability. Second, penetration of the exogenous antioxidant to the site of ROS generation (e.g., mitochondria) or damage (e.g., nuclear DNA) is likely to be poor. Finally, ROS involvement in physiological systems such as neutrophil regulation is crucial, so any nonspecific antioxidant activity may be detrimental. Their therapeutic role in oxygen toxicity or diseases known to involve ROS is therefore far from fully clarified.

Normobaric Hyperoxia

The commonest indication for oxygen enrichment of the inspired gas at normal atmospheric pressure is the prevention of arterial hypoxaemia ('anoxic anoxia') caused either by hypoventilation (page 322) or by venous admixture (page 142). Increasing the $F_{I_{O_2}}$ may also be used to mitigate the effects of hypoperfusion ('stagnant hypoxia'). The data in Table 25.1 show that there will be only marginal improvement in oxygen delivery (page 154), but it may be critical in certain situations. 'Anaemic anoxia' will be only partially relieved by oxygen therapy, but, because the combined oxygen is less than what is seen in a subject with normal haemoglobin concentration, the effect of additional oxygen carried in solution will be relatively more important.

Clearance of gas loculi in the body may be greatly accelerated by the inhalation of oxygen, which greatly reduces the total partial pressure of the dissolved gases in the venous blood (Table 25.2). This results in the capillary blood having additional capacity to carry away gas dissolved from the loculi. Total gas partial pressures in venous blood are always slightly less than atmospheric, and this is critically important in preventing the accumulation of air in potential spaces such as the pleural cavity, where the pressure is subatmospheric. Oxygen is therefore useful in the treatment of air embolism (page 346) and pneumothorax (page 361).

The most important clinical conditions in which oxygen has been identified as the sole precipitating cause are retrolental fibroplasia and pulmonary oxygen toxicity, although there are many other clinical situations where excess oxygen has adverse effects.

Increasing the Inspired Oxygen Concentration[16]

Many systems exist for increasing the inspired oxygen concentration, and an understanding of these is crucial for effective therapy.

TABLE 25.2 Normal Arterial and Mixed Venous Blood Gas Partial Pressure

	kPa		mmHg	
	Arterial Blood	Venous Blood	Arterial Blood	Venous Blood
Breathing Air				
P_{O_2}	13.3	5.2	98	39
P_{CO_2}	5.3	6.1	40	46
P_{N_2}	76.0	76.0	570	570
Total gas partial pressure	94.6	87.3	708	655
Breathing Oxygen				
P_{O_2}	80.0	6.4	600	48
P_{CO_2}	5.3	6.1	40	46
P_{N_2}	0	0	0	0
Total gas partial pressure	85.3	12.5	640	94

Fixed Performance Devices

These allow the delivery of a known concentration of oxygen, independent of the patient's respiratory system; that is, the oxygen concentration delivered is unaffected by respiratory rate, tidal volume and inspiratory flow rate. Methods may be divided into low-flow (closed) or high-flow (open) delivery systems.

Closed delivery systems include a seal between the apparatus delivering the flow of gas and the patient's airway. Airtight seals may be obtained with cuffed tracheal or tracheostomy tubes or, at low airway pressures, with a tight-fitting facemask or laryngeal mask airway. These devices should give complete control over the composition of the inspired gas. Any closed delivery system requires the use of a breathing system that provides suitable separation of inspired and expired gases to prevent rebreathing and does not present significant resistance to breathing. Alternatively, the oxygen level may be controlled in the patient's gaseous environment. The popularity of oxygen tents declined because of their large volume and high rate of leakage, which made it difficult to attain and maintain a high oxygen concentration unless the volume was reduced, and a high gas flow rate was used. In addition, the fire hazard cannot be ignored. These problems are minimized when the patient is an infant, and oxygen control within an incubator is a satisfactory method of administering a precise oxygen concentration. A similar system is used with the hood ('space helmet') in critical care environments in which the patient's head is enclosed within a small, clear respirable atmosphere.

Open delivery systems make no attempt to provide an airtight seal; instead they provide a high flow of gas which can vent to atmosphere between the mask and the face, thus preventing the inflow of air. The required flow of air/oxygen mixture needs to be in excess of the peak inspiratory flow rate. For normal resting ventilation this is approximately 30 $L.min^{-1}$, but in patients with respiratory distress it may be considerably greater.

Oxygen may be passed through the jet of a Venturi to entrain air. Venturi-based devices are a convenient and highly economical method for preparing high flows of oxygen mixtures in the range of 25% to 40% concentration. For example, 3 $L.min^{-1}$ of oxygen passed through the jet of a Venturi with an entrainment ratio of 8:1 will deliver 27 $L.min^{-1}$ of 30% oxygen. Higher oxygen concentrations require a lower entrainment ratio, and therefore a higher oxygen flow to maintain an adequate total delivered flow rate. With an adequate total flow rate of the air/oxygen mixture, the Venturi mask need not fit the face with an airtight seal. The high flow rate escapes round the cheeks as well as through the holes in the mask, and room air is effectively excluded. Numerous studies have indicated that the Venturi mask gives good control over the inspired oxygen concentration that is mostly unaffected by variations in the ventilation of the patient, except at high oxygen concentrations.

Variable Performance Devices

Simple disposable oxygen masks and nasal catheters aim to blow oxygen at or into the air passages. The oxygen is mixed with inspired air to give an inspired oxygen concentration that is a complex function of the geometry of the device, the oxygen flow rate, the patient's ventilation and whether the patient is breathing through their mouth or nose. The effective inspired oxygen concentration is impossible to predict, and may vary within very wide limits. These devices cannot be used for oxygen therapy when the exact inspired oxygen concentration is critical, but are useful in many other situations such as recovery from routine anaesthesia. With simple oxygen masks a small inspiratory reservoir will store fresh gas during expiration for use during inspiration, which will tend to increase the inspired oxygen concentration, but, again, in a somewhat unpredictable fashion.

With a device such as a nasal catheter or prongs, the lower the ventilation, the greater the fractional contribution of the fixed flow of oxygen to the inspired gas mixture. There is thus an approximate compensation for hypoventilation, with greater oxygen concentrations delivered at lower levels of ventilation. Arterial Po_2 may then be maintained in spite of a progressively falling ventilation, but this will do nothing to prevent the rise in Pco_2, which may reach a dangerous level without the development of low oxygen saturations.

High-Flow Nasal Therapy

High-flow nasal therapy (HFNT) is variably described as high-flow nasal oxygen or high-flow nasal cannulae in the literature. Ideally warmed and humidified gases are delivered at oxygen concentrations of 21% to 100% at flows of up to 60 $L.min^{-1}$, benefitting patients by the avoidance of mucosal drying and inspissation of secretions in the airway. It is more acceptable to patients than conventional high-flow oxygen masks or helmets, and so compliance with the therapy is generally good.[17] HFNT delivers high oxygen concentrations, generates positive pressure in the pharynx and reduces dead space and rebreathing by purging carbon dioxide from the upper airway.[18] HFNT can be delivered to patients who are either spontaneously breathing or who are apnoeic.

HFNT has been demonstrated to confer clinical benefit across a range of conditions and situations, for example, in patients with acute respiratory failure,[19] in those undergoing elective or emergency awake fibre-optic intubation, during airway surgery[20] or during emergency intubation in critically ill patients.[21] It may also have a role in the perioperative setting to reduce the incidence of postoperative pulmonary complications, or in the management of chronic disease, for example, by reducing the number of exacerbation days in patients with COPD.[22]

The positive pressure produced by HFNT is greatest in expiration, that is, it is not a constant pressure, in contrast to that generated during continuous positive airway pressure (page 377). The pressure generated is also variable, as it is affected by factors such as whether the mouth is open or closed, as well as nasal pathology or variations in anatomy, but has been found by one study to increase by 1 cmH$_2$O for each 10 L.min^{-1} increase in HFNT flow rate across a range of 30 to 50 L.min^{-1}.[23] Despite the variation and inconsistency of the pressure generated, the increase in end-expiratory pressure is sufficient to benefit patients with respiratory failure. HFNT improves respiratory system mechanics by reducing the work of breathing, increasing dynamic lung compliance and decreasing inspiratory resistance.[24,25] In the spontaneously breathing patient with respiratory failure, the effect of HFNT on carbon dioxide clearance offers particular benefit.

During apnoea, HFNT is applied with the aim of maintaining arterial oxygenation in patients who are not receiving any tidal ventilation to facilitate airway manipulation, for example intubation or airway surgery. Oxygenation may be maintained for prolonged periods of time under these circumstances because of the mass movement of oxygen into the lungs (page 132). However, of note, a slower increase in carbon dioxide level is observed during apnoea with HFNT compared with when no HFNT is used, or when HFNT is used at lower flow rates.[26] Carbon dioxide clearance during apnoea is the subject of ongoing research, but studies suggest that a number of mechanisms are important, including gas mixing from turbulence, cardiogenic oscillations and molecular diffusion.[27]

Clinical Effects of Normobaric Hyperoxia

Retinopathy of Prematurity[27]

Previously known as retrolental fibroplasia, retinopathy of prematurity (RP) was first described in 1942, and soon afterwards it was established that hyperoxia was a major aetiological factor. Oxygen use in neonates was strictly curtailed, but resulted in an increase in morbidity and mortality attributable to hypoxia. Thereafter oxygen was carefully titrated in the hope of steering the narrow course between the Scylla of hypoxia and the Charybdis of RP. The same balance between oxygenation and RP continues today, with uncertainty about the optimal target oxygen saturation to use in premature neonates.[28] RP develops in two phases. In phase 1 there is delayed vascular development of the retina with avascular peripheral areas, and in phase 2 there is vasoproliferation leading to intravitreal angiogenesis. These abnormalities are believed to result from changes in Po$_2$ affecting the activity of hypoxia-inducible factor (page 276), and in particular its effect on vascular growth factors at this crucial stage of eye development for humans. Antioxidants such as vitamin E have showed some promise for treatment of RP, but often with unacceptable side effects, and current therapeutic strategies are therefore aimed at inhibiting vascular growth factors.

Pulmonary Oxygen Toxicity

Pulmonary tissue Po$_2$ is the highest in the body. In addition, a whole range of other oxidizing substances may be inhaled, including common air pollutants and the constituents of cigarette smoke (Chapter 20). The lung is therefore the organ most vulnerable to oxygen toxicity, and a range of defence mechanisms have developed. Overall antioxidant activity from both enzymes and other endogenous antioxidants is very high in the fluid lining of the respiratory tract. Extracellular SOD is abundant in pulmonary airway tissues, and abnormalities in its regulation may contribute to some lung diseases. Type II alveolar epithelial cells, which produce surfactant (page 16), are believed to also incorporate vitamin E into the surfactant lipids.[29]

Pulmonary oxygen toxicity is unequivocal and lethal in laboratory animals such as the rat. Humans seem to be far less sensitive, but there are formidable obstacles to investigation of both human volunteers and patients. Study of oxygen toxicity in the clinical environment is complicated by the presence of the pulmonary pathology that necessitated the use of oxygen.

Symptoms[30]

High concentrations of oxygen cause irritation of the tracheobronchial tree, which gives rise initially to a sensation of retrosternal tightness. Continued exposure leads to chest pain, cough and an urge to take deep breaths. Reduced vital capacity is the first measurable change in lung function, occurring after about 24 hours of normobaric 100% oxygen. Oxygen exposure beyond this point leads to the widespread structural changes described next, which ultimately give rise to acute lung injury and possibly irreversible changes in lung function.

Cellular Changes[31]

Electron microscopy has shown that, in rats exposed to 1 atm of oxygen, the primary change is in the capillary endothelium, which becomes vacuolated and thin. Permeability is increased, and fluid accumulates in the interstitial space. At a later stage, in monkeys, the epithelial lining is lost over large areas of the alveoli. This process affects the type I cell (page 10) and is accompanied by proliferation of the type II cell, which is relatively resistant to oxygen. The alveolar/capillary membrane is greatly thickened, partly because of the substitution of type II for type I cells and partly because of interstitial accumulation of fluid.

Limits of Survival

Pulmonary effects of oxygen vary greatly between different species, probably because of different levels of provision of defences against ROS. Most strains of rat will not survive for much more than 3 days in 1 atm of oxygen. Monkeys generally survive oxygen breathing for about 2 weeks, and humans are probably even more resistant. Oxygen tolerance in humans has been investigated,[32] but these studies are based on reduction in vital capacity, and so on, which is a very early stage of oxygen toxicity. There is an approximately inverse relationship between Po$_2$ and duration of tolerable exposure. Thus 20 hours of 1 atm had a similar effect to 10 hours of 2 atm or 5 hours of 4 atm.

Pulmonary oxygen toxicity seems to be related to P_{O_2} rather than inspired concentration. Early American astronauts breathed 100% oxygen at a pressure of about one-third of an atmosphere for many days (Table 17.1) with no apparent ill effects. There is abundant evidence that prolonged exposure to this environment does not result in demonstrable pulmonary oxygen toxicity, thus establishing a P_{O_2} of 34 kPa (255 mmHg) as a safe level. It also confirms that the significant factor is partial pressure and not concentration. In contrast, the concentration of oxygen rather than its partial pressure is the important factor in absorption collapse of the lung (see later).

Pulmonary Absorption Collapse

Whatever the uncertainties about the susceptibility of humans to pulmonary oxygen toxicity, there is no doubt that high concentrations of oxygen in zones of the lung with low ventilation/perfusion ratios will result in collapse. This occurs routinely during anaesthesia (page 251), and may be demonstrated in healthy volunteers. A few minutes of breathing oxygen at residual lung volume results in radiological evidence of collapse, a reduced arterial P_{O_2} and retrosternal pain on attempting a maximal inspiration.[33]

Bleomycin Lung Toxicity

Bleomycin is an intravenous cytotoxic drug used for chemotherapy of germ-cell tumours, and has been known for decades to cause severe and sometimes fatal pulmonary toxicity. Its cytotoxic action includes binding to both DNA and an iron molecule, which is then oxidized to its Fe^{3+} state, releasing ROS that damage the DNA. Bleomycin in the circulation initially damages pulmonary capillary endothelial cells, causing leakage of fluid into the interstitial space, where the drug gains access to type 1 alveolar cells vulnerable to ROS damage, resulting in lung injury.[34] Animal studies have demonstrated the critical role of ROS by showing that SOD mimetic molecules can attenuate the lung damage.[35] Lung toxicity has been reported as occurring in 2.8% to 6.3% of patients treated with the drug with predictors of this complication including older age, renal impairment and total dose of bleomycin used.[36] The role of supplemental oxygen in exacerbating lung toxicity and the duration after treatment when patients are at risk are controversial, with conflicting reports from heterogeneous case series. One possible explanation for the lack of clear findings is that hyperoxia simply exacerbates preexisting lung damage, irrespective of whether this is clinically apparent or subclinical, as indicated by reduced pulmonary-diffusing capacity.[34] It therefore still seems sensible to minimize oxygen exposure for any patient who has been treated with bleomycin, with most clinicians currently adopting target oxygen saturations to guide the $F_{I_{O_2}}$, as described next.

Hyperoxia in the Perioperative Period

The ease with which the $F_{I_{O_2}}$ can be increased during anaesthesia often leads to the continued use of a high $F_{I_{O_2}}$ in the perioperative period, despite little evidence of clinical benefit for an $F_{I_{O_2}}$ of 0.8 or greater.[37] Postulated beneficial effects of a high $F_{I_{O_2}}$ in the perioperative period include lower rates of postoperative nausea and vomiting (PONV), surgical pain and surgical site infection. Most studies compare $F_{I_{O_2}}$ values of 0.3 to 0.4 with those of 0.6 to 0.8.[38]

PONV. Hyperoxia has been proposed to reduce PONV, purportedly from improved oxygen delivery to the gut mucosa. Results from trials and meta-analyses have shown conflicting results, with the largest of these finding that hyperoxia was only beneficial in patients at high risk of PONV who received no prophylactic drugs, giving a 'number needed to treat' of 15 patients for one patient to benefit.[38]

Surgical site infection and pain. Robust evidence to support the theory that hyperoxia helps to prevent surgical site infection is lacking. The suggested mechanism is the increased tissue P_{O_2} resulting from hyperoxia, which then improves ROS availability, thus facilitating the killing of pathogens by neutrophils. However, a Cochrane review in 2016 of 28 randomized trials[39] including 7537 patients concluded that insufficient evidence exists to support the use of a higher $F_{I_{O_2}}$ in the perioperative period. A recent trial of 5749 operations concluded that an $F_{I_{O_2}}$ of 0.8 versus 0.3 had no effect on the incidence of major infections and healing-related complications following major intestinal surgery lasting over 2 hours.[40] Postoperative pain seems to be similarly unaffected by $F_{I_{O_2}}$.[41]

In addition, morbidity and mortality may be adversely affected in the perioperative period by a higher $F_{I_{O_2}}$. In particular, adverse effects on the myocardium and pulmonary function have been suggested. A review of the cardiovascular effects of hyperoxia during and after cardiac surgery indicated that hyperoxia may compromise cardiovascular performance because of oxidative stress.[42] The proposed mechanism is that hyperoxia induces vasoconstriction, disrupts the microcirculation and can contribute to diastolic dysfunction. In turn this leads to decreased cardiac output and increased myocardial injury. An intraoperative $F_{I_{O_2}}$ of 0.8 versus 0.3 causes a greater degree of atelectasis perioperatively, and is associated in a dose-dependent manner with higher rates of major postoperative pulmonary complications.[43] The administration of an $F_{I_{O_2}}$ of 0.8 in the perioperative period has also been found to be associated with significantly increased long-term mortality in patients undergoing cancer surgery, although causality is not proven.[44]

Hyperoxia in Acute Medicine

In clinical practice the administration of oxygen to acutely ill patients has become almost ubiquitous, both in hospital and community settings. Prevention of dangerous hypoxia is always the first priority, and hypoxia must be treated in spite of the various hazards associated with the use of oxygen. The now widespread availability of pulse oximetry has led to many guidelines challenging this reflex administration of emergency oxygen therapy, instead suggesting that oxygen should be targeted at a predetermined oxygen saturation, with suggested values of 94% to 98% in most acutely ill patients or 88% to 92% for those at risk of hypercapnia.[16] A recent meta-analysis including over 16 000 patients found that, compared with a more conservative strategy, a liberal approach to oxygen therapy (mean oxygen saturation levels of 96.4%) increased in-hospital mortality amongst acute medical patients across a range of acute conditions including acute myocardial infarction (AMI), stroke, sepsis and cardiac arrest. Supplemental oxygen may therefore become unfavourable above saturations of 94% to 96%.[45] When these targets are not achievable by increasing inspired oxygen alone, it is important to remember that oxygen delivery can also be increased by improving cardiac output and haemoglobin levels.

Clinical situations where the routine use of oxygen is now being challenged include:

- *Exacerbations of COPD.* The mechanisms of the adverse effects are described on page 333. Uncontrolled use of oxygen is associated with increased mortality in these patients.[37]
- *AMI.* There is some evidence that oxygen therapy in the first few hours after AMI does not improve survival, and may be associated with poorer outcomes.[46] Supplemental oxygen therapy has been associated with a higher incidence of reinfarction and greater infarct size.[47] A large randomized clinical trial of patients with suspected AMI who were not hypoxaemic (SaO_2 ≥90%) did not show improved outcomes at a year for those managed with ambient air versus supplemental oxygen administered via a facemask at 6 L.min^{-1} for 6 to 12 hours.[48] Hyperoxia causes vasoconstriction of systemic blood vessels, an effect inhibited by vitamin C, suggesting a mechanism involving ROS.[49] The same is true for coronary blood flow, and the effect may be more pronounced in diseased arteries that are already under oxidative stress.
- *Acute ischaemic stroke.* There is some evidence that hyperoxia causes an increased mortality in patients following severe ischaemic stroke who require artificial ventilation.[50] Hyperoxia is known to reduce cerebral blood flow, and the same vasoconstrictor effect described earlier is believed to be the cause of the worse outcomes following stroke.
- *Cardiopulmonary resuscitation (CPR).* During CPR (page 393) 100% oxygen should be administered to maximize the oxygen content in the poor circulation generated by cardiac compressions. However, at the return of spontaneous circulation (ROSC) it has been shown that the FiO_2 used impacts subsequent patient survival, with an odds ratio of 1.8 (confidence interval [CI] 1.5–2.2) for death in patients receiving hyperoxia (PaO_2 >40 kPa, 300 mmHg).[51] Once the ROSC is established well enough for a pulse oximeter to give a reliable reading, FiO_2 should be titrated to a normal level.

Hyperoxia in Critical Care

A study in 1967 of patients who died after prolonged artificial ventilation found more structural pulmonary abnormalities (fibrin membranes, oedema and fibrosis) in those who had received 100% oxygen.[52] However, the higher concentrations of oxygen would probably have been used in the patients with more severe defects in gas exchange, and it is therefore difficult to distinguish between the effects of oxygen itself and the conditions which required its use. More recently, adverse clinical outcomes associated with hyperoxia have prompted debate regarding the optimal level of target oxygen saturation or Po_2 in critical care. A 2017 multicentre retrospective study of over 14 000 intensive care patients found that hyperoxia (PO_2 ≥26.6 kPa, 200 mmHg) was associated with increased mortality and fewer ventilator-free days (Figure 25.6).[53] However, a much larger study found no adverse effects of hyperoxia once adjustments for comorbidities were made.[54] Further work is needed to define whether hyperoxia is indeed a marker or cause of poorer outcomes, and, if so, the duration and level of hyperoxia at which this becomes significant. There is a certainly a current move away from the liberal use of supplemental oxygen and hyperoxia in the critical care setting, with a trend towards more precise control of arterial oxygenation, a 'permissive hypoxaemia' strategy[55] and an appreciation that inspired oxygen in artificially ventilated patients should be titrated to a target oxygen saturation, as already advocated in other acutely ill patients, as described above.[56]

Hyperbaric Hyperoxia

Oxygen Convulsions (The Paul Bert Effect)

It is well established that exposure to oxygen at a partial pressure in excess of 2 ATA may result in convulsions, usually preceded by a variety of nonspecific neurological symptoms such as headache and visual disturbances. This limits the depth to which closed-circuit oxygen apparatus can be used. It is interesting that the threshold for oxygen convulsions is close to that at which brain tissue Po_2 is likely to be sharply increased (Table 25.1). The relationship to cerebral tissue Po_2 is supported by the observation that an elevation of Pco_2 lowers the threshold for convulsions. High Pco_2 increases cerebral blood flow, therefore raising the tissue Po_2 relative to the arterial Po_2. Hyperventilation and anaesthesia each provide limited protection.

Convulsions result from poorly understood changes in cellular interactions between γ-aminobutyric acid (GABA) and nitric oxide. Because GABA is an inhibitory neurotransmitter, it is not unreasonable to suggest that a reduced level might result in convulsions. Nitric oxide sensitizes neurones to the toxic effects of GABA in hypoxia, and is also involved in hyperoxic convulsions. Nitric oxide inhibitors delay the onset of convulsions in hyperoxia,[57] but paradoxically, the same effect is seen with some nitric oxide donors. Whatever the role of nitric oxide, the final common pathway seems to

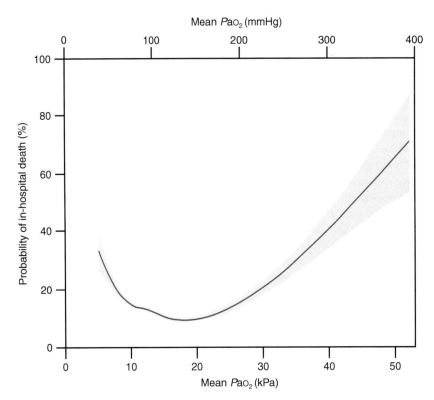

• **Fig. 25.6** Adjusted probability of in-hospital death by mean arterial PO_2 amongst 14 441 intensive care patients (From reference 52, with permission of the publishers of *Critical Care Medicine*.)

be mediated by disturbed calcium fluxes and increased cyclic-GMP concentration.[57]

Incidence

Hyperbaric oxygen used therapeutically, as described later, involves intermittent exposure to less than 3 ATA, and carries little risk of oxygen convulsions. At 2 ATA, a large series reported no convulsions in over 12 000 treatments.[58] Treatment for carbon monoxide poisoning is associated with a greater incidence of convulsions because of the higher pressures used (normally 2.8–3.0 ATA) and the toxic effects of carbon monoxide on the brain. In this case, 1% to 2% of patients experience convulsions.

Therapeutic Effects of Hyperbaric Oxygen

Administration of short periods of very high PO_2 may bring about therapeutic effects by a variety of mechanisms, as follows.

Effect on PO_2. Hyperbaric oxygenation is the only way arterial PO_2 values in excess of 90 kPa (675 mmHg) may be obtained. Tissues are not exposed to the PO_2 present in the chamber; terms such as 'drenching the tissues with oxygen' have been used, but are meaningless. In fact, the simple calculations shown in Table 25.1, supported by experimental observations, show that large increases in venous, and presumably therefore minimum tissue, PO_2 do not occur until the PO_2 of the arterial blood is of the order of 270 kPa (2025 mmHg), when the whole-tissue oxygen requirements can be met from the dissolved oxygen. However, the relationship between arterial and tissue PO_2 is highly variable

(page 119), and hyperoxia-induced vasoconstriction in the brain and other tissues limits the rise in venous and tissue PO_2. Direct access of ambient oxygen will increase PO_2 in superficial tissues, particularly when the skin is breached.

Effect on PCO_2. An increased haemoglobin saturation of venous blood reduces its buffering power and carbamino carriage of carbon dioxide, possibly resulting in carbon dioxide retention. The increase in tissue PCO_2 from this cause is unlikely to exceed 1 kPa (7.5 mmHg). However, in the brain this might result in a significant increase in cerebral blood flow, causing a secondary rise in tissue PO_2.

Vasoconstriction. As described earlier, high PO_2 causes vasoconstriction, which may be valuable for reduction of oedema in the reperfusion of ischaemic limbs and in burns (see later discussion).

Angiogenesis. The growth of new blood vessels is improved when oxygen is increased to more than 1 ATA pressure, although the mechanism by which angiogenesis is stimulated is uncertain. When normoxia follows a period of hypoxia, ROS are produced, and these are known to stimulate the production of a variety of growth factors that initiate angiogenesis.[59] The same mechanism may occur during hyperbaric oxygenation.

Antibacterial effect. For many years oxygen was believed to play a role in bacterial killing by the formation of ROS, particularly in polymorphs and macrophages, although this has recently been refuted (page 289). However, oxygen still has a direct toxic effect on microorganisms, particularly on anaerobic bacteria, and relief of hypoxia improves the performance of polymorphs.

Boyle's law effect. The volume of gas spaces within the body is reduced inversely to the absolute pressure according to Boyle's law (page 415). This effect is additional to that resulting from reduction of the total partial pressure of gases in venous blood (Table 25.2)

Clinical Applications of Hyperbaric Oxygenation Therapy

In practice, hyperbaric oxygen therapy (HBOT) means placing a patient into a chamber at 2 to 3 ATA and providing apparatus to allow them to breathe 100% oxygen, normally a tight-fitting facemask. Treatment is usually for about 1 to 2 hours, and repeated daily for up to 30 days. Since its first use in 1960, enthusiasm for hyperbaric oxygenation has waxed and waned, and its use is still confined to relatively few centres. Clear indications of its therapeutic value have been slow to emerge from controlled trials, which are admittedly very difficult to conduct in the conditions for which benefit is claimed. In particular, a proper 'control' group of patients must undergo a sham treatment in a hyperbaric chamber, which has been used in very few trials. The most commonly accepted indications are as follows.

Infection is the most enduring field of application of hyperbaric oxygenation, particularly anaerobic bacterial infections. High partial pressures of oxygen increase the production of ROS, which are cidal not only to anaerobes but also to aerobes. The strongest indications are for clostridial myonecrosis (gas gangrene), refractory osteomyelitis and necrotizing soft tissue infections, including cutaneous ulcers. Bacteriostatic effects have also been demonstrated against species of *Escherichia* and *Pseudomonas*.

Gas or air embolus and decompression sickness are unequivocal indications for hyperbaric therapy, and the rationale of treatment was considered earlier and in Chapter 17.

Carbon monoxide poisoning may occur from exposure to automobile exhaust fumes, fires and defective heating appliances. Indications for hyperbaric oxygenation following carbon monoxide poisoning include loss of consciousness, neurological deficits, ischaemic cardiac changes, significant metabolic acidosis or carboxyhaemoglobin (COHb) levels of more than 25%, and the aim is to reduce both mortality and neurological sequelae in survivors.[60,61] The original rationale for therapy, increased rate of dissociation of COHb, seems simple when the half-life of COHb is approximately 4 to 5 hours while breathing air and only 20 minutes with hyperbaric oxygen. However, breathing 100% oxygen at normal pressure reduces the half-life of COHb to just 40 minutes; therefore in many cases, by the time transport to a hyperbaric chamber is achieved, COHb levels will already be considerably reduced. Other potential benefits of hyperbaric oxygen are believed to derive from minimizing the effects of carbon monoxide on cytochrome *c* oxidase and reducing lipid peroxidation by neutrophils to attenuate the immune-mediated and inflammatory sequelae.[61]

Wound healing is improved by hyperbaric oxygenation, even when used intermittently. It is particularly useful when ischaemia contributes to the ineffective healing, for example, in diabetes mellitus or peripheral vascular disease. The mechanisms involve improved tissue oxygen levels probably resulting from direct diffusion of oxygen into the affected superficial tissues and increased release of growth factors.[62]

In the early 1980s there was great interest in the therapeutic value of hyperbaric oxygenation in multiple sclerosis. However, a review of 14 controlled trials concluded that hyperbaric oxygen cannot be recommended for the treatment of multiple sclerosis.[63]

Overall, HBOT is a considered a safe and well-tolerated therapy when used under the direction of experienced and licensed treatment facilities.[62]

References

1. Ershler WB. A gripping reality: oxidative stress, inflammation, and the pathway to frailty. *J Appl Physiol.* 2007;103:3-5.
2. Webster NR, Nunn JF. Molecular structure of free radicals and their importance in biological reactions. *Br J Anaesth.* 1988;60:98-108.
3. Dweik RA. Nitric oxide, hypoxia, and superoxide: the good, the bad, and the ugly! *Thorax.* 2005;60:265-267.
4. Zorov DB, Juhaszova M, Sollott SJ. Mitochondrial reactive oxygen species (ROS) and ROS-induced ROS release. *Physiol Rev.* 2014;94:909-950.
5. Marriott HM, Jackson LE, Wilkinson TS, et al. Reactive oxygen species regulate neutrophil recruitment and survival in pneumococcal pneumonia. *Am J Respir Crit Care Med.* 2008;177:887-895.
6. Harrison R. Structure and function of xanthine oxidoreductase: Where are we now? *Free Radic Biol Med.* 2002;33:774-797.
7. Sturrock JE, Nunn JF. Chromosomal damage and mutations after exposure of Chinese hamster cells to high concentrations of oxygen. *Mutat Res.* 1978;57:27-31.
8. Sallmyr A, Fan J, Datta K, et al. Internal tandem duplication of FLT3 (FLT3/ITD) induces increased ROS production, DNA damage, and misrepair: implications for poor prognosis in AML. *Blood.* 2008;111:3173-3182.
9. Speit G, Dennog C, Radermacher P, et al. Genotoxicity of hyperbaric oxygen. *Mutat Res.* 2002;512:111-119.
10. Salvemini D, Riley DP, Cuzzocrea S. SOD mimetics are coming of age. *Nat Rev Drug Discov.* 2002;1:367-374.
11. Kinnula VL, Crapo JD. Superoxide dismutases in the lung and human lung diseases. *Am J Respir Crit Care Med.* 2003;167:1600-1619.
12. Holowatz LA. Ascorbic acid: what do we really NO? *J Appl Physiol.* 2011;111:1542-1543.
13. McKeever TM, Lewis SA, Smit HA, et al. The association of acetaminophen, aspirin, and ibuprofen with respiratory disease and lung function. *Am J Respir Crit Care Med.* 2005;171:966-971.
14. Ghio AJ, Fracica PJ, Young SL, et al. Synthetic surfactant scavenges oxidants and protects against hyperoxic lung injury. *J Appl Physiol.* 1994;77:1217-1223.
15. Laitano O, Bumsoo A, Patel N, et al. Pharmacological targeting of mitochondrial reactive oxygen species counteracts diaphragm weakness in chronic heart failure. *J Appl Physiol.* 2016;120:733-742.
*16. **O'Driscoll BR, Howard LS, Earis J. BTS guideline for oxygen use in adults in healthcare and emergency settings. *Thorax.* 2017;72:i1-i90.**

17. Ashraf-Kashani N, Kumar R. High flow nasal oxygen therapy. *Br J Anaesth Educ*. 2017;17:63-67.

18. Pinkham M, Burgess R, Mündel T, et al. Nasal high flow reduces minute ventilation during sleep through a decrease of carbon dioxide rebreathing. *J Appl Physiol*. 2019;126:863-869.

19. Rochwerg B, Granton D, Wang DX, et al. High flow nasal cannula compared with conventional oxygen therapy for acute hypoxemic respiratory failure: a systematic review and meta-analysis. *Intensive Care Med*. 2019;45:563-572.

20. Badiger S, John M, Fearnley R, et al. Optimizing oxygenation and intubation conditions during awake fibreoptic intubation using a high-flow nasal oxygen-delivery system. *Br J Anaesth*. 2015;115:629-632.

21. Chanques G, Jaber S. Nasal high-flow preoxygenation for endotracheal intubation in the critically ill patient? *Maybe*. *Intensive Care Med*. 2019;45:532-534.

22. Hernandez G, Roca O, Colinas L. High-flow nasal cannula support therapy: new insights and improving performance. *Crit Care*. 2017;21:62-73.

23. Parke RL, McGuinness SP. Pressures delivered by nasal high flow oxygen during all phases of the respiratory cycle. *Respir Care*. 2013;58:1621-1624.

24. Delorme M, Bouchard PA, Simon M, et al. Effects of high-flow nasal cannula on the work of breathing in patients recovering from acute respiratory failure. *Crit Care Med*. 2017;45:1981-1988.

25. Mauri T, Turrini C, Eronia N, et al. Physiologic effects of high-flow nasal cannula in acute hypoxemic respiratory failure. *Am J Respir Crit Care Med*. 2017;195:1207-1215.

26. Patel A, Nouraei SAR. Transnasal humidified rapid-insufflation ventilatory exchange (THRIVE): a physiological method of increasing apnoea time in patients with difficult airways. *Anaesthesia*. 2015;70:323-329.

27. Hartnett ME, Penn JS. Mechanisms and management of retinopathy of prematurity. *N Engl J Med*. 2012;367:2515-2526.

28. The BOOST II United Kingdom, Australia, and New Zealand Collaborative Groups. Oxygen saturation and outcomes in preterm infants. *N Engl J Med*. 2013;368:2094-2104.

29. Kolleck I, Sinha P, Rüstow B. Vitamin E as an antioxidant of the lung. Mechanisms of vitamin E delivery to alveolar Type II cells. *Am J Respir Crit Care Med*. 2002;166:S62-S66.

30. Montgomery AB, Luce JM, Murray JF. Retrosternal pain is an early indicator of oxygen toxicity. *Am Rev Respir Dis*. 1989;139:1548-1550.

31. Weibel ER. Oxygen effect on lung cells. *Arch Intern Med*. 1971;128:54-56.

32. Clark JM, Lambertsen CJ, Gelfand R, et al. Effects of prolonged oxygen exposure at 1.5, 2.0, or 2.5 ATA on pulmonary function in men (Predictive studies V). *J Appl Physiol*. 1999;86:243-259.

33. Nunn JF, Williams IP, Jones JG, et al. Detection and reversal of pulmonary absorption collapse. *Br J Anaesth*. 1978;50:91-100.

34. Mathes DD. Bleomycin and hyperoxia exposure in the operating room. *Anesth Analg*. 1995;81:624-629.

35. Tanaka K-I, Azuma A, Miyazaki Y, et al. Effects of lecithinized superoxide dismutase and/or pirfenidone against bleomycin-induced pulmonary fibrosis. *Chest*. 2012;142:1011-1019.

36. O'Sullivan JM, Huddart RA, Norman AR, et al. Predicting the risk of bleomycin lung toxicity in patients with germ-cell tumours. *Ann Oncol*. 2003;14:91-96.

37. O'Driscoll BR, Decalmer S. Oxygen: friend or foe in peri-operative care? *Anaesthesia*. 2013;68:8-12.

38. Hovaguimian F, Lysakowski C, Elia N, et al. Effect of intraoperative high inspired oxygen fraction on surgical site infection, postoperative nausea and vomiting, and pulmonary function. Systematic review and meta-analysis of randomized controlled trials. *Anesthesiology*. 2013;119:303-316.

*39. **Wetterslev J, Meyhoff CS, Jørgensen LN, et al. The effects of high perioperative inspiratory oxygen fraction for adult surgical patients – (review). *Cochrane Database Syst Rev*. 2015;(6):CD008884.**

40. Kurz A, Kopyeva T, Suliman I. Supplemental oxygen and surgical site infections: an alternating intervention controlled trial. *Br J Anaesth*. 2018;120:117-126.

41. Cohen B, Ahuja S, Schacham YN, et al. Intraoperative hyperoxia does not reduce postoperative pain: subanalysis of an alternating cohort trial. *Anesth Analg*. 2019;128:1160-1166.

42. Spoelstra-de Man A, Smit B, Oudemans-van Straaten H, et al. Cardiovascular effects of hyperoxia during and after cardiac surgery. *Anaesthesia*. 2015;70:1307-1319.

43. Staehr-Rye AK, Meyhoff CS, Scheffenbichler FT, et al. High intraoperative inspiratory oxygen fraction and risk of major respiratory complications. *Br J Anaesth*. 2017;119:140-149.

44. Meyhoff C, Jorgensen L, Wetterslev, et al. Increased long term mortality after a high perioperative inspired oxygen fraction; follow up of a randomized clinical trial. *Anesth Analg*. 2012;115:849-854.

45. Chu D, Kim L, Young P, et al. Mortality and morbidity in acutely ill adults treated with liberal versus conservative oxygen therapy (IOTA): A systematic review and meta-analysis. *Lancet*. 2018;391:1693-1703.

46. Cabello JB, Burls A, Emparanza JI, et al. Oxygen therapy for acute myocardial infarction. *Cochrane Database Syst Rev*. 2010;(6):CD007160.

47. Stub G, Smith K, Bernard S, et al. Air versus oxygen in ST-segment-elevation myocardial infarction. *Circulation*. 2015;131:2143-2150.

48. Hofmann R, James SK, Jernberg T, et al. Oxygen therapy in suspected acute myocardial infarction. *N Engl J Med*. 2017;377:1240-1249.

49. Ranadive SM, Joyner MJ, Walker BG, et al. Effect of vitamin C on hyperoxia-induced vasoconstriction in exercising skeletal muscle. *J Appl Physiol*. 2014;117:1207-1211.

50. Rincon F, Kang J, Maltenfort M, et al. Association between hyperoxia and mortality after stroke: A multicenter cohort study. *Crit Care Med*. 2014;42:387-396.

51. Kilgannon JH, Jones AE, Shapiro NI, et al. Association between arterial hyperoxia following resuscitation from cardiac arrest and in-hospital mortality. *JAMA*. 2010;303:2165-2171.

52. Nash G, Blennerhassett JB, Pontoppidan H. Pulmonary lesions associated with oxygen therapy and artificial ventilation. *N Engl J Med*. 1967;276:368-374.

53. Helmerhorst H, Arts D, Schultz M, et al. Metrics of arterial hyperoxia and associated outcomes in critical care. *Crit Care Med*. 2017;45:187-195.

54. Villar J, Kacmarek R. Oxygen: Breath of life or kiss of death? *Crit Care Med*. 2017;45:368-369.

55. Martin DS, Grocott MPW. Oxygen therapy in critical illness: precise control of arterial oxygenation and permissive hypoxemia. *Crit Care Med*. 2013;41:423-432.

*56. **Martin DS. Oxygen therapy: is the tide turning? *Crit Care Med*. 2014;42:1553-1554.**

57. Wang WJ, Ho XP, Yan YL, et al. Intrasynaptosomal free calcium and nitric oxide metabolism in central nervous system toxicity. *Aviat Space Environ Med*. 1998;69:551-555.

58. Hill RK. Is more better? A comparison of different clinical hyperbaric treatment pressures—a preliminary report. *Undersea Hyperb Med*. 1993;20(suppl):12.

59. Maulik N, Das DK. Redox signalling in vascular angiogenesis. *Free Radic Biol Med*. 2002;33:1047-1060.

60. Rose JJ, Nouraie M, Gauthier MC, et al. Clinical outcomes and mortality impact of hyperbaric oxygen therapy in patients with carbon monoxide poisoning. *Crit Care Med*. 2018;46:e649-e655.

61. Rose JJ, Wang L, Xu Q, et al. Carbon monoxide poisoning: pathogenesis, management, and future directions of therapy. *Am J Respir Crit Care Med*. 2017;195:596-606.

*62. **Choudhury R. Hypoxia and hyperbaric oxygen therapy: a review. *J Int Gen Med*. 2018;11:431-442.**

63. Kleijnen J, Knipschild P. Hyperbaric oxygen for multiple sclerosis. Review of controlled trials. *Acta Neurol Scand*. 1995;91:330-334.

26

Comparative Respiratory Physiology

COAUTHOR KATHERINE LUMB BVSC MSC MRCVS

KEY POINTS

- The animal kingdom contains a myriad of solutions to the challenge of respiratory gas exchange, such as integument respiration, external or internal gills in water or a tracheae system or lung for breathing air.
- Factors affecting respiratory system design include the breathing medium (water or air), body temperature and activity level (metabolic rate), with homeothermic (warm-blooded) animals requiring more efficient systems and air to breathe to obtain sufficient oxygen.
- Circulatory systems for gas transport vary, from 'open' systems containing haemolymph in primitive animals, to single circulations in fish with gills and other organs in series, to the dual circulation for the lungs and body of homeotherms.

- There are only three types of oxygen-binding molecule in the entire animal kingdom, all based on a metal atom bound to a protein, with the familiar haemoglobin being the most common, although this exists in many different functional forms.
- Mammals have adapted to extreme environments that challenge respiration to its limits, such as living in underground burrows, at high altitude and in the marine environment where spectacular depths and durations of dive can be tolerated.
- Thoroughbred horses have been selectively bred to exercise efficiently and can generate almost double the exercise capacity of a human, although the adaptations to allow this also make them more vulnerable to some lung diseases such as exercise-induced pulmonary haemorrhage.

Until now this book has only considered respiration in a single species. Elsewhere in the animal kingdom there is wide variation in respiratory system design to accommodate the varying environments and lifestyles of the millions of different species. This chapter provides the briefest of outlines of these different systems in the major phyla of the animal kingdom (Table 26.1). The respiratory system that has evolved in humans works well enough for us, but compared with many other animals its design flaws and limitations become apparent, and the examples in this chapter of extreme physiological adaptations in animals illustrate this. Conversely, some animals have significant limitations placed on them by their respiratory systems, so the pathophysiologies of common respiratory conditions in veterinary practice are also described.

Designs of Respiratory System

The primary function of a respiratory system is the transport of oxygen and carbon dioxide to and from their point of use and production in cells. There are three ways by which gas molecules may be moved:

1. *Diffusion*. This has been considered in detail in Chapter 8, and describes the movement of gas from an area with a high partial pressure to an area with a lower partial pressure, with the rate affected by molecular size and temperature. Diffusion of gases dissolved in liquids is further complicated by its solubility in the liquid (page 112) and is significantly slower than its diffusion within a gas mixture. For example, at 20°C oxygen in water diffuses 200 000 times slower than oxygen in air.

2. *Mass movement*. This can occur in gases or liquids. In gas mixtures mass movement describes movement of gas in response to a total pressure difference, for example, tidal ventilation into lungs or movement of air into an insect's tracheal system during flying. In liquids, mass movement of the liquid in which the gas is dissolved can occur, for example, when oxygen-containing water flows through the gills of fish.

3. *Facilitated mass movement*. This describes a system in which liquid is altered to improve its gas-carrying capacity, for example, by the addition of a molecule such as haemoglobin (Hb) to improve carriage of both oxygen and carbon dioxide.

Structural Designs for Gas-Exchange Apparatus

These are illustrated in Figure 26.1 and may be classified as follows:

Integument respiration. Gas exchange by diffusion across the animal's body surface is feasible on a small scale and

TABLE 26.1 **Animal Kingdom Taxonomy and Some Features of Their Respiratory Systems**

Phylum	Class	Examples	Gas Exchange	Respiratory Circulation	Oxygen Carrier
Annelida	Segmented worms	Earthworm	Diffusion across integument	Closed circulation, multiple hearts, sub-cutaneous capillaries for gas exchange	Monomeric Hb, both intracellular and extracellular
Arthropoda	Chelicerata	Spiders, horseshoe crabs	Tracheae and book lungs	Open circulation, multiple hearts, no role in respiratory gas transport	Extracellular Hb or Hc in haemolymph
	Myriapoda	Centipedes, millipedes	Tracheae	Open circulation, multiple hearts, no role in respiratory gas transport	Extracellular Hc
	Crustacea	Shrimp, lobster, crabs	Internal gills, located in branchial chambers above each leg	Open circulation, some valve systems to direct flow into a circular pattern	Extracellular Hc
	Hexapoda	Insects	Tracheae	Open circulation, multiple hearts, no role in respiratory gas transport	None (Hb in larval stage)
Brachiopoda	Articulata	Lamp shells	Diffusion across mantle surface	Open circulation	Hc in pink blood cells in coelomic fluid
Chordata	Amphibia	Frogs, salamanders	Multimodal: gills as larvae, lungs and skin as adults	Dual system, two atria and single ventricle	Hb as trimers (deoxygenated) or tetramers (oxygenated)
	Reptilia	Reptiles	Primitive lungs	Dual system, variable heart structure with three or four chambers	Tetrameric Hb
	Aves	Birds	—	Dual system, four-chamber heart	Tetrameric Hb
	Mammalia	Mammals	—	Dual system, four-chamber heart	Tetrameric Hb
	Chondrichthyes	Cartilaginous fish, e.g., sharks	Gills	Single circulation, with gills and body tissues in series	Monomeric Hb in jawless fish; tetrameric in others
	Osteichthyes	Bony fish	Gills	Single circulation, with gills and body tissues in series	Tetrameric Hb
Cnidaria		Jellyfish, anemones	Diffusion, metabolically active cells on the body surface	None	None
Echinodermata		Starfish, sea urchins	Diffusion across integumental papullae	Water vascular system	Dimeric Hb (deoxygenated), tetrameric Hb (oxygenated)
Mollusca	Gastropoda	Slugs, snails	Diffusion, via integument or air-containing mantle chamber	Open circulation	Hc
	Cephalopoda	Octopus, squid	Internal gills, water flow generated by locomotion or currents	Closed circulation, one main heart and multiple 'gill hearts'	Hc
	Bivalvia	Clams, oysters, mussels	Internal gills, water flow generated by cilia	Open circulation	Tetrameric or dimeric Hb (some species = Hc)
Platyhelminthes		Flatworms	Diffusion	None	None
Porifera		Sponges	Diffusion, facilitated by water flow through an atrium generated by flagella	None	None

Table includes only those animals discussed in this chapter. *Hb*, Haemoglobin; *Hc*, haemocyanin.

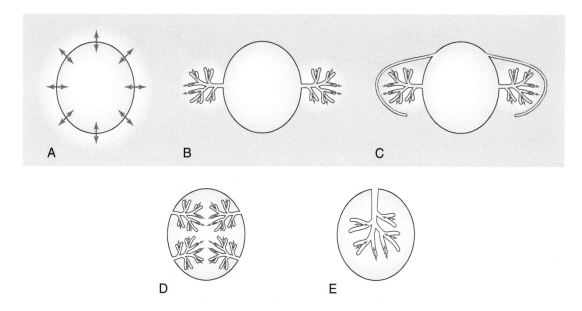

• **Fig. 26.1** Structural designs for gas-exchange systems. **(A)** Diffusion across the cell membrane directly into the cytoplasm. **(B)** External gills, through which blood flows for gas exchange. **(C)** Internal gills, in which the gas-exchange mechanism is covered by a protective operculum. **(D)** Insect tracheal system, in which gas is conducted along passages into close proximity with tissue. **(E)** Lungs, in which air is taken into the body and a circulatory system transports gases to and from the tissues. Blue indicates aquatic environments, and yellow indicates respiration in air, although there are exceptions to these general rules.

is normally the only method available to single-cell organisms. For diffusion alone to support respiration the organism must either live in water or have a wet surface in which the gases can dissolve before diffusing across the cell wall. Many larger and more complex animals, for example, amphibians, use integument respiration as an adjunct to other gas-exchange strategies.

External gills. Gills are organs of gas exchange in aquatic animals. The simplest design is for gills to protrude out of the body into the surrounding water. The gas-exchange surface area is normally maximized by a branching structure of the gills, which may simply contain cytoplasm or fluid or, in more complex animals, blood vessels. For efficient exchange of gases across gills the diffusion barrier needs to be as thin as possible, thus external gills are inevitably fragile structures and prone to damage from the animal's environment.

Internal gills. For larger animals in which external gills are impractical, the gills are covered by a protective structure usually referred to as an operculum. With this protection the gills can be larger and structurally better designed to maximize gas exchange.

Tracheal system. Insects use a system of body cavity tubes into which air diffuses directly to the tissues. This is an efficient system except for the size limitations described later.

Lungs. A lung refers to an internal structure into which air is transported by mass movement to allow gas exchange. Because air has lower viscosity and contains more oxygen than water, mass transport for respiration is easier, thus air breathing allows a smaller gas-exchange area to support a greater metabolic demand. Gas flow in the lungs of most species is tidal in nature, but in some animals, such as birds, gas flow through the lungs may be almost continuous. A drawback of lungs is the requirement to keep the gas-exchange surface wet to allow diffusion to occur, a problem that has been solved by internalization of the lungs.

For more complex animals that have a circulatory system, an important design consideration is the way in which the air or water in the external environment comes into contact with the blood (Fig. 26.2). In its simplest form, diffusion across the body surface should be sufficient because the blood is exposed to the ambient gas partial pressures, but the diffusion barrier of the integument is inevitably large compared with more specialized gas-exchange organs. In animals with tidal breathing (including humans) the carbon dioxide leaving the circulation mixes with the oxygen entering the lung (Fig. 26.2, *B*), resulting in the alveolar partial pressures of both gases being intermediate between values in blood and inspired gas. As a result, the partial pressure difference driving gas diffusion between blood and lung is lower than the difference between inspired gas and blood. A countercurrent system of gas exchange is much more efficient. If the flow of blood through the lung or gill capillaries is in the opposite direction to the flow of gas or water, then exchange of respiratory gases will be maximized, and can, in theory at least, result in partial pressures of carbon dioxide and oxygen in blood leaving the lung or gill almost equal to those in the air or water being breathed. There will always be

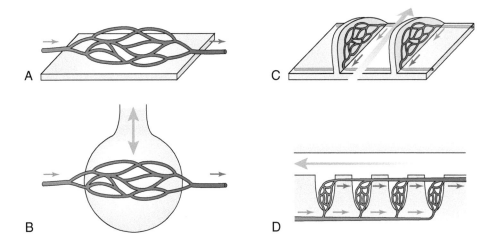

• **Fig. 26.2** Different designs for exchange of respiratory gases between air or water and blood. **(A)** Open system of exchange across skin. **(B)** 'Pool' system such as the mammalian lung with tidal ventilation of air into a blind ending alveolus. **(C)** Countercurrent mechanism of a fish gill in which blood flow through the lamella is in the opposite direction to the water flow. **(D)** Cross-current mechanism of the bird lung in which blood flows across the air capillaries along the parabronchus in the opposite direction to air flow.

some difference because of the diffusion barrier across the lung/gill membrane, but a countercurrent arrangement will always be more efficient than tidal breathing. Finally, in a cross-current design, seen in bird lungs, the anatomical arrangement of the air and blood passages is similar to a countercurrent system. Air flows through the parabronchus in the opposite direction to lung blood flow, and capillaries cross the air capillaries throughout the length of the parabronchus (Fig. 26.2, *D*). Thus the first capillaries become better oxygenated than the later ones as the oxygen level in the parabronchus falls.

Factors Affecting Respiratory System Design

Respiratory Medium for Breathing

Availability of oxygen in the surrounding medium is highly variable between different environments, as shown in Table 26.2.[1] It can be seen that air breathing is very advantageous for oxygen availability, with oxygen more abundant even at very high altitude compared with in water. Apart from altitude, other environmental factors may affect the constituents of the respiratory medium, for example, in burrowing mammals. The subterranean existence of the blind mole rat exposes it to significantly hypoxic and hypercapnic atmospheres (measured minimum oxygen 6.1% and maximum carbon dioxide 7.2%).[2] These highly active small mammals have developed a range of adaptations to thrive in this environment, including altered ventilatory responses to hypoxia and hypercapnia,[2] larger pulmonary-diffusing capacity for oxygen and greater capillary density in muscles.

For aquatic animals the situation is even more challenging, with the oxygen content varying widely according to the temperature, salinity, depth and mixing of the water. Furthermore, the quantity of oxygen-consuming biomass in the environment has a profound effect, and if high can render water

TABLE 26.2	Quantity of Oxygen in Different Respiratory Media	
Medium		**Available Oxygen (mL.L⁻¹, Sea-Level Equivalent)**

Medium	Available Oxygen ($mL.L^{-1}$, Sea-Level Equivalent)
Air: sea level	209.4
3050 m (10000 ft) altitude	144.0
6100 m (20000 ft) altitude	66.1
Freshwater 3°C	9.4
10°C	7.9
20°C	6.4
30°C	5.3
Seawater 3°C	7.4
10°C	6.3
20°C	5.2
30°C	4.4

Note: Figures show values at 1 atmosphere absolute pressure.
(Data from reference 1.)

almost totally anoxic. As a result, large areas of the Earth's oceans are mostly hypoxic, and sewage from humans and other animals on land is rendering many coastal areas more hypoxic than ever because of the increasing numbers of bacteria in the water.[3] Fish are therefore better adapted to survive in hypoxic conditions than most air-breathing animals.

Body Temperature

A majority of the kingdom *Animalia* are ectotherms, that is their body temperature is determined mostly by their environment, although ectotherms can still control their temperature by, for example, basking in the sun. Ectotherm heat production is insignificant, and their metabolic activity, and therefore respiratory requirement, is low. Only mammals and birds are homeotherms, in which endogenous metabolic heat production allows a tightly controlled constant body temperature to be maintained. The energy required to achieve this and the respiratory requirement are very high. Homeotherms therefore have all developed complex respiratory systems based on air-breathing lungs and a dual circulation.

Metabolic Rate

For homeotherms environmental temperature will affect the respiratory requirement for heat generation. A more significant effect for both endotherms and ectotherms is their activity level. For example, flying animals such as some birds and insects have significantly higher energy requirements than similar-sized members of other phyla.

Whatever design of respiratory system is used, gas exchange ultimately depends on diffusion of gases across a tissue. Estimates of gas-exchange surface area in either lungs or gills relative to body size produce generally linear relationships within groups of similar species (Fig. 26.3).[4] Homeotherms, with their greater respiratory requirements, tend to require more gas-exchange area than ectotherms. An exception to this rule is the many species of tuna, all of which are very active fish. They have adapted to become partly endothermic and are able to increase the temperature of some parts of their body, such as the muscles, to improve metabolic rate and thus appear similar to endotherms, as seen in Figure 26.3.

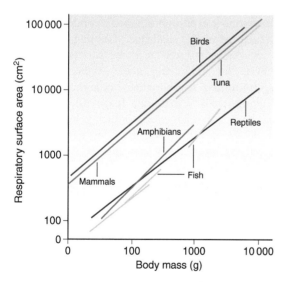

• **Fig. 26.3** Relationship between respiratory gas-exchange surface area and body mass in the animal kingdom. Note the linear relationship for most groups of animals, and the generally higher requirement for endotherms (mammals and birds). Fish species vary according to their activity levels and normal environmental temperature. (From reference 4.)

Respiratory Systems of Major Phyla

The design of respiratory systems for different groups of animals may be divided into those predominantly evolved for existing in water, air or both. However, as can be seen from the following examples, these divisions are blurred, with many examples of animals adapting one system to function perfectly well in a different environment; notable examples are land crabs and lung fish.

Aquatic Respiration

Diffusion Respiration in Small Species

Single-cell organisms of other kingdoms can all respire adequately by diffusion. A ciliated surface and locomotion through the water reduces the boundary layer where oxygen levels are low around the organism, and internal movement ('stirring') of the cytoplasm produces mass movement of respiratory gases. Theoretical calculations suggest that the maximum distance oxygen can diffuse in biological media is 0.9 mm. For small animals diffusion respiration works well enough, for example, in fish larvae before their gills have developed, although it does make entire populations of larvae susceptible to hypoxia and death if the Po_2 of the water falls.

Larger animals can use diffusion respiration by changing their body shapes, for example. small aquatic worms can be sustained by diffusion alone either by flattening the body (e.g., flatworms) or by undulating the body to increase gas exchange. In more complex animals a circulation is required which takes blood to the body surface where diffusion respiration occurs.

Much larger aquatic animals have adapted to use diffusion respiration by a variety of techniques. All Porifera species (sponges) rely solely on diffusion, and in the larger animals this is done by either pumping water through an atrium inside their body, usually using flagella, or by living in areas where natural water currents exist to prevent the formation of a hypoxic boundary layer. A further strategy to maximize diffusion respiration is illustrated by Cnidaria (e.g., jellyfish) in which all the metabolically active cells are on the animal's surface. The internal structure, furthest away from the source of oxygen, consists of mostly structural proteins such as form the jelly and which have no metabolic requirement for oxygen.

Echinodermata

Echinodermata (e.g., starfish, sea urchins) have an internal fluid-filled coelomic cavity within their body connected to an extensive 'water vascular system' around which water is circulated by cilia. As an example, in a starfish the water vascular system communicates with numerous branchial papulae on the animal's surface and the tube feet underneath, both of which are thin-walled structures that allow diffusion of gases between the coelomic fluid and the ambient water, thus functioning as numerous small external gills. The water vascular system extends up each of the five tentacles and communicates in the centre of the animal, allowing distribution of oxygenated fluid around the whole body, particularly when the animal is moving and oxygen requirement increased.

Mollusca

This large seawater-dwelling phylum is characterized by the presence of a mantle, or seawater-filled body cavity, within their structure. Depending on the species, the mantle contains varying numbers of gills, which are protected from the environment by the mollusc's body or shell. Water flow through the mantle in most classes is achieved by beating cilia, which generate water flow in the opposite direction to gill blood flow to establish a countercurrent system. In many molluscs the gill structure is in the form of sheets, with pores between adjacent layers through which cilia propel the water, thus maximizing both surface area and contact with the water. In Cephalopoda (e.g., squid, octopus), the mantle has no cilia, and water flow is generated by swimming or by external water currents.

The Gastropoda class of molluscs are land-dwelling animals (e.g., slugs, snails), and depend mostly on diffusion respiration, requiring them to live in moist habitats. Some specialized gastropods, also referred to as 'pulmonates', have developed an air-filled mantle cavity, normally within their shell. They have no gills, but a highly vascular mantle lining (a primitive lung) which supplements integumental respiration, particularly when body movements provide some mass movement of air into the mantle cavity.

Crustacea

Decapod crustaceans (e.g., crabs, shrimps, lobsters), so named because of their five pairs of legs on the thorax, are characterized by a sheet of exoskeleton covering their thorax and head called a carapace. Developmentally their gills originate with their legs and lie in the water-filled spaces between the carapace and their thorax skeleton, each occupying a single branchial chamber. Water is driven through the chambers by scaphognathites, or gill bailers, which beat rhythmically and rapidly to propel water across the gills, again in a unidirectional pattern, generating a countercurrent system with gill blood flow. In land-dwelling crabs, the same anatomical structure is retained, and the branchial chambers are ventilated in the same way but with air. Because of the high oxygen content of air compared with water (see Table 26.2), land crabs have evolved smaller gills than their aquatic relatives, and their enlarged branchial chambers have developed vascularized linings that contribute to respiratory gas exchange.

Fish

Gills in fish are arranged as a series of cartilaginous gill arches, each of which has two rows of gill filaments forming a corrugated structure through which the water flows (Fig. 26.4). Each gill filament has numerous secondary lamellae (approximately 40 per mm) protruding perpendicularly from both sides, through which blood flows in the opposite direction to the flow of water (Fig. 26.4, C) establishing a countercurrent system.

Gas-exchange efficiency is therefore dependent on the rate at which water flows across the gills, and different species have developed a wide range of strategies to control this. Buccal-opercular pumping is the most common (Fig. 26.4, C), in which the entrances to the mouth and operculum are opened and closed alternately, and the muscular walls of the cavities used to pump water across the gills. Pumping may result from generating a positive pressure in the buccal cavity, negative pressure in the opercular cavity or both, and commonly results in continuous water flow. For even greater water flow, fish may adopt 'ram' ventilation in which they swim forwards with both the mouth and opercular cavities open and rely on their forward movement to push water across the gills. For some particularly active species, such as tuna, ram ventilation is obligatory. This also results in an automated control of oxygen uptake during exercise—the faster the fish swims, the more energy and oxygen are required, which is automatically provided by the increased water flow across the gills and associated increased rate of oxygen uptake.

Gills in most aquatic animals, including fish, have many other functions apart from gas exchange, and may include feeding, excretion of water-soluble waste, acid–base balance and control of body electrolytes. As a result, the blood–gas barrier of a gill is often thicker than in a lung,[5,6] most commonly because of the required ion-exchange functions and also from the requirement for more structural cells (pillar cells) to prevent gill collapse (Fig. 25.5). This dual function of gills gives rise to the term 'osmorespiratory compromise'.[3] In freshwater fish, the gills are required to actively absorb electrolytes from the water flowing through the gills, whereas in seawater fish the gills need to excrete the excess electrolytes absorbed into the body from the surrounding hypertonic environment.

As previously described, an aquatic environment means more frequent exposure to hypoxic conditions, and fish are well-adapted to this challenge.[3] Gulping air and skimming the oxygen-rich water near the surface are behavioural methods for improving acute hypoxia. Gills contain oxygen-sensitive neuroepithelial cells that closely resemble the glomus cells in mammals (page 50), and when stimulated have a similar effect, inducing hyperventilation of the gills. Finally, if hypoxia lasts a few days, in some species gill cellular morphology can change, increasing the gas-exchange surface area.

Air-breathing fish are a reminder of the evolutionary path from which land animals developed. Gas exchange may occur either through the well-perfused walls of gas bladders or in more specialized structures, regarded as primitive lungs, although the distinction between these is rather arbitrary. Of extant species the lungfish, as the name suggests, has the most structurally advanced gas-exchange system, with its lungs containing complex ridges of cartilaginous parenchyma covered in respiratory epithelium which closely resembles the alveolar epithelium of mammals (page 10).

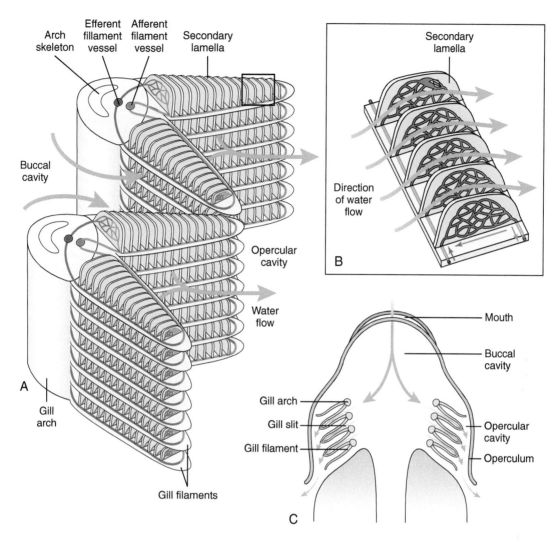

• **Fig. 26.4** Structure and function of gills in bony fish. **(A)** Structure of the gill arch, filaments and secondary lamellae, and the direction of water flow. **(B)** Water flow is in the opposite direction to blood flow through the secondary lamellae, establishing an efficient countercurrent system. **(C)** Water flows through the buccal cavity, across the gills and out through the opercular cavity, with muscular control of the openings to the cavities used to pump water through the gills when required.

Amphibia

Amphibians are the next evolutionary step away from water for vertebrates. Most species begin life as larvae in water and metamorphose into animals able to live in either air or water.[7] They are an excellent example of multimodal respiration, using gills as larvae, progressing to both lung and integument (skin) respiration as adults. Amphibian larval gills may be external (salamanders) or internal in the order Anura (frogs and toads). Adult amphibian lungs are primitive compared with mammals: salamanders, which rely heavily on skin gas exchange, may have no lungs at all, or simple air-filled sacs. In Anura species the lungs are more developed, with the lining containing multiple folds giving a honeycomb structure. Ventilation in air is by a buccal pump mechanism in which the floor of the mouth repeatedly pushes air into the lung under positive pressure; expiration is mostly passive. In amphibians the lungs are effectively an organ predominantly for oxygen uptake, with carbon dioxide excretion occurring mostly via the skin. When hibernating in cold water frogs depend purely on skin respiration for long periods of time, facilitated by their very low oxygen requirement at low temperatures.

Air Respiration

Annelida

Segmented worms, for example, earthworms, use diffusion respiration by having blood capillaries just below their body surface, which must remain wet at all times for survival. Air reaches them underground by diffusion between the soil particles, a process that is reduced when water levels in the soil become high, forcing the worms to the surface to seek air. The limited surface area available for diffusion restricts this design to small, generally low-activity animals.

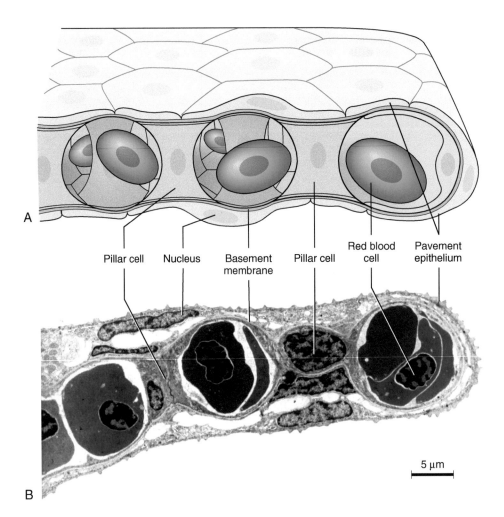

• **Fig. 26.5** Schematic drawing **(A)** and electron micrograph **(B)** showing the cellular structure of a fish gill lamella.[6] Note only a small area of contact between the capillary and the water, and a thick diffusion barrier compared with the mammalian structure shown in Fig. 1.8. This arises because of the presence of pillar cells, which are required to prevent the gill collapsing, and the overlying pavement epithelial cells, which are thicker than alveolar epithelial cells, as they are also active ion-exchange cells. Note also that fish red blood cells are nucleated. (Electron micrograph kindly provided by Professor Olson. Reproduced by permission of the publishers of the *Journal of Experimental Zoology*.)

Arthropoda

Two of the major subphyla of the arthropods, Myriapoda (e.g., centipedes, millipedes) and Hexapoda (insects), use a system of tracheae for gas exchange. Tracheae are air passages running from the animal's surface into the body tissues, and have walls containing chitin to maintain their patency. Successive divisions result in smaller and smaller tubes, ending as tracheoles with diameters of less than 0.2 µm.[7] Gas moves along the tracheae mostly by diffusion and diffuses from the tracheoles directly into the cells. The final distribution of the tracheoles matches the tissue oxygen requirements, so, for example, the highest density of tracheoles is normally found in the wing muscles of flying insects. At times of high metabolic requirement, particularly when flying, the insect's body movements cause some mass movement of air into the tracheae to supplement diffusion.

A significant design flaw of this system is loss of water vapour from the tracheae, which is minimized by the small number of surface openings, all of which are covered by spiracles which are carefully controlled to only allow the gas exchange required for the animal's metabolism at that time. Control of ventilation by spiracles also occurs with changing atmospheric oxygen concentration,[8] limiting the exposure of the tissues to hyperoxia or hypoxia, a much more effective adaptation than in vertebrates.

A trachaeal breathing system limits the size to which Arthropoda can grow. As species become larger, the proportion of their body volume occupied by tracheae increases, limiting their ultimate size. The giant insects indicated by Palaeozoic fossil records may, among other reasons, only have existed because of the higher atmospheric oxygen concentration at that time (Chapter 34).

A third subphylum of Arthropoda, Chelicerata (horseshoe crabs, spiders and scorpions), use tracheae for respiration, but some species have also developed a more specialized respiratory structure. Referred to as a 'book' lung (or gill in the horseshoe crab) after its resemblance to the pages of a book, the underside of the body hides a collection of sheets of well-perfused gas-exchanging tissue, often 'ventilated' by flapping of nearby body surface sections.

Reptilia

Most reptile species have similar lungs to the amphibians from which they evolved. They usually involve single chambers, sometimes with folds of epithelium forming vascularized septa where the gas exchange occurs. Some retain the amphibian ventilation system of buccal pumping, but most achieve ventilation by expanding their rib cage or other body structures to generate a negative pressure which draws air into the lungs. Snakes and lizards achieve this solely by expanding their rib cage, but other reptiles have a fixed rib cage and use other techniques for ventilation; for example, tortoises do this by simply extending their limbs.[7] These systems may sound inefficient compared with the mammalian lungs with which we are familiar, but it must be remembered that reptiles are ectotherms and commonly have sedentary existences, so metabolic requirements are low.

Crocodilian reptiles (e.g., crocodiles, caimans and alligators) have a more specialized respiratory system. Their lungs are ventilated by a 'hepatic piston' system involving cephalad/caudad movement of the liver within the body cavity by muscles running longitudinally from the liver ligaments to the pelvis. Furthermore, crocodilian lung structure resembles that of birds (described later) in that air flow through the gas-exchanging components is believed to be unidirectional rather than tidal.[9] How this is achieved without the complex range of air sacs used in birds is unknown, but this does provide efficient respiration, possibly explaining how in evolutionary terms the crocodilians have survived for such a long time.

Mammalia

Lung evolution from reptiles towards the mammalian system of tidal ventilation into alveoli facilitated the development of endothermic animals. The fundamental difference in lung structure is the subdivision into millions of small, very thin-walled alveoli, achieving much greater gas-exchange efficiency with a similar volume of tissue. This effect is even seen between different individual humans, explaining why populations born at high altitude develop lifelong improved oxygen transfer (page 210). Conversely, the disease emphysema (page 332) results in lung tissue developing large air spaces, returning the gas exchange efficiency to that of animals from earlier in the evolution process.

Aves (Birds)[10,11]

Many species of birds fly at high altitude; the best example is bar-headed geese that have been sighted flying over Everest and tagged flying over the Himalayas on their migration. The highest flying altitude recorded for a bird is for a Rüppell's griffon vulture that unfortunately collided with a commercial airliner at 11 285 m (37 900 ft). Compared with mammals, birds have a higher body temperature (40°C) and are generally more active, expending more energy per unit body mass. The activity of flying is strenuous, with oxygen consumption in a flying bird reaching 13 to 30 times resting values, depending on conditions. To supply this high oxygen consumption whilst at altitude requires the architecture of the avian respiratory system to be fundamentally different to that of mammals, and evolution of birds led to the development of a lung–air sac system.

Much of a bird's body volume consists of air sacs, which can be inflated or deflated by the muscles of the body cavities. The air sacs are crucial to a bird's breathing, but also have numerous other functions such as reducing body weight for flying and for voice production by the passage of air through the syrinx. Avian lungs make up a much smaller proportion of a bird's body than in mammals, and are almost rigid, being firmly fixed to the ribs. Rather than the tidal breathing used by mammals, in birds the various air sacs are used to pass gas through the lungs, in the same direction, during both inspiration and expiration, so the lungs are, in effect, simply acting as a passive gas exchanger. This is achieved with two main groups of air sacs, which vary widely between bird species, but may be approximately divided into caudal and cephalad groups (Fig. 26.6). During inspiration, inspired air passes through the larynx and syrinx into each primary intrapulmonary bronchus, from which some air enters the dorsal secondary bronchus and the remainder inflates the caudal air sacs. From the secondary bronchus air passes through the numerous parabronchi, where gas exchange occurs, and on through the ventral secondary bronchus into the cephalad air sacs. On expiration, the caudal air sacs empty into the dorsal secondary bronchus, the air passing through the lung and being expired through the primary bronchus, while the cephalad air sacs empty and the gas is expired. As a result of this pattern of breathing, there is an almost continuous flow of inspired air through the lung in a caudad to cephalad direction, whereas pulmonary blood flow is in a cephalad to caudad direction, providing an efficient cross-current gas-exchange system (Fig. 26.2).

Other features of avian physiology further increase its gas-exchange efficiency. At a microscopic level within the avian lung, the blind-ending air capillaries (equivalent to a mammalian alveolus, but more tubular in shape) that arise from the parabronchi are structurally arranged with the blood capillaries to provide a further countercurrent system (Fig. 26.2, D). The blood–gas barrier in avian lungs is also much thinner than in mammals, because the lack of repetitive movement required by tidal breathing requires less structural strength.[10] Two separate countercurrent gas-exchange systems and the reduced blood–gas barrier mean that, in birds, the P_{O_2} of inspired gas and pulmonary venous blood are almost equal. Finally, to generate the high oxygen

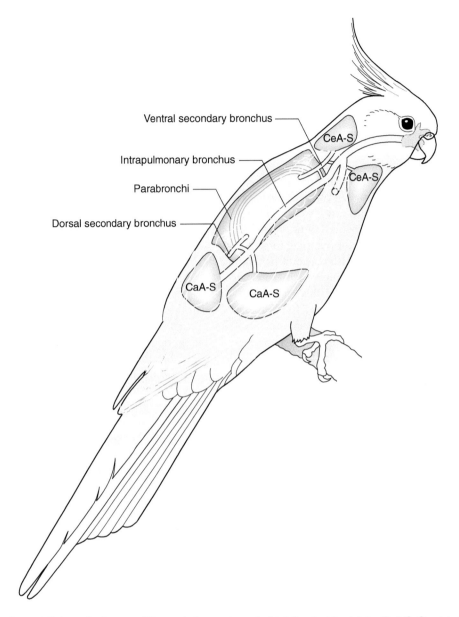

• **Fig. 26.6** Schematic diagram of the respiratory system of a bird. See text for details. *CaA-S,* Caudal air sacs; *CeA-S,* cephalad air sacs.

delivery required for exercising in a hypoxic environment, relative to body size birds have larger hearts than other animals and lack any significant hypoxic pulmonary vasoconstriction (HPV).

Carriage of Gases in Blood

Circulation Configurations

A summary of the circulatory systems of the animals previously described is shown in Table 26.1. Invertebrates mostly have an 'open' circulation which lacks blood vessels, consisting instead of fluid spaces within the body containing haemolymph. Muscle movements or one or more hearts move the fluid around the body to distribute nutrients and transport respiratory gases. Transport function in an open circulation is inefficient, and there is limited control of the fluid movement, but the system works well enough for the animals concerned.

Fish

Circulation through fish gills is in series with the systemic circulation, that is, there is no separate pulmonary circulation. Gill blood flow is therefore arterioarterial rather than arteriovenous. This has two consequences. First, pumping blood through gill capillaries increases the total vascular resistance massively and results in poor blood flow to the tissues, a problem overcome in some species by the use of auxiliary hearts. Second, the delicate gas-exchange gill structures are exposed to full systemic arterial pressure, requiring them to be more robust than low-pressure mammal or bird lungs, resulting in a thicker gas-exchange membrane. These two factors explain why, for permanent residence as air breathers on land, it was necessary to evolve a dual circulation.

Amphibians

Multimodal respiration requires an adaptable circulatory system. A single ventricle supplies both the systemic and pulmonary circulations, although the latter also includes the skin blood supply, which is a major respiratory organ in amphibians. When underwater, pulmonary blood flow can be significantly reduced, and despite having only a single ventricle its structure somehow allows functionally selective distribution of oxygenated blood to the required organs.

Reptiles

Most reptiles have a similar heart structure to amphibians, although there is normally an incomplete septum in the single ventricle, dividing it into two separate regions to better direct blood flow. However, unless the ventricle is completely separated into two chambers, the pulmonary and systemic arterial pressures will be the same. The relative blood flow to the two circulations and the oxygenation of systemic blood will therefore be determined by their vascular resistances. In reptiles, pulmonary vascular resistance and ventilation perfusion matching are controlled by the autonomic nervous system, and many species also have a HPV reflex.[12] Crocodilians and pythons have completed the evolution into a four-chambered heart and true dual circulation.

Birds and Mammals

As previously described, the increased oxygen requirements of endothermy necessitate a thinner and larger area of gas-exchange tissue. This is only feasible if a separate low-pressure high-flow pulmonary circulation is developed. The details of an example of this strategy are described in Chapter 6.

Oxygen-Carrying Molecules

As already described for humans in Chapter 10, oxygen is carried in blood in both physical solution and in combination with Hb. For one species, the Antarctic ice fish, dissolved oxygen is sufficient, and its blood contains no oxygen-carrying molecules. By living in cold water where oxygen levels are high (Table 26.2), leading a mostly sedentary existence to minimize oxygen requirement and having a large heart that sustains a permanently high cardiac output, Hb is not required. But for all other species, dissolved oxygen alone is insufficient, and oxygen-binding molecules have evolved. There are only three of these across the entire animal kingdom, all based on a metal atom bound to a protein. They may be extracellular, located in tissues, blood or haemolymph or intracellular, in blood cells.

Haemerythrin

Despite its name this molecule contains no haem group, instead containing a di-iron oxygen binding site attached to a protein. Haemerythrin (Hr) is normally contained within nucleated cells referred to as 'pink blood cells' found in the coelomic fluid of the Sipuncula phylum of marine worms and many brachiopods. In some brachiopods which live in the intertidal zone it is believed that Hr acts as a store of oxygen lasting up to 2 hours while the animal is outside of its normal seawater environment.

Haemocyanin

Haemocyanin is a similarly erroneously named molecule that contains no iron, but instead uses two copper atoms directly bound to a protein chain for oxygen carriage, and occurs in numerous species within the phyla Arthropoda and Mollusca (see Table 25.1). These protein chains are very large, are normally extracellular and appear colourless when deoxygenated, becoming blue when oxygenated. In different species the copper–protein complexes bind together into hexameric or decameric complexes.

Haemoglobin

Tetrameric Hb structure and function has been described in Chapter 10, and is the most common form of Hb, although some species have monomeric or dimeric molecules. The combination of two α and two β chains of human HbA is also the most common form in other animals. This apparent structural uniformity of Hb in the animal kingdom does not lead to functional uniformity. Different physiological milieu of differing species, particularly relating to body temperature and blood pH, mean that an identical Hb molecule in the two species will have quite different functional characteristics. Furthermore, Hb molecules do subtly vary in structure, particularly with respect to the position and number of histidine side chains[13] which are crucial for buffering hydrogen ions (page 126).

All these molecules include multiple protein subunits bound into complex quaternary structures to allow cooperativity during oxygen binding (page 143), with the complexity increasing in the higher animals. Homeotherms have one of the less adaptable forms of Hb because of the relatively constant nature of blood temperature, pH, P_{CO_2}, and so on, with most other animals facing much wider variations in their physiological conditions. For example, fish Hb differs from that of mammals by displaying the Root effect,[14,15] an exaggerated form of the Bohr effect (page 146) in which hydrogen ions cause the molecule to become stabilized in the T-state. This effectively prevents cooperativity from occurring and reduces oxygen affinity to such an extent that oxygen is forced off the molecule irrespective of the local P_{O_2}. In some tissues, for example, the eyes and swim bladder of fish, active secretion of lactate deliberately induces the Root effect in the local area to provide oxygen to the tissues.

Animals at Physiological Extremes

Mammals at Altitude

Human acclimatization and adaptation to altitude have been described in detail in Chapter 16, and the evolution of bird lung structure to facilitate flying at high altitude was outlined earlier. The primary respiratory response of humans at high altitude, hyperventilation, occurs in all mammals to some extent, but animals that have lived at altitude for thousands of years have evolved multiple other adaptations as well. The South American camelids (e.g., llamas and alpacas) are one of the best examples of mammals adapted to live at high altitudes because they are found at varying altitudes, allowing comparison of different physiological adaptations.

Oxygen Carriage[16,17]

Most animals living at high altitude have evolved to improve the efficiency of Hb–oxygen binding. Increasing the affinity of Hb for oxygen, that is, shifting the oxyhaemoglobin dissociation curve to the left (page 146), will improve tissue oxygen delivery, providing the lungs can still fully oxygenate blood in the hypoxic environment. Species that live at altitude have evolved unique Hb structures, normally by the substitution of a small number of different amino acids to produce functionally improved Hb. For example, the bar-headed goose has a much lower P_{50} (page 146) than its lowlander relatives, and several mammals demonstrate the same difference between high- and low-level residents, for example, the chinchilla or guinea pig compared with the rat. Camelids and some species of frog that live at high altitude have evolved Hb molecules with fewer binding sites for 2,3,-diphosphoglycerate, increasing its oxygen affinity. Finally, some high-altitude adult species (e.g., alpacas and yaks) simply retain a large proportion of foetal Hb throughout life (page 145).[17]

Although haematocrit increases as part of acclimatization in humans, the associated increase in blood viscosity may counteract any gain in oxygen delivery, and elevated haematocrit is not a common feature of animals at high altitude. The camelid species, however, have a unique adaptation to altitude survival. Their oxygen-carrying capacity has evolved to achieve similar Hb concentrations to humans but a lower haematocrit. This is achieved through evolution of the red blood cell structure to create small, ovoid-shaped red blood cells with a particularly high intracellular Hb concentration. This adaptation allows them to maintain the same oxygen-carrying capacity as other species but with a relatively reduced haematocrit and associated blood viscosity, reducing the cardiac workload and increasing tissue blood flow.

Pulmonary Vasculature

HPV occurs in most mammals, making species living at altitude susceptible to developing pulmonary hypertension. The clinical presentation of hypoxic pulmonary hypertension was initially observed in bovine species living at high altitude. Long-term exposure to hypoxia results in remodelling of the pulmonary arterial smooth muscle (page 347), causing a progressive and irreversible increase in pulmonary arterial pressure. As in humans with secondary pulmonary hypertension (page 347), right ventricular hypertrophy follows, and eventually right-sided heart failure.[18] Known in cattle as brisket disease, right-sided heart failure induced by hypoxia at altitude occurs only in some individual animals, but can occur at quite modest elevation (1600 m, 5250 ft). It is only effectively prevented or treated by remaining at, or relocating to, lower altitude.[18] These features are strikingly similar to high-altitude pulmonary oedema affecting susceptible humans (page 213). The extent to which pulmonary hypertension occurs in other mammalian species is variable, although generally less than in cattle. One way in which the cardiovascular effects of HPV can be attenuated is by reducing cardiac output, an adaptation seen in sheep that makes them very tolerant of high altitude. Indigenous high-altitude animals (e.g., llama, yak, guinea pig) have evolved thin-walled pulmonary vessels with less smooth muscle, and are incapable of producing dangerous pulmonary hypertension.

Collateral Ventilation

The ability to collaterally ventilate lung regions is well-recognized in most mammals, occurring via interalveolar (pores of Kohn), bronchoalveolar (Lambert channels) or interbronchiolar (Martin channels) communications. The degree of collateral ventilation is high in dogs, sheep and rabbits, and almost nonexistent in cattle and pigs.[19] Healthy humans have a small amount of collateral ventilation, for example, through the pores of Kohn (page 8), although this may become much more significant in parenchymal lung disease, particularly emphysema (page 332). Significant collateral ventilation provides another mechanism by which an animal can match regional pulmonary ventilation and perfusion (Chapter 7), by allowing air to flow from regions with high ventilation to adjacent, less well-ventilated areas. Comparisons between numerous different species have found an inverse relationship between the amount of collateral ventilation and the intensity of the HPV response.[19] Cattle and pigs, who have significantly poorer collateral ventilation, must use HPV to match ventilation and perfusion requirements, leaving them susceptible to pulmonary hypertension at altitude. Dogs and sheep, however, have less need for a significant HPV response because their better-developed collateral ventilation mechanisms prevent significant ventilation/perfusion ($\dot{V}/\dot{Q}$) mismatching.

Exercising Horses[20]

Horse racing as we recognize it today began in the 17th century, and through a highly selective breeding program developed the thoroughbred racehorse as we know it today. At maximum exercise capacity this artificial selection program has produced one of the most physiologically efficient animals, originating from the ability of the thoroughbred horse to supply the majority of its energy for a race aerobically. The oxygen consumption (Vo_2) of a horse will increase up to 30 times its resting value to a Vo_{2max} of 140 mL.min^{-1}.kg^{-1}, almost double that of an elite human athlete (page 184). As in humans, Vo_2 increases linearly with increasing exercise intensity until Vo_{2max} is approached, at which point metabolism becomes anaerobic and exercise efficiency reduces.

On a weight-for-weight basis, compared with humans, an exercising horse also has significantly greater capacity for increases in ventilation, cardiac output and oxygen-diffusing capacity, although the respiratory system remains the limiting factor, as described later. In relation to body weight, the relative cardiac stroke volume generated by equine and human athletes is similar; the greater equine cardiac output capacity is generated solely through an increase in heart rate.

The mechanism of exercise hyperventilation in horses is quite different from humans. Both inspiration and expiration are enhanced by using the force produced from the movement of the equine gastrointestinal tract against the diaphragm. During extreme exercise horses maintain a 1:1 ratio of ventilation to stride during the gallop. As the animal's forelimbs impact the ground the weight of the gastrointestinal organs shifts forward and displaces the diaphragm, resulting in active expiration. The reverse then occurs as the hind limbs impact the ground, assisting inspiration.[21] Respiratory rate therefore becomes intrinsically linked to exercise intensity, and, in effect, the muscles of locomotion become secondary respiratory muscles. This locomotor–respiratory coupling occurs in many species of animal, particularly quadrupeds, and may even exist to some degree in exercising humans.[22]

There are however limitations to the efficiency of the equine respiratory tract. Horses are obligate nasal breathers with a relatively poorly designed upper respiratory tract for extreme exercise. This has little impact at rest but becomes responsible for up to 90% of air flow resistance at the high minute ventilation necessary with high-level exercise.

Despite the many efficient physiological responses, hypoxia and hypercapnia do occur during exercise in racehorses, whereas they are only rarely seen in humans (page 188). Exercise-induced arterial hypoxaemia is most consistently demonstrated by an increase in alveolar-arterial Po_2 difference (($A-a)dO_2$, page 139), and several factors are thought to contribute, including:

- $\dot{V}/\dot{Q}$ *mismatch.* This increases and accounts for around a third of the elevated ($A-a)dO_2$. Compared with humans, the effects of changes in regional ventilation on overall $\dot{V}/\dot{Q}$ matching are almost certainly attenuated by the high cardiac output seen in horses.
- *Diffusion limitation.* This becomes significant and is believed to occur because of the rapid transit time of red blood cells through the pulmonary capillary (page 115);

that is, there is insufficient time to allow complete oxygenation to occur.

- *Inadequate hyperventilation.* Compared with humans, the degree of exercise hyperventilation in horses does not fully match the metabolic demands of the muscles, and so contributes to the degree of hypoxia and hypercapnia. Instead of the comparison to humans, a more helpful comparison is between horses and ponies; the latter being the same species but without many generations of selective breeding. Hyperventilation relative to exercise is greater in ponies, and hypoxia and hypercapnia during exercise less common. It should, however, be remembered that the exercise capacity of a pony is obviously considerably lower. This highlights that, although the selective breeding of the racehorse has allowed it to achieve extreme levels of exercise performance, the ability of the muscles to consume oxygen has outstripped the capacity of the cardiorespiratory system to deliver it.

All horses do however possess further physiological adaptation that contributes to equine exercise performance. During times of metabolic stress, including severe exercise, horses can increase their haematocrit by mobilizing their huge splenic reserves of blood, in some cases doubling the haematocrit and oxygen delivery.

Diving Mammals

Diving mammals rely on breath holding for dives, and have multiple adaptations that permit them to spend remarkably long times under water and attain great depths.[23] For example, sperm whales can attain depths of 1000 m, and Weddell seals can reach 500 m and remain submerged for 70 minutes. Such feats depend on a variety of biochemical, cardiovascular and respiratory adaptations. For most diving mammals complete alveolar collapse is believed to occur at depths between 30 and 100 m,[24] effectively stopping gas exchange and preventing the development of high partial pressures of nitrogen in the lung. This complete collapse is only possible because of extremely compliant chest wall and alveoli and relatively rigid airways, allowing air to move from the alveoli into the airway as the animal dives. Repeated collapse and reinflation of lungs in most mammals is harmful (page 392) because of loss of surfactant function, but diving mammals have evolved different surfactant function (mediated by surfactant protein C; page 16) to allow repeated collapse and reexpansion.[25]

Many diving mammals also use the spleen as a reservoir for oxygenated blood during dives. In some diving species the spleen represents over 10% of body mass and contains a much more muscular capsule than in terrestrial animals. Splenic contraction is the probable cause of an increase of Hb concentration from 150 to 250 g.L^{-1} during long dives.[26] Furthermore, these animals have twice the blood volume per kilogram body weight relative to humans, and thus oxygen stored in blood for a dive is proportionately about three times that of humans.

Pathophysiology of Animal Respiratory Diseases in Veterinary Practice

Ruminants

The lung parenchyma of most ruminant species is divided into eight individual lobes, each with pronounced lobulation and separated by thick tissue septa giving rise to clear demarcations between the different lobes. This structure has evolved to minimize the risk of developing widespread pulmonary infection, with the septa acting as physical barriers to prevent infection spreading between lobes. The total alveolar surface area and alveolar capillary density of the ruminant lung are small compared with other domestic mammals of a similar size. Although the lungs are sufficient to provide the basic metabolic requirements, ruminants have a limited respiratory reserve, which is accommodated by having a generally sedentary lifestyle.

Bovine Respiratory Disease[27]

Bovine respiratory disease (BRD) describes any condition causing clinical signs associated with the bovine respiratory tract, and most commonly refers to a bacterial pneumonia. Pathogenesis involves environmental stressors (e.g., weaning of calves or movement) or a primary viral or mycobacterial challenge reducing the animal's ability to control the commensal bacteria of the upper respiratory tract.[28] Enzootic pneumonia is a common form of BRD. In young calves it is primarily caused by the proliferation of *Pasteurella multocida*, whereas in older cattle a broader range of bacteria are involved. Bacterial colonization leads to a diffuse acute pleuropneumonia, obliterating functional lung tissue and impairing gas exchange, in the same way as in humans. The clinical presentation of BRD varies from a subclinical disease through to acute, sudden death. As described previously, the structure of ruminant lungs makes them less able to tolerate loss of parenchymal tissue than other mammalian species,[28] and early signs of BRD, such as pyrexia, reduced productivity or tachypnoea require prompt treatment to prevent progression to a more serious and life-threatening disease or long-term production-limiting damage to the pulmonary tissue. It is well recognized that the development of respiratory disease in young cattle reduces their productivity throughout life, including reduced growth rates as a calf, increased time to reach sexual maturity and produce a calf themselves, overall reduced yields in dairy animals and an increased mortality, all of which have significant economic impacts.[27]

Acute Interstitial Pneumonia

Also colloquially known as 'fog fever' or 'cow asthma', this condition is seen in grazing cattle, usually when they are turned out onto fresh pastures that contain high levels of tryptophan.[29] Within the animal's rumen the tryptophan is anaerobically fermented to produce 3-methylindole (3-MI), which is absorbed from the gastrointestinal tract into the circulation. Within the club cells of the lungs 3-MI is then converted to a toxic metabolite, and as a byproduct reactive oxygen species are formed (Chapter 25). The resulting cellular damage is similar to that seen with pulmonary oxygen toxicity in other mammals, with damage to type 1 alveolar epithelial cells and later in the process proliferation of type 2 epithelial cells (page 11). Pathologically this causes the development of alveolar and interstitial oedema and emphysema. The interstitial oedema increases the thickness of the interlobular septa, causing compression of the nearby parenchymal tissue, limiting the area available for gas exchange. The clinical presentation of these pathological changes can be severe, and even the effort required to move cattle off the affected pasture can cause a further decline in lung function and gas exchange, leading to sudden death.

Vena Caval Thrombosis

Lung disease as a result of venous embolization occurs in cattle, illustrating the role of the lung as a circulation filter (page 164). Caval thromboses are most commonly observed in the caudal vena cava, but can also originate in the cranial vena cava. The most common cause of septic emboli is rupture of a hepatic abscess directly into the caudal vena cava, but they can also develop by haematogenous spread from infection within the hoof, udder or uterus in adults, or from an infected umbilicus in calves.[30] The spread of a septic embolism to the lung leads to metastatic chronic suppurative bronchopneumonia through the development of multiple pulmonary abscesses and pulmonary arteritis. Pulmonary abscesses occur early in the disease process, and attributed to the distinct lobular nature of the bovine lung may be associated with few clinical signs, as the infection remains contained within one lobe. As more regions of lung become involved through the dissemination of further emboli, respiratory distress begins to become apparent because of the loss of further pulmonary parenchyma. Pulmonary arteritis, presumably secondary to release of immune mediators from the thrombus (as seen in some forms of human pulmonary emboli; Chapter 29), is a late sign in the disease process, but gives rise to haemorrhage in the lung that is usually fatal.

Parasitic Bronchitis (Lungworm or Husk)

Parasitic bronchitis is caused by the nematode *Dictyocaulus viviparous*, and although infection is most commonly seen in cattle, it can affect other ruminants (e.g., deer). The worm follows a standard nematode lifecycle, where the larvae are ingested off the grass. The adults then develop in the lungs of the cattle and produce eggs which hatch, producing larvae which are coughed up, swallowed and passed in the faeces of the cattle back onto the pasture.

Clinical disease is most often seen in first-year grazing animals who have not had any previous exposure, often leading to widespread coughing within a group, with severely affected animals showing signs of tachypnoea and dyspnea. Although morbidity can be high, mortality is usually low, providing worm burdens are not extreme.

Clinical disease is not often observed in adult animals because of the development of a strong immune response to the parasite from sufficient low-level exposure. Vaccines are available from inactivated larvae and are often given to animals before their first grazing season to boost immunity before exposure.

Equine Respiratory Disease

Equine lung structure is very different from that of the ruminant, including only a moderate degree of lobulation and extensive collateral ventilation between adjacent lobes of lung. This makes the equids susceptible to more widespread lung disease than seen in ruminants. However, the most common equine respiratory diseases originate in the upper respiratory tract because the horse's anatomy makes it an obligate nasal breather.[20]

Upper airway obstruction (UAO) is a common condition often responsible for reduced exercise tolerance. Although it can occur in any horse, it is more often reported and investigated in racing animals because of the effect on their performance when racing. It is normally diagnosed by direct observation using an endoscope while the horse exercises. A variety of conditions contribute to UAO, including laryngeal paralysis, laryngeal hemiplegia, dorsal displacement of the soft palate, epiglottic entrapment and dorsal pharyngeal collapse. Laryngeal paralysis and hemiplegia are insidious in onset, and cause a slow but progressive obstruction leading to gradually worsening exercise hypercapnia. Other causes of UAO develop more rapidly, causing acute airway obstruction and sudden fatigue resulting in the horse coming to an abrupt stop. Increased airway resistance during exercise has no direct effect on oxygenation, but contributes to worsening hypercapnia and increases the respiratory oscillations in intrathoracic pressure, making the horse more prone to exercise-induced pulmonary haemorrhage (EIPH), described later.[31]

Inflammatory airway disease (IAD) is a widely recognized condition characterized by aseptic inflammation of the airways.[32] It occurs in any horse of any age, although most commonly in young race horses, and a typical clinical picture includes poor exercise tolerance, a cough and abnormal amounts of mucus in the airways on endoscopy.[31] Its aetiology is poorly understood, but is thought to involve primarily environmental factors, in particular inhaled organic and inorganic dusts, with a potential contribution from allergic responses and infectious agents.[32] These clinical signs mean that, in nonracing animals, early detection is difficult. However, in racing animals, IAD is important, as inflammation of the smaller airways causes air-flow obstruction to the point where gas exchange becomes impaired because of poor $\dot{V}/\dot{Q}$ matching. This leads to impaired exercise performance and progressively worsening exercise-induced hypoxaemia, although hypercapnia does not seem to be exacerbated.

EIPH is defined as 'the presence of blood within the tracheobronchial tree derived from the alveolar capillaries', and occurs almost universally throughout racing Thoroughbreds.[20] Bilateral epistaxis at the end of a race is the primary presentation of EIPH, and dynamic endoscopy is required for definitive diagnosis. In common with lung damage in humans at high altitude, EIPH is a manifestation of pulmonary blood vessel stress failure (page 213) as a result of high pulmonary blood flow, particularly when hypoxic and hyperventilating. In maximally exercising horses the pressure within the pulmonary arteries and capillaries can reach levels close to 80 to 100 mmHg. The pathophysiology of EIPH is unclear, but the most likely explanation is that the combination of very high pulmonary capillary pressure and significantly negative intrathoracic pressure results in a damaging capillary transmural pressure. These changes may be compounded in racing horses by vascular remodelling of pulmonary veins occurring predominantly in the caudodorsal lung region.[33] Disruption of the alveolar-capillary structure occurs, with bleeding into the alveoli and airways and an immediate decline in gas-exchange efficiency as lung regions lose their ventilation. Although EIPH is known to occur very rarely in humans,[20] the reason for horses being so susceptible is not clear. The most likely explanation is the unique combination in an exercising horse of a huge cardiac output associated with very low intrathoracic pressures because of their susceptibility to airway obstruction. The evolution from a pony to a Thoroughbred racehorse is a spectacular demonstration of selective breeding to improve physiological performance, but this has come at a substantial cost in terms of susceptibility to respiratory disease.

References

1. Weiss RF. The solubility of nitrogen, oxygen and argon in water and seawater. *Deep-Sea Res.* 1970;17:721-735.
2. Tomasco IH, Del Río R, Iturriaga R, et al. Comparative respiratory strategies of subterranean and fossorial octodontid rodents to cope with hypoxic and hypercapnic atmospheres. *J Comp Physiol.* 2010;180:877-884.
3. Nilsson GE. *Respiratory Physiology of Vertebrates. Life with and Without Oxygen.* Cambridge, UK: Cambridge University Press; 2010.
4. Perry SF. Recent advances and trends in the comparative morphometry of vertebrate gas exchange organs. *Adv Compar Environ Physiol.* 1990;6:45-71.
5. West JB. Comparative physiology of the pulmonary circulation. *Compar Physiol.* 2011;1:1525-1539.
6. Olson KR. Vascular anatomy of the fish gill. *J Exp Zool.* 2002;293:214-231.
7. Sherwood L, Klandorf H, Yancey PH. *From Genes to Organisms. Animal Physiology.* Andover, UK: Cengage; 2013.
8. Harrison J, Frazier MR, Henry JR, et al. Responses of terrestrial insects to hypoxia or hyperoxia. *Respir Physiol Neurobiol.* 2006;154:4-17.
9. Farmer CG, Sanders K. Unidirectional airflow in the lungs of alligators. *Science.* 2010;327:338-340.
10. West JB, Watson RR, Fu Z. The human lung: did evolution get it wrong? *Eur Respir J.* 2007;29:11-17.
11. Lague SL. High-altitude champions: birds that live and migrate at altitude. *J Appl Physiol.* 2017;123:942-950.

12. Skovgaard N, Wang T. Local control of pulmonary blood flow and lung structure in reptiles: Implications for ventilation perfusion matching. *Respir Physiol Neurobiol*. 2006;154:107-117.

13. Berenbrink M. Evolution of vertebrate haemoglobins: Histidine side chains, specific buffer value and Bohr effect. *Respir Physiol Neurobiol*. 2006;154:165-184.

14. Berenbrink M. Historical reconstructions of evolving physiological complexity: O_2 secretion in the eye and swimbladder of fishes. *J Exp Biol*. 2007;210:1641-1652.

15. Brauner CJ, Harter TS. Beyond just hemoglobin: red blood cell potentiation of hemoglobin-oxygen unloading in fish. *J Appl Physiol*. 2017;123:935-941.

16. Storz JF, Moriyama H. Mechanisms of haemoglobin adaptation to high altitude hypoxia. *High Alt Med Biol*. 2008;9:148-157.

17. Weber RE. High-altitude adaptations in vertebrate hemoglobins. *Respir Physiol Neurobiol*. 2007;158:132-142.

18. Malherbe CR, Marquard J, Legg DE, et al. Right ventricular hypertrophy with heart failure in Holstein heifers at elevation of 1,600 meters. *J Vet Diag Invest*. 2012;24:867-877.

19. Delaunois L. Anatomy and physiology of collateral respiratory pathways. *Eur Respir J*. 1989;2:893-904.

*20. **Hopkins SR. The lung at maximal exercise: insights from comparative physiology. *Clin Chest Med*. 2005;26:459-468.**

21. Attenburrow DP. Time relationship between the respiratory cycle and limb cycle in the horse. *Equine Vet J*. 1982;14:69-72.

22. Perry SF, Similowski T, Klein W, et al. The evolutionary origin of the mammalian diaphragm. *Respir Physiol Neurobiol*. 2010;171:1-16.

23. Butler PJ, Jones DR. Physiology of diving of birds and mammals. *Physiol Rev*. 1997;77:837-895.

24. Bostroma BL, Fahlmana A, Jonesa DR. Tracheal compression delays alveolar collapse during deep diving in marine mammals. *Respir Physiol Neurobiol*. 2008;161:298-305.

25. Foot NJ, Orgeig S, Daniels CB. The evolution of a physiological system: The pulmonary surfactant system in diving mammals. *Respir Physiol Neurobiol*. 2006;154:118-138.

26. Qvist J, Hill RD, Schneider RC. Hemoglobin concentrations and blood gas tensions of free-diving Weddell seals. *J Appl Physiol*. 1986;61:1560-1569.

27. Van Der Fels-Klerx HJ, Martin SW, Nielen M, et al. Effects on productivity and risk factors of Bovine Respiratory Disease in dairy heifers; a review for the Netherlands. *Neth J Agric Sci*. 2002;50:27-45.

28. Rice JA, Carrasco-Medina L, Hodgins DC, et al. Mannheimia haemolytica and bovine respiratory disease. *Anim Health Res Rev*. 2007;8:117-128.

29. Loneragan GH, Gould DH, Mason GL. Association of 3-methyleneindolenine, a toxic metabolite of 3-methylindole, with acute interstitial pneumonia in feedlot cattle. *Am J Vet Res*. 2001;62:1525-1530.

30. Braun U. Clinical findings and diagnosis of thrombosis if the caudal vena cava in cattle. *Vet J*. 2008;175:118-125.

31. Sánchez A, Couëtil LL, Ward MP, et al. Effect of airway disease on blood gas exchange in racehorses. *J Vet Intern Med*. 2005;19:87-92.

32. Couëtil LL, Hoffman AM, Hodgson J, et al. Inflammatory airway disease in horses. *J Vet Intern Med*. 2007;21:356-361.

33. Stack A, Derksen FJ, Williams KJ, et al. Lung region and racing affect mechanical properties of equine pulmonary microvasculature. *J Appl Physiol*. 2014;117:370-376.

PART III

Physiology of Pulmonary Disease

27

Ventilatory Failure

KEY POINTS

- Ventilatory failure occurs when alveolar ventilation becomes too low to maintain normal arterial blood gas partial pressures.
- There are many causes, involving the respiratory centre, the respiratory muscles or their nerve supply and abnormalities of the chest wall, lung or airways.

- Modest increases in the inspired oxygen concentration will correct hypoxia because of ventilatory failure but may worsen hypercapnia.

Definitions

Respiratory failure is defined as a failure of maintenance of normal arterial blood gas partial pressures. Hypoxia as a result of cardiac and other extrapulmonary forms of shunting are excluded from this definition. Respiratory failure may be subdivided according to whether the arterial P_{CO_2} is normal or low (type 1) or elevated (type 2). The mean normal arterial P_{CO_2} is 5.1 kPa (38.3 mmHg), with 95% limits (2 standard deviations [SD]) of $\pm$ 1.0 kPa (7.5 mmHg). The normal arterial P_{O_2} is more difficult to define because it decreases with age (page 148) and is strongly influenced by the concentration of oxygen in the inspired gas. Mechanisms that contribute to respiratory failure include ventilatory failure (reduced alveolar ventilation) and venous admixture as a result of either pure intrapulmonary shunt or ventilation perfusion mismatch (Chapter 7).

Ventilatory failure is defined as a pathological reduction of the alveolar ventilation below the level required for the maintenance of normal alveolar gas partial pressures. Because arterial P_{O_2} (unlike arterial P_{CO_2}) is so strongly influenced by shunting, the adequacy of ventilation is conveniently defined by the arterial P_{CO_2}, although it is also reflected in end-expiratory P_{CO_2} and P_{O_2}. This chapter is concerned mainly with pure ventilatory failure; other causes of respiratory failure are described in Chapters 28–31.

Pattern of Changes in Arterial Blood Gases

Figure 27.1 shows, on a P_{O_2}/P_{CO_2} diagram, the typical patterns of deterioration of arterial blood gases in respiratory failure. The pale blue area indicates the normal range of values with increasing age corresponding to a leftward shift. Pure ventilatory failure in a young person with otherwise normal lungs would result in changes along the broken line. Chronic obstructive pulmonary disease (COPD), the most common cause of predominantly ventilatory failure, occurs in older people, and the observed pattern of change is shown within the upper orange arrow in Figure 27.1. The limit of survival, while breathing air, is reached at a P_{O_2} of about 2.7 kPa (20 mmHg) and P_{CO_2} of 11 kPa (83 mmHg). The limiting factor is not P_{CO_2} but P_{O_2}. This prevents the rise of P_{CO_2} to higher levels, except when the patient's inspired oxygen concentration is increased. It may also be raised above 11 kPa by the inhalation of carbon dioxide. In either event, a P_{CO_2} in excess of 11 kPa may be considered an iatrogenic disorder. The green arrow in Figure 27.1 shows the pattern of blood gas changes caused by shunting or pulmonary venous admixture (Chapter 7).

In general, the arterial P_{O_2} indicates the severity of respiratory failure (assuming that the patient is breathing air), whereas the P_{CO_2} indicates the differential diagnosis between ventilatory failure and shunting, as shown in Figure 27.1. In respiratory disease it is, of course, common for ventilatory failure and shunting to coexist, and the relative contribution of each mechanism will determine whether type 1 or 2 respiratory failure develops.

Time Course of Changes in Blood Gases in Acute Ventilatory Failure

Although the upper arrow in Figure 27.1 shows the effect of established ventilatory failure on arterial blood gases, short-term deviations from this pattern occur in acute ventilatory failure. This is because the time courses of changes

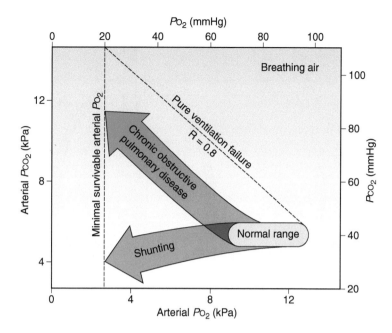

• **Fig. 27.1** Pattern of deterioration of arterial blood gases in chronic obstructive pulmonary disease and pulmonary shunting. The pale blue area indicates the normal range of arterial blood gas partial pressures from 20 to 80 years of age. The oblique broken line shows the theoretical changes in alveolar Po_2 and Pco_2 resulting from pure ventilatory failure. In chronic obstructive pulmonary disease, the arterial Po_2 is always less than the value that would be expected in pure ventilatory failure at the same Pco_2 value. Discussion of shunting is found in Chapter 7, and further discussion of chronic obstructive pulmonary disease in Chapter 28.

of Po_2 and Pco_2 in response to acute changes in ventilation are quite different.

Body stores of oxygen are small, amounting to about 1550 mL while breathing air. Therefore, following a step change in the level of alveolar ventilation, the alveolar and arterial Po_2 rapidly reach the new value and the half-time for the change is only 30 seconds (see page 157 and Fig. 10.18). In contrast, the body stores of carbon dioxide are very large: of the order of 120 L. Therefore, following a step change in the level of alveolar ventilation, the alveolar and arterial Pco_2 only slowly attain the value determined by the new alveolar ventilation. Furthermore, the time course is slower following a reduction of ventilation than an increase (see Fig. 9.11), and the half-time of rise of Pco_2 following a step reduction of ventilation is of the order of 16 minutes.

The practical point is that, during the early phase of acute hypoventilation, there may be a low Po_2 while the Pco_2 is increasing but is still within the normal range. Thus the pulse oximeter may, under certain circumstances such as when breathing air, give an earlier warning of hypoventilation than the capnograph. This breaks the rule that the Pco_2 is the essential index of alveolar ventilation, and it may be erroneously believed that the diagnosis is shunting rather than hypoventilation.

Causes of Ventilatory Failure[1]

The causes of ventilatory failure may be conveniently considered under the headings of the anatomical sites where they arise. These sites are indicated in Figure 27.2. Lesions or malfunctions at sites A to E result in a reduction of input to the respiratory muscles. Dyspnoea may not be apparent, and the diagnosis of ventilatory failure may be easily overlooked. Lesions or malfunctions at sites G to J result in evident dyspnoea, and no one is likely to miss the diagnosis of hypoventilation. The various sites will now be considered individually.

1. *The respiratory neurones of the medulla* are depressed by hypoxia and also by very high levels of Pco_2, probably of the order of 40 kPa (300 mmHg), but at a lower Pco_2 in the presence of some drugs (see later). Reduction of Pco_2 below the apnoeic threshold results in apnoea in the unconscious subject, but usually not in the conscious subject. Loss of respiratory sensitivity to carbon dioxide occurs in various types of long-term ventilatory failure, particularly COPD, and this is discussed further on page 333. A wide variety of drugs may cause central apnoea or respiratory depression (page 55), including opioids, barbiturates and most anaesthetic agents, whether intravenous or inhalational. The respiratory neurones may also be affected by a variety of neurological conditions such as raised intracranial pressure, stroke, trauma or neoplasm.

2. *The upper motoneurones* serving the respiratory muscles are most likely to be interrupted by trauma. Only complete lesions above the third or fourth cervical vertebrae will affect the phrenic nerve and result in total apnoea.[2] However, fracture dislocations of the lower cervical

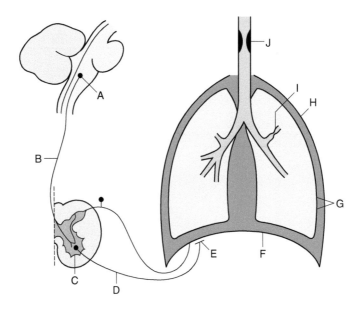

• **Fig. 27.2** Summary of sites at which lesions, drug action or malfunction may result in ventilatory failure. A, Respiratory centre; B, upper motor neuron; C, anterior horn cell; D, lower motor neuron; E, neuromuscular junction; F, respiratory muscles; G, altered elasticity of lungs or chest wall; H, loss of structural integrity of chest wall and pleural cavity; I, increased resistance of small airways; J, upper airway obstruction.

vertebrae are relatively common, and result in loss of action of the intercostal and expiratory muscles, while sparing the diaphragm. Upper motoneurones may be involved in various disease processes, including tumours, demyelination and, occasionally, syringomyelia.

3. *The anterior horn cell* may be affected by various diseases, of which the most important is poliomyelitis. Fortunately this condition is now rare in the developed world, but it can produce any degree of respiratory involvement up to total paralysis of all respiratory muscles.

4. *Lower motoneurones* supplying the respiratory muscles are prone to normal traumatic risks, and in former times the phrenic nerves were surgically interrupted for the treatment of pulmonary tuberculosis. Today the most common causes of phrenic nerve damage are iatrogenic injury following surgery in the chest or compression by intrathoracic tumours.[2] The later stages of motoneurone disease may cause ventilatory failure at this level. Idiopathic polyneuritis (Guillain–Barré syndrome) remains a relatively common neurological cause of ventilatory failure. The syndrome results from an immune-mediated aetiology and is characterized by a rapidly ascending motor nerve paralysis, which in 20% to 30% of patients progresses to quadriplegia and respiratory muscle paralysis. With modern ventilatory support and immunotherapy around 75% of sufferers make a complete neurological recovery, but unfortunately 3% to 7% of patients still die of the condition or its complications.[3]

5. *Neuromuscular junction* function is impaired by several causes, including botulism, neuromuscular blocking drugs used in anaesthesia, organophosphorus compounds and nerve gases. However, myasthenia gravis is by far the most common cause of ventilatory failure at this site; marked respiratory muscle weakness occurs in 15% to 20% of cases.[4] Myasthenia gravis is an autoimmune disease in which the acetylcholine receptors on the neuromuscular junction are destroyed, leading to progressive weakness. Administration of an anticholinesterase drug such as edrophonium increases acetylcholine concentration at the neuromuscular junction and causes an immediate improvement in symptoms. Plasma exchange, intravenous immunoglobulins or thymectomy are effective current therapies.

6. *The respiratory muscles* are rarely entirely responsible for ventilatory failure, but they often contribute to reduced alveolar ventilation in a variety of respiratory diseases. For example, the efficiency of contraction of the respiratory muscles is severely impaired by the hyperinflation that normally accompanies COPD. In these patients, although the curvature of the diaphragm may remain normal, the zone of apposition is reduced (see Figs 5.1 and 5.2), and the resultant shortening of diaphragmatic muscle fibres significantly impairs their function. Unilateral diaphragmatic paralysis is usually asymptomatic, but bilateral paralysis leads to significant dyspnoea, particularly when supine, when the diaphragmatic contribution to breathing is greater (page 64).[2] The respiratory muscles may also become fatigued as a result of working against excessive impedance, but this is not thought to occur until very late in the course of most acute respiratory problems. Patients who require critical care commonly develop a polyneuropathy or myopathy of the respiratory muscles, particularly if sepsis is the underlying cause of their multiorgan failure. Activation of cytokines and malnutrition are believed to be contributing mechanisms. Furthermore, following a long period of

artificial ventilation, respiratory muscles develop 'disuse atrophy'. These factors all make weaning from ventilation difficult (page 385). Cardiac failure may result in respiratory muscle weakness because of reduced blood supply, often coupled with low-compliance lungs because of pulmonary oedema (Chapter 29).

Assessment of respiratory muscle strength is described on page 71.

7. *Loss of elasticity of the lungs or chest wall* is a potent cause of ventilatory failure. It may arise within the lungs (e.g., pulmonary fibrosis or acute lung injury), in the pleura (e.g., empyema; page 363), in the chest wall (e.g., kyphoscoliosis) or in the skin (e.g., contracted burn scars in children). It is frequently forgotten that seemingly mild pressures applied to the outside of the chest may seriously embarrass the breathing and even result in total apnoea. A sustained pressure of only 6 kPa (45 mmHg or a depth of 2 ft of water) is sufficient to prevent breathing. This can occur when crowds get out of control and people fall on top of one another, or when either children or adults become accidentally buried under sand or other heavy materials.

8. *Loss of structural integrity of the chest wall* may result in ventilatory failure, for example, from multiple fractured ribs. A condition known as flail chest arises when multiple ribs are broken in two places, allowing the middle, 'flail', rib section to move independently of the anterior and posterior 'fixed' sections. Movement of the flail segment is then determined by changes in intrathoracic pressure; with spontaneous breathing, a paradoxical respiratory movement of the flail segment develops, which if large enough will compromise tidal volume. Flail chest may need to be treated by artificial ventilation, although conservative treatment with good analgesia, sometimes assisted by rib fixation, is becoming more common.

Closed pneumothorax causes interference with ventilation in proportion to the quantity of air in the chest and is described on page 361.

9. *Small airway resistance* remains the commonest and most important cause of ventilatory failure. The physiology of diseases affecting airway resistance is described in Chapter 28, and will not be further discussed here. However, the relationship between airway resistance and ventilatory failure is a complex subject, which is considered later. In the clinical field, airway resistance is less frequently measured, but is most often inferred from measurement of ventilatory capacity.

10. *Upper airway obstruction* occurs in a wide range of conditions such as airway and pharyngeal tumours, upper respiratory tract infections, inhaled foreign bodies and tumour or bleeding in the neck causing external compression of the airway. Stridor is common and should quickly alert the clinician to the cause of respiratory distress. A smaller airway diameter in babies and children makes them more susceptible than adults to upper airway obstruction, as airway oedema from infections such as croup or epiglottitis quickly causes dramatic stridor. The excellent ability of the respiratory system to overcome increased airway resistance (page 37) is such that ventilatory failure is normally a late development.

Increased Dead Space

Very rarely, a large increase in the respiratory dead space may cause ventilatory failure. Minute volume may be normal or increased, but the alveolar ventilation is reduced, and the patient presents with a high $P\mathrm{co_2}$. An increase in the arterial/end-expiratory $P\mathrm{co_2}$ gradient (more than 2 kPa or 15 mmHg) indicates an increase in the alveolar dead space. This condition may be caused by ventilation of large unperfused areas of lung (e.g., an air cyst communicating with the bronchus), pulmonary emboli or pulmonary hypotension. External or apparatus dead space also tends to reduce alveolar ventilation and may be added either intentionally or accidentally.

Relationship Between Ventilatory Capacity and Ventilatory Failure

Tests for the measurement of ventilatory capacity are described on page 71. However, a severe reduction in ventilatory capacity does not necessarily mean that a patient will be in ventilatory failure. Figure 27.3 shows the lack of correlation between forced expiratory volume in 1 s (FEV_1) and arterial $P\mathrm{co_2}$ in the grossly abnormal range of $FEV1_1$ 0.3 to 1 L from a series of patients with COPD.

It should again be stressed that the usual tests of ventilatory capacity depend on the expiratory muscles, whereas the work of breathing is normally achieved by the action of inspiratory muscles.

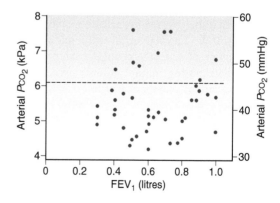

• **Fig. 27.3** Lack of correlation between arterial $P\mathrm{co_2}$ and forced expiratory volume in one second (FEV_1) in 44 patients with chronic obstructive pulmonary disease. The broken line indicates the upper limit of normal for $P\mathrm{co_2}$. (Data from Nunn JF, Milledge JS, Chen D, et al. Respiratory criteria of fitness for surgery and anaesthesia. *Anaesthesia.* 1988;43:543-551.)

Metabolic Demand and Ventilatory Failure

In renal failure, protein intake is a major factor in the onset of uraemia. Similarly, in ventilatory failure, the onset of hypoxia and hypercapnia is directly related to the metabolic demand. Just as patients with renal failure benefit from a low-protein diet, those with a severe reduction of ventilatory capacity protect themselves by limiting the exercise they perform.

As COPD progresses, the ventilatory capacity decreases, and the minute volume of breathing required for a particular level of activity increases. The increased ventilatory requirement is because both the dead space and the oxygen cost of breathing increase. The patient is thus trapped in a pincer movement of decreasing ventilatory capacity and increasing ventilatory requirement. As the jaws of the pincer close, there is first a limitation on heavy exercise, then on moderate exercise and so on until the patient is dyspnoeic at rest. At any time his or her work capacity is limited by the fraction of his ventilatory capacity that he or she is able to maintain for a given level of oxygen uptake.

The complex interaction between these factors is demonstrated in Figure 27.4, where the upper part shows the normal state. Assuming that an untrained subject can comfortably maintain a minute volume equal to about 30% of his or her maximal breathing capacity (MBC) without dyspnoea, he or she has a reserve of ventilatory capacity that is adequate for rest and a power output of 100 W. However, a power output of 200 W requires a minute volume that exceeds a third of his MBC, and he or she becomes aware of his or her breathing at this level of exercise.

Figure 27.4, *B*, shows moderately severe COPD with the following changes:

1. MBC reduced from 150 to 60 L.min^{-1}.
2. Dead space/tidal volume ratio increased from 30% to 40%.
3. Oxygen cost of breathing increased by 10% for each level of activity.

Factors 2 and 3 together result in an increased minute volume for each level of activity. Again, on the assumption that dyspnoea will not be apparent until the minute volume is 30% of MBC, the reserve of ventilation is now sufficient for rest, but 100 W of power output will result in dyspnoea. Finally, in Figure 27.4, *C*, the changes have progressed to the point where resting minute volume exceeds 30% of MBC and the patient is dyspnoeic at rest.

Breathlessness[5]

Breathlessness or dyspnoea has been defined as 'a subjective experience of breathing discomfort that consists of qualitatively distinct sensations that vary in intensity'.[6] This definition applies to both the awareness of breathing during severe exercise in the healthy subject and the dyspnoea of a patient with respiratory failure or heart failure. In the first case the sensation is normal and to be expected. However, in the latter, it is pathological and should be considered as a symptom.

The Origin of the Sensation

Hypoxia and hypercapnia may force the patient to breathe more deeply, but they are not per se responsible for the sensation of dyspnoea, which arises from the ventilatory response rather than the stimulus itself. Patients with respiratory paralysis caused by poliomyelitis did not usually complain of dyspnoea in spite of abnormal blood gases. Dyspnoea is now regarded as a similar physiological condition to pain.[7] Like pain, dyspnoea includes a distressing perception usually referred to as 'air-hunger,' which seems to result more from hypercapnia than from the work of breathing.[8] Some patients have dyspnoea at relatively low levels of work of breathing, whereas others show no dyspnoea at high levels of work. Functional imaging of the brain also shows that the cortical areas activated by dyspnoea are close to regions activated by pain.[9] Finally, as for pain, there is undoubtedly a psychological component to the sensation of breathlessness, involving both affective and emotional responses.[7] Dyspnoea arising from respiratory disease, particularly acutely, is often associated with anxiety and panic, which exacerbate the symptom. Conversely, many patients with primary psychological complaints such as panic disorder present with dyspnoea in the absence of any respiratory disease. As a result of this variable combination of physiological and emotional components, quantifying dyspnoea is best done with a multidimensional instrument.[10]

An early suggestion for the origin of dyspnoea was an 'inappropriateness' between the tension generated in the respiratory muscles and the resultant shortening of the muscle fibres. This sensory input from respiratory muscle afferents would indicate to the brain that breathing was in some way hindered, and probably gives rise to the 'work/effort' sensation (breathing takes work or effort) of dyspnoea.[7] The theory has since been widened to include other sensory receptors in the respiratory system, again suggesting that dyspnoea results from a mismatch between motor output and sensory input in the respiratory centre.[1] These theories seem to fit observations made during breath holding (page 54), which provide some insight into the origin of the sensation of breathlessness, as blood gas partial pressures are by no means the only factor limiting breath-holding time. Other nervous system origins for dyspnoea include the respiratory centre, where a drive to breathe that is not matched by an adequate response from the respiratory muscles can lead to an air hunger sensation (urge to breathe, starved for air).[7]

It cannot be said that the problem of breathlessness is completely understood at the present time.[1,6,7] The origin seems to be multifactorial, and the mechanisms of its generation are clearly complex.

Treatment of Breathlessness

Optimal treatment of the underlying disease process causing the dyspnoea is clearly the first approach to managing the symptom. However, in the later stages of many respiratory diseases, and in almost all patients with malignancy, breathlessness becomes an intractable and distressing

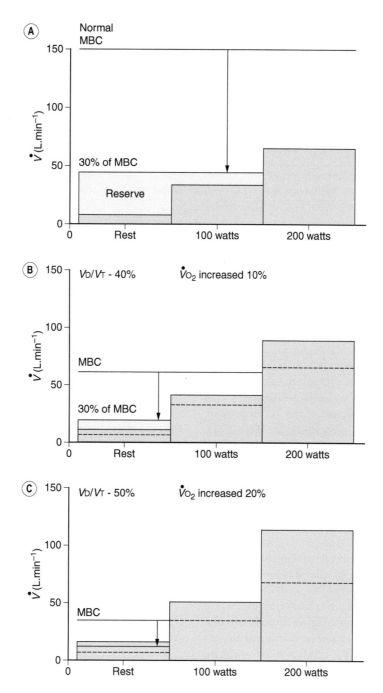

• **Fig. 27.4** Relationship between maximal breathing capacity *(MBC)* and ventilatory requirements at rest and work at 100 and 200 W. The tips of the arrows indicate 30% of MBC, which can usually be maintained without dyspnoea. Ventilatory reserve is between this level and the various ventilatory requirements. **(A)** Normal; **(B)** moderate loss of ventilatory capacity with some increase in oxygen cost of breathing; **(C)** severe loss of ventilatory capacity with considerable increase in the oxygen cost of breathing, leaving no ventilatory reserve even at rest. Broken lines in parts **(B)** and **(C)** show the normal levels of minute ventilation from **(A)**.

problem. Palliation of breathlessness is now recognized as a valuable form of therapy, and offers further insight into the multifactorial nature of the symptom.[11,12] The type of sensation described by an individual patient may guide the best form of therapy (Table 27.1). Simple measures such as a fan blowing on the face or acupuncture are effective. Breathing oxygen relieves dyspnoea in many patients, even some who

are not hypoxic,[11] and high-flow nasal therapy (page 292) or noninvasive ventilation ([NIV]; page 376) may also be helpful. Opioids are effective, whether exogenous or endogenous as a result of exercising.[13] Whether this opioid effect is mediated by reducing the respiratory drive (and so air hunger) or by simply altering the patient's perception of his or her breathlessness is unknown.

TABLE 27.1	Different Subtypes of Dyspnoea, Their Potential Physiological and Pathological Origins and Possible Methods for Symptomatic Treatment		
Subtype	Physiological Origin	Example of Disease	Possible Treatment to Alleviate Symptom
Air hunger	Chemoreflex activity	Pulmonary hyperinflation (COPD, late phase of asthma attack)	NIV, CPAP, bronchodilators
Increased work of breathing	Activity of cerebral motor cortex	Muscle weakness (neuromuscular diseases)	NIV
Chest tightness	Stimulation of slowly adapting receptors in large airways	Bronchospasm (early phase of asthma attack)	Bronchodilators
Rapid breathing, tachypnoea	Stimulation of pulmonary C fibres	Interstitial lung disease, pulmonary venous congestion	Opioids, high-flow nasal therapy (page 292)

COPD, Chronic obstructive pulmonary disease; *CPAP*, continuous positive airway pressure; *NIV*, noninvasive ventilation.
(From reference 12.)

Principles of Therapy for Ventilatory Failure

Many patients lead normal lives with arterial $P\text{CO}_2$ levels as high as 8 kPa (60 mmHg). Higher levels are associated with increasing disability, largely because of the accompanying hypoxaemia when the patient is breathing air (Fig. 27.1). Treatment may be divided into symptomatic relief of hypoxaemia and attempts to improve the alveolar ventilation.

Treatment of Hypoxaemia Caused by Hypoventilation by Administration of Oxygen

Hypoxia must be treated as the first priority, and administration of oxygen is the fastest and most effective method.

The relationship between alveolar $P\text{O}_2$ and alveolar ventilation is explained on page 137 and illustrated in Figure 10.2. If other factors remain constant, an increase in inspired gas $P\text{O}_2$ will result in an equal increase in alveolar gas $P\text{O}_2$. Therefore only small increases in inspired oxygen concentration are required for the relief of hypoxia caused by hypoventilation. Figure 27.5 shows the rectangular hyperbola relating $P\text{CO}_2$ and alveolar ventilation (as in

Fig. 9.9), but superimposed are the concentrations of inspired oxygen required to restore a normal alveolar $P\text{O}_2$ for different degrees of alveolar hypoventilation. It is seen that 30% is sufficient for the degree of alveolar hypoventilation resulting in an alveolar $P\text{CO}_2$ of 13 kPa (almost 100 mmHg). Clearly this is an unacceptable $P\text{CO}_2$; therefore 30% can be regarded as the upper limit of inspired oxygen concentration to be used in the palliative relief of hypoxia because of ventilatory failure, without attempting to improve the alveolar ventilation.

The use of very high concentrations of inspired oxygen will prevent hypoxia even in gross alveolar hypoventilation, which carries the risk of dangerous hypercapnia. Although this is a strong contraindication to the use of high concentrations of oxygen under these circumstances, the effect may be even worse in patients with COPD, in whom oxygen therapy often leads to hypercapnia (page 333). Recognition of this potential problem unfortunately resulted in a tendency to withhold oxygen for fear of causing hypercapnia. The rule is that hypoxia must be treated first, because hypoxia kills quickly, whereas hypercapnia kills slowly. However, it must always be remembered that administration of oxygen to a patient with ventilatory failure will do nothing to improve the $P\text{CO}_2$, and may make it worse.

Improvement of Alveolar Ventilation

The only way to reduce arterial $P\text{CO}_2$ is to improve alveolar ventilation. The first line of therapy is to improve ventilatory capacity by treatment of the underlying cause, while simultaneously providing carefully controlled oxygen therapy and avoiding the use of drugs that depress breathing.

The second line is chemical stimulation of breathing. Doxapram stimulates breathing via an action on the peripheral chemoreceptors (page 56), and is effective in treating exacerbations of COPD, but only for the first few hours after admission to hospital.

The third line of treatment is by NIV, followed by the final option of artificial ventilation, both of which are

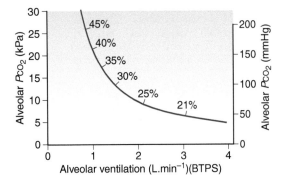

• **Fig. 27.5** Alveolar $P\text{CO}_2$ as a function of alveolar ventilation at rest. The percentages indicate the inspired oxygen concentration that is then required to restore normal alveolar $P\text{O}_2$. *BTPS*, body temperature and pressure, saturated.

described in Chapter 32. It is difficult to give firm guidelines for the institution of artificial ventilation, and the arterial $P\text{co}_2$ should not be considered in isolation. Nevertheless, a $P\text{co}_2$ in excess of 10 kPa (75 mmHg) that cannot be reduced by other means in a patient who is deemed recoverable is generally considered as a firm indication. However, artificial ventilation may be required at much lower levels of $P\text{co}_2$ if there is actual or impending respiratory fatigue as a result of increased work of breathing. This may be difficult to diagnose or predict. Although it is now recognized that intense activity by the respiratory muscles results in fatigue, as in the case of other skeletal muscles under similar conditions, it is also thought that ventilatory failure from this cause occurs only very late in the course of most respiratory diseases.

References

1. Laghi F, Tobin MJ. Disorders of the respiratory muscles. *Am J Respir Crit Care Med.* 2003;168:10-48.
2. McCool FD, Tzelepis GE. Dysfunction of the diaphragm. *N Engl J Med.* 2012;366:932-942.
3. Willison HJ, Jacobs BC, van Doorn PA. Guillain-Barré syndrome. *Lancet.* 2016;388:717-727.
4. Alshekhlee A, Miles JD, Katirji B, et al. Incidence and mortality rates of myasthenia gravis and myasthenic crisis in US hospitals. *Neurology.* 2009;72:1548-1554.
5. Ekström MP, Abernethy AP, Currow DC. The management of chronic breathlessness in patients with advanced and terminal illness. *BMJ.* 2015;350:g7617.
6. Parshall MB, Schwartzstein RM, Adams L, et al. An official American Thoracic Society statement: Update on the mechanisms, assessment, and management of dyspnea. *Am J Respir Crit Care Med.* 2012;185:435-452.
*7. Laviolette L, Laveneziana P, on behalf of the ERS Research Seminar Faculty. Dyspnoea: a multidimensional and multidisciplinary approach. *Eur Respir J.* 2014;43:1750-1762.
8. Banzett RB, Pedersen SH, Schwartzstein RM, et al. The affective dimension of laboratory dyspnea: air hunger is more unpleasant than work/effort. *Am J Respir Crit Care Med.* 2008;177:1384-1390.
9. von Leupoldt A, Dahme B. Cortical substrates for the perception of dyspnea. *Chest.* 2005;128:345-354.
10. Banzett RB, Moosavi SH. Measuring dyspnoea: new multidimensional instruments to match our 21st century understanding. *Eur Respir J.* 2017;49:1602473.
11. Booth S, Wade R. Oxygen or air for palliation of breathlessness in advanced cancer. *J R Soc Med.* 2002;96:215-218.
*12. Pisani L, Hill NS, Pacilli AMG, et al. Management of dyspnea in the terminally ill. *Chest.* 2018;154:925-934.
13. Mahler DA, Murray JA, Waterman LA, et al. Endogenous opioids modify dyspnoea during treadmill exercise in patients with COPD. *Eur Respir J.* 2009;33:771-777.

28

Airways Disease

KEY POINTS

- Whatever the cause, airway narrowing leads to expiratory flow limitation, gas trapping and hyperinflation of the lung, which manifests itself as breathlessness.
- Asthma involves intermittent, reversible airway obstruction caused by airway inflammation and bronchial smooth muscle contraction, both as a result of mediators released from mast cells and eosinophils.
- Chronic obstructive pulmonary disease is progressive, with a poorly reversible airway narrowing caused by airway inflammation and loss of lung tissue elasticity, mostly as a result of smoking-induced activation of airway neutrophils.
- Cystic fibrosis is an inherited disease in which abnormal chloride transport in the airway impairs the normal pulmonary defence mechanisms, leading to chronic and destructive pulmonary infections.

This chapter considers the physiological changes seen in the three most common diseases of the pulmonary airways: asthma, chronic obstructive pulmonary disease (COPD) and cystic fibrosis (CF). The first two of these have many clinical and physiological features in common, and together constitute the vast majority of respiratory disease seen in clinical practice.

Asthma

It is estimated that 4.3% of people have asthma worldwide,[1] with a prevalence that has increased by approximately 50% per decade. In industrially developed countries the increasing prevalence is believed to have now levelled off at 10% to 15% of the population, and may be decreasing in some countries.[2] Meanwhile asthma prevalence is increasing rapidly in developing countries as lifestyles change. The prevalence of asthma amongst children in the developed world increased two- to threefold in the last 50 years.[3] Although the worldwide prevalence is no longer increasing, hospital admissions for asthma continue to rise. Fortunately, improved treatments mean that deaths attributable to asthma have been falling consistently since the 1980s,[4] but the years of life lost because of asthma remains considerably higher in low sociodemographic index countries.[1]

Clinical Features

Asthma causes recurrent episodes of chest 'tightness', wheezing, breathlessness and coughing as a result of airway narrowing from a combination of inflammation of the small airways and contraction of bronchial smooth muscle in the lower airway. In an acute episode of asthma there are three closely related phases.

Bronchoconstriction occurs early in an asthma 'attack'. This is particularly prominent in allergic asthma, when, within minutes of exposure to an allergen, wheezing develops. Narrowing of small airways occurs because of contraction of airway smooth muscle (ASM) in response to the cellular mechanisms described in the next section. Bronchoconstriction in different regions of the lung may not be uniform, and two different scanning techniques have shown that, in many patients with asthma, ventilation becomes heterogeneous, with clusters of poorly ventilated lung regions (Fig. 28.1).[5,6] This might be expected to cause maldistribution of ventilation and perfusion, but a further study showed that blood flow to the poorly ventilated areas is also reduced,[7] presumably illustrating the efficiency of hypoxic pulmonary vasoconstriction (page 80). It is not clear why only some asthmatic patients develop ventilation defects; one possible explanation is asymmetric airway branching patterns in susceptible subjects.[8] What is more clear is that heterogeneity of bronchoconstriction is associated with more severe clinical disease[5] and has significant implications for inhaled therapy, as these studies suggest that most of an inhaled drug will be deposited in the better-ventilated regions rather than where it is most needed.

With more severe bronchoconstriction airway closure begins to occur during expiration, gas trapping occurs, and the lungs become hyperinflated. Eventually the patient is

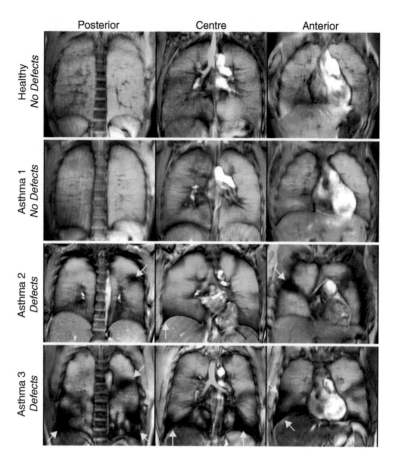

Posterior   Centre   Anterior

Healthy
No Defects

Asthma 1
No Defects

Asthma 2
Defects

Asthma 3
Defects

• **Fig. 28.1** Hyperpolarized ³He magnetic resonance imaging (MRI) scans of the lung following inhaled methacholine challenge. Ventilation distribution (*blue*) is superimposed on a standard MRI of the thorax, showing three coronal slices for each subject. The arrows show the ventilation defects in two of the subjects with asthma, which are not present in a different patient with asthma or the healthy control subject. (Reproduced from reference 5 with permission of the authors and BMJ Publishing Group Ltd.)

attempting to breath in when the lungs are almost at total lung capacity, and a sensation of inspiratory dyspnoea results, even though the defect is with expiration. Physiological effects of hyperinflation are described on page 332.

Bronchoconstriction may quickly subside, either spontaneously or with treatment, but more commonly progresses to a late-phase reaction.

Late-phase reactions are characterized by inflammation of the airway, and develop a few hours after the acute bronchoconstriction. Airway obstruction continues, and cough with sputum production develops. Asthma precipitated by respiratory tract infection may 'bypass' the acute bronchoconstriction phase, and the onset of symptoms is then more gradual.

Airway hyperresponsiveness (AHR) describes the observation that asthmatic subjects become wheezy in response to a whole range of stimuli that have little effect on normal individuals. Stimuli include such things as cold air, exercise, pollution (page 241) or inhaled drugs, and occur via the neural pathways present in normal lungs (page 34). Methacholine or histamine can be used to measure AHR accurately by determining the inhaled concentration that gives rise to a 20% reduction in forced expiratory volume in 1 second (FEV_1).

Asthma Phenotypes[9]

The term 'asthma' includes a wide spectrum of illnesses, varying from a wheezy 6-month-old baby with a viral infection to a young adult with repeated episodes of wheezing or an older patient with chronic lung disease. Asthma is therefore not a single disease, but more a heterogeneous group of underlying disease processes with a variety of presentations, physiological characteristics and patient outcomes. As a result, the concept of asthma phenotyping has emerged, which involves integrating biological and clinical features with the ultimate goal of providing more personalized therapy. Commonly used clinical phenotypes include:

• *Allergic asthma.* Onset usually in childhood, associated with a history of atopy, with sputum examination typically showing eosinophilic inflammation.
• *Nonallergic asthma.* Adult onset, not associated with allergic triggers of bronchospasm; sputum examination may reveal neutrophilia, eosinophilia or few inflammatory cells.
• *Late-onset asthma.* Presents in adult life, more commonly in women; manifests as nonallergic wheezing.

- *Asthma with fixed airflow limitation.* Patients with long-standing asthma develop fixed airflow limitation, thought to be secondary to airway remodelling.
- *Asthma with obesity.* This is described on page 202.

Cellular Mechanisms of Asthma[10]

Many cell types are involved in the pathophysiology of asthma. A summary of the interactions between these cells in allergic asthma is shown in Figure 28.2, which also shows the principal cytokines that facilitate communication between the cells.

Mast cells are plentiful in the walls of airways and alveoli, and also lie free in the lumen of the airways. where they may

be recovered by bronchial lavage. Mast cell activation is the main cause of the immediate bronchospasm seen in allergic asthma. The surface of the mast cell contains a large number of binding sites for the immunoglobulin IgE. Activation of the cell results from antigen bridging of only a small number of these receptors, and may also be initiated by complement fractions C3a, C4a and C5a and substance P, physical stimulation and many drugs and other organic molecules.

The triggering mechanism of the mast cell is thus extremely sensitive, and is mediated by an increase in inositol triphosphate and intracellular calcium ions. Within 30 seconds of activation, there is degranulation, with discharge of a range of preformed mediators listed in Table 28.1. Histamine acts directly on H_1 receptors in the bronchial smooth muscle

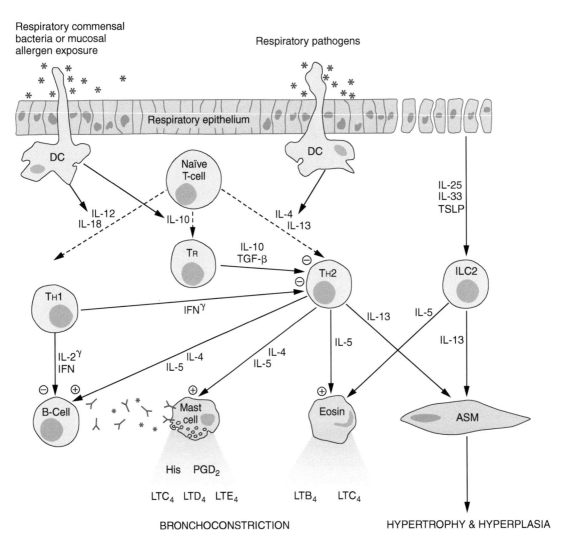

* Allergen or antigen
Y Immunoglobulin

• **Fig. 28.2** Inflammatory cells involved in the pathogenesis of allergic asthma, and the main cytokines by which they communicate with each other. For details see text. The immune pathways shown are based on a combination of animal and human studies. IL-25 and IL-33 are released when airway epithelium is damaged, as shown on the right of the figure. *ASM,* Airway smooth muscle cell; *B-cell,* B-lymphocyte; *DC,* dendritic (antigen-presenting) cell; *Eosin,* eosinophil; *ILC2,* natural type-2 helper cell; *IL,* interleukin; *IFN,* interferon; *Th2 and Th1,* subtypes of T-lymphocyte helper cells; *TGF,* transforming growth factor; *Treg,* regulatory lymphocyte; *TSLP,* thymic stromal lymphopoietin.

TABLE 28.1	Mediators Released from Mast Cells when Activated by Immunoglobin E		
Preformed Mediators	**Newly Generated Mediators**	**Cytokines**
Histamine	Prostaglandin D_2	Interleukins 3, 4, 5, 6 and 13
Heparin	Thromboxane A_2	Granulocyte/macrophage-colony stimulating factor
Serotonin	Leukotrienes C_4, D_4 and E_4	Tumour necrosis factor
Lysosomal enzymes:		Platelet-activating factor
Tryptase		
Chymase		
β-Galactosidase		
β-Glucuronidase		
Hexosaminidase		

fibres to cause contraction, on other H_1 receptors to increase vascular permeability and on H_2 receptors to increase mucous secretion. The granules also contain proteases, mainly tryptase, which can detach epithelial cells from the basement membrane, resulting in desquamation and possibly activating neuronal reflexes causing further bronchospasm.

The second major event after mast cell activation is the initiation of synthesis of arachidonic acid derivatives (see Fig. 11.3). The most important derivative of the cyclooxygenase pathway is the prostaglandin PGD_2, which is a bronchoconstrictor, although its clinical significance is still not clear. The lipoxygenase pathway results in the formation of leukotriene (LT) C_4, from which two further leukotrienes, LTD_4 and LTE_4, are formed (see Fig. 3.10).

Finally, mast cells also release a variety of cytokines. Interleukin-5 (IL-5) and granulocyte/macrophage colony-stimulating factor (GM-CSF) are chemotactic for eosinophils, and IL-4 stimulates IgE production by B-lymphocytes, amplifying the activation of mast cells.

Eosinophils are freely distributed alongside mast cells in the submucosa, and are believed to be the principal cell involved in the late-phase reaction of asthma. In particular, they release LTB_4 and LTC_4, which are potent bronchoconstrictors with a prolonged action. They are attracted to the area by GM-CSF, which is released by many inflammatory cells, before being activated by IL-5 originating from mast cells and lymphocytes.

Lymphocytes have an important role in the control of mast cell and eosinophil activation.[11] Activated B-lymphocytes are responsible for production of the antigen specific IgE needed to cause mast cell degranulation. B-cells are in turn controlled by various subsets of T-'helper' lymphocytes.

Th2 cells are important proinflammatory cells in asthma, promoting both bronchospasm and inflammation by stimulation of mast cells, eosinophils and B-lymphocytes. The Th2 cell is nonspecific in its response, and relies on stimulation by IL-4 and IL-13 from dendritic (antigen-presenting) cells (DCs) both for its generation from naive T-cells and its subsequent activation to produce its own proinflammatory cytokines. The airway epithelium contains many DCs which have toll-like receptors, as do the epithelial cells themselves (page 167).[12] Once activated by their specific antigen, the DCs migrate to lymphoid tissue

in the lungs to control the division of naive lymphocytes into their various subtypes.

Th1 cells are also generated from naive T-cells in lymphoid tissue in response to cytokines released by activated DCs. Th1 cells normally act as antiinflammatory cells by producing interferon and IL-2, which inhibit the activity of Th2 and B-cells.

The relative activity of the opposing effects of Th1 and Th2 lymphocytes was, until recently, believed to play an important role in the development and severity of asthma. However, this convenient explanation, based mainly on studies in animals, is now thought to be an oversimplification of the situation in humans, particularly with respect to the generation of Th1 cells. The third subtype of T-lymphocyte involved in immune regulation of the lung are regulatory T-cells (Tregs),[13] which are again generated from naive T-cells, this time in response to IL-10 released by activated DCs. Activation of the DCs to produce the antiinflammatory cytokines IL-10, IL-12 and IL-18 is believed to occur in response to antigens from respiratory tract commensal bacteria or from exposure to high levels of allergens. Tregs exert an antiinflammatory effect by secretion of IL-10 and transforming growth factor β, which modify the activities of both Th1 and Th2 cells. Finally, a recently described fourth regulatory T-cell (group 2 innate lymphoid cell) has been described which is generated in response to IL-25 and IL-33 released by damaged epithelial cells. These cells reside within the epithelium and produce large amounts of IL-5, which further activates eosinophils and, more importantly, IL-13, which leads to AHR and airway remodelling, including goblet cell hyperplasia.[14,15]

Neutrophils are important contributors to the nonallergic phenotypes of asthma, and when activated lead to airway narrowing and inflammation. A different series of cytokines to those already described are involved, with predominantly IL-6 activating Th1 and Th17 lymphocytes, which in turn release a variety of forms of IL-17 to activate neutrophils.[10,16]

Causes of Airway Obstruction in Asthma

Airway Smooth Muscle

Stimulation of bronchial smooth muscle by the substances shown in Figure 28.2 and Table 28.1 explains some of the airway narrowing seen in asthma, particularly during the acute and early stages. During deliberately induced bronchoconstriction ASM cells in asthmatic subjects also respond differently to stretching (by taking a deep inspiration) compared with in nonasthmatic subjects. In the normal lung deep inspiration causes ASM relaxation which ameliorates the bronchoconstriction, whereas in asthmatic subjects the ASM fails to respond or even contracts, exacerbating the bronchoconstriction.[17]

Inflammation

Airway narrowing during the late-phase response, or in severe asthma, results from inflammation of the airway. Many cytokines released during asthma have effects on blood vessel permeability, causing oedema of the epithelium and basement membrane. This airway narrowing because of oedema may be exacerbated by rostral fluid shifts when supine, for example, at night.[18] Protease enzymes break down normal epithelial architecture, generating defects in the epithelial barrier, leading to further inflammation and eventually detachment of the epithelium from the basement membrane. Finally, hypersecretion of mucus and impaired mucociliary clearance are both recognized features of asthma. These changes in the thickness of the airway lining translate into a significant reduction in airway cross-sectional area, and thus a large increase in resistance.

Mucus, inflammatory cells and epithelial debris cause obstruction of small airways, compound flow limitation and prevent an effective cough.

Airway Remodelling[19]

Repeated activation of inflammatory pathways inevitably leads to attempts by the body to repair the tissue concerned. In the lung, this results in morphological changes to both the ASM and the respiratory epithelium. Hypertrophy and hyperplasia of ASM cells[20] cause thickening of the airway wall, even when the muscle is relaxed (Fig. 28.3), and exacerbates the airway narrowing that occurs with muscle contraction because a lesser degree of muscle shortening now causes a greater reduction in the airway lumen. Epigenetic changes occur in ASM cells in asthma, most commonly by acetylation or methylation of histone proteins, which consequently modifies the expression of the genes within ASM cells.[21] Goblet cell hyperplasia also occurs, worsening the hypersecretion of mucus seen with airway inflammation. Finally, in asthmatic patients, there is thickening of the lamina reticularis of the epithelial basement membrane and changes to the extracellular matrix, ultimately resulting in collagen deposition and long-term loss of lung function. Most of these structural changes are stimulated by Th2 cytokines, particularly IL-13 (Fig. 28.2). The clinical significance of airway remodelling in asthma is unknown, but

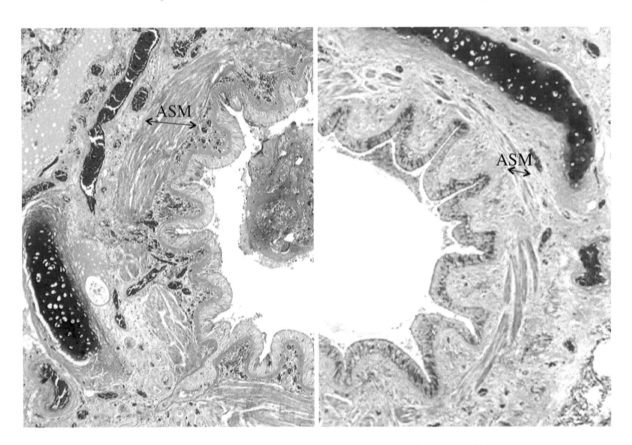

• **Fig. 28.3** Histological section of a bronchiole from a patient with chronic asthma (left) and a healthy patient (right). Note the thickened layer of airway smooth muscle (ASM), the irregular mucosal folding and the debris in the airway. (Reproduced from reference 21 with permission of the authors and the American Thoracic Society. Copyright © 2019 American Thoracic Society.)

remodelling is believed to be responsible for the long-term decline in lung function seen in some asthma patients. Widespread ASM hyperplasia is more common in fatal cases of asthma,[20] and measures of ASM mass may in future be useful to predict which patients will develop severe asthma later in life.[22] Airway remodelling may begin before asthma becomes severe or is even diagnosed at all, but unfortunately, effective drugs to reverse the structural changes are as yet to be discovered.[19]

Aetiology of Asthma[23]

Genetics

Asthma, along with other allergic diseases, has a substantial genetic component, with several genomic regions known to be linked with developing the disease or its progeression.[24] Environmental factors invariably contribute to the development of clinical disease, but genetic susceptibility to asthma is strong. Two reasons explain this observation. First, the genes for most of the cytokines involved in asthma are found close together on chromosome 5, and asthmatic patients may have increased expression of these. Second, human lymphocyte antigens (HLAs), which are involved in sensitization of DCs to specific antigens, are part of the major histocompatibility complex allowing immunological 'self-recognition', and so are inherited. It is possible that some HLA types are particularly active in the processing of common allergens, and thus the stimulation of Th2 cells or the suppression of Treg cells.

Genome-wide scans of patients have identified several genetic loci linked to different phenotypes of asthma. These genes facilitate asthma development by many different mechanisms, for example, by affecting the barrier function of the airway mucosa and so changing the interaction between allergens or pathogens and the immune cells in the airway. The most widely studied example of a gene affecting asthma is *ADAM33*, (A Disentegrin And Metalloprotease protein),[25] which encodes a large family of proteins with diverse functions, including the control of cell–cell and cell–matrix interactions. In lung tissue, the ADAM33 protein is found in smooth muscle and fibroblasts, but not epithelial cells, indicating its possible role in airway remodelling in asthma.

Allergy

Changes in living conditions are believed to have contributed to the increase in asthma prevalence. In the developing world, population shifts from rural to urban environments have reduced exposure to parasitic infections and increased exposure to other allergens, and it seems likely that the extensive immunoglobin (Ig)E and mast cell systems that formally inactivated parasites now respond to urban allergens. In the developed world, changes in living conditions have resulted in a dramatic increase in allergen exposure, in particular house dust mite ((HDM); *Dermatophagoides pteronyssinus*), domestic animals and fungi. Asthma is more common in affluent families, and correlates with exposure to HDM, which thrives in warm, humid houses with extensive carpeting and bedding. These conditions are ideal for the HDM and its food supply of shed skin flakes. Simply inhaling allergens is only part of the explanation of how allergen exposure may cause asthma, and maternal allergen exposure during pregnancy may also play a role. Despite decades of research across the world, the contribution of HDM allergy to causing asthma remains controversial.[26]

Infection

Viral respiratory tract infections cause wheezing in many patients with asthma, and account for over half of the acute exacerbations of asthma. The most likely pathogen in adults is the 'common cold' rhinovirus. In infants, respiratory syncytial or some subtypes of rhinovirus are associated with developing asthma in later life, but causation has not yet been established.[27] Viral infection gives rise to an immune response involving many cells and cytokines, but T-lymphocytes are particularly important and undergo both virus-specific and generalized activation. Inevitably, Th2 activity is increased giving rise to wheeze and airway inflammation by the mechanisms described earlier (Fig. 28.2). In addition, stimulation of allergic mechanisms in susceptible individuals continues for some time after the viral symptoms have subsided. For example, after a simple rhinovirus infection, allergen-induced histamine production and eosinophil-induced late-phase reactions remained increased for 4 to 6 weeks.[28]

Hygiene Hypothesis

This hypothesis to explain the rising incidence of asthma claims that in the clean, hygienic developed world children now are exposed to fewer infections or other environmental antigens. It is known that some infections may have a protective role in preventing the initiation of asthma in early childhood. Children who are exposed to more infections in early life, such as those with older siblings or those living on farms, are less likely to develop allergic disease. This led to a suggestion that lower infection rates in the population at large and effective immunization programmes may have contributed to the rising incidence of asthma. Measles virus, *Mycobacterium tuberculosis*, respiratory and gastrointestinal commensal bacteria, some respiratory viral infections and hepatitis A virus all have the potential to reduce asthma development by modification of the lymphocyte subtypes shown in Figure 28.2. Other microorganisms to which the modern human is now less commonly exposed, termed 'old friends' by the authors,[29] include lactobacilli from untreated dairy products, saprophytic mycobacteria found in mud and helminths (worms). All three are known to promote activity of Treg cells, potentially protecting against the development of asthma. For many of these microorganisms exposure to the entire microbe is not required, and beneficial immune responses may be gained from exposure to antigens found in the dust and dirt of the environment,[30] for example, the lipopolysaccharides which are abundant in dust samples from small, family-based farms.[31]

Smoking and Air Pollution

Tobacco smoking, including passive smoking and maternal smoking, is associated with developing asthma, and is discussed in Chapter 20. Trends in air pollution have not generally followed trends in asthma incidence over recent decades, the levels of many pollutants declining whilst asthma becomes more common. However, there is now evidence that exposure to traffic pollution may increase both the incidence and severity of asthma in children (page 240),[32] and similar data are emerging for adults.[33] There is little doubt that, in patients who already have asthma, exposure to many forms of air pollution exacerbates their symptoms.

Obesity

The role of obesity in adult and childhood asthma is described in Chapter 15.

Paracetamol (Acetaminophen)

Depletion of glutathione in the lung (page 290) leading to increased oxidative stress or a reduced interferon-mediated inflammatory response to virus infections are both potential mechanisms to explain a link between asthma and paracetamol.[34] Several large cohort studies have demonstrated an association between paracetamol use and the development of asthma. This of course does not prove causation, and other explanations exist, for example, children who have frequent infections may be given paracetamol more often. However, given that the increasing use of paracetamol in children has followed a similar timescale to the rising incidence in childhood asthma, further research may eventually reveal a relatively simple contributor to the current childhood asthma epidemic.

Aspirin and Asthma[35]

The involvement of arachidonic acid derivatives in the normal control of bronchial smooth muscle (see Table 3.2 and page 170) predicts that drugs blocking these pathways may influence the airways of asthma patients. This is indeed the case with aspirin and the closely related nonsteroidal antiinflammatory drugs, which sometimes cause bronchospasm in asthma patients. Amongst the general population of patients with asthma 7.2 % exhibit aspirin-exacerbated respiratory disease (AERD),[35] but when provocation with oral aspirin is performed 21% of patients develop a reduction in FEV_1.[36] Many asthmatic patients who are sensitive to aspirin have a characteristic clinical presentation. Typically, AERD develops in patients at around 30 years of age, is preceded for a few years by rhinitis and nasal polyps, in two-thirds of patients is associated with a history of atopy and occurs in slightly more female than male patients.

Mechanism of Aspirin Sensitivity

Inhibitors of the cyclooxygenase (COX) pathway in the airway will reduce synthesis of the bronchodilator prostaglandin PGE_2, but this cannot alone account for AERD.

Loss of mast cell inhibition by PGE_2 also causes increased release of histamine and leukotrienes (see Fig. 3.10), which give rise to most of the symptoms of AERD. Multiple isoforms of COX exist (page 170), and COX-1 is responsible for most cases of AERD. Coxibs, a group of drugs that specifically inhibit COX-2, seem to be safe for use in AERD patients. The analgesic effects of paracetamol are mediated by inhibition of COX-3, and a small subset of patients with AERD develop bronchospasm in response to paracetamol. This sensitivity to paracetamol usually involves only a mild reaction in response to high doses of the drug, and occurs in less than 2% of asthmatic patients.[35,36]

Principles of Therapy[1]

Detailed guidelines on the treatment of asthma are published in many countries, and are beyond the scope of this book. Except for mild asthma, treatment has now moved away from the traditional bronchodilator inhaler 'when needed' approach of the past. The emphasis is now on continuous treatment with drugs and other strategies aimed at preventing exacerbations and suppressing airway inflammation. Therapeutic approaches are discussed next.

Bronchodilators remain a common treatment for relief of acute bronchospasm. The β_2-adrenoceptor agonists (page 35) are widely used, and now include wider use of longer-acting drugs, although concerns remain about the mortality for patients using these drugs in the long term.[37] In the emergency treatment of life-threatening asthma intravenous bronchodilators are more useful because small tidal volumes or ventilation defects may prevent inhaled drugs from reaching their target site, although there are significant side effects from intravenous β_2-agonists in such sick patients. Other bronchodilator drugs include inhibitors of LT receptors on bronchial smooth muscle (page 36), blocking the effects of LTC_4, LTD_4 and LTE_4. They are effective in treating asthma, including the bronchospasm seen in the late-phase reaction, and may be particularly useful in patients with exercise-induced asthma or AERD.

Steroids,[38] either inhaled or oral, are an invaluable method of prophylaxis and treatment in asthma. Steroids act on a glucocorticoid receptor found in the cytoplasm of cells, following which the receptor–drug complex can enter the nucleus and regulate the transcription of numerous genes. By a combination of direct and indirect effects on transcription, steroids inhibit the synthesis of a wide range of inflammatory proteins, including cytokines, adhesion molecules and inflammatory receptors. Around one-third of patients with asthma have a poor therapeutic response to steroids, and this may be caused by a genetic variant of the glucocorticoid-induced transcript 1 gene.[39]

Other therapeutic approaches for asthma include allergen avoidance. This is an attractive strategy for the prevention of asthma in patients with known allergies, but effective reduction of allergen load is difficult. Many studies have failed to demonstrate a clinical benefit of allergen load reduction, although moving to altitude where low humidity significantly reduces HDM numbers or implementing fastidious allergen reduction techniques within the home have been shown to help.[40]

'Biologic' drugs include numerous monoclonal antibodies active against the cytokines involved in asthma pathogenesis (Fig. 28.2), opening up the possibility in the future of more accurately targeted therapies aimed at specific underlying abnormalities of airway immunity.[10,41,42]

Chronic Obstructive Pulmonary Disease

Clinical features of COPD are similar to those of asthma, with wheeze, cough and dyspnoea, but the air flow limitation is poorly reversible with bronchodilators. Much older patients are affected by COPD than asthma, and the progressive nature of the process leads to more serious interruption of normal activities, and eventually respiratory failure (page 317). COPD is currently the third leading cause of death in the world, and is estimated to affect 10% of people aged over 45 years.[43,44] Although in some developed countries the incidence has stabilized, the rapid rise in smoking in the developing world in recent decades means COPD rates there are rising at alarming rates.[45] Mortality rates from COPD are declining, but the increasing prevalence means that the number of people dying from the disease worldwide is almost static.[46] There is a strong association between COPD and cardiovascular disease, partly because of shared risk factors (e.g., smoking) and partly because of systemic inflammation and oxidative stress.[47]

Unlike asthma, where airway obstruction is usually intermittent, COPD is characterized by progressive chronic air flow limitation along with intermittent exacerbations, particularly in winter. These exacerbations vary from a slight worsening of symptoms to a life-threatening deterioration, are usually caused by viral or bacterial infections and are associated with increased airway resistance and hyperinflation leading to dyspnoea.[48]

Both asthma and COPD are characterized pathologically by airway narrowing and inflammation, but the causes and clinical course of the two diseases are quite different. Improved understanding of the pathology of COPD and asthma has uncovered a variety of major differences between the two, as shown in Figure 28.4. It is believed that around 10% of patients have a mixture of the two disease processes, now called asthma-COPD overlap.[49] This term is not a diagnosis; it describes a heterogeneous group of patients with widely varied pathology who require an individualized approach to therapy, as treating them as having either asthma or COPD alone results in poor management.[50]

Aetiology of Chronic Obstructive Pulmonary Disease

Smoking is the major aetiological factor in COPD (page 237). The accelerated decline in FEV_1 seen with smoking is shown in Figure 20.1, and the 15% to 20% of smokers who develop COPD probably represent an extreme response to this effect of tobacco smoke. This susceptibility to tobacco smoke is likely to be genetic.[51] Smokers who have developed COPD have different patterns of expression of oxidant/antioxidant pathway genes compared with smokers who have not developed COPD.[52] For example, levels of surfactant proteins A and D are reduced in smokers with COPD, and this reduction is linked to inflammation and lung fibrosis. Nicotine activates signaling pathways in vitro, leading to a decrease in the expression of these surfactant proteins, allowing specific signaling pathways to be identified and investigated.[53] Additionally, loss

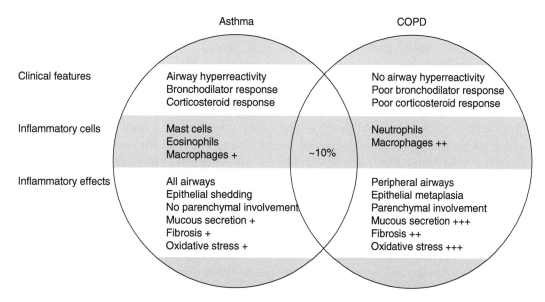

• **Fig. 28.4** Clinical and pathological differences between chronic obstructive pulmonary disease (COPD) and asthma, leading to 'asthma-COPD overlap'. (From Barnes PJ. Mechanisms in COPD. Differences from asthma. *Chest.* 2000;117:10S-14S, by permission of the author and publishers.)

of the distal-to-proximal phenotype of small airway epithelium is found in adult smokers, an observation reproducible in vitro by exposing small airway epithelial basal cells to epidermal growth factor, a factor up-regulated in smokers.[54] Attempts to identify the specific genes responsible for susceptibility to COPD in smokers are at an early stage.[55,56] A potential contender is the *FAM13A* gene, which is frequently found to be associated with COPD.[57] Excessive activity of the FAM13A protein is thought to promote the degradation of the ubiquitous intracellular molecule β-catenin, which is critical to airway and alveolar cell repair mechanisms in response to injuries,[58] for example, by cigarette smoke.

There is now an acknowledgement that lung development in early life also influences the likelihood of developing COPD independently of smoking.[56,59] Factors such as prematurity, maternal smoking during pregnancy and childhood exposure to infections and air pollution all affect lung development to such an extent that the peak FEV_1 attained in early adulthood (see Fig. 20.1) is lower. Irrespective of the subsequent rate of decline of FEV_1, a value less than 80% of predicted at age 40 years leads to a substantially greater risk of developing COPD.[60]

The cellular mechanisms underlying airway inflammation in COPD relate to the disease's strong association with smoking, with activation of neutrophils and macrophages (page 239) rather than the eosinophils and mast cells seen in asthma. Neutrophil activation, in response to stimulation by IL-17,[61] causes the release of several protease enzymes which degrade pulmonary elastin, leading to the loss of lung tissue elasticity—a characteristic feature of COPD. Smoking also induces oxidative stress in the airways which is exacerbated in patients with COPD by reactive oxygen species generated by activated inflammatory cells and cytokines.[62] These pathological changes have been likened to accelerated ageing of the lungs, opening potential new therapeutic options.[43]

The role of obesity in patients with COPD is described in Chapter 15.

Three pathophysiological changes give rise to COPD: emphysema, mucous hypersecretion of larger airways and small airway obstruction.

Emphysema

Emphysema is defined as permanent enlargement of airspaces distal to the terminal bronchiole accompanied by destruction of alveolar walls. The process begins by enlargement of normal interalveolar holes, followed by destruction of the entire alveolar septum, and potentially also involves structural damage to terminal bronchioles.[63] Both ventilation and perfusion ($\dot{V}$ and $\dot{Q}$) of the emphysematous area are reduced, although some mismatch still occurs, normally resulting in lung areas with $\dot{V}/\dot{Q}$ ratios greater than one (see Fig. 7.9, *C*) which, if widespread, will contribute to alveolar dead space (page 99). The loss of alveolar surface area with emphysema impairs pulmonary-diffusing capacity and reduces the surface forces at the air–water interface (page 14), resulting in highly compliant lung tissue. As

emphysema becomes more widespread collateral ventilation between adjacent lung regions develops. This may have beneficial effects in preventing emphysematous lung from collapsing when airway obstruction occurs, as ventilation can continue from the adjacent lung tissue.[64] This strategy is an effective way of matching $\dot{V}$ and $\dot{Q}$ in many animal species (page 310). Unfortunately, in humans collateral ventilation also limits the success of techniques aimed at treating emphysema by isolating affected lung regions (page 402). Finally, the loss of elastic tissue contained within the alveolar septa reduces the elastic recoil of the pulmonary tissue contributing to the closure of small airways, particularly during expiration.

Current views on the cellular defect responsible for emphysema involve the relationship between protease and antiprotease activity in the lung. These enzymes are normally released following activation of neutrophils (e.g., neutrophil elastase) or macrophages in response to tobacco smoke or infection. A deficiency of the most well-known antiprotease, α_1-antitrypsin, is a significant risk factor for early development of emphysema (page 167). Disturbances of other protease–antiprotease systems, such as the matrix metalloproteases group of enzymes, are also involved in the generation of emphysema, as these proteases are normally involved in remodelling of the extracellular lung matrix. Proteases with activity against elastin are likely to be responsible for generating emphysema. Elastin deposition in the lung occurs early in life, and is minimal beyond late adolescence. Later, any pulmonary elastin lost through disease is likely to be replaced with collagen, so reducing lung elasticity and probably explaining the general decline in lung recoil throughout life.

Airway Obstruction

Narrowing of small airways plays a major role in COPD, but its aetiology is controversial. Part of the expiratory air flow limitation results from emphysema, as described previously, and the remainder is because of changes in the airway wall itself. Inflammatory changes in small airways are ubiquitous in COPD, and there is extensive remodelling of airway components, including epithelial cell hyperplasia and collagen deposition in the adventitia (outer layer) of the airway wall.[19] In some terminal bronchioles these changes lead to thickening of the airway wall, while other bronchioles are destroyed, resulting in an overall decline in small airway numbers, the combination of which results in irreversible and clinically significant obstruction.[65]

Large airway disease consists of goblet cell hyperplasia, mucosal oedema and production of excessive amounts of mucus, a key component of chronic bronchitis.[66] Recurrent respiratory tract infections and smoking undoubtedly contribute, and a chronic productive cough is the result. This feature of COPD is not always present, and its contribution to overall airway obstruction is variable.

Hyperinflation

Air flow limitation in small airways results from a combination of airway narrowing and loss of elastic recoil of lung tissue. The latter is of major importance in maintaining the patency of airways less than 1 mm in diameter (page 6), which lack supporting cartilage in their walls. Expiratory flow limitation leads to prolonged expiratory time constants in affected lung units and incomplete expiration (gas trapping). Lung volume is therefore forced to increase, and the patient becomes dyspnoeic, particularly during any situation that requires a greater minute volume, such as exercise. Hyperinflation of the lung will, in theory, tend to oppose expiratory airway closure (see Fig. 3.5), but it also causes a significant reduction in the efficiency of the respiratory muscles. In particular, the diaphragm becomes displaced caudally, reducing the zone of apposition (see Fig. 5.1), and in severe disease is flattened, causing much of the muscle activity to either oppose the opposite side of the diaphragm or pull the lower ribcage inwards rather outwards (see Fig. 5.2). In time, lung hyperinflation becomes permanent, with expansion of the chest wall (barrel chest) and irreversible flattening of the diaphragm.

Respiratory Muscles in Chronic Obstructive Pulmonary Disease

The diaphragm, and to a lesser extent the intercostal muscles, is abnormal in patients with COPD. The fibre type shifts towards fatigue-resistant type 1 fibres (page 66), and the contractile mechanisms of the fibres become less efficient.[59] Whether these changes result from the chronic stretching of the diaphragm caused by hyperinflation, from systemic inflammation as a result of the COPD or from lack of physical activity by the patient is unknown, but the effect is to further impair the ventilatory capacity.

Principles of Therapy[44]

As for asthma, detailed guidelines for the treatment of COPD are published, this time on a global rather than national scale.[67] Nonmedical procedures used to treat emphysema are described on page 402.

Smoking Cessation (page 239)

This is central to all forms of treatment for COPD. The long-term benefit in terms of the progressive decline in lung function depends on the age at which permanent smoking cessation occurs (see Fig. 20.1). Patients with COPD have often been heavy smokers for a considerable number of years, and smoking cessation may therefore need great determination and support. Patients usually only become permanent nonsmokers after multiple attempts at quitting, although nicotine replacement and other drug therapies may improve this poor success rate.

Medical Treatment[68]

Inhaled bronchodilators may be used. Their efficacy depends on the reversibility of the airways disease in each patient. Both β_2-agonists and anticholinergic drugs (page 35 et seq) are used, usually with long-acting drugs which seem to be effective at reducing the frequency and severity of COPD exacerbations. Corticosteroids tend not to be as effective for treating COPD as they are for asthma. The inflammatory cells involved are different (Fig. 28.2), and may be less susceptible to steroid suppression. Nevertheless, some patients benefit from using a steroid as well as the two bronchodilators. This so-called 'triple therapy' may be particularly effective if delivered with ultrafine particle inhalers (median diameter <2 μm) to provide better drug delivery to the small airways (page 166).[69] These drugs are effective at improving symptoms, and so quality of life, and reducing the frequency of exacerbations, but have no effect on the long-term decline in lung function seen with COPD or long-term survival.[70]

Long-Term Supplemental Oxygen[71]

At low inspired concentrations for 15 to 18 hours a day, oxygen improves survival in patients with severe COPD associated with hypoxia. Thresholds for the Sa_{O_2} that merits oxygen therapy vary between countries, but are around 88%, with oxygen flows aiming to increase this to greater than 90%. There is no evidence to support using nocturnal oxygen therapy to slow the development of pulmonary hypertension from nocturnal desaturations.

Pulmonary Rehabilitation[72]

This is now a key part of treating COPD, and the term embraces a combination of patient education and support alongside a regular, supervised exercise programme. At least five sessions of 30 minutes of physical activity per week are recommended, with two to three of these under the supervision of a healthcare worker, and continued for at least 6 weeks, preferably longer. There is good evidence that these interventions increase exercise capacity and reduce dyspnoea symptoms. However, the long-term benefits are less clear,[73] and the focus has now moved on to management of those patients who decline to join, or do not complete, a rehabilitation programme.[74]

Oxygen Therapy in Chronic Obstructive Pulmonary Disease[75]

Respiratory failure is common in patients with COPD, particularly during exacerbations, and may be either type 1 or type 2 (page 316). Which pattern occurs in an individual patient depends on the relative contributions of airway disease, emphysema and loss of lung elasticity, along with their chemoreceptor sensitivities to oxygen and carbon dioxide. Whatever the type of their respiratory failure, administration of oxygen to patients with severe COPD can lead to hypercapnia. Two main mechanisms are believed to be responsible.

Ventilatory depression by oxygen is seen in patients with type 2 respiratory failure who may be relying on their hypoxic drive to maintain ventilation. If this is abolished, for example, by the achievement of a normal or high arterial P_{O_2}, hypoventilation may result. However, studies investigating oxygen-induced hypercapnia in COPD have failed to find consistent changes in minute ventilation during either periods of stable respiratory symptoms or acute exacerbations. Reduction in minute ventilation in response to oxygen was either too small to explain adequately the changes in P_{CO_2}, or only transient, returning towards baseline ventilation after a few minutes. Nevertheless, in one of these reports,[76] of 22 subjects studied, two developed severe respiratory depression leading to dangerous hypercapnia after just 15 minutes of breathing 100% oxygen. A small proportion of patients with COPD therefore seem to be susceptible to oxygen-induced respiratory depression.

Altered ventilation perfusion relationships with oxygen have been proposed to explain hypercapnia seen in COPD patients in whom minute ventilation remains essentially unchanged.[76,77] Alveolar P_{O_2} is known to contribute to hypoxic pulmonary vasoconstriction (page 80) and help to minimize $\dot{V}/\dot{Q}$ mismatch. Administration of oxygen may therefore abolish hypoxic pulmonary vasoconstriction in poorly ventilated areas, increasing blood flow to these areas and reducing blood flow to other lung regions with normal or high $\dot{V}/\dot{Q}$ ratios. These areas will then contribute further to alveolar dead space causing an increase in arterial P_{CO_2} (page 99).

Which of these mechanisms predominates in an individual patient is impossible to predict. Whatever the cause there is now widespread agreement that uncontrolled oxygen therapy in patients with exacerbations of COPD is potentially harmful, with increasing F_{IO_2} in the prehospital stage of treatment associated with increased mortality.[78] Administration of oxygen to patients with COPD must therefore be undertaken with great care, and always titrated to oxygen saturation (page 295).

Cystic Fibrosis[79]

CF is an autosomal recessive genetic disorder affecting Caucasian individuals, of whom 1 in 25 carry the gene. The disease affects approximately 1 in 3000 births, and abnormal CF genes can be identified prenatally. Prediction of phenotype from genetic screening is complex because there is a wide spectrum of clinical disease, the severity of which is determined by environmental factors (e.g., smoking) and genetic modifiers of the abnormal CF gene. Mortality from CF remains high, but has been improving for some years, and the anticipated life expectancy for a person born with CF in the year 2000 is now 50 years.[80] Although the number of CF births is constant, improved survival means that the prevalence of CF is increasing steadily.

CF affects epithelial cell function in many body systems, but gastrointestinal and respiratory functions are the most important; this chapter discusses only the latter. Abnormalities of pulmonary airway defence mechanisms lead to lifelong colonization of the CF lung with bacteria. Recurrent airway infection produces hypersecretion of mucus, cough

and, over many years, destruction of normal lung architecture, including bronchiectasis.

Aetiology of Cystic Fibrosis

Biochemical Abnormality

The gene responsible for CF is located on chromosome 7 and codes for a protein named cystic fibrosis transmembrane conductance regulator (CFTR) found in epithelial cells. The CFTR protein has multiple functions, primarily as a membrane-bound active chloride channel, but with other potential roles including bicarbonate–chloride exchange, control of sodium and water transport and regulation of epithelial cell permeability through an effect on tight junctions.[81] CFTR therefore plays a major role in controlling salt concentration in epithelial secretions. Sweat production is influenced by CFTR function, allowing measurement of the sodium concentration in sweat to remain a relatively simple investigation for diagnosis,[82] as it is over twice normal in CF patients.

The CFTR comprises three types of protein subunit, which are assembled in a complex series of posttranslational modifications.[83] A ring of membrane-spanning domains form a channel through the lipid bilayer of the cell wall (Fig. 28.5). Attached to the intracellular aspect of these are two nucleotide-binding domains (NBDs) that use adenosine triphosphate (ATP) when the channel is activated. Finally, a single regulatory domain protein is loosely attached to the NBDs and can move away from them to 'open' the channel and allow chloride to pass into or out of the cell (Fig. 28.5). Intracellular protein kinase A activates the channel by binding to the regulatory domain of CFTR, whereas ATP provides the energy and is dephosphorylated by the NBDs. Over 1000 different mutations of the CF gene have been identified, and can result in absent or insufficiently functional CFTR protein, a misfolded CFTR protein which is quickly degraded, an abnormal protein which is degraded before it can be incorporated into the membrane or protein which is appropriately positioned in the membrane but nonfunctional.[84] In normal subjects the CFTR protein also acts by inhibiting nearby epithelial sodium channels, a link which is believed to be defective in CF, further impairing the regulation of airway-lining fluid (ALF; page 166).

Causes of Lung Disease

The sequence of events by which abnormal CFTR function leads to pulmonary pathology remains controversial. Abnormalities of the airway-lining fluid and mucus result in poor defences against inhaled pathogens because of impaired mucociliary clearance. Bacterial colonization occurs early in the disease process, and CF patients have an exaggerated inflammatory response to a variety of airway pathogens.[85] A cycle becomes established in which bacterial infection leads to airway inflammation, mucus production and more infection, associated with progressive lung tissue damage. Abnormal CFTR function may adversely affect the

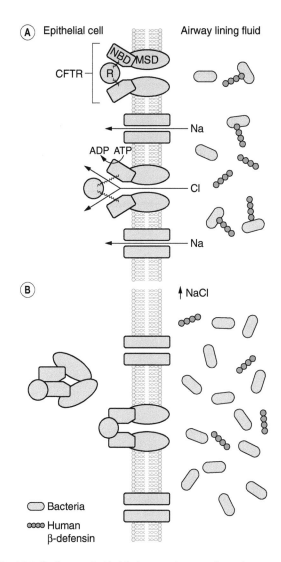

A Epithelial cell   Airway lining fluid

CFTR

NBD MSD

R

Na

ADP ATP

Cl

Na

B

↑ NaCl

Bacteria

Human β-defensin

• **Fig. 28.5** Sodium and chloride transport across the pulmonary epithelial cell wall in cystic fibrosis. **(A)** Normal lung. Cystic fibrosis transmembrane regulator *(CFTR)* chloride channel in the closed (upper) and open (lower) positions, showing movement of the regulator domain *(R)*. Sodium transport follows chloride via passive sodium channels because of altered transmembrane potentials. Bacteria in the airway lining fluid may be inactivated by human β-defensin. **(B)** Cystic fibrosis. The CFTR proteins are defective, so do not locate in the membrane, or are nonfunctional when they do. Sodium and chloride concentrations are therefore abnormally high in the airway, which may inactivate human β-defensin or alter airway-lining fluid function, allowing bacterial proliferation. *ADP,* Adenosine 5′-diphosphate; *ATP,* adenosine triphosphate; *MSD,* Membrane-spanning domain; *NBD,* nucleotide-binding domain.

ability of the airway to remove inhaled pathogens by a variety of mechanisms, as follows.

Salt-defensin hypothesis. The human lung produces a variety of endogenous antibiotics, of which the most studied is human β-defensin (HBD), which may play an important role in preventing pulmonary infection. Consisting of a 64–amino acid peptide, HBD has been shown to be inactivated by increased sodium chloride concentrations

or low pH, so allowing proliferation of bacteria in CF lungs (Fig. 28.5).[86]

Inflammation first hypothesis. This proposes that airway inflammation is the primary event in CF lungs, possibly caused by abnormal cell signalling by the CFTR-deficient epithelial cells.[87] Inflammation may originate from dysregulated innate immune function in the respiratory epithelium, leading to colonization with pathogens early in the course of the disease.[88]

Cell-receptor hypothesis. In normal lung, the CFTR found on epithelial cells, along with a range of cell surface glycoproteins, binds many bacterial pathogens as part of the normal process for killing inhaled microorganisms. Low pH around epithelial cells from CF lung inhibits the binding of lung pathogens found in CF.

Depleted airway lining fluid hypothesis.[89] Despite the altered sodium and chloride transport in CF lung epithelial cells, the 'sol', or periciliary layer of the ALF (page 165) is believed to be isotonic. However, the volume of periciliary fluid is reduced, and this disturbs the physical linkage between the cilia and the periciliary and mucous layers of ALF, effectively preventing the normal clearance of the ALF. The mucous layer becomes abnormally deep, which inhibits the function of endogenous antimicrobial systems such as HBD, lactoferrin and lysozyme, and also creates a layer of hypoxic mucus in which anaerobic bacteria can thrive.

Principles of Therapy[90]

Conventional treatment primarily involves assisting the clearance of airway secretions by physiotherapy, postural drainage and exercise. The mucous layer in patients with CF is not usually highly viscous, but is abnormally tenacious or adhesive, and so difficult to clear.[91] The tenacity of the mucus results in part from degradation of the numerous inflammatory cells found in infected airways, and it is DNA from these cells that can aggregate and further increase viscosity. Treatment with inhaled recombinant human DNase will break down DNA molecules or, more recently, inhaled poly-L-lysine will compact the molecules in the sputum,[91] and both have been shown to improve sputum clearance. Antibiotic therapy, for both infective exacerbations and maintenance therapy, is now used for all patients, and is believed to be the main reason for improved survival in CF.

Drug treatment.[92] Drugs have now been developed that can correct some of the defects in the CFTR protein. In the G551D mutation, which affects only 5% of CF patients, the CFTR protein localizes correctly in the membrane but has a defective opening of the channel gate. Ivacaftor is a drug which partially corrects the defect, and in clinical use leads to significant improvements in the clinical picture. Around half of CF patients are homozygous for the F508del mutation in which CFTR posttranslational folding is incomplete, causing the protein to remain attached to the endoplasmic reticulum. Lumacaftor administration partially corrects the abnormal folding, and so increases the amount of CFTR located in the membrane, but the protein is still functionally abnormal, and its activity can be further enhanced by also adding ivacaftor, with good clinical results.[93] Other drugs continue to be developed.[94]

Lung transplantation is a recognized treatment for CF, and is described in Chapter 33.

Correcting the Abnormal Cystic Fibrosis Transmembrane Conductance Regulator

Gene therapy held great potential ever since the CF gene was identified in 1989, but unfortunately this potential has not been realized. A normal *CFTR* gene can be produced, but the problem arises in incorporating the gene into the airway cells and stimulating its expression into functioning CFTR protein in vivo. Gene delivery either in liposomes or viral vectors has been attempted, but the functional effect is poor, with only transient or small changes in CFTR expression. A more promising strategy is the recent development of drugs which can improve CFTR production or function in some of the specific mutations causing CF, and there have been encouraging early clinical results.[95]

References

1. Papi A, Brightling C, Pedersen SE, et al. Asthma. *Lancet.* 2018; 391:783-800.
2. Sears MR. Trends in the prevalence of asthma. *Chest.* 2014; 145:219-225.
3. Anderson HR, Gupta R, Strachan DP, et al. 50 years of asthma: UK trends from 1955 to 2004. *Thorax.* 2007;62:85-90.
4. Wijesinghe M, Weatherall M, Perrin K, et al. International trends in asthma mortality rates in the 5- to 34-year age group. A call for closer surveillance. *Chest.* 2009;135:1045-1049.
*5. Svenningsen S, Kirby M, Starr D, et al. **What are ventilation defects in asthma?** *Thorax.* **2014;69:63-71.**
6. Dame Carroll JR, Magnussen JS, Berend N, et al. Greater parallel heterogeneity of airway narrowing and airway closure in asthma measured by high-resolution CT. *Thorax.* 2015;70:1163-1170.
7. Harris RS, Winkler T, Tgavalekos N, et al. Regional pulmonary perfusion, inflation, and ventilation defects in bronchoconstricted patients with asthma. *Am J Respir Crit Care Med.* 2006;174:245-253.
8. Leary D, Winkler T, Braune A, et al. Effects of airway tree asymmetry on the emergence and spatial persistence of ventilation defects. *J Appl Physiol.* 2014;117:353-362.
9. Moore WC, Meyers DA, Wenzel SE, et al. Identification of asthma phenotypes using cluster analysis in the Severe Asthma Research Program. *Am J Respir Crit Care Med.* 2010;181: 315-323.
10. Chung KF. Targeting the interleukin pathway in the treatment of asthma. *Lancet.* 2015;386:1086-1096.
11. Moldaver DM, Larché M, Rudulier CD. An update on lymphocyte subtypes in asthma and airway disease. *Chest.* 2017;151:1122-1130.
12. Renz H. Asthma protection with bacteria—science or fiction? *Thorax.* 2011;66:744-745.
13. Stelmaszczyk-Emmel A. Regulatory T cells in children with allergy and asthma: it is time to act. *Respir Physiol Neurobiol.* 2015;209: 59-63.
14. Cosmi L, Annunziato F. Group 2 innate lymphoid cells are the earliest recruiters of eosinophils in lungs of patients with allergic asthma. *Am J Respir Crit Care Med.* 2017;196:666-668.
15. Tanabe T, Rubin BK. Airway goblet cells secrete pro-inflammatory cytokines, chemokines, and growth factors. *Chest.* 2016;149: 714-720.
16. Lindén A, Dahlén B. Interleukin-17 cytokine signalling in patients with asthma. *Eur Respir J.* 2014;44:1319-1331.
17. Hulme KM, Salome CM, Brown NJ, et al. Deep inspiration volume and the impaired reversal of bronchoconstriction in asthma. *Respir Physiol Neurobiol.* 2013;189:506-512.
18. Bhatawadekar SA, Inman MD, Fredberg JJ, et al. Contribution of rostral fluid shift to intrathoracic airway narrowing in asthma. *J Appl Physiol.* 2017;122:809-816.
*19. Hirota N, Martin JG. **Mechanisms of airway remodeling.** *Chest.* **2013;144:1026-1032.**
20. James AL, Elliot JG, Jones RL, et al. Airway smooth muscle hypertrophy and hyperplasia in asthma. *Am J Respir Crit Care Med.* 2012;185:1058-1064.
21. Kaczmarek KA, Clifford RL, Knox AJ. Epigenetic changes in airway smooth muscle as a driver of airway inflammation and remodeling in asthma. *Chest.* 2019;155:816-824.
22. Oliver BGG, Black J. Asthma: airways that are hyperactive by design. *Am J Respir Crit Care Med.* 2016;193:596-598.
23. Weiss ST, Litonjua AA, Vitamin D. Vitamin D, the gut microbiome, and the hygiene hypothesis. How does asthma begin? *Am J Respir Crit Care Med.* 2015;191:492-493.
24. Steinke JW. Can genes control asthmatic lung function patterns? *Am J Respir Crit Care Med.* 2016;194:1439-1451.
25. Holgate ST, Holloway JW. Is big beautiful? The continuing story of ADAM33 and asthma. *Thorax.* 2005;60:263-264.
26. Von Hertzen L, Haahtela T. Con: house dust mites in atopic diseases. Accused for 45 years but not guilty? *Am J Respir Crit Care Med.* 2009;180:113-119.
27. Camargo Jr CA. Human rhinovirus, wheezing illness, and the primary prevention of childhood asthma. *Am J Respir Crit Care Med.* 2013;188:1281-1282.
28. Calhoun WJ, Dick EC, Schwartz LB, et al. A common cold virus, rhinovirus 16, potentiates airway inflammation after segmental antigen bronchoprovocation in allergic subjects. *J Clin Invest.* 1994;94:2200-2208.
29. Rook GAW, Adams V, Hunt J, et al. Mycobacteria and other environmental organisms as immunomodulators for immunoregulatory disorders. *Springer Semin Immunopathol.* 2004;25:237-255.
30. Weber J, Illi S, Nowak D, et al. Asthma and the hygiene hypothesis. Does cleanliness matter? *Am J Respir Crit Care Med.* 2015;191:522-529.
31. Chatila TA. Innate immunity in asthma. *N Engl J Med.* 2016; 375:477-479.
32. Sbihi H, Koehoorn M, Tamburic, et al. Asthma trajectories in a population-based birth cohort impacts of air pollution and greenness. *Am J Respir Crit Care Med.* 2017;195:607-613.
33. Young MT, Sandler DP, DeRoo LA, et al. Ambient air pollution exposure and incident adult asthma in a nationwide cohort of U.S. women. *Am J Respir Crit Care Med.* 2014;190:914-921.
34. Holgate ST. The acetaminophen enigma in asthma. *Am J Respir Crit Care Med.* 2011;183:147-151.
*35. White AA, Stevenson DD. **Aspirin-exacerbated respiratory disease.** *N Engl J Med.* **2018;379:1060-1070.**
36. Jenkins C, Costello J, Hodge L. Systematic review of prevalence of aspirin induced asthma and its implications for clinical practice. *BMJ.* 2004;328:434-437.
37. Dixon AE. Long-acting β-agonists and asthma: the saga continues. *Am J Respir Crit Care Med.* 2011;184:1220-1221.
38. Gerber AN. Glucocorticoids and airway smooth muscle: Some answers, more questions. *Am J Respir Crit Care Med.* 2013;187:1040-1041.

39. Drazen JM. A step toward personalized asthma treatment. *N Engl J Med.* 2011;365:1245-1246.

40. Platts-Mills TAE, Woodfolk JA. Mite avoidance as a logical treatment for severe asthma in childhood. Why not? *Am J Respir Crit Care Med.* 2017;196:119-121.

41. Bardin PG, Price D, Chanez P, et al. Managing asthma in the era of biological therapies. *Lancet Respir.* 2017;5:376-378.

42. McGregor MC, Krings JG, Nair P, Castro M. Role of biologics in asthma. *Am J Respir Crit Care Med.* 2019;199:433-445.

43. Barnes PJ. Senescence in COPD and its comorbidities. *Annu Rev Physiol.* 2017;79:517-539.

44. Rabe KF, Watz H. Chronic obstructive pulmonary disease. *Lancet.* 2017;389:1931-1940.

45. Viegi G, Pistelli F, Sherrill DL, et al. Definition, epidemiology and natural history of COPD. *Eur Respir J.* 2007;30:993-1013.

46. Burney PGJ, Patel J, Newson R, et al. Global and regional trends in COPD mortality, 1990–2010. *Eur Respir J.* 2015;45:1239-1247.

47. Maclay JD, MacNee W. Cardiovascular disease in COPD: Mechanisms. *Chest.* 2013;143:798-807.

48. Aaron SD. Management and prevention of exacerbations of COPD. *BMJ.* 2014;349:g5237.

49. Barnes PJ. Asthma-COPD overlap. *Chest.* 2016;149:7-8.

50. Hynes G, Pavord ID. Asthma-like features and chronic obstructive pulmonary disease. *Am J Respir Crit Care Med.* 2016;194:1308-1309.

51. Morse D, Rosas IO. Tobacco smoke–induced lung fibrosis and emphysema. *Annu Rev Physiol.* 2014;76:493-513.

52. Pierrou S, Broberg P, O'Donnell RA, et al. Expression of genes involved in oxidative stress responses in airway epithelial cells of smokers with chronic obstructive pulmonary disease. *Am J Respir Crit Care Med.* 2007;175:577-586.

53. Zhou W, Liu S, Hu J, et al. Nicotine reduces the levels of surfactant proteins A and D via Wnt/ β-catenin and PKC signalling in human airway epithelial cells. *Respir Physiol Neurobiol.* 2015;221:1-10.

54. Yang J, Zuo W, Fukui T, et al. Smoking-dependent distal-to-proximal repatterning of the adult human small airway epithelium. *Am J Respir Crit Care Med.* 2017;196:340-352.

55. Boezen HM, Mannino DM. The future of nature versus nurture in understanding chronic obstructive pulmonary disease. *Am J Respir Crit Care Med.* 2013;188:891-892.

*56. Martinez FD. Early-life origins of chronic obstructive pulmonary disease. *N Engl J Med.* 2016;375:871-878.

57. Jiang Z, Lao T, Qiu W, et al. A chronic obstructive pulmonary disease susceptibility gene, FAM13A, regulates protein stability of β-catenin. *Am J Respir Crit Care Med.* 2016;194:185-197.

58. Skronska-Wasek W, Mutze K, Baarsma HA, et al. Reduced frizzled receptor 4 expression prevents WNT/β-catenin–driven alveolar lung repair in chronic obstructive pulmonary disease. *Am J Respir Crit Care Med.* 2017;196:172-185.

*59. Mattes J, Gibson PG. The early origins of COPD in severe asthma: the one thing that leads to another or the two things that come together? *Thorax.* 2014;69:789-790.

*60. Lange P, Celli B, Agustí A, et al. Lung-function trajectories leading to chronic obstructive pulmonary disease. *N Engl J Med.* 2015;373:111-122.

61. Bozinovski S, Vlahos R. Multifaceted role for IL-17A in the pathogenesis of chronic obstructive pulmonary disease. *Am J Respir Crit Care Med.* 2015;191:1213-1214.

62. Kirkham PA, Barnes PJ. Oxidative Stress in COPD. *Chest.* 2013;144:266-273.

63. Mitzner W. Emphysema—a disease of small airways or lung parenchyma? *N Engl J Med.* 2011;365:1637-1639.

64. Cetti EJ, Moore AJ, Geddes DM. Collateral ventilation. *Thorax.* 2006;61:371-373.

65. MacNee W, Murchison JT. Small airway disease or emphysema: which is more important in lung function and FEV1 decline? An old story with a new twist. *Am J Respir Crit Care Med.* 2016;194:129-130.

66. Wedzicha JA. Airway mucins in chronic obstructive pulmonary disease. *N Engl J Med.* 2017;377:986-987.

67. Vogelmeier CF, Criner GJ, Martinez FJ, et al. Global strategy for the diagnosis, management, and prevention of chronic obstructive lung disease 2017 report. GOLD executive summary. *Am J Respir Crit Care Med.* 2017;195:557-582.

68. Celli BR. Pharmacological therapy of COPD. Reasons for optimism. *Chest.* 2018;154:1404-1415.

69. Papi A, Vestbo J, Fabbri L, et al. Extrafine inhaled triple therapy versus dual bronchodilator therapy in chronic obstructive pulmonary disease (TRIBUTE): a double-blind, parallel group, randomised controlled trial. *Lancet.* 2018;391:1076-1084.

70. Aaron SG. Reaching for the holy grail of chronic obstructive pulmonary disease outcomes can medications modify lung function decline? *Am J Respir Crit Care Med.* 2018;197:2-3.

*71. Lacasse Y, Tan A-YM, Maltais F, et al. Home oxygen in chronic obstructive pulmonary disease. *Am J Respir Crit Care Med.* 2018;197:1254-1264.

72. Spruit MA, Singh SJ, Garvey C, et al. An official American Thoracic Society/European Respiratory Society statement: key concepts and advances in pulmonary rehabilitation. *Am J Respir Crit Care Med.* 2013;188:e13-e64.

73. Evans RA, Steiner MC. Pulmonary rehabilitation: the lead singer of COPD therapy but not a "one-man band". *Chest.* 2017;152:1103-1105.

74. Singh SJ, Steiner MC. Pulmonary rehabilitation; what's in a name? *Thorax.* 2013;68:899-901.

75. O'Driscoll BR, Howard LS, Earis J, et al. BTS guideline for oxygen use in adults in healthcare and emergency settings. *Thorax.* 2017;72:i1-i90.

76. Aubier M, Murciano D, Milic-Emili J, et al. Effects of the administration of O_2 on ventilation and blood gases in patients with chronic obstructive pulmonary disease during acute respiratory failure. *Am Rev Respir Dis.* 1980;122:747-754.

77. Crossley DJ, McGuire GP, Barrow PM, et al. Influence of inspired oxygen concentration on deadspace, respiratory drive, and $Paco_2$ in intubated patients with chronic obstructive pulmonary disease. *Crit Care Med.* 1997;25:1522-1526.

78. Wijesinghe M, Perrin K, Healy B, et al. Pre-hospital oxygen therapy in acute exacerbations of chronic obstructive pulmonary disease. *Intern Med J.* 2011;41:618-622.

79. Elborn JS. Cystic fibrosis. *Lancet.* 2016;388:2519-2531.

80. Dodge JA, Lewis PA, Stanton M, et al. Cystic fibrosis mortality and survival in the UK: 1947–2003. *Eur Respir J.* 2007;29:522-526.

81. Csanády L, Vergani P, Gadsby DC. Structure, gating, and regulation of the CFTR anion channel. *Physiol Rev.* 2019;99:707-738.

82. Simmonds NJ, Bush A. Diagnosing cystic fibrosis: what are we sweating about? *Thorax.* 2012;67:571-573.

83. McClure ML, Barnes S, Brodsky JL, et al. Trafficking and function of the cystic fibrosis transmembrane conductance regulator: a complex network of posttranslational modifications. *Am J Physiol Lung Cell Mol Physiol.* 2016;311:L719-L733.

84. Rogan MP, Stoltz DA, Hornick DB. Cystic fibrosis transmembrane conductance regulator intracellular processing, trafficking, and opportunities for mutation-specific treatment. *Chest.* 2011;139:1480-1490.

85. Zemanick ET, Accurso FJ. Cystic fibrosis transmembrane conductance regulator and Pseudomonas. *Am J Respir Crit Care Med.* 2014;189:763-765.

86. Stoltz DA, Meyerholz DK, Welsh MJ. Origins of cystic fibrosis lung disease. *N Engl J Med.* 2015;372:351-362.

87. Cohen-Cymberknoh M, Kerem E, Ferkol T, et al. Airway inflammation in cystic fibrosis: molecular mechanisms and clinical implications. *Thorax*. 2013;68:1157-1162.

88. Stick SM, Kicic A, Ranganathan S. Of pigs, mice, and men: understanding early triggers of cystic fibrosis lung disease. *Am J Respir Crit Care Med*. 2016;194:784-785.

89. Haq IJ, Gray MA, Garnett JP, et al. Airway surface liquid homeostasis in cystic fibrosis: pathophysiology and therapeutic targets. *Thorax*. 2016;71:284-287.

90. Heltshe SL, Cogen J, Ramos KJ, et al. Cystic fibrosis: the dawn of a new therapeutic era. *Am J Respir Crit Care Med*. 2017;195:979-984.

91. Rubin BK. Faster, higher, stronger. *Am J Respir Crit Care Med*. 2013;188:634-635.

92. Gentzsch M, Mall MA. Ion channel modulators in cystic fibrosis. *Chest*. 2018;154:383-393.

93. Davis PB. Another beginning for cystic fibrosis therapy. *N Engl J Med*. 2015;373:274-276.

94. Grasemann H. CFTR modulator therapy for cystic fibrosis. *N Engl J Med*. 2017;377:2085-2087.

95. Massie J, Castellani C, Grody WW. Carrier screening for cystic fibrosis in the new era of medications that restore CFTR function. *Lancet*. 2014;383:923-925.

29

Pulmonary Vascular Disease

KEY POINTS

- Pulmonary oedema occurs when increases in pulmonary capillary pressure or the permeability of the alveolar/capillary membrane cause fluid to accumulate in the interstitial space and alveoli.
- Pulmonary embolism, with either thrombus or air, partially occludes the pulmonary circulation, causing an increase in alveolar dead space and pulmonary arterial hypertension.
- Pulmonary hypertension most commonly results from long-term hypoxia or elevated left atrial pressure and involves reduced nitric oxide production and remodelling of the pulmonary blood vessels.

Pulmonary Oedema

Pulmonary oedema is defined as an increase in pulmonary extravascular water, which occurs when transudation or exudation exceeds the capacity of the lymphatic drainage. In its more severe forms, there is free fluid in the alveoli.

Anatomical Factors

The pulmonary capillary endothelial cells abut against one another at fairly loose junctions which are of the order of 5 nm wide. These junctions permit the free passage of quite large molecules, including albumin. On their luminal surface endothelial cells are lined by endothelial glycocalyx (EG), which is a complex layer of macromolecules bound to the cell surface that acts as a passive barrier to large molecules and water, controlling permeability of the endothelium (see later).[1,2] The endothelial cell and EG barrier allows some macromolecules to pass through, and pulmonary lymph contains albumin at about half the concentration in plasma. Alveolar epithelial cells are connected by tight junctions at their alveolar surface, with a gap of only about 1 nm. Under normal circumstances the tightness of these junctions prevents the escape of large molecules, such as albumin, from the interstitial fluid into the alveoli. However, the proteins that make up the tight junction are not simply passive structural units, and can, for example, in response to nitric oxide, be modified and allow an increase in permeability across the tight junction.[3]

The lung has a well-developed lymphatic system draining the interstitial space through a network of channels around the bronchi and pulmonary vessels towards the hilum. Lymphatic vessels are seen in the juxtaseptal alveolar region (see later discussion) and are commonly found in association with bronchioles. Down to airway generation 11 (see Table 1.1), the lymphatics lie in a potential space around the air passages and vessels, separating them from the lung parenchyma. In the hilum of the lung, the lymphatic drainage passes through several groups of tracheobronchial lymph glands, where they receive tributaries from the superficial subpleural plexus. Most of the lymph from the left lung usually enters the thoracic duct, whereas the right side drains into the right lymphatic duct.

The normal lymphatic drainage from human lungs is astonishingly small—only about 10 mL per hour. However, lymphatic flow can increase up to 10 times this value when transudation into the interstitial space is increased. This presumably occurs when pulmonary oedema is threatened, but it cannot be conveniently measured in humans.

Pulmonary Fluid Dynamics

For intravascular fluid to enter the alveoli it must traverse three barriers. First, it must move from the microcirculation into the interstitial space (across the EG and endothelium), second through the interstitial space and finally from the interstitial space into the alveoli (across the epithelium; Fig. 29.1).

Fluid Exchange Across the Endothelium[4]

This is promoted by the hydrostatic pressure difference between capillary and interstitial space but counteracted by the osmotic pressure of the plasma proteins. The balance of pressures is normally sufficient to prevent any appreciable transudation, but it may be upset in a wide variety of pathological circumstances.

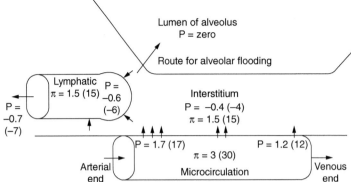

P = Hydrostatic pressure (kPa or cmH₂O) – relative to atmosphere
π = Protein osmotic pressure (kPa or cmH₂O)

• **Fig. 29.1** Normal values for hydrostatic and plasma protein osmotic pressures in the pulmonary microcirculation and interstitial space.

It is customary to display the relationship between fluid flow and the balance of pressures in the form of the Starling equation. For the endothelial barrier this is as follows:

$$\dot{Q} = K[(P_C - P_{IS}) - \Sigma(\Pi_C - \Pi_{IS})],$$

$\dot{Q}$ is the flow rate of transudated fluid which, in equilibrium, will be equal to the lymphatic drainage.

K is the hydraulic conductance (i.e., flow rate of fluid per unit pressure gradient across the endothelium).

P_C is the hydrostatic pressure in the pulmonary capillary.

P_{IS} is the hydrostatic pressure in the interstitial space.

Σ is the reflection coefficient, in this case applying to albumin. It is an expression of the permeability of the endothelium to the solute (albumin). A value of unity indicates total reflection corresponding to zero concentration of the solute in the interstitial fluid. A value of zero indicates free passage of the solute across the membrane and, with equal concentrations on both sides of the membrane, the solute could exert no osmotic pressure across the membrane. This normally applies to the crystalloids in plasma.

Π_C is the osmotic pressure the solute exerts within the pulmonary capillary.

Π_{IS} is the osmotic pressure the solute exerts in the interstitial space.

Under normal circumstances in humans, the pulmonary lymph flow $\dot{Q}$ is about 10 mL per hour, with a protein content about half that of plasma. The pulmonary microvascular pressure (P_C) is in the range of 0 to 2 kPa (0–15 mmHg) relative to atmosphere, depending on the vertical height in the lung field. Furthermore, there is a progressive decrease in capillary pressure from its arterial to its venous end because approximately one-half the pulmonary vascular resistance is across the capillary bed (see Figs 6.2 and 29.1). In this context, it is meaningless to think of a single value for the mean pulmonary capillary pressure.

The hydrostatic pressure in the interstitial space (P_{IS}) of the lung is not easy to measure, but from animal studies was measured as approximately −0.40 to −1.25 kPa (−4 to −12.5 cmH₂O).[5] In the excised lung there was no vertical gradient in interstitial pressures such as might have been expected from the effect of gravity, but this was observed when measurements were made with the chest and pleura intact.[5]

The reflection coefficient for albumin (Σ) in the healthy lung is about 0.5. The overall osmotic pressure gradient between blood and interstitial fluid is about 1.5 kPa (11.5 mmHg). Thus there is a fine balance between forces favouring and opposing transudation. There is a considerable safety margin in the upper part of the lung, where the capillary hydrostatic pressure is lowest. However, in the dependent part of the lung, where the hydrostatic pressure is highest, the safety margin is slender.

Like many physiological principles that are several decades old the Starling equation model for capillary fluid movements is an oversimplification. In particular, the EG plays a vital, but incompletely understood, role.[1,2] For example, in lung tissue the hydraulic conductance for the endothelium–EG complex is probably not constant, as assumed in the Starling equation, and may vary in different lung regions, with different inflation pressures or at different vascular pressures. Damage to the EG structure by a variety of pathological processes will then result in greater permeability to water and other molecules, leading to oedema.

Fluid Dynamics Within the Interstitial Space

The interstitial space does not simply act as a passive conduit for fluid transfer to the lymphatics. Proteoglycan and hyaluron molecules are present in the pulmonary interstitial space of animals, and they function like a gel to absorb water to minimize increase in interstitial pressure and prevent hydration of other extracellular structures such as collagen. Regional differences in the properties of these molecules are believed to be responsible for the establishment of a pressure gradient between the septal interstitial space and the juxtaseptal region where lymphatic channels originate. This gradient may promote, and allow some control of, fluid flow from the endothelium to the lymphatics in the normal lung.

With increased fluid transfer across the endothelium, the interstitial space can accommodate large volumes of water with only small increases in pressure, and the interstitial compliance is high. About 500 mL can be accommodated in the interstitial space and lymphatics of the human lungs with a rise of pressure of only about 0.2 kPa (2 cmH$_2$O). Eventually, the capacity of the molecules to absorb water is exceeded, and the proteoglycan structure breaks down, possibly leading to disturbances of nearby collagen molecules and therefore basement membrane function, producing alveolar oedema.

Fluid Exchange Across the Alveolar Epithelium[6]

The permeability of this barrier to gases is considered in Chapter 8. It is freely permeable to gases, water and hydrophobic substances, but virtually impermeable to albumin. Fluid is actively cleared from the alveoli in normal human lungs.[2] For methodological reasons, most studies of this system have involved type II alveolar epithelial cells, but the same processes are believed to occur in type I cells and in club cells in the distal airways. On the alveolar side of the cells, the cell membrane contains epithelial sodium channels[7] and cystic fibrosis transmembrane regulator channels (page 334), which actively pump sodium and chloride ions, respectively, into the cell. On the interstitial border of the cells, chloride moves passively out of the cell, and the Na$^+$/K$^+$-ATPase channel actively removes sodium from the cell. Water from the alveolus follows these ion transfers down an osmotic gradient into the interstitial space. Aquaporins are found in human alveolar epithelial cells, suggesting that transcellular water movement may be facilitated by these water channel proteins, but their role in lungs remains unclear, and paracellular water movement probably is more important.[6]

A small amount of active clearance of fluid from the alveoli occurs under normal circumstances, but these systems become vital when pulmonary oedema threatens. Active removal of alveolar fluid by alveolar epithelial cells increases within 1 hour of the onset of oedema.[8] Stimulation of β$_2$-adrenoceptors by catecholamines increases the affinity of existing Na$^+$/K$^+$-ATPase channels for sodium and causes new channels to be incorporated into the cell membrane from intracellular endosomal stores. After a few hours, a variety of hormones[8] (e.g., thyroxine, aldosterone, glucocorticoids) and cytokines (e.g., tumour necrosis factor) induce the transcription of new Na$^+$/K$^+$-ATPase channels and increase fluid clearance. These mechanisms are important both for minimizing the severity of pulmonary oedema and clearing oedema fluid once the precipitating cause has resolved.

Stages of Pulmonary Oedema

There is presumably a prodromal stage in which pulmonary lymphatic drainage is increased, but there is no increase in extravascular water. This may progress to the following stages.

Stage I: Interstitial Pulmonary Oedema

In its mildest form there is an increase in interstitial fluid, but without passage of oedema fluid into the alveoli. With the light microscope this is first detected as cuffs of distended lymphatics, typically '8'-shaped around the adjacent branches of the bronchi and pulmonary artery (Fig. 29.2). There is fluid accumulation in the alveolar septa. but this is confined to the 'service' side of the pulmonary capillary which contains the stroma, leaving the geometry of the 'active' side unchanged (see page 8 and Fig. 1.8). Thus gas exchange is better preserved than might be expected from the overall increase in lung water.

Physical signs are generally minimal in stage I, except perhaps for mild dyspnoea, particularly with exercise. The alveolar/arterial Po$_2$ gradient is normal or only slightly increased.

Stage II: Crescentic Filling of the Alveoli

With further increase in extravascular lung water, interstitial oedema of the alveolar septa is increased, and fluid begins to pass into some alveolar lumina. It first appears as crescents in the angles between adjacent septa, at least in lungs which have been fixed in inflation (Fig. 29.2). The centre of the alveoli and most of the alveolar walls remain clear, and gas exchange is not grossly abnormal, but dyspnoea at rest is likely, and the characteristic butterfly shadow may be visible on the chest radiograph.

Stage III: Alveolar Flooding

In the third stage, there is quantal alveolar flooding. Some alveoli are totally flooded, whereas others, frequently adjacent, have only the crescentic filling or else no fluid at all in their lumina. It seems that fluid accumulates up to a point at which a critical radius of curvature results in surface tension, sharply increasing the transudation pressure gradient. This produces flooding on an all-or-none basis for each individual alveolus. Because of the effect of gravity on pulmonary vascular pressures (page 77), alveolar flooding tends to occur in the dependent parts of the lungs. Rales can be heard during inspiration, and the lung fields show an overall opacity superimposed on the butterfly shadow.

Clearly there can be no effective gas exchange in the capillaries of an alveolar septum which is flooded on both sides, and blood flow through these alveoli constitutes shunt. This results in an increased alveolar/arterial Po$_2$ gradient and hypoxaemia, which may be life-threatening. Blood flow to the oedematous lung regions is slightly reduced by hypoxic pulmonary vasoconstriction (page 80), possibly in conjunction with interstitial swelling causing capillary narrowing, but the shunt commonly remains substantial.

Hypercapnia is not generally a problem. In less severe pulmonary oedema, there is usually an increased respiratory drive, due partly to hypoxaemia and partly to stimulation of vagal nociceptors (page 48). As a result the Pco$_2$ is usually normal or somewhat decreased.

Stage IV: Froth in the Air Passages

When alveolar flooding is extreme, the air passages become blocked with froth, which moves to and fro with breathing. This effectively stops all gas exchange and is rapidly fatal unless treated.

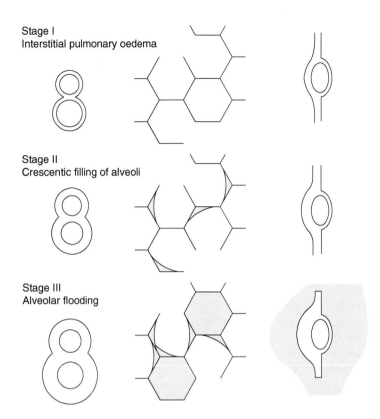

Stage I
Interstitial pulmonary oedema

Stage II
Crescentic filling of alveoli

Stage III
Alveolar flooding

• **Fig. 29.2** Schematic diagram of the stages in the development of pulmonary oedema. On the left is shown the development of the cuff of distended lymphatics around the branches of the bronchi and pulmonary arteries. In the middle is the appearance of the alveoli by light microscopy (fixed in inflation). On the right is the appearance of the pulmonary capillaries by electron microscopy. The active side of the capillary is to the right. See text for details.

Aetiology of Pulmonary Oedema

On the basis of the Starling equation, it is possible to make a rational approach to the aetiology of pulmonary oedema. There are three groups of aetiological factors, classified according to their effect on components of the Starling equation.

Increased Capillary Pressure (Haemodynamic Pulmonary Oedema)

This group comprises the commonest causes of pulmonary oedema. There is an elevation of the hydrostatic pressure gradient across the pulmonary capillary wall, until it exceeds the osmotic pressure of the plasma proteins. Interstitial fluid accumulates until it overwhelms the ability of the interstitial space to absorb fluid and transport it to the lymphatics. Fluid then begins to enter the alveoli and will initially be actively removed by the alveolar epithelial cells until this system is also overwhelmed. The oedema fluid has a protein content which is less than that of normal pulmonary lymph or plasma. Apart from transudation in accord with the Starling equation, severe pulmonary capillary hypertension may result in loss of structural integrity (see later).

Causes of an increase in pulmonary capillary pressure are numerous:

- Absolute hypervolaemia may result from excessive or rapid administration of blood or other plasma expanders or from acute renal failure.

- Relative pulmonary hypervolaemia may result from redistribution of the circulating blood volume into the lungs, for example, from the use of the Trendelenburg position or vasopressor drugs that constrict only the systemic circulation redirecting blood into the pulmonary circulation.

- Raised pulmonary capillary pressure will inevitably result from an increase in pulmonary venous pressure, which may occur from any form of left heart failure. In this situation the severe exercise-induced dyspnoea is believed to result from increased dead space secondary to reduced pulmonary blood flow.[9]

- Increased pulmonary blood flow may raise the pulmonary capillary pressure sufficiently to precipitate pulmonary oedema. This may result from a left-to-right cardiac shunt, anaemia or, rarely, as a result of exercise.

Increased Permeability of the Capillary/ Endothelial Glycocalyx/Alveolar Barrier (Permeability Oedema)

This group comprises the next commonest causes of pulmonary oedema. The mechanism is the loss of integrity of the capillary/EG/alveolar barrier, allowing albumin and other macromolecules to enter the alveoli. The osmotic pressure gradient which opposes transudation is then lost. The oedema fluid has a protein content that approaches that of plasma.

'Stress failure' of the pulmonary capillaries occurs when the pulmonary capillary pressure is increased in the range of 3 to 5 kPa (30–50 cmH$_2$O). Discontinuities appear in the capillary endothelium and type I alveolar epithelial cells, whereas the basement membrane often remains intact. This seems to result in increased permeability and leakage of protein into the alveoli. High-altitude pulmonary oedema (page 213) is an example of this mechanism.

Decreased Osmotic Pressure of the Plasma Proteins

The Starling equation indicates that the osmotic pressure of the plasma proteins is a crucial factor opposing transudation. Although seldom the primary cause of pulmonary oedema, a reduced plasma albumin concentration is very common in the seriously ill patient, and it must inevitably decrease the microvascular pressure threshold at which transudation commences.

Other Causes of Pulmonary Oedema

Neurogenic pulmonary oedema may follow head injuries or other cerebral lesions. The existence of pulmonary venous sphincters has provided a possible mechanism for neurogenic pulmonary oedema. Constriction of these sphincters, either the result of circulating adrenaline or a neural response, could cause an abrupt increase in pulmonary capillary pressure. A study of neurogenic pulmonary oedema in humans supported this hypothesis by demonstrating that the oedema fluid often has a low protein content suggesting a haemodynamic mechanism (see previous discussion).

Negative pressure pulmonary oedema occurs when a patient attempts to overcome severe airway obstruction by generating extreme negative intrathoracic pressures.[10] The low-protein nature of oedema fluid in these patients also suggests its origin is simply the increased hydrostatic pressure gradient between capillary and interstitial space. Fortunately, once the airway obstruction is resolved the oedema usually resolves within hours.

Reexpansion pulmonary oedema is described on page 361, and pulmonary oedema following lung resection on page 407.

Principles of Therapy

Immediate treatment aims to restore the arterial Po$_2$ to normal values. The inspired oxygen concentration should be increased up to 100% if necessary. Sitting the patient up is a simple way to reduce central blood volume. Treatment of the underlying cause of pulmonary oedema follows directly from the Starling equation and an understanding of the aetiology.

Haemodynamic Pulmonary Oedema

Treatment aims to reduce left atrial pressure. Depending on the aetiology, treatment is directed towards improvement of left ventricular function and/or reduction of blood volume. The latter may be quickly and easily achieved by peripheral vasodilatation. Drugs that predominantly dilate the capacitance (venous) system, such as nitrates or angiotensin-converting enzyme inhibitors, will be most effective. This mechanism is probably also responsible for the beneficial effects of furosemide and diamorphine in the acute situation. Diuretics act more slowly but are useful for long-term treatment. Essentially the patient is titrated to the left along his or her Frank–Starling curve (Fig. 29.3). In addition, the curve is moved upwards and to the left, if this is possible, using positive inotropes as an adjunct to correction of left ventricular malfunction, for example, from ischaemia.

Permeability Pulmonary Oedema

Treatment should be directed towards restoration of the integrity of the capillary/EG/alveolar barrier. Unfortunately, no particularly successful measures are available towards this end. It is, however, important to minimize left atrial pressure, even though this is not the primary cause of the oedema. Attempts may be made to increase the plasma albumin concentration if it is reduced.

Artificial Ventilation and Positive End-Expiratory Pressure

Severe pulmonary oedema causes degrees of hypoxia that may quickly be lethal. Trachaeal intubation and positive pressure ventilation is therefore commonly required, and the results are often spectacular. Froth in the airways may be aspirated, and any areas of atelectasis occurring along with the oedema improved. Artificial ventilation is often combined with positive end-expiratory pressure (PEEP), resulting in further improvements in arterial Po$_2$. It was originally thought that the positive pressure drove the fluid back into the circulation, but evidence that extravascular lung water is reduced by PEEP is contradictory, with few human studies. Animal studies of pulmonary oedema indicate that, by increasing the lung volume, the capacity of the interstitial space to hold liquid is increased.[11] Similarly, with haemodynamic pulmonary oedema in animals, PEEP does not alter the total amount of lung water, but a greater proportion is in the extraalveolar interstitial space, and lymphatic drainage is increased.[12] With haemodynamic pulmonary oedema positive pressure ventilation has beneficial effects on the function of the failing heart (page 389), and it is probably this effect, rather than any effect on the lungs, that causes the clinical benefit in humans.

Measurement of Extravascular Lung Water

Measurement of lung water in the intact subject is difficult. Two techniques are described for use in patients. A double indicator method uses the same techniques as for the measurement of pulmonary or central blood volume by dye dilution, but with two indicators. One indicator is chosen to remain within the circulation (usually indocyanine green), whereas the other diffuses into the interstitial fluid (usually 'coolth', i.e., cold saline). Extravascular lung water is then derived as the difference between the volumes as

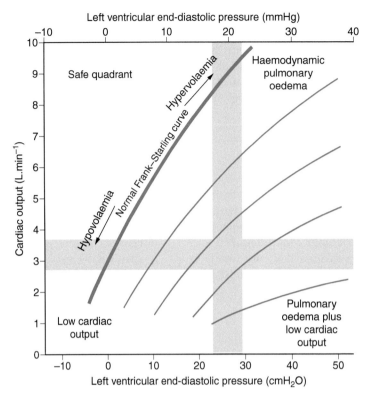

• **Fig. 29.3** Quadrant diagram relating cardiac output to left ventricular end-diastolic pressure. The thick blue curve is a typical normal Frank–Starling curve. To the right are shown curves representing progressive left ventricular failure. *Top left* is the safe quadrant, which contains a substantial part of the normal curve, but much less of the curves representing ventricular failure. *Top right* is the quadrant representing normal cardiac output but raised left atrial pressure, attained at the upper end of relatively normal Frank–Starling curves (e.g., hypervolaemia). There is a danger of haemodynamic pulmonary oedema. *Bottom left* is the quadrant representing normal or low left atrial pressure but low cardiac output, attained at the lower end of all curves (e.g., hypovolaemia). The patient is in shock. *Bottom right* is the quadrant representing both low cardiac output and raised left atrial pressure. There is simultaneous danger of pulmonary oedema and shock, and the worst Frank–Starling curves hardly leave this quadrant.

measured with the two indicators. The single indicator method also uses coolth as the indicator, and relies on analysis of the shape of the indicator decay curve to assess both intrathoracic blood and total water volumes, because the curves for these two compartments decay at different rates. Both methods have been validated against ex vivo techniques and are suitable for use in critical care.

Pulmonary Embolism

The pulmonary circulation may be occluded by embolism, which may be gas, thrombus, fat, tumour or foreign body. The architecture of the microvasculature is well adapted to minimize the effects of embolism. Large numbers of pulmonary capillaries tend to arise at right angles from metarterioles, and there are abundant anastomoses throughout the microcirculation. This tends to preserve circulation distal to the impaction of a small embolus. Nevertheless, a large pulmonary embolus is a serious and potentially lethal condition.

Thromboembolism

The most common pulmonary embolus consists of detached venous thromboses from veins in the thigh and the pelvic venous plexuses. Smaller thrombi are filtered in the lungs without causing symptoms, but larger emboli may impact in major vessels, typically at a bifurcation forming a saddle embolus. There may be a catastrophic increase in pulmonary vascular resistance with acute right heart failure or cardiac arrest.

Diagnosis of Pulmonary Thromboembolus[13]

Massive pulmonary thromboembolus causes sudden cardiac arrest and death, with many only being diagnosed at autopsy[14] and around 15% of symptomatic cases proving rapidly fatal. Conversely, small pulmonary emboli are common and completely asymptomatic, with the incidence varying between different patient groups but occurring in around 3% of patients having computed tomography (CT) scans.[15] For patients with intermediate-sized emboli, a combination of pleuritic chest pain, dyspnoea and tachypnoea is indicative of pulmonary embolus. Changes in the electrocardiogram following pulmonary embolus reflect disturbed right-sided cardiac function secondary to elevated pulmonary arterial pressure, are generally nonspecific and typically only occur after a large embolism. Measurement of fibrin D-dimer indicates degradation of fibrin somewhere in the body, and may help to exclude pulmonary embolism if the value is low. A variety of imaging techniques are available, with CT scanning now regarded as the investigation of choice for diagnosis of pulmonary thromboembolism (Fig. 29.4). Pulmonary radioisotope perfusion or ventilation–perfusion scans may detect smaller emboli not seen with CT scanning, but the technique has low sensitivity.[13]

Pathophysiology

Three mechanisms give rise to the physiological changes seen in pulmonary embolism. First is physical occlusion of the pulmonary vascular system. Second, platelet activation within the thrombus leads to release of 5-hydroxytryptamine (5-HT, serotonin) and thromboxane A_2, causing a further increase in pulmonary vascular resistance. Finally, the right ventricle commonly is unable to overcome the raised pulmonary vascular resistance, and cardiac output falls, eventually culminating in right heart failure.

The primary respiratory lesion is an increase in alveolar dead space with an increased arterial/end-tidal $P\text{CO}_2$ gradient. Carbon dioxide elimination is therefore reduced, and if ventilation remains unchanged arterial $P\text{CO}_2$ slowly climbs, until elimination is restored in spite of the large dead space. However, in awake patients hypercapnia is unusual because hyperventilation is almost always present, and arterial $P\text{CO}_2$ is usually below the normal range. The cause of respiratory stimulation is unclear, but may involve stimulation of nociceptors as in air embolism (see later), or hypoxia if present.

Arterial $P\text{O}_2$ is also decreased. This results from derangement of normal ventilation/perfusion ($\dot{V}/\dot{Q}$) relationships. Initially, although cardiac output remains normal, partial obstruction of the pulmonary circulation results in excessive blood flow to those lung regions that are still perfused, giving a low $\dot{V}/\dot{Q}$ ratio in these areas. When cardiac output begins to decrease as a result of a failing right ventricle pulmonary perfusion will fall below normal levels and low

mixed venous oxygen content will exacerbate the abnormal $\dot{V}/\dot{Q}$ relationships (page 103). Elevated right atrial pressures, as a consequence of pulmonary hypertension, may cause right-to-left intracardiac shunting through an unsuspected patent foramen ovale (page 164).

Bronchospasm is a well-recognized complication, and has been attributed to the 5-HT released from platelets and also to local hypocapnia in the part of the lung without effective pulmonary circulation. Pulmonary compliance may be reduced with large pulmonary emboli, but the mechanism of this change is unknown. Pulmonary infarction, which might be expected to occur, is rarely a problem. The lung can obtain oxygen directly from air within the airways and alveoli, from backflow along pulmonary veins and from the bronchial circulation. Only when these sources are also impaired does infarction occur, for example, when localized pulmonary oedema or pulmonary haemorrhage into the airways occurs in conjunction with embolism.

Principles of Therapy[13]

Anticoagulation with intravenous heparin is the mainstay of treatment, and prevents further clot from forming, either in lung or elsewhere, and allows endogenous fibrinolysis to proceed. If right ventricular dysfunction occurs or haemodynamic instability is present because of a low cardiac output, thrombolytic therapy may also be used. Thrombolysis aims to reperfuse lung tissue, but carries a high risk of bleeding complications and is safer if performed with lower doses delivered by a central catheter directly into the pulmonary circulation.[16] Thrombus removal is reserved for patients with significant pulmonary embolism who have a high predicted mortality.

Air Embolism

An embolus may arise from pneumothorax or pulmonary barotrauma but is most commonly iatrogenic. In neurosurgery, the usual cause of air embolism is the use of the sitting position for posterior fossa surgery. A subatmospheric venous pressure at the operative site allows air to enter dural veins, which are held open by their structure. In open cardiac surgery, it is almost impossible to remove all traces of air from the cardiac chambers before closing the heart. Some small degree of air embolism is almost inevitable in all types of intravenous therapy, but catastrophic air embolism can occur when compression bags are used to accelerate the flow rate of intravenous fluids or blood bags that accidentally already contain air.

Detection of Air Embolism

Early diagnosis of air embolism is essential in neurosurgery, and there are three principal methods in routine use. Bubbles in circulating blood give a very characteristic sound with a precordial Doppler probe. The method is, if anything, too sensitive, because a shower of very small bubbles produces a particularly large signal. The simplest method is based on the end-expired carbon dioxide concentration,

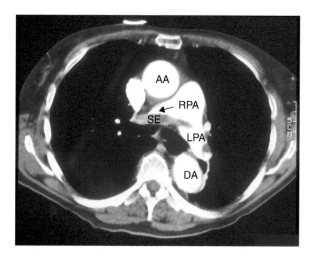

• **Fig. 29.4** Spiral computed tomographic scan of a pulmonary thromboembolus. Intravenous contrast injected immediately before scanning makes the blood vessels appear white. Emboli then appear as darker areas within the blood vessel lumen. Saddle embolus *(SE)* situated mainly in the right pulmonary artery *(RPA)*. *AA*, Ascending aorta; *DA*, descending aorta; *LPA*, left pulmonary artery.

which is easily measured from capnography. Many factors influence the end-expiratory concentration (page 130), but a sudden decrease is likely to be either cardiac arrest or air embolism. Transoesophageal echocardiography is an efficient method of detecting air embolism and, furthermore, it is the only practicable method of detecting paradoxical air embolism (see later).

Pathophysiology of Air Embolus

Provided there is no major intracardiac right-to-left shunt, small quantities of air are filtered out by the lungs where they are gradually excreted, and little harm results. Alveolar dead space is increased according to the proportion of the pulmonary circulation that is occluded. The resultant increase in arterial/end-expiratory P_{CO_2} gradient is the basis of detection of air embolism by capnography as previously described. Pulmonary arterial pressure is increased by a large embolus caused by the right ventricle working against an increased pulmonary vascular resistance.

Massive air embolism (probably in excess of 100 mL) may cause cardiac arrest by accumulation in the right ventricle, where compression of the air bubble prevents ventricular ejection of blood. Treatment then requires aspiration of air through a cardiac catheter, which is difficult.

Paradoxical Air Embolism

Rarely, there may be passage of air emboli from the right to left heart without an overt right-to-left shunt. This is important because air then enters the systemic arterial circulation where there may be embolism and infarction, particularly of the brain. It is possible to pass a probe through such a foramen ovale in over 25% of the adult population (page 164), but paradoxical embolism does not usually occur because pressure is slightly higher in the left atrium than in the right. However, under many circumstances, such as following pulmonary embolism, right atrial pressure may be elevated to the point that a right-to-left shunt occurs.

Fat Embolism

Fracture of long bones or major orthopaedic surgery may be associated with fat embolism.[17] This term is not strictly correct, as the features of 'fat embolism syndrome' result from release of bone marrow microemboli. Some degree of fat embolism occurs in almost all patients having hip and knee replacement surgery, but clinical sequelae occur in less than 1% of these.

Microscopic intravascular bone marrow fragments promote intravascular coagulation and platelet adherence, particularly under the conditions of venous stasis present during surgery, and so develop into larger 'mixed' emboli. There is initially an increase in physiological dead space, but this is soon accompanied by an increase in shunt. Release of inflammatory mediators in the lung causes bronchospasm, increases capillary permeability and leads to localized pulmonary oedema.[17]

Lipid seems to pass through the pulmonary circulation to invade the systemic circulation. Surface forces between blood and lipid are much less than between blood and air, and so would not offer the same hindrance to passage through the lungs. In the systemic circulation, fat emboli cause characteristic petechiae in the anterior axillary folds, and there is often evidence of cerebral involvement.

Amniotic Fluid Embolism[18,19]

Amniotic fluid embolism occurs rarely during delivery, affecting around 1.7 in 100 000 births in the UK, but it is fatal in 19% of cases. Death normally results from cardiovascular disturbances and haemorrhage secondary to coagulopathy. Pulmonary vascular resistance is increased, but animal studies indicate that pulmonary hypertension is only transient, returning to normal after just a few minutes. Disseminated intravascular coagulation soon occurs, leading to a profound coagulopathy and major haemorrhage. The reasons for the effect on the pulmonary circulation remain unclear. Amniotic fluid and foetal cells in the circulation may not cause cardiovascular changes, and an immune-mediated response involving mast cell degranulation or complement activation is thought to be the most likely source of vasoactive mediators causing the clinical syndrome.[19]

Pulmonary Hypertension

Pulmonary arterial hypertension (PAH), defined as a mean pulmonary artery pressure of greater than 25 mmHg, initially presents with progressive dyspnoea, but ultimately leads to right heart failure (cor pulmonale) and death.[20,21] Three-year survival rates from diagnosis are between 55% and 73%.[22] There are many causes which are classified as either primary or secondary (Table 29.1). The latter is much more common and is therefore considered first.

Secondary Pulmonary Arterial Hypertension

Respiratory disease. Pulmonary vascular resistance is increased by almost any pulmonary disease that results in chronic hypoxia (Table 29.1). Similar changes occur with residence at high altitude or intermittent hypoxia caused, for example, by sleep apnoea (Chapter 14). The change is initially temporary and reversible, but progresses to become permanent as pulmonary vasculature remodelling occurs (see later).

Left heart disease. Valvular disease of the left heart leads to an elevation of pressure in the left atrium and pulmonary veins. Increases in pulmonary capillary pressure from this tend to be long-term, and again lead to remodelling of the pulmonary circulation. A low cardiac output, either from the original valvular heart disease or the resulting right heart failure, results in reduction of mixed venous P_{O_2}, which then causes further increases in pulmonary vascular resistance.

TABLE 29.1 Causes of Pulmonary Hypertension

Primary	Secondary		
	RESPIRATORY	CARDIAC	OTHER
Primary pulmonary hypertension	COPD	Left heart failure	Sleep apnoea
Hepatopulmonary syndrome	Emphysema	Valvular disease	Lupus
	Pulmonary fibrosis	Congenital disease	Scleroderma
	Cystic fibrosis		Rheumatoid arthritis
	Chronic embolism		HIV infection
			Vasculitis
			High altitude
			Schistosomiasis

COPD, Chronic obstructive pulmonary disease; *HIV*, human immunodeficiency virus.

Respiratory and left-heart disease account for 97% of cases in resource-rich countries, but in resource-limited regions over half of cases result from congenital and rheumatic heart disease, schistosomiasis and residence at high altitude.[23]

Treatment should first be directed towards improving the underlying condition, particularly if this is causing chronic or intermittent hypoxia. Long-term administration of oxygen, during the day and during sleep, is beneficial and recommended for any patient with hypoxia and PAH.[21] Pulmonary vasodilator therapy is discussed in the next section.

Primary Pulmonary Arterial Hypertension

PAH occurring in the absence of hypoxia is termed primary PAH and has a prevalence of approximately 127 per 100 000 population.[23] It is a progressive disease which normally presents in early adulthood. There is a familial contribution to primary PAH, and it may rarely be associated with advanced liver disease or the use of some older appetite-suppressant drugs or current recreational drugs such as metamphetamine.[24] Prognosis is poor, with most patients dying within 3 years of diagnosis.

Pathophysiology of Vascular Remodelling

The disease is characterized by proliferation of endothelial cells, hypertrophy of pulmonary arterial smooth muscle and thrombosis within pulmonary vessels. As the process progresses, fibrosis develops in both the intima and adventitia of the vessels,[25] rendering them permanently inelastic. Abnormal endothelial function is believed to be where the primary defect occurs, and a range of inflammatory pathways are activated, which leads to activation of fibroblasts and macrophages.[26] Endothelin (page 84) is likely to be implicated because levels are known to be elevated in patients with pulmonary hypertension, and endothelin is known to be a powerful proliferative cytokine.[27] Another likely contributor is hypoxia-inducible factor (page 276) activation, as this initiates a host of inflammatory pathways and cellular remodelling in pulmonary arteries.[25]

Treatment[20,21]

In recent years a variety of drugs have been developed that lower pulmonary arterial pressures (page 83), all of which are now used for treating PAH. Prostacyclin and its analogues are the mainstays of PAH therapy, particularly now that implantable parenteral devices[28] and orally active agents are becoming available. Many different drugs that slow or reverse remodelling are now under development.[29] Endothelin receptor antagonists are also now in routine use, and have been shown to both improve symptoms and prolong survival.[30] Primary PAH remains a common indication for lung transplantation (Chapter 33).

Hepatopulmonary Syndrome

Hepatopulmonary syndrome (HPS) describes the combination of liver disease, pulmonary vascular dilatation and impaired oxygenation.[31] In this syndrome the pulmonary circulation becomes abnormally dilated. Pulmonary capillary diameter at rest is normally less than 7 μm, although with physiological increases in cardiac output, for example, during exercise, this may increase up to 15 μm. In HPS pulmonary capillaries can be as large as 100 μm in diameter, and pulmonary arteriovenous or portopulmonary shunts may develop. Hypoxia is therefore the result of widespread areas with low $\dot{V}/\dot{Q}$ ratios, including shunts. With a high cardiac output state, which is common in liver failure, a diffusion barrier also develops when a large blood flow passes through dilated pulmonary capillaries, leaving insufficient time for diffusion of oxygen into the blood (Chapter 8).

Pulmonary capillary dilatation in HPS results from excessive nitric oxide (NO) production. What stimulates the excess NO production is unknown, with contenders including production of endothelin-1 or tumour necrosis factor alpha (TNFα). Excessive production of carbon monoxide by the haemoxygenase system has also been implicated, as carboxyhaemoglobin levels are high in patients with HPS.[32]

Treatment of HPS with NO antagonists has shown variable results, although using a TNFα antagonist may be useful for its prevention. Liver transplantation reverses the syndrome, although the time taken for the lung to recover is variable.

References

*1. Collins SR, Blank RS, Deatherage LS, et al. The endothelial glycocalyx: emerging concepts in pulmonary edema and acute lung injury. *Anesth Analg.* 2013;117:664-674.

2. Woodcock TE, Woodcock TM. Revised starling equation and the glycocalyx model of transvascular fluid exchange: an improved paradigm for prescribing intravenous fluid therapy. *Br J Anaesth.* 2012;108:384-394.

3. Bhattacharya J. The alveolar water gate. *Am J Physiol Lung Cell Mol Physiol.* 2004;286:L257-L258.

4. Simmons S, Erfinanda L, Bartz C, et al. Novel mechanisms regulating endothelial barrier function in the pulmonary microcirculation. *J Physiol.* 2019;597(4):997-1021.

5. Miserocchi G, Negrini D, Gonano C. Direct measurement of interstitial pulmonary pressure in in situ lung with intact pleural space. *J Appl Physiol.* 1990;69:2168-2174.

6. Matthay MA. Resolution of pulmonary edema thirty years of progress. *Am J Respir Crit Care Med.* 2014;189:1301-1308.

7. Eaton DC, Helms MN, Koval M, et al. The contribution of epithelial sodium channels to alveolar function in health and disease. *Annu Rev Physiol.* 2009;71:403-423.

8. Crandall ED, Matthay MA. Alveolar epithelial transport. Basic science to clinical medicine. *Am J Respir Crit Care Med.* 2001;162:1021-1029.

9. Kee K, Stuart-Andrews C, Ellis MJ, et al. Increased dead space ventilation mediates reduced exercise capacity in systolic heart failure. *Am J Respir Crit Care Med.* 2016;193:1292-1300.

10. Bhattacharya M, Kallet RH, Ware LB, et al. Negative-pressure pulmonary edema. *Chest.* 2016;150:927-933.

11. Gee MH, Williams DO. Effect of lung inflation on perivascular cuff fluid volume in isolated dog lung lobes. *Microvasc Res.* 1979;17:192-196.

12. Mondéjar EF, Mata GV, Cardenas A, et al. Ventilation with positive end-expiratory pressure reduces extravascular lung water and increases lymphatic flow in hydrostatic pulmonary oedema. *Crit Care Med.* 1996;24:1562-1567.

13. Takach Lapner S, Kearon C. Diagnosis and management of pulmonary embolism. *BMJ.* 2013;346:f757.

14. Wiener RS, Schwartz LM, Woloshin S. When a test is too good: how CT pulmonary angiograms find pulmonary emboli that do not need to be found. *BMJ.* 2013;347:f3368.

15. Klok FA, Huisman MV. Management of incidental pulmonary embolism. *Eur Respir J.* 2017;49:1700275.

16. Howard LS. Thrombolysis for PE: less is more? *Thorax.* 2018; 73:412-413.

17. Hofmann S, Huemer G, Salzer M. Pathophysiology and management of the fat embolism syndrome. *Anaesthesia.* 1998;53 (suppl 2):35-37.

18. Tuffnell D, Knight M, Plaat F. Amniotic fluid embolism—an update. *Anaesthesia.* 2011;66:3-6.

19. Metodiev Y, Ramasamy P, Tuffnell D. Amniotic fluid embolism. *Br J Anaesth Educ.* 2018;18:234-238.

*20. Kiely DG, Elliot CA, Sabroe I, et al. Pulmonary hypertension: diagnosis and management. *BMJ.* 2013;346:f2028.

21. Galiè N, Humbert M, Vachiery JL, et al. 2015 ESC/ERS Guidelines for the diagnosis and treatment of pulmonary hypertension. *Eur Respir J.* 2015;46:903-975.

22. Oudiz RJ. Death in pulmonary arterial hypertension. *Am J Respir Crit Care Med.* 2013;188:269-270.

23. Rich S, Haworth SG, Hassoun PM, et al. Pulmonary hypertension: the unaddressed global health burden. *Lancet Respir Med.* 2018;6:577-579.

24. Orcholski ME, Yuan K, Rajasingh C, et al. Drug-induced pulmonary arterial hypertension: a primer for clinicians and scientists. *Am J Physiol Lung Cell Mol Physiol.* 2018;314:L967-L983.

25. Dorfmüller P, Humbert M. Progress in pulmonary arterial hypertension pathology: Relighting a torch inside the tunnel. *Am J Respir Crit Care Med.* 2012;186:210-212.

26. Stenmark KR, Tuder RM, El Kasmi KC. Metabolic reprogramming and inflammation act in concert to control vascular remodeling in hypoxic pulmonary hypertension. *J Appl Physiol.* 2015;119:1164-1172.

27. Pepke-Zaba J, Morrell NW. The endothelin system and its role in pulmonary arterial hypertension (PAH). *Thorax.* 2005;60:443-444.

28. Brown LM. Expanded drug delivery modalities in the treatment of pulmonary arterial hypertension. *Chest.* 2016;150:3-4.

29. Hensley MK, Levine A, Gladwin MT, et al. Emerging therapeutics in pulmonary hypertension. *Am J Physiol Lung Cell Mol Physiol.* 2018;314:L769-L781.

30. Pulido T, Adzerikho I, Channick RN, et al. Macitentan and morbidity and mortality in pulmonary arterial hypertension. *N Engl J Med.* 2013;369:809-818.

31. Rodriguez-Roisin R, Krowka MJ. Hepatopulmonary syndrome—a liver-induced lung vascular disorder. *N Engl J Med.* 2008;358:2378-2387.

32. Arguedas MR, Drake BB, Kapoor A, et al. Carboxyhemoglobin levels in cirrhotic patients with and without hepatopulmonary syndrome. *Gastroenterology.* 2005;128:328-333.

30

Diseases of the Lung Parenchyma and Pleura

KEY POINTS

- Lung collapse occurs either from compression of lung tissue or by absorption of gas from lung units with occluded or severely narrowed airways.
- Many forms of interstitial lung disease exist, varying from purely inflammatory conditions (alveolitis) to those involving progressive fibrosis with minimal lung inflammation.
- Lung fibrosis arises from an imbalance between the cellular systems responsible for inflammation and tissue repair.

- Lung cancer is a common malignancy which is difficult to treat effectively and is mostly preventable by avoiding tobacco smoke and radon exposure.
- Pleural effusion, infection and pneumothorax remain common occurrences, and can all impair respiratory function in the short or long term.

Pulmonary Collapse

Pulmonary collapse may be defined as an acquired state in which the lungs or part of the lungs become airless. Atelectasis is strictly defined as a state in which the lungs of a newborn have never been expanded, but the term is widely used as a synonym for regional pulmonary collapse.

Collapse may be caused by two different mechanisms. The first of these is loss of the forces opposing the elastic recoil of the lung, which then decreases in volume to the point at which airways are closed and gas is trapped behind the closed airways. The second is obstruction of airways at normal lung volume, which may be attributed to many different causes. This also results in trapping of gas behind the obstructed airway. Whatever the cause of the airway closure, there is rapid absorption of the trapped gas because the total partial pressure of gases in mixed venous blood is always less than atmospheric (see Table 25.2). This generates a subatmospheric pressure more than sufficient to overcome any force tending to hold the lung expanded.

Pulmonary collapse during anaesthesia is described in Chapter 21.

Loss of Forces Opposing Retraction of the Lung

The lungs are normally prevented from collapse by the outward elastic recoil of the rib cage and any resting tone of the diaphragm. The pleural space normally contains no gas, but, if a small bubble of gas is introduced, its pressure is

subatmospheric (see Fig. 2.4). Pulmonary collapse because of loss of forces opposing lung retraction may be considered as follows.

1. *Voluntary reduction of lung volume.* It seems unlikely that voluntary reduction of lung volume below closing capacity will cause overt collapse of the lung in a subject breathing air. However, in older subjects, there is an increase in the alveolar/arterial Po_2 gradient, suggesting trapping of alveolar gas (see Fig. 21.10).

2. *Excessive external pressure.* Ventilatory failure is the more prominent aspect of an external environmental pressure in excess of about 6 kPa (60 cmH$_2$O), which is not communicated to the airways (page 319). However, some degree of pulmonary collapse could also occur, and this is a normal consequence of the great depths attained by diving mammals while breath holding (page 311). An approximately normal lung volume is maintained during conventional diving operations when respired gas is maintained at the surrounding water pressure, although this does not occur with surface diving or snorkelling (page 221).

3. *Loss of integrity of the rib cage.* Multiple rib fractures may impair the elastic recoil of the rib cage to the point at which partial lung collapse results. This depends entirely on the extent of the injury to the rib cage, but multiple adjacent ribs fractured in two places will usually result in collapse. However, extensive trauma to the rib cage also causes interference with the mechanics of breathing, which is generally more serious than collapse.

349

4. *Intrusion of abdominal contents into the chest.* Extensive atelectasis results from a congenital defect of the diaphragm. Abdominal contents may completely fill one-half of the chest with total atelectasis of that lung. In adults, similar changes may occur with a large hiatus hernia, or ascites may push the diaphragm into the thoracic cavity. Paralysis of one side of the diaphragm causes the diaphragm to lie higher in the chest, with a tendency to basal collapse on that side.

5. *Space occupation of the pleural space.* Air introduced into the pleural space (pneumothorax) reduces the forces opposing retraction of the lung, and this is a potent cause of collapse (see Fig. 30.5, *A*). The same effect occurs when the pleural space is occupied by an effusion, empyema or haemothorax. Pleural disease is discussed on page 360 et seq.

6. *Hypergravity.* Increased pressure on dependent lung regions as a result of the extreme gravitational forces experienced in military aircraft also causes lung collapse.

Absorption of Trapped Gas

Absorption of alveolar gas trapped beyond obstructed airways may be the consequence of reduction in lung volume by the mechanisms described previously. However, it is the primary cause of collapse when there is total or partial airway obstruction at normal lung volume. Obstruction is commonly attributed to secretions, pus, blood or tumour, but may be caused by local bronchospasm or airway oedema.

Gas trapped beyond the point of airway closure is absorbed by the pulmonary blood flow. The total of the partial pressures of the gases in mixed venous blood is always less than atmospheric (see Table 25.2), although pressure gradients for the individual component gases between alveolar gas and mixed venous blood may be quite different.

The Effect of Respired Gases

If the patient has been breathing 100% oxygen before obstruction the alveoli will contain only oxygen, carbon dioxide and water vapour. Because the last two together normally amount to less than 13.3 kPa (100 mmHg), the alveolar P_{O_2} will usually be in excess of 88 kPa (660 mmHg). However, the P_{O_2} of the mixed venous blood is unlikely to exceed about 6.7 kPa (50 mmHg), so the alveolar/mixed venous P_{O_2} gradient will be of the order of 80% of an atmosphere. Absorption collapse will thus be rapid, and there will be no nitrogen in the alveolar gas to maintain inflation. This has important implications during anaesthesia, when 100% oxygen is commonly administered (page 251).

The situation is much more favourable in a patient who has been breathing air, as most of the alveolar gas is then nitrogen, which is at a partial pressure of only about 0.5 kPa (4 mmHg) below that of mixed venous blood. Alveolar nitrogen partial pressure rises above that of mixed venous blood as oxygen is absorbed, and eventually the nitrogen will be fully absorbed. Collapse must eventually occur, but the process is much slower than in the patient who has been breathing oxygen. Fig. 30.1 shows a computer simulation of the time required for collapse with various gas mixtures.[1] Nitrous oxide/oxygen mixtures may be expected to be absorbed almost as rapidly as 100% oxygen. This is partly because nitrous oxide is much more soluble in blood than

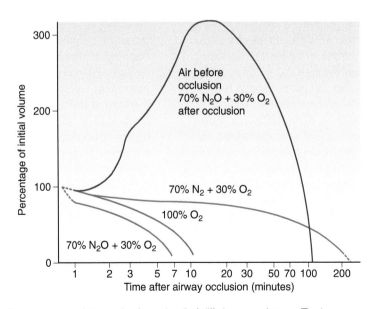

• **Fig. 30.1** Predicted rates of absorption from alveoli of differing gas mixtures. The lower curves show the rate of absorption of the contents of sections of the lung whose air passages are obstructed, resulting in sequestration of the contents. The upper curve shows the expansion of the sequestered gas when nitrous oxide is breathed by a patient who has recently developed regional airway obstruction whilst breathing air. In all other cases, it is assumed that the inspired gas is not changed after obstruction has occurred. Similar considerations apply to closed gas cavities elsewhere in the body. (Reproduced from reference 1 by permission of the publishers of *Anaesthesia*.)

nitrogen, and partly because the mixed venous partial pressure of nitrous oxide is usually much less than the alveolar partial pressure, except after a long period of inhalation.

When the inspired gas composition is changed after obstruction and trapping occur, complex patterns of absorption may ensue. The inhalation of nitrous oxide, after airway occlusion has occurred while breathing air, results in temporary expansion of the trapped volume (Fig. 30.1). This is caused by large volumes of the more soluble nitrous oxide passing from blood to alveolus in exchange for smaller volumes of the less soluble nitrogen passing in the reverse direction. This phenomenon also applies to any closed airspace in the body, such as closed pneumothorax, gas emboli, bowel and the middle ear with a blocked pharyngotympanic (Eustachian) tube. It is potentially dangerous and may contraindicate the use of nitrous oxide as an anaesthetic.

Magnitude of the Pressure Gradients

It needs to be stressed that the forces generated by the absorption of trapped gases are very large. The total partial pressure of gases in mixed venous blood is normally 87.3 kPa (655 mmHg). The corresponding pressure of the alveolar gases is 95.1 kPa (713 mmHg), allowing for water vapour pressure at 37°C. The difference, 7.8 kPa (58 mmHg or 78 cmH$_2$O), is sufficient to overcome any forces opposing

recoil of the lung. Absorption collapse after breathing air may therefore result in drawing the diaphragm up into the chest, reducing rib cage volume or displacing the mediastinum. If the patient has been breathing oxygen the total partial pressure of gases in the mixed venous blood is barely one-tenth of an atmosphere, and absorption of trapped alveolar gas generates enormous forces.

Effect of Reduced Ventilation/Perfusion Ratio

Absorption collapse may still occur in the absence of total airway obstruction, provided the ventilation/perfusion ($\dot{V}/\dot{Q}$) ratio is sufficiently low. Older subjects, as well as those with a pathological increase in scatter of $\dot{V}/\dot{Q}$ ratios, may have substantial perfusion of areas of lung, with $\dot{V}/\dot{Q}$ ratios in the range of 0.01 to 0.1. This shows as a characteristic 'shelf' in the plot of perfusion against $\dot{V}/\dot{Q}$ (Fig. 30.2). These grossly hypoventilated areas are liable to collapse if the patient breathes oxygen (Fig. 30.2, B). If the $\dot{V}/\dot{Q}$ ratio is less than 0.05, ventilation even with 100% oxygen cannot supply the oxygen that is removed (assuming the normal arterial/mixed venous oxygen content difference of 5 mL.dL^{-1}). As the $\dot{V}/\dot{Q}$ ratio decreases below 0.05, so the critical inspired oxygen concentration necessary for collapse also decreases (Fig. 30.2, C). The flat part of the curve between $\dot{V}/\dot{Q}$ ratios of 0.001 and 0.004 means that small

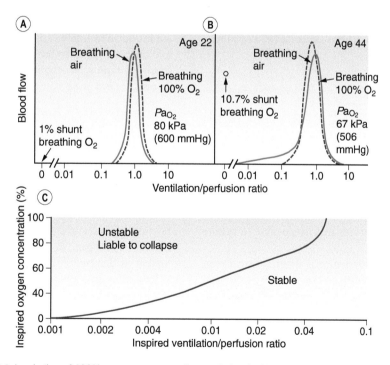

• **Fig. 30.2** Inspiration of 100% oxygen causes collapse of alveoli with very low ventilation/perfusion ($\dot{V}/\dot{Q}$) ratios. **(A)** The minor change in the distribution of blood flow (in relation to $\dot{V}/\dot{Q}$) when a young subject breathes oxygen. Collapse is minimal, and a shunt of 1% develops. **(B)** The changes in an older subject with a 'shelf' of blood flow distributed to alveoli with very low $\dot{V}/\dot{Q}$ ratios. Breathing oxygen causes collapse of these alveoli, and this is manifested by disappearance of the shelf and development of an intrapulmonary shunt of 10.7%. **(C)** The inspired oxygen concentration relative to the inspired $\dot{V}/\dot{Q}$ ratio that is critical for absorption collapse. (From Wagner PD, Laravuso RB, Uhl RR, et al. Continuous distributions of ventilation-perfusion ratios in normal subjects breathing air and 100% O$_2$. *J Clin Invest.* 1974;54:54-68, by permission of the publishers of the *Journal of Clinical Investigation*; and Dantzker DR, Wagner PD, West JB. Instability of lung units with low $\dot{V}$A/$\dot{Q}$ ratios during O$_2$ breathing. *J Appl Physiol.* 1975;38:886-895, by permission of the publishers of *Journal of Applied Physiology.*)

differences in inspired oxygen concentration in the range of 20% to 30% may be very important in determining whether collapse occurs or not. In lung regions with these very low $\dot{V}/\dot{Q}$ ratios collapse is therefore likely to occur, but still not inevitable—a modelling study suggests that lung recoil is crucial for maintaining airway patency even with apnoeic ventilation of the alveoli.[2]

Diagnosis of Pulmonary Collapse

The diagnosis may be made on physical signs of decreased air entry and chest dullness, but reliance is usually placed on chest radiography. Pulmonary opacification is seen, along with indirect signs of thoracic volume loss, such as displacement of interlobular fissures, raised diaphragms and displaced hilar or mediastinal structures.[3,4] In the upright position, collapse is commonest in the basal segments, often concealed behind the cardiac shadow unless the exposure is appropriate. Areas of atelectasis are clearly seen with computed tomography (CT; see Fig. 21.9).

Collapse results in a reduction in pulmonary compliance, but the value of this in diagnosis is limited by the wide scatter of normal values. A sudden reduction in compliance may give an indication of collapse, provided, of course, that control measurements were available before collapse. Collapse also reduces the functional residual capacity and arterial P_{O_2}. However, in a patient with impaired oxygenation a reduction in arterial P_{O_2} cannot distinguish between the three very common conditions of collapse, consolidation or oedema of the lungs.

Principles of Therapy

Therapy depends on the physiological abnormality. Factors opposing the elastic recoil of the lung should be removed wherever possible. For example, pneumothorax, pleural effusion and ascites may be corrected. In other cases, particularly impaired integrity of the chest wall, it may be necessary to treat the patient with artificial ventilation. Reexpansion of collapsed lung often requires high pressures to be applied (page 251), but it is usually possible to restore normal lung volume.

When collapse is caused by regional airway obstruction, the most useful methods in both treatment and prevention are by chest physiotherapy (page 375), combined when necessary with tracheobronchial toilet, through either a tracheal tube or a bronchoscope.

Voluntary maximal inspirations are effective in clearing areas of absorption collapse and this manoeuvre is the basis of the 'incentive spirometer', which is used to prevent postoperative lung collapse.

With artificial ventilation a logical approach is hyperinflation of the chest or an artificial 'sigh'. Some ventilators were designed to provide an intermittent 'sigh', but evidence of its efficacy was never found. Current strategies to prevent pulmonary collapse during artificial ventilation are described in Chapter 32.

Pulmonary Consolidation (Pneumonia)

Inflammation of areas of lung parenchyma, usually because of infection, can lead to the accumulation of exudate within the alveoli and small airways, causing consolidation. Areas of consolidation may be patchy, and referred to as bronchopneumonia, or confined to discrete areas of the lung, forming lobar pneumonia. Pulmonary collapse frequently occurs in conjunction with pneumonia as a result of airway narrowing in surrounding lung areas. Clinical features of pyrexia, cough and dyspnoea occur with signs of consolidation such as bronchial breathing, chest dullness and inspiratory crackles, although physical signs may be absent in bronchopneumonia. Diagnosis again relies on chest radiography, where consolidation appears as pulmonary shadowing, sometimes accompanied by an 'air bronchogram'. With resolution of the infection, cough becomes more productive, and the lung returns to normal within a few weeks.

The most common cause of community-acquired pneumonia is the *Streptococcus pneumoniae* (pneumococcus) bacterium which is responsible for around one-third of cases worldwide.[5] Vaccination programmes against some serotypes of bacteria that cause pneumonia, and improved testing for viruses may be leading to an increased recorded incidence of viral pneumonia.[5,6] Recent years have seen the emergence of some particularly virulent viral pneumonias, the latest of which are Middle East respiratory syndrome and COVID-19 (**Co**rona **vi**rus **d**isease 2019). The coronaviruses responsible are found in animals and mutate frequently, allowing them to cross host species to become highly contagious to humans, causing a rapidly progressive and lethal pneumonia in some victims.[7]

Effects on Gas Exchange

Patients with pneumonia are commonly hypoxaemic. Consolidated areas of lung behave in a similar fashion to collapse, forming an intrapulmonary shunt through which mixed venous blood flows. In addition, there is an increase in areas with low $\dot{V}/\dot{Q}$ ratios (<0.1), but the contribution of these areas to impaired oxygenation is believed to be small because of hypoxic pulmonary vasoconstriction. Administration of oxygen to patients with pneumonia causes a further widening of the scatter of $\dot{V}/\dot{Q}$ ratios, implying a reduction in hypoxic pulmonary vasoconstriction, but nevertheless results in a considerable improvement in arterial P_{O_2}. Compared with collapsed lung, consolidation is commonly associated with a worse pulmonary shunt and therefore more severe hypoxia. Many of the inflammatory mediators released as part of the response to infection act as local pulmonary vasodilators, in effect overriding hypoxic pulmonary vasoconstriction.

Pathophysiology[8–10]

Airway inflammation was described in detail in Chapter 28. Invasion of the lower respiratory tract with viruses and bacteria leads to further inflammatory changes characterized by migration of neutrophils from the circulation into the lung tissue. Depending on the pathogen involved, the stimulus for this migration may originate from the lung epithelial cells or alveolar macrophages. Chemokines released from these cells initiate neutrophil margination, and a range of proinflammatory cytokine pathways begin. Once in the lung tissue and activated, neutrophils are highly effective killers of the invading pathogen (page 368). As part of this process an inflammatory exudate develops leading to consolidation of the lung tissue. The exudate is a complex mixture of invading organisms, inflammatory cells (dead and alive), immunoglobulins and other immune mediators, fluid transudate from increased capillary permeability and products resulting from destruction of lung tissue as a result of protease activity.

Margination of Neutrophils[11]

Before a neutrophil can contribute to the inflammatory response it must stick to the blood vessel wall (margination), migrate across the endothelium, interstitium and epithelium and become activated, ready to contribute to pathogen removal (see Fig. 31.2). These activities are controlled by an extensive series of cytokines in a very similar fashion to airway inflammation (see Fig. 28.2). Lymphocytes again play an important role, but in parenchymal inflammation macrophages have an important control function instead of the eosinophils and mast cells involved in airway inflammation.

Neutrophil margination has been extensively studied in the systemic circulation. Selectins expressed on the surface of endothelial cells transiently bind the neutrophil causing it to roll along the blood vessel wall. Eventually, different adhesion molecules on the endothelial cell (e.g., intercellular adhesion molecule-1) bind to specific receptors on the neutrophil surface (e.g., β_2-integrins CD11/CD18), causing a firmer adhesion to the endothelium. Once 'caught' by the endothelial cell, cytokines are released, and neutrophil activation begins. The way in which neutrophils are marginated in the lung differs from elsewhere in the body.[12] Adhesion to endothelial cells occurs predominantly in the pulmonary capillary, rather than in venules as in the systemic circulation. Selectin-induced rolling of neutrophils may not occur. Adhesion is facilitated by a slow transit time for neutrophils across pulmonary capillaries. Human neutrophils are of similar size to red blood cells, but are much less deformable, so neutrophils take up to 120 seconds to traverse a pulmonary capillary compared with less than 1 seconds for a red blood cell. Inflammatory mediators may cause changes to the biomechanical properties of neutrophils, in particular, a stiffening of the cell that will further impede its movement through the pulmonary capillary. Once adhered to the pulmonary capillary wall neutrophils may become flattened, leaving some of the capillary lumen available for blood flow. In this position, emigration into the pulmonary tissue begins, and the neutrophil moves through small holes in the capillary basal laminae, guided by chemokines released from epithelial cells and possibly assisted by fibroblasts in the interstitial space (Fig. 30.3).[13]

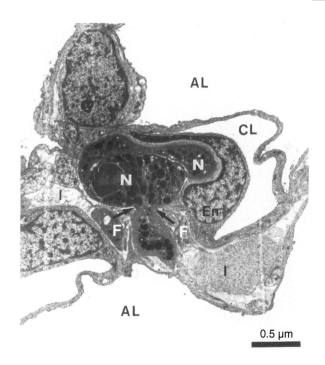

• **Fig. 30.3** Neutrophil emigration in rabbit lung during streptococcal pneumonia. This electron micrograph shows that the neutrophils *(N)*, which are normally the same diameter as a pulmonary capillary, are elongated, so leaving capillary lumen *(CL)* partly patent. These neutrophils have already emigrated from the capillary lumen across the endothelium *(En)*, and one is now passing into the interstitium *(I)* through a small hole in the capillary basement membrane *(arrows)*. The pseudopod of the neutrophil is in close contact with fibroblasts *(F)*, which may be guiding the neutrophil through the defect in the basement membrane. *AL*, Alveolar lumen. (Figure kindly provided by Professor D.C. Walker. Reproduced from reference 13 by permission of the author and publishers of *Microvascular Research*.)

Interstitial Lung Disease and Pulmonary Fibrosis

Diffuse pulmonary inflammation occurs in a wide variety of conditions, which are summarized in Table 30.1. Pneumonitis may simply resolve, as in pneumonia, leaving no permanent damage, but with long-term inflammation varying degrees of pulmonary fibrosis develop.

Clinical features vary according to the aetiology. Pneumonitis alone (i.e., without fibrosis) may be asymptomatic at first, progressing to a cough and dyspnoea, and in severe cases gives rise to systemic symptoms such as fever. When accompanied by fibrosis, dyspnoea becomes worse, and basal inspiratory crackles are present on examination. Lung function tests show a typical restrictive pattern with similar reductions in both forced vital capacity (FVC) and forced expiratory volume in one second (FEV_1). Diffuse reticular shadows develop on chest radiography, and high-resolution CT scanning of the lungs shows either 'ground glass' appearances, which correlate with pneumonitis, or 'honeycombing', which represents more advanced fibrosis.

TABLE 30.1 Causes of Interstitial Pneumonitis and Pulmonary Fibrosis

Causes	Subgroups	Examples
Drug-induced	Anticancer	Bleomycin, busulfan, cyclophosphamide, methotrexate
	Antibiotics	Isoniazid, nitrofurantoin, sulphonamides
	Others	Amiodarone
Dust	Inorganic	Silicosis
		Asbestosis
	Organic	Farmer's lung
Infections	Viral	Viral pneumonia
		Human immunodeficiency virus
	Others	*Mycoplasma*
		Opportunistic infections
Systemic disease	Connective tissue disease	Rheumatoid arthritis, scleroderma, systemic lupus erythematosus, ankylosing spondylitis
	Others	Sarcoidosis, histiocytosis, uraemia
Miscellaneous	Acute inflammation	Acute lung injury
	Inhalation injury	Smoke, cadmium, sulphur dioxide
	Radiation lung damage	
	Cryptogenic fibrosing alveolitis	

Causes of Pulmonary Fibrosis

These have been summarized in Table 30.1.

Drug-induced fibrosis may follow lung injury induced by oxygen toxicity precipitated by, for example, bleomycin (page 294), but the mechanism of this response is poorly understood.

Inorganic dusts from occupational exposure, such as asbestos fibres (asbestosis) or silica (silicosis), for many years leads to pulmonary fibrosis. Inhaled dust particles between 1 and 3 µm in diameter reach the small airways and alveoli and are ingested by macrophages. Different dust types have variable persistence in the lung, some being rapidly cleared and others persisting within the pulmonary macrophage for many years. How the macrophage recognizes silica particles is unknown, but once ingested and incorporated into a lysosome, the silica damages the lysosomal membrane, releasing its contents into the cytosol and triggering an inflammatory reaction.[14]

Organic dusts may cause lung inflammation by an immune mechanism, a condition referred to as extrinsic allergic alveolitis. The allergen is normally derived from a fungus to which the patient has occupational exposure, giving rise to a host of disease names such as farmer's lung, malt worker's lung, and so on. Bird fancier's lung differs in that it is precipitated by exposure to immunoglobin (Ig)A derived from domestic birds. In extrinsic allergic alveolitis, pneumonitis results from activation of T-lymphocytes and IgG-mediated inflammation. If caught early enough, and avoidance measures taken, allergic alveolitis resolves completely, but with continued exposure fibrosis develops.

Systemic diseases that lead to fibrosis are numerous and the mechanisms obscure. Many of the diseases associated with lung fibrosis have an immunological basis. For example, sarcoidosis results from T-lymphocyte activation in response to an unknown stimulus,[15] whereas many connective tissue diseases are known to have an autoimmune aetiology. These immune changes are therefore likely to cause activation of the pulmonary inflammatory cells described next.

Radiation lung damage[16] is seen following radiotherapy for tumours in or near the chest. Radiation pneumonitis develops over several weeks following radiotherapy, whereas fibrosis may take up to 2 years to develop. Cellular radiation damage occurs when cell division occurs, so susceptible cells in the lung are those with the greatest rate of turnover. Thus radiation injury begins with damage to type II pneumocytes and capillary endothelial cells, which results in altered surfactant and interstitial pulmonary oedema (page 341), respectively. A cascade of inflammatory cell activation will then follow, often proceeding to fibrosis.

Idiopathic pulmonary fibrosis (IPF)[17] includes all cases of pulmonary fibrosis in which no cause can be found. It is the most common type of pulmonary fibrosis, occurs more commonly in males and with increasing age and is of uncertain aetiology. Diagnosis requires exclusion of all the other causes of lung fibrosis, and either CT scanning or lung biopsy. The prognosis is poor, with a median survival of 3.8 years in patients aged 65 or over when diagnosed.[18] Previously regarded as a primarily inflammatory disease, IPF is now seen more as a fibrotic response secondary to abnormal activation of alveolar epithelial cells.

Cellular Mechanisms of Pulmonary Fibrosis[19–21]

Inflammation anywhere in the body is naturally succeeded by a cellular healing process that involves the laying down of new collagen. The lung is no exception, and pulmonary fibrosis is a result of excessive deposition of collagen in the lung extracellular matrix.

In pulmonary fibrosis the initial disease process is diverse (Table 30.1) and may cause changes in either type I or type II alveolar epithelial cells, pulmonary macrophages, neutrophils or T-lymphocytes. Interactions between these cells produce numerous cytokines, which amplify the inflammatory response and initiate cellular repair mechanisms. Once these repair mechanisms are established, apoptosis occurs in the inflammatory cells and tissue repair proceeds. Transforming growth factor-β (TGF-β) and vascular endothelial growth factor A are the principal cytokines involved in stimulating tissue repair, with TGF-β probably acting as the final common pathway for most mechanisms leading to fibrosis.[22] Caveolin-1, which is a structural protein forming caveoli on the plasma membrane of many cells, is believed to be the endogenous regulator of TGF-β activity. Myofibroblasts are the cells responsible for repairing the extracellular matrix in lung tissue; this matrix forms the scaffolding on which new lung tissue is formed. Once myofibroblasts have completed their task, they too undergo apoptosis.

In most causes of pulmonary fibrosis this well-controlled sequence of events is abnormal. The activity of acute inflammatory cells may not subside once the stimulus has been removed, and prolonged stimulation of repair mechanisms occurs, or the normal mechanisms that terminate myofibroblast activity may be defective. For example, in IPF the normal ageing process in alveolar epithelial cells and fibroblasts contributes to their abnormal responses which promote fibrosis.[18] Around one-third of the risk of developing IPF is genetic, with seven known genes that contribute,[23] the most important being *MUC5B* which codes for an airway mucin glycoprotein (page 165). How an abnormality of mucin leads to such severe lung disease is unknown, but probably relates to a lifetime of dysregulated innate immunity to common pathogens. These abnormalities are then compounded by repeated minor injuries at a cellular level (e.g., tobacco smoke, infections) which damage alveolar epithelial cells, allowing proteins to enter the alveolus and form a protective matrix or 'wound clot'. This stimulates bronchiolar and alveolar epithelial cells to proliferate in an attempt to repair the tissue, and this proliferation becomes excessive, releasing numerous cytokines and growth factors which attract fibroblasts to the region. There is even some evidence from animal studies that alveolar epithelial cells can be stimulated by TGF-β to transform into mesenchymal cells and eventually into fibroblasts.[20]

Similar to emphysema (page 332), excessive myofibroblast activity leads to a reduction in the amount of elastin present. Synthesis of elastin in normal lung is minimal in adults, and although there is some evidence of increased production in pulmonary fibrosis, the elastic fibres formed are abnormal and probably nonfunctional. Loss of elasticity by this mechanism causes collapse of both alveolar and small airway walls, leading to a reduction in compliance and the area available for gas exchange.

Principles of Therapy[18,24,25]

Where feasible, removal of the stimulant for lung inflammation or fibrosis is vital, including smoking cessation. Although this may not halt the development of fibrosis, for example, following irradiation, it may limit the degree of pulmonary damage that occurs. Drug treatments for IPF have advanced greatly in recent years. Pirfenidone is a drug with a variety of antifibrotic actions including inhibiting the effects of TGF-β, reducing fibroblast proliferation and impairing collagen synthesis. Nintedanib is a tyrosine kinase inhibitor with activity against fibroblast growth factor. Early results from trials of these drugs suggest they can slow the progress of the fibrosis, reduce the frequency of hospitalization with respiratory problems and, when used in combination, prolong life expectancy. Lung transplantation (page 407) remains the best current treatment to extend survival in IPF.

Lung Cancer

At the start of the 20th century lung cancer was a rare disease, but by the end of the century improved longevity and greater exposure to environmental carcinogens has led to lung cancer becoming one of the most common preventable causes of death in the world.[26,27] Improvements in the success rates for treatment of lung cancer have been less than for malignancies in other organs, and the overall 5-year survival rate for lung cancer remains poor at less than 16% in most countries. It is estimated that 1.6 million people worldwide die of lung cancer each year.[28]

Epidemiology

Occupational exposure to lung carcinogens such as asbestos was one of the earliest causative factors for lung malignancy to be identified, with several other occupational agents subsequently linked with lung cancer such as arsenic, cadmium, beryllium and silica. Coexisting lung disease and diet have also been shown to be linked with the development of lung cancer. The role of these factors in causing lung cancer is, however, now known to be insignificant compared with exposure to environmental radon and the overwhelming role of tobacco smoke.

Tobacco

Tobacco smoking (Chapter 20) is responsible for three-quarters of lung cancers worldwide and 90% of lung cancers in countries where smoking is common, and, on a population scale, lung cancer rates mirror smoking rates with an approximate lag time of 20 years. Both the number of cigarettes smoked per day and the duration of being a smoker are positively correlated with the risk of developing lung cancer, although the latter is the stronger association. Quitting smoking has the predictable opposite effect, with the risk of developing lung cancer decreasing with every year of continued abstinence, although the risk never falls as low as that for a lifetime nonsmoker.

Smoking prevalence amongst men was at a peak approximately 20 years before the peak for women, so at present the lung cancer incidence in men is declining, whereas in women the incidence continues to increase. The greater incidence of lung cancer in women is not caused solely by differences in smoking prevalence, but on a dose-for-dose basis women also seem to be more susceptible to the carcinogens found in cigarette smoke, with an odds ratio of between 1.2 and 1.7 compared with men for developing lung cancer with equivalent smoking habits.[29]

Most of the carcinogens in tobacco smoke are found amongst the 3500 compounds that make up the particulate phase, or 'tar', of cigarette smoke (page 236), and their mechanism of carcinogenesis is described later.

Radon

The second most important cause of lung cancer is environmental exposure to radon gas.[30] Radon is part of the natural decay series of uranium (Fig. 30.4), and both elements are ubiquitous in the soil and rocks of the world, although in widely varying concentrations. Radon gas is approximately eight times heavier than air, and therefore tends to accumulate in the cellars and basements of dwellings, making it an important indoor pollutant. There is concern that current drives to make homes more energy-efficient to reduce our impact on global warming may be increasing our exposure to radon.[31] The highest concentrations are found in mines, in particular uranium mines; therefore miners are the group most exposed to radon, and an association between this occupation and lung cancer has been described for centuries. Residential exposure to radon may account for 10% of deaths from lung cancer or make an even greater contribution to the relatively rare cases of lung cancer in nonsmokers.[32]

Radon is an inert gas, so when inhaled into the lung there will be no chemical reaction with other molecules, and with a molecular weight of 222 its diffusion within the alveolus (page 113) and absorption into the blood will both be slow. Most inhaled radon will therefore be exhaled in the same breath, but the most common environmental isotope, ^{222}Rn, has a half-life of only 3.8 days, so while in the airway some of the radon will decay. The decay products are mostly solids which may be deposited in the airways, and also have short half-lives (Fig. 30.4). As a result, inhaled radon and its progeny are a source of large quantities of alpha irradiation. In comparison with beta and gamma radiation the alpha particle, made up of two protons and two neutrons, contains an enormous amount of energy, and is therefore more harmful to biological molecules. For a subatomic particle, an alpha particle has a large mass, and when travelling at around 15000 km.s^{-1} this equates to a large kinetic energy. The strong positive charge of the alpha particle causes the electron shells of nearby atoms to

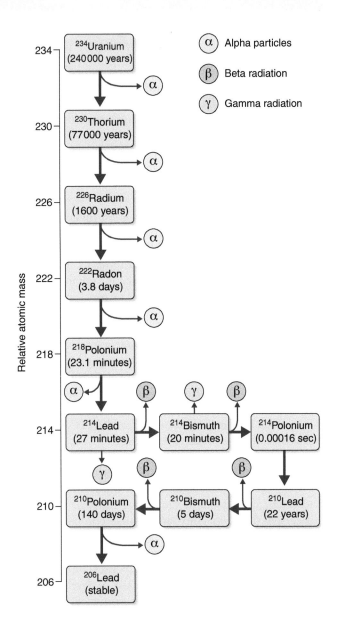

• **Fig. 30.4** Decay series of ^{234}uranium to stable ^{206}lead. An inhaled ^{222}radon molecule will decay to ^{210}lead within minutes, releasing three alpha and two beta particles in the process.

rapidly slow the particle, dissipating its energy in a much smaller area than other forms of radiation. Alpha particles travel only a few centimetres in air, and probably only 30 to 50 μm in living tissue. It is unknown whether the alpha particles released in the lung by radon inhalation can penetrate deeply enough into the airway epithelium to damage the rapidly dividing epithelial stem cells, which are far more likely to be a source of a malignancy than superficial, nondividing cells. An alternative explanation is that the radioactive progeny of radon are absorbed by other pulmonary cells such as macrophages and carried deeper into lung tissue.

Carcinogenesis of Lung Cancer

Radiation

There are three postulated mechanisms by which an alpha particle may initiate malignancy. First, when individual cells are traversed by a single alpha particle only 20% die, and the molecular damage in the survivors doubles their gene mutation rate.[33] Second, the cells surrounding those hit by the alpha particle are damaged by molecular products released from the directly hit cell, an observation known as the bystander effect. Third, much of the positive charge of an alpha particle is neutralized in tissue by removal of electrons from the abundant and nearby water molecules, initiating the production of a range of reactive oxygen species (Chapter 25).

Tobacco Smoke Carcinogens

Tobacco smoke contains 44 known human carcinogens, but two groups are of significance to the formation of lung cancer, polycyclic aromatic hydrocarbons and nitrosamines. As for radiation, much of the molecular damage is caused by the carcinogens generating reactive oxygen species. The normal defence mechanisms (page 289) are overwhelmed, and DNA, RNA, lipids and protein molecules are damaged by oxidation reactions. Many tobacco carcinogens also directly react with DNA either by causing methylation of bases within the DNA or simply by forming adducts between themselves and the DNA molecule. These various chemical changes to the DNA molecule will either interfere with transcription immediately or induce mutations when the DNA replicates during subsequent cell divisions, explaining why rapidly dividing cells are more susceptible to malignant change.

Molecular Mechanisms of Carcinogenesis

To appreciate how the various molecular injuries bring about malignant change it is useful to review the normal biochemical systems that produce functioning proteins within a cell from the genes within the cell nucleus, and the normal phases of the cell cycle. Transcription of genes in eukaryotic cells has several complex stages:

1. *Exposure of the gene.* The human genome is large, and the vast amount of DNA that makes up this genome needs to be highly compacted to fit within the cell nucleus. The double helix of the DNA molecule is wrapped tightly around histone protein complexes, and these nucleosomes are linked together by DNA strands before further histone protein interactions compress the nucleosomes into a compact structure termed chromatin. Most of the genes that may be required are therefore not accessible to transcription proteins, and the nucleosomes must first be rearranged to expose the required gene.

2. *Transcription.* Numerous proteins, referred to as transcriptional factors, are required to control and initiate transcription from the gene by binding to the required promoter region. In conjunction with less specific RNA polymerase proteins a single strand of pre-mRNA chain is then produced as the entire complex moves along the gene.

3. *Posttranscriptional processing.* The pre-mRNA undergoes considerable processing before it is suitable for translation. Methylation of RNA nucleotides near the ends of the chain makes the molecule more stable, varying amounts of redundant RNA are cleaved from the end of the molecule to better delineate the terminal sequence of the RNA, and large sections of redundant RNA (introns) are spliced from the molecule and the sections required for the protein production (exons) joined together and the final mRNA molecule formed.

4. *Translation.* Eukaryotic ribosomes consist of two subunits which must first dissociate before reforming as an initiation complex with the mRNA molecule, an initial tRNA and a methionine molecule. Elongation of the peptide chain then begins with individual tRNA molecules delivering each amino acid and one GTP molecule providing the energy for each addition. When the end of the translatable RNA sequence is reached, a series of release factors are activated which complete the peptide chain and release it from the ribosome before dissociating the mRNA, tRNA and ribosome subunit proteins from each other.

5. *Protein modifications.* Proteins that ultimately reside in the cytoplasm are produced by free ribosomes, whereas proteins destined either for export from the cell or placement in the cell membrane are produced in the ribosomes bound to endoplasmic reticulum. Many sections of the initial peptide chain include 'signal peptides' that guide the posttranscriptional processing of proteins, for example, by facilitating correct folding of the peptide chain or by binding the protein to the correct transporter systems within the cell.

As part of the normal cell cycle, all cells pass through various stages of division:

- G0: The cell is quiescent, that is, it is metabolically active, performing its normal functions and not moving through the cell cycle towards division.
- G1: the cell is preparing for division by producing the macromolecules required.
- S: synthesis phase when the DNA content of the cell is replicating.
- G2: preparation for mitosis when the cell organelles are arranged ready for physical division.
- M: mitosis when the cell divides.

Regulation of progression between these phases, particularly G1 to S and G2 to M, is controlled by a complex group of proteins called cyclin-dependent kinases (CDKs). These proteins may, for example, be required to 'hold' the cell in the S phase until all the DNA has been replicated, and failure of this system will lead to premature replication of the cell, producing two progeny each with an abnormal DNA complement. Much of the activity of CDK is posttranscriptional, that is, new CDK molecules are not being produced. Instead, control of the protein is exerted by phosphorylation and dephosphorylation of the various CDK components, with the degree of phosphorylation affecting the structure, and therefore activity, of the CDK. Alteration of a single base pair in the gene for a CDK will change a single amino acid of the CDK molecule, fundamentally disturbing the regulation of cell division.

A further way in which molecular damage within a cell may promote malignant change is via apoptosis or programmed physiological cell death. Apoptosis is regulated by many of the same genes responsible for control of cell division, so abnormalities of these systems may also prolong the life of a cell beyond its normal physiological term, contributing to tumour growth.

Considering the continuous bombardment with toxic chemicals and radiation that airway cells receive and the myriad steps at which the production and function of a protein could be harmed, and cell division disturbed, it seems surprising that not everybody develops a lung malignancy. Many cells will be killed by the radiation or tobacco constituents, but the resulting tissue damage is quickly repaired, and although in the long term this repeated inflammation and repair cycle may itself damage lung tissue (see Fig. 20.1), lung cancer does not result. Even more cells will be damaged, but the body's extensive and incompletely understood cellular repair mechanisms prevent malignancy developing. For a cell to become malignant, the cellular damage must fundamentally alter the cell's passage through the cell cycle or progress towards apoptosis in such a way that tissue growth becomes uncontrolled, which is the fundamental characteristic of a malignant cell.

The immune system has a role in preventing the development of cancer. Cell-mediated immunity involves T-lymphocytes recognizing the body's own cells via the major histocompatibility (MHC) antigens present on the surface of all cells. In cancer cells, the damage to DNA and its transcription into proteins may produce abnormal or absent MHC proteins or may cause the cell to display other abnormal peptide molecules that the T-lymphocytes recognize as abnormal. An example is the presence on the cell surface of a malignant cell of peptide chains that are similar enough to those displayed by cells infected with a virus to cause the T-lymphocyte to attack the cell. By this mechanism we are protected against the formation of clinically apparent cancers, and differences in immune responsiveness may explain why some individuals are more vulnerable to developing malignancies.

Target Genes for Pulmonary Carcinogenesis

Genetic changes play a significant role in lung cancer development. Whole exome sequencing from cancer cells of patients who smoked shows an average of 8 to 10 mutations per million base pairs.[34] Abnormal functioning of two groups of genes contributes to causing lung cancer—oncogenes and tumour suppressor genes. Oncogenes involved include the following:

- *ras* genes code for a G-protein involved in signal transduction of growth factor receptors on the cell surface. Mutations of the *ras* gene in lung cancer stimulate excessive cell growth even with normal levels of growth factor.
- *myc* genes encode transcription factors that are involved in controlling the transition of cells from the G0 to G1 phases of cell division, and although the *myc* gene is of normal structure in lung cancer it is overexpressed, amplifying its effect.

- the *bcl-2* oncogene is normally involved in controlling cell division in the embryo or in adult stem cells; it also has a role in controlling the timing of apoptosis. This gene is also overexpressed in some lung cancers, facilitating cell proliferation and delaying apoptosis.

The physiological function of tumour suppressor genes is to respond to stress signals within a cell. Thus if a cell undergoes a period of hypoxia or oxidative stress or incurs damage to its DNA, these genes are activated and will either delay progress through the cell cycle to allow time for damage to be repaired, or hasten apoptosis to prevent further cellular dysfunction.

Tumour suppressor genes involved in lung cancer include the following:

- *p53* activation, depending on the circumstances, holds the cell in the G1 phase or induces apoptosis. A wide range of *p53* mutations occur in lung cancer, including deletions and altered splicing of the pre-mRNA.
- the *RB* gene codes for one of the proteins involved in controlling transition from the G1 to S phase of cell division. Mutation of the *RB* gene probably produces a protein structure that is only slightly altered, but unable to be phosphorylated as required to hold the cell in the G1 phase, allowing cell division to progress too rapidly.

Better understanding of the genetic basis of lung cancer and the availability of genetic sequencing tests in clinical practice should lead to improved survival from the disease, although realization of this ambition has been limited thus far.[34-36]

Clinical Aspects

Unfortunately, in a majority of patients, lung cancer has already spread beyond the primary tumour by the time symptoms develop. This remains the main reason for the continued poor outcomes for lung cancer treatment compared with many other malignancies. Therefore, there is a desperate need for a useable screening test for lung cancer. Analysis of biomarkers from exhaled breath condensate is under investigation, but has not yet been evaluated on a large scale.[37] Low-dose CT has been shown to be better than repeated chest radiographs, but the scans identify a large number of lung lesions, most of which are benign, all of which must be further investigated. Despite this, low-dose CT screening is now recommended in individuals between 55 and 74 years of age with a 30 pack-year smoking history who are current smokers or have quit within the last 15 years.[38]

Pathology

Lung cancers can be divided into small cell lung cancer (SCLC) and nonsmall cell lung cancer (NSCLC), which is further divided into squamous cell carcinoma and adenocarcinoma. Squamous cell carcinomas account for around one-third of lung cancers, and mostly arise from central airways, often growing peribronchially to cause airway narrowing without necessarily being visible from within the airway lumen. They tend to be slow growing and metastasize late, and in the periphery of the lung may undergo central necrosis and cavitation. Adenocarcinomas also account for around one-third of lung cancers, but predominantly arise in the periphery of the lung, are faster growing than squamous cell carcinomas and metastasize early via the blood or lymphatics. Finally, the NSCLC tumours include a range of different pathological malignancies, all of which share highly malignant characteristics including early spread via the lymphatic system.

Clinical Features[39]

Cough is the most common symptom of lung cancer, occurring in most patients at some stage of their disease, although cough is such a common complaint in smokers that this remains a very nonspecific symptom. A cough arises from the lung cancer normally by direct irritation of the airway wall, either from within the lumen or from the peribronchial tissue and is typically positional as the tumour presses on the airway in specific postures. Haemoptysis is the second commonest symptom, occurring in half of patients, and varying from staining of expectorated sputum to massive haemoptysis if the tumour erodes into a major thoracic vessel. Wheezing as a result of small airway occlusion by a peripheral lung tumour occurs in around 10% of patients and may be misdiagnosed as adult onset asthma. Narrowing of larger airways causes stridor, although this is only believed to occur when the cross-sectional airway is reduced by more than 75%. Dyspnoea, chest pain and chest infections (usually distal to an airway obstructed by tumour) are other pulmonary symptoms resulting from lung tumours. Finally, any lung cancer, but particularly NSCLC, may present with the symptoms and signs of distant metastases.

Principles of Therapy

A detailed description of the complex subject of treating lung cancer is beyond the scope of this book, and detailed reviews are available.[26,28,39,40] There are three main therapeutic options, and their use is dependent on many factors, of which the two most important are the type of tumour and the stage at which the disease presents:

1. *Surgery.* Lung resection is described in Chapter 33. Resection of the tumour, a lobe of lung or an entire lung is normally done for NSCLC tumours that have not spread beyond the lung or local lymph nodes. For SCLC diagnosed at an early stage lung resection may be performed with the intention of curing the patient, but chemotherapy and radiotherapy are also used for the more malignant SCLC tumours, as distant spread must be assumed to have occurred at diagnosis.

2. *Chemotherapy.* All anticancer drugs must affect malignant cells in such a way as to induce apoptosis or necrosis. A summary of the drugs used most commonly for treatment of lung cancer, and their mechanism of action and common side effects, is shown in Table 30.2.

    Chemotherapy may be used as an adjuvant treatment for patients having surgical management, or may be used as the mainstay of treatment in more advanced NSCLC. Some form of chemotherapy is invariably used for treatment of SCLC. Chemotherapy is normally given in multiple short courses, mostly to allow the patient to recover from the inevitable toxicity (Table 30.2). Also, this pattern of administration may increase the efficacy of the cytotoxic drugs, as repeated hits by the drug encourage the malignant cells to all become aligned in the same phase of the cell cycle. Chemotherapy alone is unlikely to ever be curative. A 1-cm lung cancer is estimated to contain 10^9 malignant cells. If a dose of chemotherapy kills 99.9% of those cells, then 10^6 still remain after the treatment, and this number will increase during the recovery period between treatments. Thus many treatments are required, with the associated toxicity, and in theory it is not possible to kill every malignant cell. However, given that the immune system is also known to have significant cytotoxic abilities, chemotherapy can reduce the tumour cell burden to such an extent that T-lymphocytes may completely remove the cancer.

TABLE 30.2   Examples of Chemotherapeutic Agents Used for Treatment of Lung Cancer

Group	Mechanism of Action	Toxicity	Examples
Alkylating agents	Alkylation of DNA, RNA and proteins	Myelosuppression Nausea and vomiting	Cyclophosphamide, ifosfamide
Platinum analogues	Cross-linking of DNA strands	Nausea and vomiting Nephrotoxicity	Cisplatin, carboplatin
Microtubular inhibitors	Inhibition of microtubulin—arrest of mitosis or induction of apoptosis	Neurotoxicity Myelosuppression	Vincristine, vinblastine, paclitaxel, docetaxel
Topoisomerase inhibitors	Inhibits DNA unwinding and breakage–reunion reactions	Myelosuppression Alopecia Myocardial toxicity	Etoposide, doxorubicin, irinotecan, topotecan
Antimetabolites	Analogue of cytidine—halts DNA replication	Myelosuppression	Gemcitabine

Improved understanding of the interaction between tumour cells and the immune system is driving the development of numerous new therapeutic molecules for lung cancer, broadly referred to as immunotherapy. Monoclonal antibodies active against harmful molecules produced by cancer cells such as programmed cell death protein 1 have shown clinical benefits in some patients.[28] In future, targeted immune therapy using vaccination will hopefully be even more convenient and effective.[41]

3. *Radiotherapy.* Treatment with radiotherapy is indicated either as an adjunct to surgery for localized spread of NSCLC, in combination with chemotherapy for advanced NSCLC, or for treatment of SCLC. Considering that radiation is responsible for causing a proportion of lung cancers it may appear surprising that the same form of energy is used in its treatment. For therapeutic use the same molecular mechanisms of radiation damage are used to kill malignant cells rather than to subtly damage them to induce malignancy, as previously described. The aim of radiotherapy is to focus the most intense area of radiation energy on the tumour while minimizing radiation exposure to nearby normal tissue, although collateral tissue damage is inevitable and results in considerable toxicity from radiotherapy. The recent development of stereotactic body radiation therapy has allowed more targeted delivery of radiation to lung tumours and may provide an alternative curative therapy for patients with small tumours who cannot have surgery.

A major determinant of the sensitivity of a tumour cell to killing by radiation is the Po_2 in the cell when it is irradiated, with most mammalian tumour cells requiring two to three times more radiation to cause cell death when hypoxic. This observation supports the hypothesis that much of the molecular damage induced by radiation is mediated via reactive oxygen species. Animal studies have demonstrated that many solid tumours have hypoxic centres, an observation which is believed to result from an inability of angiogenesis to keep pace with the rapidly growing tumour and leaving some regions with no blood supply. Positron emission tomography may be used to detect hypoxic tissue within tumours, and in a study of patients with NSCLC 48% of the tumour volume was found to be hypoxic, with a majority of tumours containing areas with an estimated Po_2 below 0.27 kPa (2 mmHg), a level at which radiation sensitivity would be poor.[42]

Pleural Disease

Physiology of the Pleural Space[43]

Two pleural layers exist: the first lines the inside of the thoracic cavity (parietal pleura) including the diaphragm, and the second (visceral pleura) covers the lung from the hilum outwards, including the major and minor pulmonary fissures. The opposing elastic forces of lung and chest wall (Chapter 2) cause a pressure of 3 to 5 cmH$_2$O below atmospheric to exist in the pleural space. The pleural space facilitates mechanical coupling between the chest wall and

the lungs, and to do this efficiently, that is with minimal loss of energy, there should be minimal friction between the two structures. The visceral and parietal pleura must therefore slide easily against each other, and this is achieved by the presence of a small amount of pleural fluid and a layer of surfactant molecules on the surface of the mesothelial cells lining both pleural membranes.

An average 70-kg human has a total pleural surface area of 4000 cm^2 containing approximately 18 mL of pleural fluid,[44] which is an ultrafiltrate of plasma containing only small amounts of protein (approximately 1 g.dL^{-1}). Pleural fluid production is determined by the same Starling's forces that determine movement of fluid across capillary walls (page 339). In the parietal pleura, which is supplied by the systemic circulation, the negative intrapleural pressure results in an increased hydrostatic pressure gradient, favouring fluid movement out of the capillary, but the pleural mesothelial cells are less permeable to protein than systemic capillaries, producing an oncotic gradient that opposes fluid movement out of the capillary. The net effect in parietal pleura is a gradient of about 6 cmH$_2$O for fluid to move from the capillary into the pleural space. The blood supply of the visceral pleura derives from the bronchial circulation or the pulmonary circulation, both of which drain to the low pressure pulmonary venous system, and the hydrostatic pressure gradient is therefore much smaller than in parietal pleura, and no fluid movement is believed to occur from the visceral pleura into the pleural space. Another source of pleural fluid, particularly under pathological conditions, is direct flow from the interstitial space of the lung.

Fluid leaves the pleural space via the lymphatic system draining directly through openings, called stomata, between the parietal pleural and lymphatic channels. Stoma are up to 6 µm in diameter, permitting fluid, proteins and cells to pass through, and are probably more numerous in the caudal and diaphragmatic regions of the pleura, where pleural fluid accumulates because of gravity. Under physiological conditions pleural fluid turnover is about 0.01 mL.kg^{-1}.h^{-1}, but when excess fluid accumulates in the pleural space drainage can increase by about 28 times.

Pleural Effusion

Excessive production of pleural fluid will eventually overwhelm the ability of the lymphatic system to drain the pleural space, and fluid accumulates. There are numerous reasons for excessive pleural fluid production, and these are divided into two main groups:[43]

1. *Transudative* effusions contain fluid with a low protein concentration and arise from an increased hydrostatic pressure gradient or a low protein concentration in the blood, both of which will favour fluid transfer out of capillaries into the pleural space. Congestive heart failure, liver cirrhosis and nephrotic syndrome are common examples, and the effusions are usually bilateral as the same factors affect both pleural cavities.

2. *Exudative* effusions have high protein content, are commonly unilateral and arise because of increased permeability

of the mesothelial cells, usually caused by pathology involving the pleura such as malignancy, infection or following trauma or surgery. Pleural effusions as a result of thoracic malignancy are often caused simply by tumour cells and debris blocking the stomata.

Investigation of pleural effusions requires care to avoid unnecessary drainage of the effusion with the associated possibility of introducing an infection. Provided the patient's serum protein levels are normal, then the protein level in the effusion fluid will differentiate between exudates and transudates, and cytology of the cells in the effusion fluid will allow relatively easy diagnosis in 60% of malignant effusions.

Reexpansion of lung following drainage of a pleural effusion can result in pulmonary oedema of the expanded lung, and it is suggested that no more than 1 L of fluid should be removed at one time. There is some evidence that recently expanded lung tissue has a leaky microvasculature,[45] caused either by physical loss of integrity of the tight junctions between endothelial cells or by the generation of negative interstitial hydrostatic pressures favouring movement of fluid out of the capillary (page 340). It remains unclear whether the likelihood of pulmonary oedema occurring relates to the volume of fluid removed or the amount of negative pressure created by its removal. A study of 185 patients found that reexpansion pulmonary oedema only occurred in 2.7% of patients and was unrelated to the volume of fluid removed, provided that the intrathoracic pressure was not allowed to fall below $-20 \, cmH_2O$.[46]

Pneumothorax

This occurs when air enters the pleural space either from the outside across a defect in the chest wall and parietal pleura or from the lung or mediastinum through a defect in the visceral pleura. The many causes of pneumothorax are usually divided into spontaneous and acquired aetiology and are outlined in Table 30.3.

Spontaneous pneumothorax is the most common cause,[47] and may be primary when occurring in otherwise healthy patients (Fig. 30.5, A) or secondary in patients with lung disease. Spontaneous pneumothorax is postulated to result from rupture of small, thin-walled cysts in the immediate subpleural lung tissue, referred to as blebs if less than 2 cm in diameter or bullae if greater than 2 cm (Fig. 30.5, B). Blebs or bullae are seen in most patients presenting with a primary spontaneous pneumothorax, but are also present in 6% of the normal healthy population, so their role in causing pneumothorax remains controversial.[48] Whatever the cause, varying degrees of collapse of a lung will inevitably impair gas exchange, and arterial hypoxaemia occurs in three-quarters of patients with a pneumothorax on presentation, with the hypoxaemia being worse with larger pneumothoraces or underlying lung disease.

Tension Pneumothorax

Occasionally, the defect in the lung or chest wall through which air gains entry to the pleural space forms a valve mechanism, and a tension pneumothorax occurs. During inspiration, air is sucked into the pleural space but cannot leave the pleura during expiration. A large pneumothorax develops, and increased respiratory effort reduces intrapleural pressure further, until the pressure in the affected hemithorax remains above atmospheric throughout almost the entire respiratory cycle, because air is only drawn into the pleura during peak inspiratory effort. Ventilation of the lung on the affected side ceases, the lung collapses, and extensive shunt and severe hypoxaemia occur. A more dramatic effect is the shift of the mediastinum away from the pneumothorax, which causes a sudden and catastrophic reduction in venous return and therefore cardiac output. Insertion of a cannula into the affected hemithorax relieves the pressure, creates an open pneumothorax and invariably saves the patient's life.

Principles of Therapy for Spontaneous Pneumothorax

Treatment of a pneumothorax depends on whether it is primary or secondary, its size and the patient's symptoms. For example, no intervention is required for a primary

TABLE 30.3	Common Causes of Pneumothorax			
	Spontaneous		**Acquired**	
Primary	Rupture of subpleural bleb	Iatrogenic	Central venous access Lung biopsy Postlaparoscopy Blunt trauma ± rib fracture
Secondary	Bullous disease (COPD) Cystic fibrosis Asthma Lung cancer Lung metastasis Oesophageal rupture Marfan syndrome *Pneumocystis* pneumonia Lung abscess	Traumatic Barotrauma	Penetrating trauma Artificial ventilation (Chapter 32)

COPD, Chronic obstructive pulmonary disease.

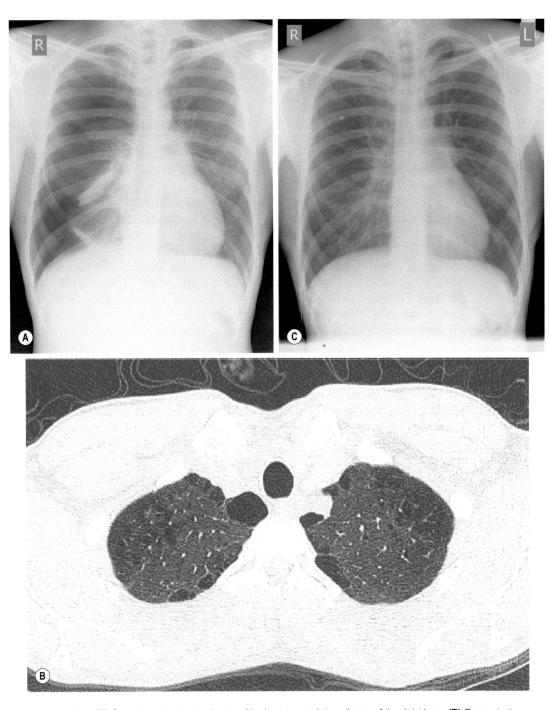

• **Fig. 30.5** **(A)** Spontaneous pneumothorax with almost complete collapse of the right lung. **(B)** Computed tomography scan of the lung apices in the same patient showing multiple lung blebs. **(C)** The pneumothorax has been treated by the insertion of a chest drain, with complete reexpansion of the lung.

pneumothorax in a patient who is not breathless and in whom the rim of air between the lung and chest wall on a chest radiograph is less than 2 cm wide.[49] For larger or symptomatic pneumothoraces aspiration of air is performed and the chest radiograph reviewed to confirm lung expansion. If this is unsuccessful, then a chest drain is placed, complete lung reexpansion is confirmed (Fig. 30.5, *C*), the drain is left in place until there is no further air leak and the lung is allowed to fully expand for 24 hours. If the lung fails

to reexpand with a chest drain in situ, or an air leak persists for days, then surgery is usually required. During surgery any visible blebs or bullae at the lung apex are resected, and a pleurodesis (page 402) performed, following which the lung is reexpanded under direct vision.

Absorption of Air from the Pleural Space

For small asymptomatic pneumothoraces, or following treatment as previously described, complete resolution of a closed pneumothorax requires air to be reabsorbed from the pleura. How quickly this occurs depends on the partial pressure gradients of the various gases between the pleura and the circulation, in particular, the venous blood where partial pressures are lowest (see Table 25.2). Two phases of gas reabsorption will theoretically occur: phase 1, when gases in the pleura come into equilibrium with the venous blood, and phase 2, when the gas is absorbed. For phase 1, the cause of the pneumothorax is important in that the gas entering the pleura may be either air from the outside or alveolar gas from the lung. When ambient air, which is likely to be dry, enters the pleural space the first change to occur is a small increase in volume as water vapour humidifies the gas. Oxygen will be absorbed into the blood and carbon dioxide will diffuse into the pleural space, but these two volume changes should be approximately equal and cause little change in volume.

For partial pressures, the loss of oxygen from the pleural air is partially offset by the gain of water vapour and carbon dioxide, but overall the nitrogen partial pressure increases slightly, and some nitrogen will slowly be absorbed into the circulation. When alveolar gas, which is already humidified and contains carbon dioxide, enters the pleural space the only change will be the absorption of a small amount of oxygen and a slight reduction in the volume of the pneumothorax, and therefore lung reexpansion. In patients breathing oxygen at the time of a pneumothorax (originating from the lung) the situation is, in theory, more favourable, as the alveolar gas is now almost entirely oxygen, and most of the pneumothorax will be quickly absorbed into the bloodstream. A similar phenomenon has been observed if the pneumothorax involves carbon dioxide entering the pleural space during laparoscopic surgery (technically a capnothorax), following which complete resolution occurred within 2 hours.[50] In both these situations nitrogen from the blood will diffuse into the pleural space, but this process is very slow compared with oxygen or carbon dioxide absorption.

In phase 2 of reabsorption of a pneumothorax, the partial pressures of each gas in the pleural space are in equilibrium with the venous blood. Fortunately the subatmospheric total gas partial pressure of venous blood (Table 25.2) maintains small gradients that facilitate slow reabsorption of the pneumothorax. A further theoretical benefit of breathing oxygen may be obtained during phase 2 of pneumothorax reabsorption. The greater the inspired oxygen concentration the lower the blood P_{N_2}, increasing the rate of diffusion of nitrogen from the pleura into the blood.

These theoretical considerations are harder to demonstrate in practice. Although not investigated for some years, there is agreement that absorption of gas from a pneumothorax is slow; the most widely quoted estimate is that 1.8% of the hemithorax volume is absorbed per day.[51] This means that a small pneumothorax occupying 15% of hemithorax volume will take approximately 10 days to resolve fully. Animal studies have shown a dose-dependent reduction in the time taken for a pneumothorax to resolve with increasing inspired oxygen fraction, with the duration approxi-

mately halved by breathing 50% oxygen compared with air.[52] Small studies in humans found that during periods breathing an unspecified high oxygen concentration resolution of the pneumothorax was approximately three to four times faster than when breathing air.[53]

Empyema

Empyema thoracis is a condition resulting from bacterial infection of the normally sterile pleural space. Almost two-thirds of patients with pneumonia develop a 'simple', non-infected pleural effusion by direct movement of interstitial fluid from the infected lung tissue into the pleural space. In around 10% of these effusions bacterial spread from the underlying pneumonia follows, and an empyema develops. Other, less common, causes of empyema include its development as a complication of trauma, thoracic surgery, pneumothorax or diagnostic thoracocentesis. The bacterial infection of the pleural fluid follows the normal stages of inflammation, with influx of white cells eventually causing the formation of pus. In empyema, deposition of fibrin begins early and is aggressive, and within a few weeks a thick layer of collagen (referred to as 'rind' or 'peel') is deposited on both pleural spaces. If left untreated the process continues until pleural fibrosis causes contraction of the chest wall and lung (fibrothorax).

A restrictive pattern of reduced lung function occurs with FEV_1 and FVC values of half predicted normal being typical. Early intervention with antibiotics, fibrinolysis or chest drainage may limit the progression of the fibrotic process.[54] However, if these less invasive therapies fail or restrictive lung disease is already apparent, more extensive intervention is required in the form of surgical drainage or decortication, in which the peel formed on the pleura, particularly the parietal layer, is stripped off to allow the underlying lung to reexpand.

References

1. Webb SJS, Nunn JF. A comparison between the effect of nitrous oxide and nitrogen on arterial Po₂. *Anaesthesia*. 1967;22:69-81.
2. Butler JP, Malhotra A, Loring SH. Revisiting atelectasis in lung units with low ventilation/perfusion ratios. *J Appl Physiol*. 2019;126:782-786.
3. Ray K, Bodenham A, Paramasivam E. Pulmonary atelectasis in anaesthesia and critical care. *Contin Educ Anaesth Crit Care Pain*. 2014;14:236-245.
4. Marini JJ. Acute lobar atelectasis. *Chest*. 2019;155:1049-1058.
5. Prina E, Ranzani OT, Torres A. Community-acquired pneumonia. *Lancet*. 2015;386:1097-1108.
*6. **Ruuskanen O, Lahti E, Jennings LC, et al. Viral pneumonia. *Lancet*. 2011;377:1264-1275.**
7. Zumla A, Hui DS, Perlman S. Middle East respiratory syndrome. *Lancet*. 2015;386:995-1007.
8. Mizgerd JP. Acute lower respiratory tract infection. *N Engl J Med*. 2008;358:716-727.
9. Quinton LJ, Mizgerd JP. Dynamics of lung defense in pneumonia: resistance, resilience, and remodeling. *Annu Rev Physiol*. 2015;77:407-430.
*10. **Quinton LJ, Walkey AJ, Mizgerd JP. Integrative physiology of pneumonia. *Physiol Rev*. 2018;98:1417-1464.**

11. Liew PX, Kubes P. The neutrophil's role during health and disease. *Physiol Rev.* 2019;99:1223-1248.

12. D'Ambrosio D, Mariani M, Panina-Bordignon P, et al. Chemokines and their receptors guiding T lymphocyte recruitment in lung inflammation. *Am J Respir Crit Care Med.* 2001;164:1266-1275.

13. Walker DC, Behzad AR, Chu F. Neutrophil migration through preexisting holes in the basal laminae of alveolar capillaries and epithelium during streptococcal pneumonia. *Microvasc Res.* 1995;50:397-416.

14. Leung CC, Yu ITS, Chen W. Silicosis. *Lancet.* 2012;379:2008-2018.

15. Spagnolo P, Rossi G, Trisolini R, Sverzellati N, Baughman RP, Wells AU. Pulmonary sarcoidosis. *Lancet Respir Med.* 2018;6:389-402.

16. Movsas B, Raffin TA, Epstein AH, et al. Pulmonary radiation injury. *Chest.* 1997;111:1061-1076.

17. Richeldi L, Collard HR, Jones MG. Idiopathic pulmonary fibrosis. *Lancet.* 2017;389:1941-1952.

18. Lederer DJ, Martinez FJ. Idiopathic pulmonary fibrosis. *N Engl J Med.* 2018;378:1811-1123.

19. Thannickal VJ, Toews GB, White ES, et al. Mechanisms of pulmonary fibrosis. *Annu Rev Med.* 2004;55:395-417.

20. Fernandez IE, Eickelberg O. New cellular and molecular mechanisms of lung injury and fibrosis in idiopathic pulmonary fibrosis. *Lancet.* 2012;380:680-688.

21. Kulkarni T, de Andrade J, Zhou Y, et al. Alveolar epithelial disintegrity in pulmonary fibrosis. *Am J Physiol Lung Cell Mol Physiol.* 2016;311:L185-L191.

22. Atamas SP. Vascular endothelial growth factor in idiopathic pulmonary fibrosis. An imbalancing act. *Am J Respir Crit Care Med.* 2017;196:409-411.

23. Evans CM, Fingerlin TE, Schwarz MI, et al. Idiopathic pulmonary fibrosis: a genetic disease that involves mucociliary dysfunction of the peripheral airways. *Physiol Rev.* 2016;96:1567-1591.

24. Adegunsoye A, Strek ME. Therapeutic approach to adult fibrotic lung diseases. *Chest.* 2016;150:1371-1386.

25. Maher TM. Combination therapy and the start of a new epoch for idiopathic pulmonary fibrosis? *Am J Respir Crit Care Med.* 2018;197:283-284.

26. Reck M, Heigener DF, Mok T, et al. Management of non-small-cell lung cancer: recent developments. *Lancet.* 2013;382:709-719.

27. Malhotra J, Malvezzi M, Negri E, La Vecchia C, Boffetta P. Risk factors for lung cancer worldwide. *Eur Respir J.* 2016;48:889-902.

*28. **Hirsch FR, Scagliotti GV, Mulshine JL, et al. Lung cancer: current therapies and new targeted treatments. *Lancet.* 2017;389:299-311.**

29. Zang EA, Wynder EL. Differences in lung cancer risk between men and women: Examination of the evidence. *J Natl Cancer Inst.* 1996;88:183-192.

30. Gray A, Read S, McGale P, et al. Lung cancer deaths from indoor radon and the cost effectiveness and potential of policies to reduce them. *BMJ.* 2009;338:215-218.

31. Woodward A. Cutting household ventilation to improve energy efficiency. A warning about radon and lung cancer. *BMJ.* 2014;348:f7713.

32. Ruano-Ravina A, Kelsey KT, Fernández-Villar A, et al. Action levels for indoor radon: different risks for the same lung carcinogen? *Eur Respir J.* 2017;50:1701609.

33. Hei TK, Wu L-J, Liu S-X, et al. Mutagenic effects of a single and an exact number of particles in mammalian cells. *Proc Natl Acad Sci U S A.* 1997;94:3765-3770.

34. Swanton C, Govindan R. Clinical implications of genomic discoveries in lung cancer. *N Engl J Med.* 2016;374:1864-1873.

*35. **Nana-Sinkam SP, Powell CA. Molecular biology of lung cancer. Diagnosis and management of lung cancer, 3rd ed: American College of Chest Physicians evidence-based clinical practice guidelines. *Chest.* 2013;143(suppl):e30S-e39S.**

36. Hiley CT, Le Quesne J, Santis G, et al. Challenges in molecular testing in non-small-cell lung cancer patients with advanced disease. *Lancet.* 2016;388:1002-1011.

37. López-Sánchez LM, Jurado-Gámez B, Feu-Collado N, et al. Exhaled breath condensate biomarkers for the early diagnosis of lung cancer using proteomics. *Am J Physiol Lung Cell Mol Physiol.* 2017;313:L664-L676.

38. Kauczor H-U, Bonomo L, Gaga M, et al. ESR/ERS white paper on lung cancer screening. *Eur Respir J.* 2015;46:28-39.

*39. **Neal RD, Sun F, Emery JD, et al. Lung cancer. *BMJ.* 2019;265:I1725.**

40. Baldwin DR, White B, Schmidt-Hansen M, et al. Diagnosis and treatment of lung cancer: summary of updated NICE guidance. *BMJ.* 2011;342:d2110.

41. Chee J, Robinson BWS, Holt RA, et al. Immunotherapy for lung malignancies from gene sequencing to novel therapies. *Chest.* 2017;151:891-897.

42. Rasey JS, Koh W, Evans ML, et al. Quantifying regional hypoxia in human tumors with positron emission tomography of [^{18}F]fluoromisonidazole: a pretherapy study of 37 patients. *Int J Radiat Oncol Biol Phys.* 1996;136:417-428.

43. Feller-Kopman D, Light R. Pleural disease. *N Engl J Med.* 2018;378:740-751.

44. Zocchi L. Physiology and pathophysiology of pleural fluid turnover. *Eur Respir J.* 2002;20:1545-1558.

45. Wilkinson PD, Keegan J, Davies SW, et al. Changes in pulmonary microvascular permeability accompanying reexpansion oedema: evidence from dual isotope scintigraphy. *Thorax.* 1990;45:456-459.

46. Feller-Kopman D, Berkowitz D, Boiselle P, et al. Large-volume thoracentesis and the risk of reexpansion pulmonary edema. *Ann Thorac Surg.* 2007;84:1656-1662.

47. Bintcliffe O, Maskell N. Spontaneous pneumothorax. *BMJ.* 2014;348:g2928.

48. Baumann MH. To bleb or not to bleb? *Chest.* 2007;132:1110-1112.

49. Tschopp J-M, Bintcliffe O, Astoul P, et al. ERS task force statement: diagnosis and treatment of primary spontaneous pneumothorax. *Eur Respir J.* 2015;46:321-335.

50. Karayiannakis AJ, Anagnostoulis S, Michailidis K, et al. Spontaneous resolution of massive right-sided pneumothorax occurring during laparoscopic cholecystectomy. *Surg Laparosc Endosc Percutan Tech.* 2005;15:100-103.

51. Flint K, Al-Hillawi AH, Johnson NM. Conservative management of spontaneous pneumothorax. *Lancet.* 1984;323:687-688.

52. England GJ, Hill RC, Timberlake GA, et al. Resolution of experimental pneumothorax in rabbits by graded oxygen therapy. *J Trauma.* 1998;45:333-334.

53. Chadha TS, Cohn MA. Noninvasive treatment of pneumothorax with oxygen inhalation. *Respiration.* 1983;44:147-152.

54. Davies CWH, Gleeson FV, Davies RJO. BTS guidelines for the management of pleural infection. *Thorax.* 2003;58(suppl 2):18-28.

31

Acute Lung Injury

KEY POINTS

- Acute lung injury is lung inflammation that develops in response to a variety of both pulmonary and generalized acute diseases.
- The clinical features of acute lung injury vary from mild, self-limiting dyspnoea to rapidly progressive and fatal respiratory failure.
- Widespread pulmonary inflammation causes increased permeability of the alveolar capillary membrane, leading to

flooding and collapse of alveoli and severely impaired gas exchange.
- Artificial ventilation in severe acute lung injury is challenging, though a 'protective ventilation' strategy using small tidal volumes and moderate levels of positive end-expiratory pressure is beneficial.

Acute lung injury (ALI) describes a characteristic form of parenchymal lung disease, and represents a spectrum of severity from short-lived dyspnoea to a rapidly terminal failure of the respiratory system, when the term acute respiratory distress syndrome (ARDS) is used. There are many synonyms for ALI, including acute respiratory failure, shock lung, respirator lung, pump lung and Da Nang lung.

Clinical Aspects of Acute Lung Injury[1,2]

Definition

There is no single diagnostic test, and confusion has arisen in the past from differing diagnostic criteria. This has complicated comparisons of incidence, mortality, aetiology and efficacy of therapies. To address this problem, European–American consensus conferences produced the following widely accepted definitions in 1994.[3]

ALI diagnosis required the presence of four criteria:
1. Acute onset of impaired oxygenation.
2. Severe hypoxaemia defined as a Pa_{O_2} to $F_{I_{O_2}}$ ratio of 40 or less (Pa_{O_2} in kPa) or 300 or less (Pa_{O_2} in mmHg).
3. Bilateral diffuse infiltration on the chest radiograph consistent with pulmonary oedema.
4. Absence of left atrial hypertension.

ARDS was defined in almost identical terms, except that the impairment of gas exchange was worse, with a Pa_{O_2} to $F_{I_{O_2}}$ ratio of 26.7 or less kPa or 200 or less mmHg.

These criteria were widely accepted and extremely helpful in researching ALI, though for ARDS there were concerns over the definition of 'acute', the effect of ventilator settings on Pa_{O_2} to $F_{I_{O_2}}$ ratio and the poor reliability of chest radiograph interpretation. In 2012 these concerns were addressed with updated diagnostic criteria for ARDS, referred to as the Berlin definition, which also, for the first time, introduced three different grades of hypoxia (Table 31.1).[4] Although generally accepted as an improvement on its predecessor, the Berlin definition similarly does not relate to the typical histopathological picture seen in a patient's lungs, with the usual features of ARDS, diffuse alveolar damage, being absent in some patients who meet the diagnostic criteria.[5]

Predisposing Conditions and Risk Factors for Acute Lung Injury

Although the clinical and histopathological features of ALI are remarkably consistent, they have been described as the sequel to a large range of predisposing conditions (Table 31.2). There are, however, very important differences in the progression of ALI and its response to treatment, depending on the underlying cause and associated pathology. Nevertheless, recognition of the predisposing conditions is crucially important for predicting which patients are at risk and making an early diagnosis.

The conditions listed in Table 31.2 are not equally likely to proceed to ALI. Studies have consistently identified sepsis as the condition most likely to result in development of ALI, with pneumonia, pancreatitis, trauma and transfusion-related ALI (TRALI) also being common contributors. The last of these, TRALI, is unusual in that it occurs 50 times more often in critically ill patients than other hospitalized patients, making transfusion of blood products particularly

TABLE 31.1	The Berlin Definition of Acute Respiratory Distress Syndrome[4]			
Timing	Within 1 week of a known clinical insult or new or worsening respiratory symptoms			
Chest imaging[a]	Bilateral opacities—not fully explained by effusions, lobar/lung collapse or nodules			
Origin of oedema	Respiratory failure not fully explained by cardiac failure or fluid overload Need objective assessment (e.g., echocardiography) to exclude hydrostatic oedema if no risk factor present			
Oxygenation:	Pa_{O_2} in kPa:		Pa_{O_2} in mmHg:	End-expiratory pressure:
Mild	$26.7 < Pa_{O_2} : FI_{O_2} \leq 40.0$		$200 < Pa_{O_2} : FI_{O_2} \leq 300$	With PEEP or CPAP ≥ 5 cmH$_2$O
Moderate	$13.3 < Pa_{O_2} : FI_{O_2} \leq 26.7$		$100 < Pa_{O_2} : FI_{O_2} \leq 200$	With PEEP ≥ 5 cmH$_2$O
Severe	$Pa_{O_2} : FI_{O_2} \leq 13.3$		$Pa_{O_2} : FI_{O_2} \leq 100$	With PEEP ≥ 5 cmH$_2$O

[a]Based on chest radiograph or computed tomography.

TABLE 31.2	Some Predisposing Conditions for Acute Lung Injury (ALI)	
Direct Lung Injury		**Indirect Lung Injury**
Common:		**Common:**
Pneumonia		Sepsis
Aspiration of gastric contents		Severe nonthoracic trauma
		TRALI
Less Common:		**Less Common:**
Lung contusion		Acute pancreatitis
Near-drowning		Cardiopulmonary bypass
Inhalation of toxic gases or vapours		Severe burns
Fat or amniotic fluid embolus		Drug overdose
Reperfusion oedema e.g., following lung transplantation		Disseminated intravascular coagulation

TRALI, Transfusion-related acute lung injury.

hazardous in patients who are already at risk of ALI.[6] Overall, 25% of patients with a single risk factor develop ARDS, but this rises to 42% with two factors and 85% with three.

Age does not seem to affect the likelihood of developing ALI, but it may be more common in men than women and less common in some racial groups.[7] ARDS also occurs in children, with an incidence of 1.8% described in a study of almost 150 000 patients under 18 admitted to an intensive care unit following a traumatic injury.[8]

Pulmonary and Extrapulmonary Acute Lung Injury

Patients with ALI should be broadly divided into two separate groups. Pulmonary ALI results from clinical conditions that cause direct lung injury, whereas extrapulmonary ALI follows indirect lung injury (Table 31.2). These two subgroups of ALI have been shown to differ with respect to pathological mechanisms, appearances on chest radiographs and computed tomography (CT) scans, abnormalities of respiratory mechanics and response to ventilatory strategies.[9]

Incidence and Mortality

In the past, the lack of accepted definitions of lung injury led to widely varying estimates of the incidences of ALI and ARDS. Despite more consistent diagnostic criteria in recent years, the estimated incidence of ALI remains variable at 5 to 7 cases per year per 100 000 individuals in Europe and 34 per 100 000 in the United States.[10] The reasons for this variation in estimates of the incidence of ALI is unknown, but the incidence may be decreasing. Around 70% of cases of ALI are severe enough to be classified as ARDS. There is, however, considerable agreement that mortality from ARDS is high: 2 decades ago in excess of 50% of patients died, whatever the criteria of diagnosis. Outcome has improved in recent years, with studies indicating a decline in mortality rate from 35% in 1996 to just over 28% in 2013.[11] In children under 18 years old a mortality of 20% is reported, although this did not improve over the decade of study data collection.[8] Significant long-term disability is common in survivors, although this does not usually involve the respiratory system, which seems to recover well.[2]

Clinical Course

Four phases may be recognized in the development of severe ALI. In the first the patient is dyspnoeic and tachypneic, but there are no other abnormalities. The chest radiograph is normal at this stage, which lasts for about 24 hours. In the second phase there is hypoxaemia, but the arterial P_{CO_2} remains normal or subnormal. There are minor abnormalities of the chest radiograph. This phase may last for 24 to 48 hours. Diagnosis is easily missed in these prodromal stages and is very dependent on the history of one or more predisposing conditions. Identification of patients in this stage of ALI is becoming increasingly important as we gain a greater understanding of interventions which can worsen or improve the chances or progressing to ARDS.[12]

It is only in phase three that the diagnostic criteria of ALI become established. There is significant arterial hypoxaemia caused by an increased alveolar/arterial Po_2 gradient, and the arterial Pco_2 may be slightly elevated. The lungs become stiff, and the chest radiograph shows the characteristic bilateral diffuse infiltrates. Ventilatory support is usually instituted at this stage.

The fourth phase is often terminal and comprises massive bilateral consolidation with unremitting hypoxaemia even when ventilated with very high inspired oxygen concentrations. Dead space is substantially increased, and the arterial Pco_2 is only with difficulty kept in the normal range.

Not every patient passes through all these phases, and the condition may resolve at any stage. It is difficult to predict whether the condition will progress, and there is currently no useful laboratory test, although animal studies have identified biomarkers for alveolar fluid clearance which may be associated with resolution of ALI.[13] Serial observations of the chest radiograph, the alveolar/arterial Po_2 gradient and the function of other compromised organs are the best guides to progress.

Pathophysiology[2]

Alveolar/Capillary Permeability

This is increased substantially throughout the course of ALI. Increased permeability may be demonstrated at the bedside by the measurement of extravascular lung water (page 344), which in patients with ARDS is commonly double the normal value of 3 to 7 mL.kg^{-1}.[14]

Maldistribution of Ventilation and Perfusion[15]

CT scans of patients with ARDS show that opacities representing collapsed areas are distributed throughout the lungs in a heterogeneous manner, but predominantly in the dependent regions.[16] Following a change in posture, the opacities move to the newly dependent zones within a few minutes. The most conspicuous functional disability is the shunt (Fig. 31.1), which is usually so large (often >40%) that increasing the inspired oxygen concentration cannot produce a normal arterial Po_2 (see the iso-shunt chart, Fig. 7.13). CT scans of patients with ALI also demonstrate substantial areas of lung overdistension. These areas contribute to the increased dead space, which may exceed 70% of tidal volume and requires a large increase in minute volume to attempt to preserve a normal arterial Pco_2. Both shunt and dead space correlate strongly with the noninflated lung tissue seen with CT (Fig. 31.1).

Lung Mechanics

In established ARDS, lung compliance is greatly reduced, and the static compliance of the respiratory system (lungs + chest wall) is of the order of 300 mL.kPa^{-1} (30 mL. cmH$_2$O^{-1}). Patients with pulmonary and extrapulmonary

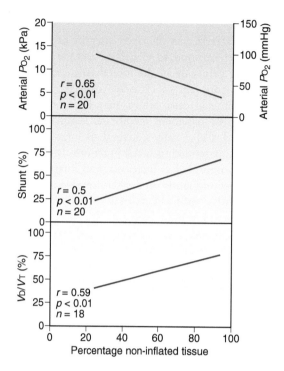

• **Fig. 31.1** Relationship of arterial Po_2, shunt and physiological dead space (V_D/V_T) to the percentage of noninflated lung tissue seen by computed tomography in patients with acute respiratory distress syndrome, artificially ventilated with positive end-expiratory pressure of 0.5 kPa (5 cmH$_2$O). (From Gattinoni L, Pesenti A, Bombino M, et al. Relationships between lung computed tomographic density, gas exchange, and PEEP in acute respiratory failure. *Anesthesiology.* 1988;69:824-832.)

forms of ARDS (see previous discussion) have different abnormalities of respiratory system mechanics. Respiratory system compliance is reduced to a similar extent in both groups, but the abnormality is mostly with lung compliance when lung disease is the cause, and chest wall compliance with extrapulmonary causation.

Functional residual capacity is reduced by collapse and increased elastic recoil.

Mean total resistance to airflow is increased to around 1.5 to 2 kPa.L^{-1}.s (15–20 cmH$_2$O.L^{-1}.s), or about three times that of anaesthetized patients with normal lungs, measured by the same technique. Using the model shown in Figure 3.4, about two-thirds of the total resistance in patients with ARDS could be assigned to viscoelastic resistance of tissue, although the airway resistance was still about twice normal.

Mechanisms of Acute Lung Injury

Histopathology

Although of diverse aetiology, the histological appearances of ARDS are remarkably consistent, and this lends support for ARDS being considered a discrete clinical entity. Histological changes at autopsy may be divided into the following two stages.

Acute Stage

This is characterized by damaged integrity of the blood–gas barrier, often referred to as diffuse alveolar damage. The changes are primarily in the interalveolar septa, and electron microscopy shows extensive damage to the type I alveolar epithelial cells, which may be totally destroyed. Meanwhile the basement membrane is usually preserved, and the endothelial cells still tend to form a continuous layer with apparently intact cell junctions. Endothelial permeability is nevertheless increased, and interstitial oedema is found, predominantly on the 'service' side of the capillary as seen in other forms of pulmonary oedema (page 341). Protein-containing fluid leaks into the alveoli, which also contain red blood cells, leukocytes and strands of fibrin. Intravascular coagulation is common, and, in patients with septicaemia, capillaries may be completely plugged with leukocytes and the underlying endothelium damaged.

Fibroproliferative Stage

Attempted repair of lung structure predominates in this phase. Within a few days of the onset of ARDS, there is a thickening of endothelium, epithelium and the interstitial space. The type I epithelial cells are destroyed and replaced by type II cells, which proliferate but do not differentiate into type I cells as usual. They remain cuboidal and about ten times the thickness of the type I cells they have replaced. This appears to be a nonspecific response to damaged type I cells and is similar to that which results from exposure to high concentrations of oxygen (page 293). The interstitial space is expanded by oedema fluid, fibres and a variety of proliferating cells. In the same way as for other causes of pulmonary fibrosis, extracellular matrix remodelling begins (page 355). Fibrosis commences after the first week, and ultimately fibrocytes predominate: extensive fibrosis is seen in resolving cases. Recent work suggests that fibroproliferative changes may be more a result of the artificial ventilation used to treat the patients rather than from the ARDS disease process itself,[17] and improved ventilation strategies have reduced the likelihood of patients progressing to this phase.[18]

Cellular Mechanisms[19]

The diversity of predisposing conditions suggests that there may be several possible mechanisms, at least in the early stages of development of ALI, but the end result is remarkably similar. In all cases, lung injury seems to begin with damage to the alveolar/capillary membrane. This is followed by progressive inflammation leading to alveolar epithelial cell injury, alveolar transudation, pulmonary vasoconstriction and capillary obstruction.

Cells that are capable of damaging the alveolar capillary membrane include neutrophils, basophils, macrophages and platelets. Damage may be inflicted by a large number of substances, including bacterial endotoxin, reactive oxygen species, proteases, thrombin, fibrin, fibrin degradation products, arachidonic acid metabolites and innumerable

proinflammatory cytokines. It seems improbable that any one mechanism is responsible for all cases of ALI. It is more likely that different mechanisms operate in different predisposing conditions and in different animal models of ALI.

Neutrophils have a key role in human ALI.[20] Although ALI can still be induced in neutrophil-depleted animals, patients with ARDS have large numbers of neutrophils and associated cytokines in bronchoalveolar lavage fluid samples. Neutrophil activation may occur in response to a large number of substances, some of which are illustrated in Figure 31.2. Which of these are important in ALI is unknown, but likely to depend on the predisposing condition; for example, complement component C5a is known to be involved in sepsis-related ALI. Margination of neutrophils from the pulmonary capillary into the lung parenchyma is the first stage of neutrophil activation and has been described on page 353. During margination and once in the interstitium, the neutrophil is 'primed', that is, stimulated to produce preformed mediators ready for release, and to establish the bactericidal contents of their lysosomes. Finally, stimulation results from a whole host of cytokines, some derived from other inflammatory cells (macrophages, lymphocytes or endothelial cells) and some

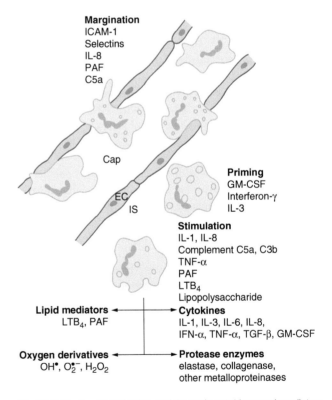

Margination
ICAM-1
Selectins
IL-8
PAF
C5a

Cap

EC
IS

Priming
GM-CSF
Interferon-γ
IL-3

Stimulation
IL-1, IL-8
Complement C5a, C3b
TNF-α
PAF
LTB₄
Lipopolysaccharide

Lipid mediators ←
LTB₄, PAF

Cytokines
IL-1, IL-3, IL-6, IL-8,
IFN-α, TNF-α, TGF-β, GM-CSF

Oxygen derivatives ←
OH•, O₂•⁻, H₂O₂

Protease enzymes
elastase, collagenase,
other metalloproteinases

• **Fig. 31.2** Neutrophil activation and the main cytokines and mediators involved. This takes place in three stages. *Margination*, when neutrophils adhere to the capillary *(Cap)* wall and migrate between endothelial cells *(EC)* into the interstitial space *(IS)*; *priming*, when the cells generate preformed mediators and lysosomal contents; and *stimulation*, when neutrophils release the various mediators shown. The scheme shown is based on studies of both systemic and pulmonary inflammation. Neutrophil margination may occur by different mechanisms in pulmonary capillaries (see page 353).

from other neutrophils, amplifying the process. Stimulation causes release of a whole host of inflammatory mediators (Fig. 31.2) and is also associated with inappropriate release of lysosomal contents. Instead of being released into phagocytic vesicles containing bacteria, they come into direct contact with the endothelium, which is thereby damaged.

Four groups of substances released from neutrophils (see Fig. 31.2) are considered to contribute to lung damage:
1. Cytokines. Neutrophils are capable of producing numerous cytokines, most of which are proinflammatory. Tumour necrosis factor alpha (TNFα) and interleukin-1β (IL-1β) have widespread proinflammatory effects, including activation of endothelial cells to upregulate the intercellular adhesion molecule and selectins, which facilitate margination of further inflammatory cells (page 353). Complement component C5a, platelet-activating factor (PAF) and IL-8 accelerate margination. Granulocyte macrophage colony-stimulating factor and IL-3 contribute to priming of further neutrophils along with interferon-γ released from other inflammatory cells. Finally, IL-1, IL-8 and TNFα all exert positive feedback on neutrophils, causing further stimulation. Transforming growth factor beta is the principal antiinflammatory cytokine produced by neutrophils, and is responsible for fibroblast stimulation and the development of pulmonary fibrosis (page 355).
2. Protease enzymes lead to extensive tissue damage in the lung. The most damaging is elastase which, unlike its name suggests, is very nonspecific, with proteolytic activity against collagen, fibrinogen and many other proteins as well as elastin. Matrix metalloproteinases are more specific for individual substrates such as collagen.
3. Reactive oxygen species and related compounds (see Chapter 25) are powerful and important bactericidal agents, which also have the capacity to damage the endothelium by lipid peroxidation and other means. In addition, they inactivate α_1-antitrypsin, an important antiprotease enzyme (page 167).
4. Lipid-derived mediators include prostaglandins, thromboxanes and leukotrienes (LT), but LTB_4 and PAF are the most important in ALI. These two act in the same way as other cytokines to amplify neutrophil activation, and, in addition, PAF damages endothelial cells directly and promotes intravascular coagulation.

Therapeutic strategies for ALI that target neutrophil activity have shown mixed results, one possible explanation being that neutrophils are also involved in lung repair once the disease process resolves, making the timing of their inhibition crucial.[20]

Macrophages, alveolar epithelial cells and monocytes have all been implicated in regulating neutrophil influx into the alveoli during ALI, though their individual roles remain unclear.[21] Macrophages are already present in the normal alveolus (page 11), but their numbers increase greatly in ALI. They produce a wide range of bactericidal agents and cytokines similar to those of the neutrophil.

Platelets are present in the pulmonary capillaries in large number in ARDS. Aggregation in the capillary is associated with increased capillary hydrostatic pressure.

Along with giving rise to pulmonary oedema, many of the mediators released by these inflammatory cells have other effects that contribute to the pulmonary changes seen in ALI. For example, arachidonic acid metabolites cause pulmonary venoconstriction, which will raise pulmonary capillary pressure and compound the effect of increased permeability. Accumulation of platelets and neutrophils along with intravascular coagulation will occlude pulmonary vessels, producing pulmonary hypertension and unperfused lung units. It has also been noted that many plasma proteins and nonsurfactant lipids such as cholesterol can antagonize the action of surfactant. Surfactant production and release are also both impaired by ALI, possibly as a result of altered alveolar expansion patterns which normally influence surfactant release.[19] Reduced surfactant function increases the surface forces in the alveolus and encourages fluid transudation (page 16). Finally, mechanisms that normally clear fluid from alveoli (page 341) are impaired in ARDS because of the effects of neutrophil cytokines on the ion channels responsible or from direct damage to alveolar epithelial cells.[22]

The potential contribution to ALI of lung damage secondary to artificial ventilation is described on page 392.

Principles of Therapy[2,10,23,24]

Early identification of ALI results in more prompt treatment of the underlying causes and allows supportive treatment to be instituted earlier.[25] This approach aims to prevent progression to ARDS and the need for artificial ventilation, and is proving an effective strategy in reducing both its incidence and mortality.[26] Studies of noninvasive ventilation (NIV; page 376) in early ALI have found conflicting results, with some showing high NIV failure rates and greater mortality when NIV was used.[27] The mode of administering NIV may also affect its efficacy, with helmet or high-flow nasal therapy being better than facemask delivery in patients with ALI.[27]

Once ARDS becomes established, artificial ventilation is normally required. Optimal management of the cardiovascular system and fluid balance[28] is a vital component of ALI treatment, as any increase in pulmonary capillary pressure (e.g., from fluid overload) exacerbates pulmonary oedema and further impairs oxygenation.

Artificial Ventilation in Acute Respiratory Distress Syndrome

General principles of artificial ventilation and the resulting physiological effects are described in detail in Chapter 32. In this section, only the problems associated with ventilation of patients with ARDS are described. Artificial ventilation in most critically ill patients is now focused on supporting, rather than replacing, the activity of the respiratory muscles to minimize the weakness that occurs while artificially ventilated (page 67). Ventilator-induced diaphragm dysfunction in ARDS is clearly described, and primarily caused by disuse atrophy: the greater the period of mechanical ventilation, the greater the degree of injury. Maintaining inspiratory effort during ventilation can help to attenuate diaphragm injury, but the practicalities of integrating this with wider lung-protective ventilation strategies can be challenging.[29] For example some studies have found spontaneous ventilation in patients with ARDS to actually be harmful,[30] and that the use of muscle relaxants as part of the artificial ventilation strategy may improve clinical outcomes.[24]

Although some clinical subgroups may benefit from this strategy, other evidence suggests no benefit when compared with light sedation without routine use of neuromuscular block.[31] The optimal degree and timing of neuromuscular blockade and deep sedation is therefore uncertain, and this perhaps illustrates the pathophysiological heterogeneity of patients with ARDS.

The lungs of patients with ARDS may be conveniently divided into three hypothetical functional sections. First, there will be some 'normal' areas, usually in the nondependent region. Second, there will be areas of lung, usually in dependent regions, with such severe collapse and alveolar flooding that ventilation of these areas will be impossible. Finally, there will be an intermediate area with poorly ventilated or collapsed alveoli that are capable of being 'recruited' by appropriate artificial ventilation, with a resultant improvement in gas exchange. Though the relative amounts of each section will vary greatly according to the severity of the ARDS, there will always be some lung in the final area, and so capable of recruitment. Once receiving artificial ventilation a fourth area of lung is commonly described in nondependent regions involving overdistended lung tissue, possibly leading to volutrauma (page 392) and further lung injury.

Tidal Volume

The recognition that positive pressure ventilation can lead to lung damage led to a change in ventilatory technique used in patients with ARDS. Overdistension of alveoli by application of large tidal volumes is a significant factor in lung damage. In particular, because of the extensive areas of pulmonary collapse, a typical patient with ARDS may only have approximately one-third of the lung being ventilated. This concept that only a small portion of lung tissue is available for ventilation has for many years been referred to as the 'baby lung' concept.[32] Thus use of a normal tidal volume (10–12 mL.kg^{-1}) will, for the few alveoli being ventilated, equate to a tidal volume of three times the usual for normal healthy lungs, which equates to over 2 L in a 70-kg subject. Smaller tidal volume is a key part of the protective ventilation strategy described next, but the correct tidal volume to use in an individual patient remains controversial.

Ventilation Mode

Pressure-controlled ventilation (page 378) is the preferred technique to avoid alveolar overdistension. However, with pressure-controlled ventilation in lungs with low compliance, such as ARDS, the delivery of an adequate minute volume may be difficult. Two techniques are advocated to deal with this problem. First, inverse inspiration/expiration ratios may be used, in which expiratory time is shorter than inspiratory time, allowing the delivery of a larger tidal volume. Second, the hypercapnia that results from the inadequate minute volume may be partially ignored. Known as permissive hypercapnia, arterial $P\text{CO}_2$ is allowed to increase until the respiratory acidosis is deemed detrimental. Despite evidence from animal studies that hypercapnia may reduce lung inflammation and cell apoptosis,[33] the impact of the widespread use of this strategy in clinical practice remains controversial.[34]

Positive End-Expiratory Pressure[35]

In patients with ARDS positive end-expiratory pressure (PEEP) reduces the amount of noninflated lung tissue seen on CT scans, particularly in dependent lung regions.[36] Shunt fraction and therefore the arterial $P\text{O}_2$ (Fig. 31.3) also improve. Reduced pulmonary compliance means that cardiac output is better maintained than might be expected (page 391), with a reduction of about 20% with PEEP of 15 cmH$_2$O (Fig. 31.3).

The ideal PEEP value to use has been controversial for decades. Differing end points (shown here in parentheses) have given rise to numerous terms such as 'optimal' PEEP (lowest physiological shunt fraction), 'best' PEEP (optimal static lung compliance), 'preferred' PEEP (best oxygen delivery) and 'least' PEEP (acceptable values for arterial $P\text{O}_2$, inspired oxygen and cardiac output). High levels of PEEP should result in increased alveolar recruitment and improved oxygenation, but normal alveoli can only enlarge in response to PEEP to a certain extent, above which dramatic increases in alveolar pressure, and possible damage, occur (pages 392 et seq). Identifying this point has vexed intensivists for some time. The aim is to identify patients who have 'recruitable' lung tissue and then use the minimum PEEP level required to recruit that lung. Assuming that recruiting more lung tissue will improve oxygenation, simply setting PEEP according to the $F\text{IO}_2$ being used is a simple approach.[37] Current strategies acknowledge that ventilated patients with ARDS are a heterogenous group, and that PEEP should be customized to each individual's lung mechanics.[35] One such approach is to increase PEEP until the lower inflection of the patient's respiratory system static compliance curve is reached (point A in Fig. 31.4), which is normally between 10 and 15 cmH$_2$O. The pressure seen at the lower point of inflection is believed to represent the pressure at which most recruitable alveoli have been opened, whereas the upper inflection point (Fig. 31.4, *B*) designates the point above which overdistension of alveoli is occurring.

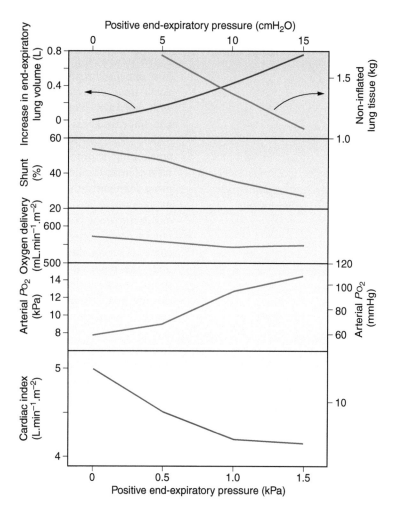

- **Fig. 31.3** Effect of positive end-expiratory pressure on various factors influencing oxygen delivery in patients with acute respiratory distress syndrome. Although arterial Po_2 is increased, cardiac output is decreased, and there is no significant change in oxygen transport. (Data on noninflated lung tissue are from Gattinoni L, Pesenti A, Bombino M, et al. Relationships between lung computed tomographic density, gas exchange, and PEEP in acute respiratory failure. *Anesthesiology.* 1988;69:824-832; remaining data from reference 36.)

Similar techniques involve titrating PEEP to driving pressure (page 393) or stress index, a measure derived from a pressure-time curve during inspiration.[35] Obese patients with a body mass index (BMI) over $35kg.m^{-2}$ are often excluded from clinical trials evaluating PEEP in ARDS. However, a recent small study of this patient group has demonstrated benefit titrating PEEP to the best respiratory system elastance following a recruitment maneuver.[38] Given the increasing prevalence of obesity, this is an area of ongoing research interest.

Finally, using imaging methods such as CT scans is seen by some as the 'gold standard' for identifying recruitable lung,[39] though not all groups have found this to be useful.[40] CT scanning is impractical to perform in unstable patients, and less invasive methods which can be performed at the bedside such as ultrasound and electrical impedance tomography (see Figure 32.7) are now being investigated.[35]

In clinical practice using higher levels of PEEP (13.2 cmH_2O) versus lower levels (8.3 cmH_2O) has been shown to improve oxygenation, but this did not result in any difference in survival.[41] Possible reasons for this lack of outcome benefit include adverse effects of the higher PEEP on the lungs or cardiovascular system, or that some patients with ALI may have very little 'recruitable' volume of lung.

Protective Ventilation Strategy

In ARDS, the ventilatory strategy used must balance the conflicting requirements of maintaining adequate gas exchange in severely diseased lungs while simultaneously avoiding damaging the lungs by the use of large tidal volumes, high airway pressures or harmful levels of inspired oxygen. Protective ventilation describes a widely advocated ventilatory strategy that may achieve the best compromise, and involves using small tidal volumes to prevent alveolar overdistension and moderate levels of PEEP to maintain alveolar recruitment. Initial tidal volumes used for ventilation should be 6 $mL.kg^{-1}$ and based on predicted body weight. A personalized level of PEEP is set as described

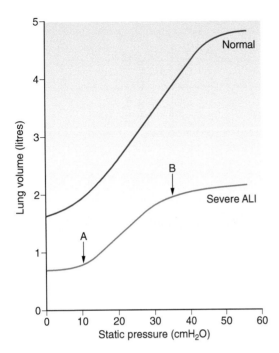

• **Fig. 31.4** Static pressure versus lung volume curves for patients receiving positive pressure ventilation. Note the severely reduced lung volume and compliance in acute lung injury *(ALI)*. Point A indicates the lower inflection of the curve, above which compliance is considerably improved. Application of a positive end-expiratory pressure of approximately 12 cmH₂O in this patient will therefore improve tidal volume relative to the ventilatory pressure required. Point B indicates the upper inflection point, above which alveolar overdistension may occur; therefore, in this patient airway pressure should ideally be maintained below 35 cmH₂O.

earlier. If plateau airway pressure exceeds 30 cmH₂O, or the inspired oxygen level required to obtain acceptable arterial $P\text{O}_2$ exceeds 0.65, then an alternative ventilatory strategy should be considered. Driving pressure (page 264) appears to be the component of protective ventilation most strongly associated with improved survival,[42,43] except in obese patients in whom there is no association.[44] This is believed to result from the chest wall rather than lung contribution to the increased driving pressure (page 199).

Protective ventilation is the only intervention in the management of ARDS that has consistently been found to improve survival. Despite this clear benefit, the use of protective ventilation in patients with ARDS is not yet universally adopted, and this results in avoidable mortality.[45]

Recruitment Manoeuvres[46]

Recruitment manoeuvres, similar to those described for atelectasis during anaesthesia (page 251), may be used in patients with ARDS. Transient, self-limiting, cardiovascular changes[47] and/or desaturation are common, but the manoeuvres do improve oxygenation, though this has not yet been proven to translate into improved outcomes. Recent work in an animal model of ARDS found that recruitment manoeuvres dislodged airway mucous into more distal airways,[48] raising the possibility that abnormal sputum clearance during artificial ventilation worsens ARDS.[49]

Prone Positioning[50]

In the ventilated patient in the prone position lung perfusion remains broadly unchanged, whereas recruitment of dorsal lung units exceeds the derecruitment in ventral areas with consistent improvement in oxygenation.[51] There are also improvements in chest wall mechanics and, in many patients, carbon dioxide clearance. Metaanalysis of prone positioning shows improvements in mortality with low rates of serious complications, suggesting it should be used more frequently than as a rescue technique for refractory hypoxaemia.[52] Proning 'dose', the number of hours per day in the prone position, varies widely, from 4 to 24 hours, but increased dose may be associated with improved outcomes. During the COVID-19 pandemic of 2020 (page 352) the reported benefit of early proning even during spontaneous ventilation led to the common usage of this therapy in an attempt to avoid the risks of intubation and artificial ventilation.

Alternative Respiratory Support Strategies[53]

Many other techniques are described as part of respiratory support for patients with ARDS who continue to have unacceptably poor gas exchange despite the use of protective ventilation. Possible interventions include:

- Muscle relaxation (see discussion)
- Inverse ratio ventilation (page 381)
- Inhaled nitric oxide (page 84)[54]
- High-frequency oscillatory ventilation (page 384)[55]
- Extrapulmonary gas exchange (page 394)[56]
- Partial liquid ventilation.[57]

Other Therapeutic Options[58]

Specific therapy for ALI is the goal of much research, which is directed particularly towards the control of sepsis and the development of antagonists to the various mediators considered earlier. In most cases it has proved difficult to demonstrate their efficacy in the clinical setting. Detailed description of these, and several other pharmacological approaches to the treatment of ALI, is beyond the scope of this book, but a summary is shown in Table 31.3.

Future Directions

Using reanalyses of earlier randomized trials, two ARDS subphenotypes have been identified: the hyperinflammatory subphenotype characterized by higher plasma concentrations of inflammatory biomarkers and a higher prevalence of sepsis, and the hypoinflammatory subphenotype, which is more common. The hyperinflammatory subphenotype is associated with greater mortality.[59] Genetic studies have also been carried out indicating an association between genotype and outcome in ARDS.[60] Whether subphenotypes or genotypes are amenable to targeted treatment strategies is as yet unclear, but indicate future areas of research interest.

TABLE 31.3 Summary of Pharmacological Interventions Suggested for the Treatment of Acute Lung Injury (ALI) or Acute Respiratory Distress Syndrome

Therapy	Examples	Proposed Mechanism
Pulmonary vasodilators	Prostacyclin	Nonspecific pulmonary vasodilator
	Nitric oxide	Regional pulmonary vasodilator (see text)
	Almitrine	Enhancement of hypoxic pulmonary vasoconstriction
Surfactant	Artificial surfactants	Replace depleted alveolar surfactant, may also have antiinflammatory properties
Antiinflammatory	Steroids	General antiinflammatory
	Ketoconazole	Inhibits thromboxane synthesis
	Ibuprofen/indomethacin	Inhibits prostaglandin production
	Prostaglandin E$_1$	Inhibits platelet aggregation, vasodilator
	Statins	Antiinflammatory and endothelial protection
	Pentoxifylline	Reduces neutrophil chemotaxis and activation
	Endotoxin/TNF/IL-1 antagonists	Inhibition of specific aspects of inflammatory response
Antioxidants	N-Acetylcysteine	Increased glutathione activity (page 290)
	Recombinant human manganese SOD	Replaces epithelial extracellular SOD (page 290)
Anticoagulants	Heparin	Reduce fibrin deposition in alveoli
Antiplatelets	Aspirin	Reduce platelet adhesion in pulmonary capillaries

All the therapies listed have been shown to have beneficial effects in in vitro or animal studies of ALI. There is insufficient evidence of improved outcome for any of the therapies listed to be recommended for routine use in human ALI.

IL-1, Interleukin-1; *SOD,* superoxide dismutase; *TNF,* tumour necrosis factor.

References

1. Wheeler AP, Bernard GR. Acute lung injury and the acute respiratory distress syndrome: a clinical review. *Lancet.* 2007;369:1553-1565.
2. MacSweeney R, McAuley DF. Acute respiratory distress syndrome. *Lancet.* 2016;388:2416-2430.
3. Bernard GR, Artigas A, Brigham KL, et al. The American-European consensus conference on ARDS: definitions, mechanisms, relevant outcomes, and clinical trial coordination. *Am J Respir Crit Care Med.* 1994;149:818-824.
*4. The ARDS Definition Task Force. **Acute respiratory distress syndrome. The Berlin definition. JAMA. 2012;307:2526-2533.**
5. Fröhlich S, Murphy N, Boylan JF. ARDS: progress unlikely with non-biological definition. *Br J Anaesth.* 2013;111:696-699.
6. Vlaar APJ, Juffermans NP. Transfusion-related acute lung injury: a clinical review. *Lancet.* 2013;382:984-994.
7. Lemos-Filho LB, Mikkelsen ML, Martin GS, et al. Sex, race, and the development of acute lung injury. *Chest.* 2013;143:901-909.
8. Killien E, Mills B, Watson RS. Morbidity and mortality among critically injured children with acute respiratory distress syndrome. *Crit Care Med.* 2019;47:e112-e119.
9. Pelosi P, D'Onofrio D, Chiumello D, et al. Pulmonary and extrapulmonary acute respiratory distress syndrome are different. *Eur Respir J.* 2003;22(suppl 42):48S-56S.
10. Thompson BT, Chambers RC, Liu KD. Acute respiratory distress syndrome. *N Engl J Med.* 2017;377:562-572.
11. Zhang Z, Spieth P, Chiumello D, et al. Declining mortality in patients with acute respiratory distress syndrome; an analysis of the acute respiratory distress network trials. *Crit Care Med.* 2019;47:315-323.
12. Coudroy R, Frat J-P, Boissier F, et al. Early identification of acute respiratory distress syndrome in the absence of positive pressure ventilation: implications for revision of the Berlin criteria for acute respiratory distress syndrome. *Crit Care Med.* 2018;46:540-546.
13. Matthay MA, Ware LB. Resolution of alveolar edema in acute respiratory distress syndrome. Physiology and biology. *Am J Respir Crit Care Med.* 2015;192:124-125.
14. Michard F. Bedside assessment of extravascular lung water by dilution methods: temptations and pitfalls. *Crit Care Med.* 2007;35:1186-1192.
*15. Radermacher P, Maggiore SM, Mercat A. **Gas exchange in acute respiratory distress syndrome. Am J Respir Crit Care Med. 2017;196:964-984.**
16. Cressoni M, Cadringher P, Chiurazzi C, et al. Lung inhomogeneity in patients with acute respiratory distress syndrome. *Am J Respir Crit Care Med.* 2014;189:149-158.
*17. Cabrera-Benitez NE, Laffey JG, Parotto M, et al. **Mechanical ventilation–associated lung fibrosis in acute respiratory distress syndrome. A significant contributor to poor outcome. Anesthesiology. 2014;121:189-198.**
18. Hendrickson CM, Crestani B, Matthay MA. Biology and pathology of fibroproliferation following the acute respiratory distress syndrome. *Intensive Care Med.* 2015;41:147-150.
19. Bhattacharya J, Matthay MA. Regulation and repair of the alveolar-capillary barrier in acute lung injury. *Annu Rev Physiol.* 2013;75:593-615.
20. Grudzinska FS, Sapey E. Friend or foe? The dual role of neutrophils in lung injury and repair. *Thorax.* 2018;73:305-307.
21. Su X. Leading neutrophils to the alveoli. Who is the guider? *Am J Respir Crit Care Med.* 2012;186:472-473.

22. Matthay MA. Resolution of pulmonary edema thirty years of progress. *Am J Respir Crit Care Med.* 2014;189:1301-1308.

*23. Fan E, Brodie D, Slutsky AS. Acute respiratory distress syndrome. Advances in diagnosis and treatment. *JAMA.* 2018;319:698-710.

24. Matthay MA, McAuley DF, Ware LB. Clinical trials in acute respiratory distress syndrome: challenges and opportunities. *Lancet Respir Med.* 2017;5:524-534.

25. Rogers AJ, Liu VX. 16 Years and counting? Time to implement noninvasive screening for ARDS. *Chest.* 2016;150:266-267.

26. Bersten AD, Cooper DJ. Better supportive care, less ARDS. Just do it? *Am J Respir Crit Care Med.* 2011;183:6-7.

27. Hill NS, Garpestad E. The bumpy road for noninvasive ventilation in acute respiratory distress syndrome coming to an end? *Am J Respir Crit Care Med.* 2017;195:9-10.

28. Seeley EJ. Fluid therapy during acute respiratory distress syndrome: less is more, simplified. *Crit Care Med.* 2015;43:477-478.

29. Schepens T, Goligher E. Lung and diaphragm protective ventilation in acute respiratory distress syndrome. *Anaesthesiology.* 2019; 130: 620-633.

30. Yoshida T, Fujino Y, Amato MBP, et al. Spontaneous breathing during mechanical ventilation risks, mechanisms, and management. *Am J Respir Crit Care Med.* 2017;195:985-992.

31. Slutsky A, Villar J. Early paralytic agents for ARDS? Yes, no and sometimes. *N Eng J Med.* 2019;380:2061-2063.

32. Gattinoni L, Marini JJ, Pesenti A, et al. The "baby lung" became an adult. *Intensive Care Med.* 2016; 42:663-673.

33. Nardelli LM, Rzezinski A, Silva JD, et al. Effects of acute hypercapnia with and without acidosis on lung inflammation and apoptosis in experimental acute lung injury. *Respir Physiol Neurobiol.* 2015;205:1-6.

*34. Barnes T, Zochios V, Parhar K. Re-examining permissive hypercapnia in ARDS. *Chest.* 2018;154:185-195.

35. Sahetya SK, Goligher EC, Brower RG. Setting positive end-expiratory pressure in acute respiratory distress syndrome. *Am J Respir Crit Care Med.* 2017;195:1429-1438.

36. Gattinoni L, D'Andrea L, Pelosi P, et al. Regional effects and mechanism of positive end-expiratory pressure in early adult respiratory distress syndrome. *JAMA.* 1993;269:2122-2127.

37. Miller RR, MacIntyre NR, Hite RD, et al. Point: should positive end-expiratory pressure in patients with ARDS be set on oxygenation? Yes. *Chest.* 2012;141:1379-1382.

38. Fumagalli J, Santiago R, Droghi M, et al. Lung recruitment in obese patients with acute respiratory distress syndrome. *Anesthesiology.* 2019;130:791-780.

39. Goligher EC, Villar J, Slutsky AS. Positive end-expiratory pressure in acute respiratory distress syndrome: When should we turn up the pressure? *Crit Care Med.* 2014;42:448-450.

40. Cressoni M, Chiumello D, Carlesso E, et al. Compressive forces and computed tomography-derived positive end-expiratory pressure in acute respiratory distress syndrome. *Anesthesiology.* 2014;121:572-581.

41. Brower RG, Lanken PN, MacIntyre N, et al. Higher versus lower positive end-expiratory pressures in patients with the acute respiratory distress syndrome. *N Engl J Med.* 2004;351:327-336.

42. Amato MBP, Meade MO, Slutsky AS, et al. Driving pressure and survival in the acute respiratory distress syndrome. *N Engl J Med.* 2015;372:747-755.

43. Aoyama H, Pettenuzzo T, Aoyama K, et al. Association of driving pressure with mortality among ventilated patients with acute respiratory distress syndrome: a systematic review and meta-analysis. *Crit Care Med.* 2018;46:300-306.

44. De Jong A, Cossic J, Verzilli D, et al. Impact of the driving pressure on mortality in obese and non-obese ARDS patients: a retrospective study of 362 cases. *Intensive Care Med.* 2018; 44:1106-1114.

45. Fan E, Brochard L. Underuse versus equipoise for low tidal volume ventilation in acute respiratory distress syndrome: is this the right question? *Crit Care Med.* 2014;42:2310-2311.

*46. Suzumura EA, Amato MBP, Cavalcanti AB. Understanding recruitment maneuvers. *Intensive Care Med.* 2016;42: 908-911.

47. Mercado P, Maizel J, Kontar L, et al. Moderate and severe acute respiratory distress syndrome: hemodynamic and cardiac effects of an open lung strategy with recruitment maneuver analyzed using echocardiography. *Crit Care Med.* 2018;46:1608-1616.

48. Li Bassi G, Comaru T, Marti D, et al. Recruitment manoeuvres dislodge mucus towards the distal airways in an experimental model of severe pneumonia. *Br J Anaesth.* 2019;122:269-276.

49. Marini JJ, Gattinoni L. Propagation prevention: a complementary mechanism for "lung protective" ventilation in acute respiratory distress syndrome. *Crit Care Med.* 2008;36: 3252-3258.

50. Scholten EL, Beitler JR, Prisk GK, et al. Treatment of ARDS with prone positioning. *Chest.* 2017;151:215-224.

51. Gattinoni L, Taccone P, Carlesso E, et al. Prone position in acute respiratory distress syndrome rationale, indications, and limits. *Am J Respir Crit Care Med.* 2013;188:1286-1293.

52. Chiumello D, Coppola S, Froio S. Prone position in ARDS: a simple maneuver still underused. *Intensive Care Med.* 2018; 44:241-243.

53. Ferguson ND, Guérin C. Adjunct and rescue therapies for refractory hypoxemia: prone position, inhaled nitric oxide, high frequency oscillation, extra corporeal life support. *Intensive Care Med.* 2018;44:1528-1531.

54. Afshari A, Brok J, Møller AM, et al. Inhaled nitric oxide for acute respiratory distress syndrome and acute lung injury in adults and children: a systematic review with meta-analysis and trial sequential analysis. *Anesth Analg.* 2011;112:1411-1421.

55. Sklar MC, Fan E, Goligher EC. High-frequency oscillatory ventilation in adults with ARDS. Past, present, and future. *Chest.* 2017;152:1306-1317.

56. Hardin CC, Hibbert K. ECMO for severe ARDS. *N Engl J Med.* 2018;378:2032-2034.

57. Kacmarek RM, Wiedemann HP, Lavin PT, et al. Partial liquid ventilation in adult patients with acute respiratory distress syndrome. *Am J Respir Crit Care Med.* 2006;173:882-889.

58. Curley GF, Laffey JG. Future therapies for ARDS. *Intensive Care Med.* 2015;41:322-326.

59. Shankar-Hari M, Fan E, Ferguson N. Acute respiratory distress syndrome (ARDS) phenotyping. *Intensive Care Med.* 2019; 45:516-519.

*60. Kuebler W. Acute respiratory distress syndrome; biomarkers, mechanisms and water channels. *Anaesthesiology.* 2019;130: 364-366.

32

Respiratory Support and Artificial Ventilation

KEY POINTS

- Noninvasive ventilation may be used to increase airway pressure and support a failing respiratory system without the need for tracheal intubation or tracheostomy.
- Intermittent positive pressure ventilation can be delivered by a variety of different techniques, many of which are coordinated with the patient's own respiratory efforts.
- Positive end-expiratory pressure increases the functional residual capacity, reduces airway resistance and may prevent or reverse lung collapse.
- Any increase in mean intrathoracic pressure, as seen during positive pressure ventilation, impairs venous return and

increases pulmonary vascular resistance, thus reducing cardiac output.
- Artificial ventilation may damage the lung by exerting excessive pressures or volumes on lung tissue, or by causing repeated opening and closure of small airways with each breath.
- A clinically useful artificial lung remains only a distant possibility, although extracorporeal systems that partially replace pulmonary gas exchange continue to evolve.

Chapters 27–31 outlined the numerous ways in which the respiratory system may fail to achieve its primary objective of gas exchange. This chapter describes the techniques available to clinicians to improve the gas exchange functions of the respiratory system, including supporting or replacing alveolar ventilation.

Respiratory Physiotherapy

In many of the respiratory diseases described in Chapters 27–31, the patient's respiratory system is often treated with physiotherapy. This is more as part of long-term management, for example, in pulmonary rehabilitation programmes (page 333), but is also a useful part of treatment of acute lung problems, such as in ventilated patients[1] and in the postoperative period. Despite extensive involvement of physiotherapists in respiratory care throughout the world, the evidence base for improved clinical outcomes as a direct result of physiotherapy interventions is weak.[2] There are multiple possible reasons for this, not least of which are a lack of suitable studies, an underappreciation of the placebo effect and the part played by physiotherapy as a component of 'care bundles', which overall have beneficial effects.

Physiology of Respiratory Interventions

The aims of respiratory physiotherapy can be broadly classified into the following three areas.

To Increase Lung Volume

Physiotherapy can help to attenuate loss of lung volume due to atelectasis, consolidation or pleural effusion. Techniques include controlled mobilization, in which patients are assisted to exercise at a level which just increases their ventilation enough to generate deep breathing without causing anxiety or excessive fatigue, in other words, learning to achieve and maintain a state of 'slight breathlessness'. Patient positioning is important for increasing lung volume (page 23) and ventilation/perfusion matching, and sitting upright is generally beneficial. Patients with pleural effusions or large intrathoracic tumours usually learn for themselves to lie with the nonaffected lung regions uppermost. Deep breathing exercises have many respiratory benefits, most of which relate to reexpansion and ventilation of dependent lung regions. Ten deep breaths per waking hour are recommended, including an end-inspiratory hold, if possible.[3] Incentive spirometry may help patients achieve the most benefit from deep breathing. These devices provide visual feedback to patients about their inspiratory flow rate and volume, allowing these to be tailored to the optimal values for lung reexpansion in individual patients. Continuous positive airway pressure (CPAP) is used to increase lung volume and is described later. Finally, intermittent positive pressure breathing may be used, in which a positive pressure is applied to the patient's airway during inspiration, followed by passive exhalation.

To Decrease the Work of Breathing

Dyspnoea can be treated by various techniques (page 320) and attempts made to alleviate patients' perception of their breathlessness by teaching them specific techniques to control their breathing. Pulmonary rehabilitation (page 333) or noninvasive ventilation (see later discussion) are two techniques that can increase respiratory muscle efficiency or workload, respectively.

To Clear Secretions

These techniques are used routinely in the care of patients with cystic fibrosis (page 335) and in other patients in whom airway secretions are increased or their clearance impaired, such as bronchiectasis or chronic obstructive pulmonary disease (COPD). Methods available include:

- Humidification of airway gases, including ensuring the patient is systemically well hydrated.
- Exercise, as previously described, which increases minute ventilation and thus expiratory flow rates. This increases the shear stress between gas flow and airway mucus, 'pulling' the mucus away from the airway (page 47). This then provokes coughing and expectoration.
- Active breathing techniques, which includes active cycle of breathing, consisting of a combination of deep breaths followed by huffs, rapid exhalations through an open glottis and mouth. This helps to move mucus along the airway. The point in the deep breath where the huff is performed may influence where in the airway the maximal effect is achieved according to the site of the 'choke point' (page 47). Autogenic drainage involves performing controlled breaths with slow, large, inspirations, an inspiratory pause and then slow prolonged exhalation through pursed lips to maintain airway patency and prevent flow-related collapse (page 32). A series of these manoeuvres are performed at progressively increasing lung volume.
- Postural drainage describes changing body position to allow gravity to contribute to drainage of secretions from specific lung regions. This is normally used in combination with the other breathing techniques described.
- Manual techniques include percussion or vibration of the chest wall, usually combined with postural drainage. They aim to improve the clearance of mucus from the airway wall and may work by changing the physical properties of mucus during a cough, by improving airway-lining fluid and ciliary activity, increasing expiratory flow rate or freeing adhesive mucus from the airway wall. The optimal frequency of vibration is unknown, but animal studies suggest this is between 10 and 15 Hz.
- Positive expiratory pressure (PEP) may be achieved by several devices, all of which impose an expiratory resistance, some of which also cause oscillations in expiratory pressure. Although PEP has been shown to prevent expiratory airway closure and reduce gas trapping, its effectiveness at improving clearance of secretions is uncertain.
- Cough facilitation remains a key component of respiratory physiotherapy, particularly in neurological conditions when muscle function is inadequate. It may be achieved manually or mechanically.

Noninvasive Ventilation

Noninvasive ventilation (NIV) is defined as respiratory support without establishing a tracheal airway. It may be achieved by either negative pressure ventilation or positive pressure ventilation via a mask or similar device.

Negative Pressure Ventilation

This requires the application of subatmospheric pressure to the trunk. It was first reported in 1864 using a subject seated in a rigid box connected to a manually operated piston, and following the development of automatic machines it was widely used during polio epidemics in the 1950s.[4] Enthusiasm for the technique has fluctuated since, but there continues to be interest in negative pressure ventilation for a small group of patients.

Animal studies comparing negative and positive pressure ventilation show that lung perfusion is the same with both modes, but that ventilation is more evenly distributed and oxygenation better with negative pressure ventilation.[5] Negative pressure ventilation continues to have a place in the management of respiratory failure resulting from neuromuscular disorders, central apnoeas or in paediatric intensive care.

A cabinet ventilator, often referred to as an *iron lung*, requires the whole body except the head to be encased in a cabinet with an airtight seal around the neck. An intermittent negative pressure is then applied in the tank, causing inspiration, with passive expiration as normal. A superimposed continuous negative pressure may also be applied, which provides the negative pressure equivalent of positive end-expiratory pressure (PEEP). In terms of the airway-to-ambient pressure gradient, cabinet ventilators are identical in principle to positive pressure ventilation, with similar effects on cardiovascular and respiratory physiology. Collapse of the extrathoracic upper airway during inspiration may occur, particularly during sleep. Vomiting or regurgitation of gastric contents exposes the patient to the danger of aspiration during the inspiratory phase.

Cuirass and jacket ventilators are a simplified form of cabinet ventilators in which the application of subatmospheric pressure is confined to the trunk or anterior abdominal wall. Function depends on a good airtight seal. They are less efficient than cabinet ventilators and suffer from the same disadvantages. However, they are much more convenient to use and may be useful to supplement inadequate spontaneous breathing.

Noninvasive Positive Pressure Ventilation

Positive pressure ventilation may be delivered using soft masks that fit over the mouth and nose or the nose only or using a clear plastic helmet that fits over the entire head (sealed around the neck). Most ventilator systems used are pressure generators, and so are 'leak-tolerant'; that is, flow automatically increases to compensate for a pressure drop because of gas leakage, but there is variation in how well this is achieved between different ventilators and ventilation modes.[6] With nasal ventilation, positive pressure in the nasopharynx normally displaces the soft palate anteriorly against the tongue, thus preventing escape of gas through the mouth.

Complications of NIV include nasal skin damage or ulceration, gastric distension, claustrophobia and discomfort. Helmet systems avoid some of these problems, but have a volume of around 10 L, which inevitably causes some rebreathing, making hypercapnia a common complication. The high volume in the helmet also results in a time delay when changing the pressure in the helmet to support ventilation or when sensing a spontaneous breath with pressure changes (see later).[7]

Techniques of ventilation are similar to invasive artificial ventilation. Ventilator modes that use patient triggering are better tolerated than controlled ventilation, particularly in awake patients. Pressure-controlled ventilation (PCV) or pressure support ventilation (PSV, see later) is commonly used along with CPAP. In bilevel positive airway pressure the ventilator pressure steps between two preset values for inspiration and expiration, and, except for the terminology used to describe the pressures, is the same as PSV with CPAP.

Ventilation may be provided continually during acute respiratory problems, or only at night for long-term respiratory disease. The use of nasal CPAP for treating sleep-disordered breathing has been described on page 197. In this case benefit occurs simply by displacing the soft palate away from the posterior pharyngeal wall. Benefit in other respiratory diseases is more difficult to explain, but in the COVID-19 pandemic of 2020 (page 352), CPAP (with pragmatic arterial blood gas targets for gas exchange) was reported to be particularly effective at preventing patients progressing to artificial ventilation. Possible mechanisms for a benefit of NIV include:

- Resting fatigued respiratory muscles
- Delivery of a higher inspired oxygen concentration by the use of a tight-fitting facemask
- Augmentation of minute ventilation to reduce hypercapnia
- Prevention or reexpansion of areas of atelectasis, as seen when using PEEP (see later)
- Reduction of cardiac preload in patients with heart failure (page 391)

Clinical Applications

NIV is now advocated for the treatment of acute respiratory failure from numerous causes,[8,9] although outcome evidence supporting its use is variable as follows:

- *COPD exacerbations* (page 331). NIV is now recommended for treatment of COPD exacerbation leading to respiratory acidosis, but not for other, less severe, exacerbations.
- *Cardiogenic pulmonary oedema.* This may be successfully treated with NIV, reducing the need for tracheal intubation and improving mortality. The mechanism of this beneficial effect is explained on page 344.
- *Acute lung injury (ALI).* NIV instituted early in the course of ALI (Chapter 31) may reduce the need for tracheal intubation, improve gas exchange and lead to improved long-term outcomes in survivors,[10] although data on mortality remains inconclusive.[11]
- *Weaning from invasive ventilation* (page 385).[12] NIV may be used to gradually wean patients from invasive ventilation, a strategy that is particularly useful in patients with COPD or obesity.

Intermittent Positive Pressure Ventilation

Phases of the Respiratory Cycle

Inspiration

During intermittent positive pressure ventilation (IPPV), the mouth (or airway) pressure is intermittently raised above ambient pressure. The inspired gas then flows into the lungs in accord with the resistance and compliance of the respiratory system. If inspiration is slow, the distribution is governed mainly by regional compliance. If inspiration is fast, there is preferential ventilation of parts of the lungs with short time constants (see Fig. 2.6). Different temporal patterns of pressure may be applied, as discussed next.

Expiration

During IPPV, expiration results from allowing mouth pressure to fall to ambient. Expiration is then passive and differs from expiration during spontaneous breathing in which diaphragm muscle tone is gradually reduced (page 43). Expiration may be impeded by the application of PEEP. In the past, expiration was sometimes accelerated by the application of a subatmospheric pressure, termed *negative end-expiratory pressure*, although this technique is no longer used. Expiration to ambient pressure is termed *zero end-expiratory pressure* (ZEEP).

If the inflating pressure is maintained for several seconds, the resulting tidal volume will be indicated by the following relationship:

$$\text{Tidal volume} = \text{sustained inflation pressure} \times \text{total static compliance.}$$

Thus for example, a sustained inflation pressure of 10 cmH$_2$O with a static compliance of 0.5 L.kPa^{-1} (50 mL.cmH$_2$O^{-1}) would result in a lung volume 500 mL above functional residual capacity (FRC).

Time Course of Inflation and Deflation

Equilibration according to the previous equation usually takes several seconds. When the airway pressure is raised during inspiration, it is opposed by the two forms of impedance: the elastic resistance of lungs and chest wall (Chapter 2) and resistance to air flow (Chapter 3). At any instant, the inflation pressure equals the sum of the pressures required to overcome these two forms of impedance. The pressure required to overcome elastic resistance equals the lung volume above FRC divided by the total (dynamic) compliance, whereas the pressure required to overcome air flow resistance equals the air flow resistance multiplied by the instantaneous flow rate.

The effect of applying a constant pressure (PCV) is shown in Figure 32.1. The two components of the inflation pressure vary during the course of inspiration, while their sum remains constant. The component overcoming air flow resistance is maximal at first and declines exponentially with air flow as inflation proceeds. The component overcoming elastic resistance increases with the lung volume. With normal respiratory mechanics in the unconscious patient, the change in lung volume should be 95% complete in about 1.5 seconds, as in Figure 32.1.

The approach of the lung volume to its equilibrium value is according to an exponential function of the wash-in type (see Appendix E). The time constant, which is the time required for inflation to 63% of the equilibrium value, equals the product of resistance and compliance. Normal values for an unconscious patient are as follows:

$$\text{Time constant} = \text{resistance} \times \text{compliance}$$
$$0.5\,s = 1\,kPa.L^{-1}.s \times 0.5\,L.kPa^{-1}$$

or

$$0.5\,s = 10\,cmH_2O.L^{-1}.s \times 0.05\,L.cmH_2O^{-1}$$

The time constant is the time that would be required to reach equilibrium if the initial inspiratory flow rate were maintained. It is sometimes more convenient to use the half-time, which is 0.69 times the time constant. The inflation curve is shown in full with further mathematical detail in Appendix E.

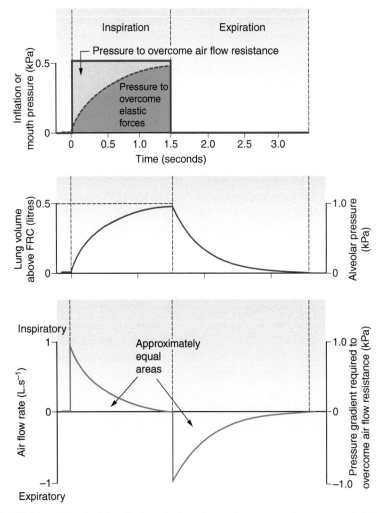

• **Fig. 32.1** Artificial ventilation by intermittent application of a constant pressure (pressure-controlled ventilation) followed by passive expiration. Inspiratory and expiratory flow rates are both exponential. Assuming that air flow resistance is constant, it follows that flow rate and pressure gradient required to overcome resistance may be shown on the same graph. Lung volume and alveolar pressure may be shown on the same graph if compliance is constant. Values are typical for an anaesthetized, supine, paralysed patient: total dynamic compliance, 0.5 L.kPa⁻¹ (50 mL.cmH₂O⁻¹); pulmonary resistance, 0.3 kPa.L⁻¹.s (3 cmH₂O.L⁻¹.s); apparatus resistance, 0.7 kPa.L⁻¹.s (7 cmH₂O.L⁻¹.s); total resistance, 1 kPa.L⁻¹.s (10 cmH₂O.L⁻¹.s); time constant, 0.5 seconds.

It is normal practice for the inspiratory phase to be terminated after 1 or 2 seconds, at which time the lung volume will still be increasing. Inflation pressure is not then the sole arbiter of tidal volume but must be considered in relation to the duration of the inspiratory phase.

If expiration is passive and mouth pressure remains at ambient, the driving force is the elevation of alveolar pressure above ambient, which is caused by elastic recoil of lungs and chest wall. This pressure is dissipated in overcoming air flow resistance during expiration. In Figure 32.1, during expiration the alveolar pressure (proportional to the lung volume above FRC) is directly proportional to expiratory flow rate, and all three quantities decline according to a wash-out exponential function with a time constant which is again equal to the product of compliance and resistance.

Effect of Changes in Inflation Pressure, Resistance and Compliance

The blue line in Figure 32.2 shows the inflation curve for the normal parameters of an unconscious paralysed patient, as listed in Table 32.1. These are the same values that were considered earlier. The basic curve is a single exponential approaching a lung volume 0.5 L above FRC with a time

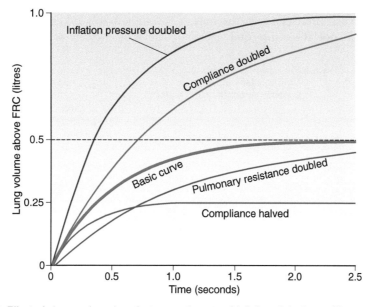

• **Fig. 32.2** Effect of changes in various factors on the rate of inflation of the lungs. Fixed relationships: final tidal volume achieved = inflation pressure × compliance; time constant = compliance × resistance. (See also Table 32.1.) *FRC,* Functional residual capacity.

TABLE 32.1 Parameters for Inflation Curves Shown in Figure 32.2

	Basic Curve	Pulmonary Resistance Doubled	Inflation Pressure Doubled	Compliance Doubled	Compliance Halved
Inflation pressure					
(kPa)	1	1	2	1	1
(cmH$_2$O)	10	10	20	10	10
Compliance					
(L.kPa^{-1})	0.5	0.5	0.5	1	0.25
(mL.cmH$_2$O^{-1})	50	50	50	100	25
Final tidal volume (L)	0.5	0.5	1	1	0.25
Pulmonary resistance					
(kPa.L^{-1}.s)	1	2	1	1	1
(cmH$_2$O.L^{-1}.s)	10	20	10	10	10
Time constant					
(s)	0.5	1	0.5	1	0.25

constant of 0.5 seconds. Changes in inflation pressure do not alter the time constant of inflation, but directly influence the amount of air introduced into the lungs in a given number of time constants. In Figure 32.2, each point on the red curve labelled 'inflation pressure doubled' is twice the height of the corresponding point on the basic curve for the same time.

Effect of Changes in Compliance and Resistance

If the compliance is doubled, the equilibrium tidal volume is also doubled. However, the time constant (product of compliance and resistance) is also doubled; therefore, the equilibrium volume is approached more slowly (Fig. 32.2). Conversely, if the compliance is halved, the equilibrium tidal volume is also halved along with the time constant.

Changes in resistance have a direct effect on the time constant of inflation, but do not affect the equilibrium

tidal volume. Thus the effect of an increased resistance on tidal volume is through the reduction in inspiratory flow rate. Within limits, this can be counteracted by prolonging inspiration or by increasing the inflation pressure and the degree of overpressure (explained later). The effects, shown in Figure 32.2, apply not only to the whole lung but also to regions that may have different compliances, resistances and time constants (page 90).

Overpressure

Increasing the inflation pressure has a major effect on the time required to achieve a particular lung volume above FRC. In Figure 32.3, the lung characteristics are the same as for the 'basic curve' in Figure 32.2. If the required tidal volume is 475 mL, this is achieved in 1.5 seconds with an inflation pressure of 10 cmH$_2$O. However, the same lung

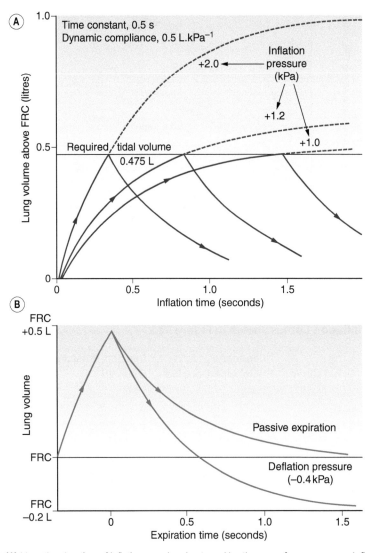

• **Fig. 32.3 (A)** How the duration of inflation may be shortened by the use of overpressure. Inflation curves are shown for +2 kPa (+20 cmH$_2$O; equilibrium 1 L), +1.2 kPa (+12 cmH$_2$O; equilibrium 0.6 L) and +1 kPa (+10 cmH$_2$O; equilibrium 0.5 L). With a required tidal volume of 0.475 L note the big reduction in duration of inflation needed when the inflation pressure is increased from 1 to 2 kPa (10–20 cmH$_2$O). **(B)** How expiration is influenced by the use of a subatmospheric pressure or 'negative phase'. Expiration may be terminated at the functional residual capacity (*FRC*) after 0.6 seconds, or may be prolonged, in which case the lung volume will fall to 0.2 L below FRC.

volume is achieved in only 0.3 seconds by doubling the inflation pressure. The application of a pressure that, if sustained, would give a tidal volume higher than that which is intended is known as overpressure; it is used extensively to increase the inspiratory flow rate to shorten the inspiratory phase. The use of a subatmospheric pressure to increase the rate of passive expiration is similar in principle but is complicated by air trapping (Fig. 32.3, *B*).

Deviations from True Exponential Character of Expiration

It is helpful to assume that the patterns of air flow previously described are exponential in character, as this greatly assists our understanding of the situation. However, there are many reasons why air flow should not be strictly exponential in character. Air flow is normally partly turbulent (see Chapter 3); therefore, resistance cannot be considered as a constant. Furthermore, as expiration proceeds, the calibre of the air passages decreases, and there is also a transition to more laminar flow as the instantaneous flow rate decreases. Approximation to a single exponential function is nevertheless good enough for many practical purposes.

Alternative Patterns of Application of Inflation Pressure

Constant pressure or square wave inflation was previously considered because it is the easiest for mathematical analysis. There are, however, a variety of pressure profiles that may be applied for IPPV. There is no convincing evidence of the superiority of one over the other, except that distribution of inspired gas is improved if there is a prolongation of the period during which the applied pressure is maximal. This permits better ventilation of the 'slow' alveoli.

Constant flow rate ventilators (volume-controlled ventilation [VCV]) are extensively used, and Figure 32.4 shows pressure, volume and flow changes in a manner analogous to Figure 32.1.

Control of Duration of Inspiration

Three methods are in general use.
1. *Time cycling* terminates inspiration after a preset time, irrespective of whether inspiration is achieved by constant pressure or constant flow generation. With constant flow generators, inspiratory time has a direct effect on the tidal volume. With constant pressure generators the relationship is more complex, as described earlier (see Fig. 32.3).
2. *Volume cycling* terminates inspiration when a preset volume has been delivered. In the absence of a leak this should guarantee the tidal volume even if the compliance or resistance of the respiratory system changes within limits.
3. *Pressure cycling* terminates inspiration when a particular airway pressure is achieved. This in no way guarantees the

tidal volume. Increased airway resistance, for example, would limit inspiratory flow rate and cause a more rapid increase in mouth pressure, thus terminating the inspiratory phase. Pressure-cycled ventilators are almost invariably flow generators.

Limitations on inspiratory duration. Whatever the means of cycling, it is possible to add a limitation on inspiratory duration, usually as a safety precaution. For example, a pressure limitation can be added to a time-cycled or a volume-cycled ventilator. This can either function as a pressure relief valve or it can terminate the inspiratory phase.

The Inspiratory to Expiratory Ratio

For a given minute volume of ventilation, it is possible to vary within wide limits the duration of inspiration and expiration and the ratio between the two. A common pattern is about 1 second for inspiration, followed by 2 to 4 seconds for expiration (inspiratory to expiratory [I:E] ratio 1:2–1:4), giving respiratory frequencies in the range of 12 to 20 breaths per minute. The problem is whether changes from this pattern confer any appreciable benefit in terms of gas exchange. Reduction of the inspiratory time to less than 1 second may cause an increase in dead space, but there is no evidence that the duration of inspiration (in the range of 0.5–3 seconds) has any appreciable effect on the alveolar/arterial P_{O_2} gradient. Thus the accepted view seems to be that 1 second is a reasonable minimal time for inspiration.

Inverse I:E ratio ventilation increases the mean lung volume and may be expected to achieve some of the advantages of PEEP as considered later. It may be achieved either by slowing the inspiratory flow rate (shallow ramp) or by holding the lung volume at the end of inspiration (inspiratory pause); the latter seems to be more logical. I:E ratios as high as 4:1 have been used, but 2:1 is generally preferable. The degree of inverse I:E ratio used is limited by the cardiovascular disturbances seen with the technique (see later discussion) and the time available for expiration. If the latter is unduly curtailed, FRC will be increased, generating so-called 'intrinsic-PEEP' (see later).

Gas redistribution during an inspiratory hold reduces the dead space (page 97), resulting in a lower P_{CO_2} for the same minute volume. This permits the use of a lower peak inflation pressure.

Clinical Use of Intermittent Positive Pressure Ventilation

The previous section classifies ventilators according to the method of gas flow generation (for example, constant flow or constant pressure generators) based on the mechanism by which the ventilator worked. Most ventilators in clinical use are now electronically controlled. These allow accurate control of gas pressure and flow throughout the ventilator circuit and can normally perform as either flow or pressure generators with various inspiratory flow patterns. In addition, they have given rise to a whole host of previously

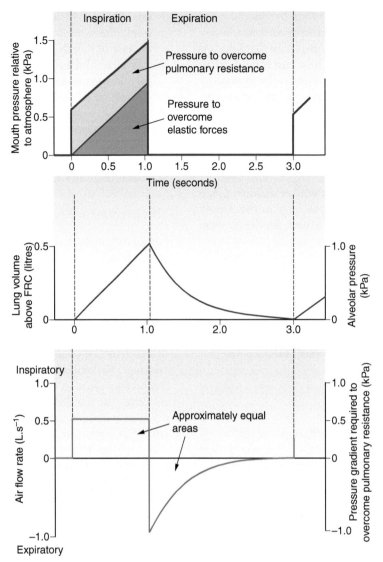

• **Fig. 32.4** Artificial ventilation by intermittent application of a constant flow (volume-controlled ventilation) with passive expiration. Note that inspiratory flow rate is constant. Assuming that pulmonary resistance is constant, it follows that a constant amount of the inflation pressure is required to overcome flow resistance. Lung volume and alveolar pressure may be shown on the same graph if compliance is constant. Values are typical for an anaesthetized, supine, paralysed patient: total dynamic compliance, 0.5 L.kPa^{-1} (50 mL.cmH$_2$O^{-1}); pulmonary resistance, 0.3 kPa.L^{-1}.s (3 cmH$_2$O.L^{-1}.s); apparatus resistance, 0.7 kPa.L^{-1}.seconds (7 cmH$_2$O.L^{-1}.s); total resistance, 1 kPa.L^{-1}.s (10 cmH$_2$O.L^{-1}.s); time constant, 0.5 seconds. *FRC*, Functional residual capacity.

impossible ventilatory techniques, a majority of which are dependent on the ventilator responding appropriately to the patient's own respiratory efforts.

Interactions Between Patient and Ventilator

For many years there have been ventilators in which the inspiratory phase could be triggered with a spontaneous breath, and mechanical ventilators could be modified to facilitate a mandatory minute volume (MMV) of ventilation, as described next. Electronic ventilators continuously monitor tidal volume, whether generated by the patient (spontaneous breath) or artificially (ventilator breath). With this information available it is a simple task to achieve, by

electronic means, a predetermined minute volume, number of breaths, and so on, by introducing extra ventilator breaths when necessary. The challenge for ventilator design in recent years has been the speed and sensitivity with which ventilators can sense, and respond to, the patient's respiratory efforts to synchronize ventilator and spontaneous breaths. Without this synchronization, a patient with any reasonable spontaneous respiratory effort begins to 'fight' against the ventilator. Some degree of asynchrony occurs in all ventilated patients,[13] and this leads to discomfort, poor gas exchange, cardiovascular disturbance and worse clinical outcomes.

There are three ways by which a ventilator may detect the onset of a spontaneous breath as follows.

Pressure Sensing

At the onset of a respiratory effort, the patient will generate a reduction in pressure within the circuit, which may be detected in the ventilator. This pressure wave travels through the circuit at approximately the speed of sound, reaching the ventilator within 12 ms, following which the pressure sensor must respond, and flow into the circuit be increased to facilitate inspiration. Overall, these events take approximately 100 ms to occur, which is undetectable by the patient. The pressure drop required to trigger inspiration is now always measured relative to circuit (not atmospheric) pressure, to allow the use of CPAP/PEEP during ventilation. The time taken to trigger the ventilator increases with decreased sensitivity settings, that is, when a greater pressure drop is required for triggering.

Flow Sensing

Detection of inspiratory flow may trigger a ventilator breath or some type of respiratory assist (see later). Most current intensive care ventilators provide a continuous base flow around the ventilator circuit of 2 to 20 L.min^{-1}. Any difference between ventilator inflow and outflow represents the patient's respiration. Flow triggering occurs in approximately 80 ms, irrespective of the sensitivity setting. A high base flow provides adequate inspiratory flow for the patient at the start of inspiration, and the flow rate is increased when the ventilator is triggered. Flow sensing can also detect the end of inspiration and is used in PSV (see later).

Neurally Adjusted Ventilatory Assist

Neurally adjusted ventilatory assist uses an oesophageal probe to measure diaphragm electromyography to coordinate the artificial breath to both the start and finish of the spontaneous breath and adjusts the airway pressure delivered to match the magnitude of diaphragmatic activity. This provides good patient–ventilator synchrony, provides tidal volume variability and reduces the risk of overventilation, but is not associated with any better gas exchange than other techniques.[14]

Improved patient–ventilator synchrony, in terms of both timing and flow patterns, potentially provides more than just greater patient comfort. There is also evidence of reduced requirements for sedation and paralysis, less disuse atrophy of respiratory muscles, shorter length of stay in intensive care and improved survival.[15,16]

Ventilatory Modes in Common Use

In addition to control mode ventilation, there are now a range of ventilation patterns. Many of these are essentially the same but have different nomenclature because of their development by rival ventilator manufacturers. In each case, when mandatory breaths are administered these may be using PCV or VCV (Figs 32.1 and 32.4, respectively). Those in common use are described next and shown graphically in Figure 32.5.

Mandatory Minute Volume

Introduced in the 1970s, MMV was a simple technique for controlling the volume of artificial ventilation so that the total of spontaneous and artificial ventilation did not fall below a preset value. If the patient was able to achieve the preset level of MMV unaided, then ventilator breaths did not occur. Achievement of the preset MMV by a rapid, shallow respiratory pattern commonly seen in intensive care patients was a major disadvantage of mechanical MMV. Electronic ventilators allow a much more complex version of MMV to be used. Referred to as adaptive support ventilation, this mode coordinates mandatory breaths with patient respiration to a greater degree than the original mechanical techniques, and includes varying both the inspiratory pressure and timing to minimize the work of breathing for the patient.[17] Most current ventilators can also provide PCV in a form which compensates for changes in compliance or resistance by automatically adjusting inspiratory flow pattern and rate to deliver a guaranteed tidal volume. This removes the risk of delivering an inadequate tidal volume and reduces the variability of driving pressure and tidal volume that occurs frequently with standard PCV.[18]

Airway Pressure Release Ventilation

Airway pressure release ventilation (Fig. 32.5, C) is a ventilation mode that differs significantly from all other forms of positive pressure ventilation and is essentially the reverse of IPPV. It consists of maintaining the breathing system at an upper airway pressure level (P_{high}) which is intermittently released to a lower airway pressure level (P_{low}), causing the patient to exhale to FRC. The pattern of the imposed breaths is similar to that of reversed I:E ratio. The patient is able to breathe spontaneously throughout the entire respiratory cycle, but most of the time this will be during P_{high}, when inspiration will start from a lung volume greater than FRC. Artificial breaths are thus within the conventional tidal range set by the patient's FRC, whereas spontaneous inspirations are usually within his or her inspiratory reserve. More frequent and longer periods at P_{low} lead to a greater minute volume, improved elimination of carbon dioxide and a lower mean airway pressure, but are also associated with greater likelihood of pulmonary collapse in injured lungs and, consequently, worsening of oxygenation. Its place in clinical practice is uncertain, with recent concerns about its safety when used in children.[19]

Synchronized Intermittent Mandatory Ventilation

Intermittent mandatory ventilation was introduced in the 1970s, followed a few years later by the ability to synchronize ventilator breaths with the patient's own respiratory effort, as described previously. The essential feature of synchronized intermittent mandatory ventilation (SIMV; Fig. 32.5, D) is to allow the patient to take a spontaneous breath between artificial breaths. This confers three major advantages. First, a spontaneous inspiration is not obstructed by a closed inspiratory valve, which helps to improve patient–ventilator synchrony. The second advantage

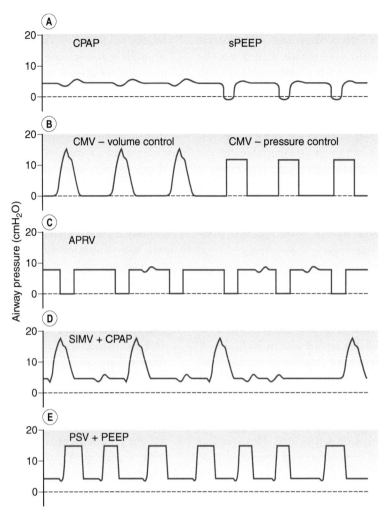

• **Fig. 32.5** Airway pressure during a variety of commonly used modes of ventilation. **(A)** Continuous positive airway pressure (*CPAP*) and true positive end-expiratory pressure applied during spontaneous breathing (*sPEEP*). **(B)** Control mode ventilation (*CMV*) showing volume and pressure-controlled inspiration. **(C)** Airway pressure release ventilation (*APRV*) with an upper airway pressure (P_{high}) of 8 cmH_2O and simultaneous spontaneous breathing. **(D)** Synchronized intermittent mandatory ventilation (*SIMV*), as for CMV except that spontaneous breathing can occur between ventilator breaths. **(E)** Pressure support ventilation (*PSV*) in which pressure-controlled breaths are triggered by the patient, who also controls the duration of each breath. In practice, many ventilators allow combinations of these modes, such as SIMV, PSV and PEEP together.

is the facilitation of weaning, which is considered in a later discussion. Third, the patient is able to breathe spontaneously at any time during prolonged ventilation; this may prevent respiratory muscle atrophy, and helps to reduce the mean intrathoracic pressure. Most ventilators now provide SIMV as a normal feature, and it is used extensively, often in conjunction with PSV (see next section).

Pressure Support Ventilation

In PSV (Fig. 32.5, *E*) a spontaneous inspiration triggers a rapid flow of gas that increases until airway pressure reaches a preselected level. Flow sensing by the ventilator is also then able to detect when the spontaneous inspiration ends, at which point the pressure support ceases and expiration occurs. The purpose is not to provide a prescribed tidal volume, but to assist the patient in making an inspiration of a pattern that lies largely within his or her own control. The level of support may be increased until the pressure is sufficient to

provide the full tidal volume (maximal pressure support) and may be gradually reduced as the patient's ventilatory capacity improves. The amount of pressure support provided does seem to be inversely related to the work of breathing.

High-Frequency Ventilation

High-frequency ventilation may be classified into the following three categories:

1. *High-frequency positive pressure ventilation (HFPPV)* is applied in the frequency range 1 to 2 Hz (60–120 breaths per minute^{-1}) and can be considered as an extension of conventional IPPV techniques. Although many conventional ventilators will operate within this frequency range, specially designed ventilators have been used.
2. *High-frequency jet ventilation (HFJV)* covers the frequency range 1 to 5 Hz. Inspiration is driven by a high-velocity stream of gas from a jet, which may or may not entrain

gas from a secondary supply. Humidification with HFJV is technically difficult, and if done properly requires equipment as complex as the ventilator itself. A unique advantage is the ability to ventilate through a narrow cannula, for example, through the cricothyroid membrane.

3. *High-frequency oscillatory ventilation (HFOV)*[20] covers the frequency range 3 to 10 Hz, and the flows are usually generated by an oscillating pump making a fourth connection to a T-piece. At these high frequencies, the respiratory waveform is usually sinusoidal, including active expiration. Tidal volumes are inevitably small and are difficult to measure.

The relationship between tidal volume and dead space during high-frequency ventilation is crucial to an understanding of the technique. It is useless to infer values for tidal volume and dead space from measurements made under other circumstances, yet it is very difficult to make direct measurements of these variables under the actual conditions of high-frequency ventilation, especially in humans.

End-expiratory pressure is inevitably raised at high frequencies, because the duration of expiration will be inadequate for passive exhalation to FRC; the time constant of the normal respiratory system is about 0.5 seconds (see earlier discussion). Therefore the use of respiratory frequencies greater than 2 Hz will usually result in 'intrinsic' PEEP, and hence an increased end-expiratory lung volume, which is likely to be a major factor promoting favourable gas exchange.

Gas flow in the airways is likely to be modified at high frequencies. The sudden reversals of flow direction are likely to set up flow patterns that blur the boundary between dead space and alveolar gas, thus improving the efficiency of ventilation. Various forms of gas movement are believed to occur during HFOV including a small amount of bulk flow, cardiogenic mixing, 'augmented dispersion' of molecules or streaming of gas flow within airways, allowing gas flow in both directions simultaneously.[21]

Clinical indications for high-frequency ventilation remain unclear. The techniques have been used mainly for weaning from artificial ventilation in adults and for respiratory support in babies.[20] There is also agreement on the special role of high-frequency ventilation for patients with bronchopleural fistula, and the technique is particularly convenient when there is no airtight junction between ventilator and the tracheobronchial tree, during surgery on the airway, for example (page 399). There is no doubt that effective gas exchange is usually possible with high-frequency ventilation, but clinical advantages over conventional artificial ventilation are less clear. Of the various techniques described, HFOV is currently the most popular in intensive care units, with continued interest in its use for patients with severe ALI (Chapter 31), but clinical trial results remain disappointing.[22] Although there are still enthusiasts, others believe that it is merely a technique in search of an application.

Weaning[23]

Two-thirds of patients who receive artificial ventilation in intensive care will be 'liberated' from the ventilator, with most of the remainder succumbing to their disease.[24] Weaning describes the process by which artificial ventilation is gradually withdrawn and the patient returned to normal respiration. In practice it is useful to think of two stages: the withdrawal of respiratory support and the removal of any artificial airway, usually a tracheal tube or tracheostomy. Only the first of these stages is considered here.

Predicting Successful Weaning

Before weaning can be attempted, the balance between ventilatory load and capacity must be favourable. Extra demands on the respiratory system may originate from increased oxygen consumption, most commonly as a result of sepsis. Reduced respiratory system compliance or increased airway resistance also impose additional loads on the respiratory system. The capacity of the respiratory system to wean depends on having adequate ventilation perfusion matching and low intrapulmonary shunt and respiratory dead space. Finally, good respiratory muscle function must be achieved (page 67), including correction of any metabolic disturbance and provision of adequate blood supply to the muscles; that is, the patient must have reasonable cardiovascular function. Numerous different measurements have been reported to predict successful weaning from ventilatory support, examples of which are shown in Table 32.2.

TABLE 32.2	Measurements Used to Assess Suitability for Weaning from Artificial Ventilation	
Measurement	**Value for Successful Weaning**
Measured on ventilator:	
$Pa_{O_2} : F_{I_{O_2}}$ ratio	>20 (Pa_{O_2} in kPa) or 150 (Pa_{O_2} in mmHg)
Resting minute volume	<10 L.min⁻¹
Negative inspiratory force	20–30 cmH₂O
PI_{max}	15–30 cmH₂O
$P_{0.1}/PI_{max}$	>0.3
Diaphragm ultrasound	Paradoxical movements
Measured during brief period of spontaneous breathing:	
Respiratory rate	<0 breaths.min⁻¹
Tidal volume	>4–6 mL.kg⁻¹
Respiratory rate:tidal volume ratio	>60 breaths.L⁻¹
RVR score	≤105 breaths.min⁻¹.L⁻¹
Blood biomarkers:	
B-type natriuretic peptide	<200 pg.mL⁻¹

PI_{max}, Maximal inspiratory pressure; $P_{0.1}$, mouth occlusion pressure 0.1 seconds after the onset of inspiration; rate:volume ratio score is respiratory rate (breaths.min⁻¹) divided by tidal volume (L) measured over 1 minute without artificial ventilation.

No single variable is a reliable enough indicator of success, and current research is focused on use of ultrasound of the diaphragm[25] and biomarkers to predict successful weaning.[26,27]

Techniques for Weaning

Recent guidelines suggest that once these predictors indicate that discontinuation of ventilation may be possible, a spontaneous breathing trial should be used.[28,29] During this trial, which should last approximately 30 minutes, the patient breathes spontaneously with only minimal respiratory support, for example 5 to 8 cmH$_2$O of CPAP, and is closely observed to ensure that respiratory pattern, patient comfort, gas exchange and cardiovascular stability are all acceptable. If this trial of spontaneous breathing fails, appropriate degrees of ventilatory support should be recommenced, and a further trial of spontaneous breathing performed at 24-hour intervals if the predictors of successful weaning remain satisfactory.

Ventilation strategies to use between trials of spontaneous breathing focus on gradual withdrawal of respiratory support using the techniques described earlier. Control mode ventilation is usually replaced by either SIMV or ACV until the patient has established adequate respiratory effort, following which the number of ventilator breaths can be gradually reduced. While breathing via an artificial airway, some respiratory support is normally required, and this is most commonly provided with PSV, the level of which can again be reduced gradually.

It is important to not place excessive reliance on modern ventilator systems to wean patients from ventilatory support. Close attention must also be paid to nutrition, psychological care such as establishment of normal night/day sleep patterns and the use of NIV (page 376) following early extubation.[30] Protocols for weaning are now widely used to ensure all of these aspects are addressed,[29] but some patients will still remain ventilated for many weeks, and specialist units now exist to care for these challenging patients.[31]

Positive End-Expiratory Pressure

A great variety of pathological conditions, as well as general anaesthesia, result in a decrease in FRC. The deleterious effect of this on gas exchange has been considered elsewhere (page 257), and it is reasonable to consider increasing the FRC by applying PEEP.

Expiratory pressure can be raised during both artificial ventilation and spontaneous breathing, and both forms are best considered together. The terminology is confusing, and this chapter adheres to the definitions illustrated in Figure 32.5. Note in particular spontaneous PEEP (sPEEP), in which a patient inhales spontaneously from ambient pressure but exhales against PEEP. This involves subjects in a considerable amount of additional work of breathing because they must raise their entire minute volume to the level of PEEP that is applied. This is undesirable, and CPAP is much preferred over sPEEP.

It is true that CPAP is more difficult to achieve than sPEEP. Biased demand valves may be used, but usually result in a pronounced dip in inspiratory pressure, increasing the total work of breathing. The simplest approach is a T-piece with a high flow of fresh gas venting through a PEEP valve at the expiratory limb throughout the respiratory phase. Electronic ventilators produce CPAP in a similar fashion by circulating high flows of gas around the ventilator circuit at the required positive pressure.

PEEP may be achieved by many techniques. The simplest is to exhale through a preset depth of water, but more convenient methods are spring-loaded valves or diaphragms pressed down by gas, a column of water or a spring. In electronic ventilators it usually achieved with fans opposing the direction of expiratory gas flow.

Intrinsic Positive End-Expiratory Pressure

If a passive expiration is terminated before the lung volume has returned to FRC, there will be residual end-expiratory raised alveolar pressure, variously known as dynamic hyperinflation, auto-PEEP or intrinsic PEEP (PEEPi).[32] The elevated alveolar pressure will not be transmitted back to the ventilator pressure sensors, so PEEPi may go undetected. Artificial ventilation with an inverse I:E ratio may result in PEEPi, but it is more commonly a result of increased expiratory flow resistance because of airway disease or retention of mucus, or from the tracheal tube (Fig. 32.6). Eventually, alveolar pressure and lung volume increase sufficiently to cause reductions in both lung compliance and airway resistance; expiratory flow rate then increases, and the degree of PEEPi stabilizes.

At first sight PEEPi may be perceived as beneficial—for example, leading to increased FRC and alveolar recruitment—and it is likely that improved gas exchange seen with an inverse I:E ratio results, at least in part, from this mechanism. However, the first hazard of PEEPi is its variability. Small changes in airway resistance, for example, with mucous retention, can lead to rapid increases in the level of PEEPi. The cardiovascular consequences of PEEPi are significant (see later) and have been described as 'applying a tourniquet to the right heart'. Finally, the presence of PEEPi will impede the ability of the patient to trigger ventilators by necessitating a greater fall in alveolar pressure to initiate respiratory support.

Application of external PEEP will, to some extent, attenuate the generation of PEEPi by maintaining airway patency in late expiration thus improving expiratory flow.

Physiological Effects of Positive Pressure Ventilation

A positive pressure in the chest cavity is a significant physiological insult that normally occurs only transiently with coughing, straining, and so on, although the pressure achieved in these situations may be very high. Most physiological effects of IPPV are related to the mean pressure throughout the

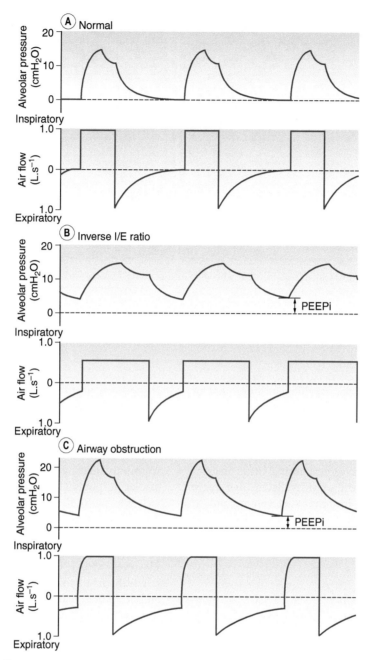

• **Fig. 32.6** Pressure and flow curves demonstrating generation of intrinsic positive end-expiratory pressure (*PEEPi*). **(A)** Normal ventilation with both alveolar pressure and airway flow returning to zero before the next breath. **(B)** Inverse I:E ratio ventilation. Although the decline in pressure and flow is normal, there is insufficient time for complete expiration to occur. **(C)** Airway obstruction. Expiratory time is normal, but the decline in pressure and flow is retarded to such an extent that expiration is again incomplete.

whole respiratory cycle, which is in turn influenced by a large number of ventilatory settings such as mode of ventilation, tidal volume, respiratory rate and I:E ratio. PEEP results in large increases in mean intrathoracic pressure. For example, IPPV in a patient with normal lungs using 10 breaths of 10 mL.kg⁻¹ and an I:E ratio of 1:2 will generate mean airway pressures of approximately 5 cmH₂O. The addition of a modest 5 cmH₂O of PEEP will therefore double the mean airway pressure, and thus the physiological insult associated with IPPV. For this reason, much research into the physiological effects of artificial ventilation has focused on PEEP.

Respiratory Effects[33]

Artificial ventilation effectively rests the respiratory muscles, and the effect of this on muscle function is described on page 67.

Distribution of Ventilation

Intermittent positive pressure ventilation results in a spatial pattern of distribution that is determined by inflation pressure, regional compliance and time constants. Based on external measurements and electrical impedance tomography,

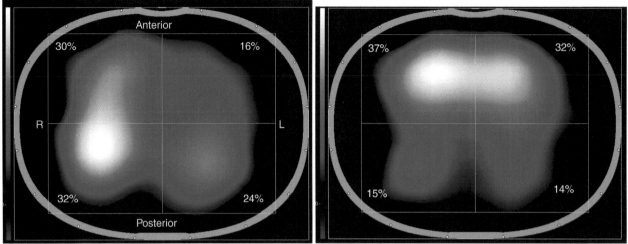

• **Fig. 32.7** Electrical impedance tomography images showing regional ventilation in a healthy subject **(A)** when awake with spontaneous breathing and **(B)** during anaesthesia with intermittent positive pressure ventilation (IPPV) using bag and mask ventilation, that is, a normal anatomical airway. The ventral redistribution of ventilation seen here does not occur when breathing spontaneously during anaesthesia and is the same irrespective of the airway used to deliver IPPV.

the distribution of inspired gas is different from that of spontaneous breathing. Compared with spontaneous breathing IPPV causes a relatively greater expansion of the rib cage and a shift of ventilation to ventral areas of lung (Fig. 32.7). This is not the case in patients with ALI, in whom the spatial distribution of gas becomes very abnormal with areas of collapse and the development of overinflated lung (page 370). Application of PEEP increases lung volume and, at high levels, reexpands collapsed alveoli, which changes the compliance of dependent lung regions, improving ventilation of these areas.

Apparatus Dead Space

Positive pressure ventilation, whether invasive or noninvasive, requires the provision of an airtight connection to the patient's airway. This inevitably involves the addition of some apparatus dead space. With orotracheal and tracheostomy tubes much of the normal anatomical dead space is bypassed, such that overall anatomical dead space may be unchanged or reduced. With NIV using facemasks, apparatus dead space may be substantial. Ventilator tubing used to deliver IPPV is normally corrugated and expands longitudinally with each inspiration. For an average ventilator circuit, this expansion may amount to 2 to 3 mL.cmH$_2$O^{-1} of positive pressure, and this volume will constitute dead space ventilation.

Physiological Dead Space

In normal lungs during anaesthesia, IPPV alone seems to have little effect on the V_D/V_T ratio compared with spontaneous breathing. There is a slight widening of the distribution of ventilation/perfusion ($\dot{V}$/$\dot{Q}$) ratios (page 95), mostly as a result of a reduction in pulmonary blood flow from depression of cardiac output (see later discussion). These

changes are normally not sufficient to alter gas exchange. The alveolar component of physiological dead space may be increased by ventilation in patients with lung injury or when mean intrathoracic pressure is high, such as with significant amounts of PEEP. Under the latter conditions, lung volume is increased to such an extent that not only does cardiac output fall but pulmonary vascular resistance rises as well (see Fig. 6.4). Perfusion to overexpanded alveoli is reduced, and areas of lung with high $\dot{V}$/$\dot{Q}$ ratios develop, constituting alveolar dead space. In healthy lungs, this effect is not seen until PEEP levels exceed 10 to 15 cmH$_2$O. However, with IPPV in ALI overdistension occurs in the relatively small number of functional alveoli (page 370), and local perfusion to these lung units is likely to be impeded.

Lung Volume

Intermittent positive pressure ventilation and ZEEP will have no effect on FRC. However, with PEEP, end-expiratory alveolar pressure will equal the level of applied PEEP, and this will reset the FRC in accord with the pressure/volume curve of the respiratory system (see Fig. 2.7). For example, PEEP of 10 cmH$_2$O will increase FRC by 500 mL in a patient with a compliance of 0.5 L.kPa^{-1} (50 mL.cmH$_2$O^{-1}). In many patients this may be expected to raise the tidal range above the closing capacity (page 31), reducing pulmonary collapse. Prevention of alveolar collapse is probably the greatest single advantage of PEEP. It will also reduce airway resistance according to the inverse relationship between lung volume and airway resistance (see Fig. 3.5). It may also change the relative compliance of the upper and lower parts of the lung (Fig. 32.8), improving the ventilation of the dependent overperfused parts of the lung.

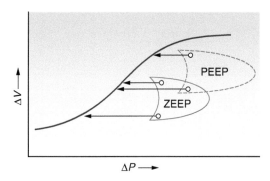

• **Fig. 32.8** Effect of positive end-expiratory pressure (*PEEP*) on the relationship between regional pressure and volume in the lung (supine position). Note that compliance is greater in the upper part of the lung with zero end-expiratory pressure (*ZEEP*) and in the lower part of the lung with PEEP, which thus improves ventilation in the dependent zone of the lung.

Arterial Po_2

Neither IPPV nor PEEP improves arterial oxygenation appreciably in patients with healthy lungs. During anaesthesia, it has been repeatedly observed that PEEP does little to improve arterial oxygenation in healthy patients. Pulmonary shunting is decreased, but the accompanying decrease in cardiac output reduces the mixed venous oxygen saturation, which counteracts the effect of a reduction in the shunt, resulting in minimal increase in arterial Po_2. There is, however, no doubt that positive pressure ventilation improves arterial Po_2 in a wide range of pathological situations. In most cases, the improvement in Po_2 relates to the mean airway pressure achieved, and, as described previously, PEEP provides an easy way of elevating airway pressures. Reexpansion of collapsed lung units, improved ventilation of alveoli with low $\dot{v}/\dot{Q}$ ratios and redistribution of extravascular lung water will all contribute to the observed improvement in oxygenation. The use of PEEP for prevention of atelectasis in anaesthesia is described on page 251, whereas its contribution to the treatment of pulmonary oedema and ALI are described on pages 344 and 370, respectively.

Pulmonary Neutrophil Retention

Neutrophils have a diameter close to that of a pulmonary capillary, and this is important in slowing their transit time through the lung to facilitate margination for pulmonary defence mechanisms (page 353). Any reduction in pulmonary capillary diameter may therefore be expected to increase pulmonary neutrophil retention, which has indeed been demonstrated in humans following a Valsalva manoeuvre or with the application of PEEP.[34] If the neutrophils trapped in this way have already been activated, for example, following cardiopulmonary bypass, then lung injury may follow.

Valsalva Effect

It has long been known that an increase in intrathoracic pressure has complex circulatory effects, characterized as the Valsalva effect, which is the circulatory response to a subject increasing his airway pressure to about $50\ cmH_2O$ against a closed glottis for about 30 seconds. The normal response is in four parts (Fig. 32.9, *A*). Initially the raised intrathoracic pressure alters the baseline for circulatory pressures, and the arterial pressure (measured relative to atmosphere) is consequently increased (phase 1). At the same time, ventricular filling is decreased by the adverse pressure gradient from peripheral veins to the ventricle in diastole, and cardiac output therefore decreases. The consequent decline in arterial pressure in phase 2 is normally mitigated by three factors—tachycardia, increased systemic vascular resistance (afterload) and an increase in peripheral venous pressure—which tend to restore the venous return. As a result of these compensations, the arterial pressure normally settles to a value fairly close to the level before starting the Valsalva manoeuvre. When the intrathoracic pressure is restored to normal, there is an immediate decrease in arterial pressure because of the altered baseline. Simultaneously the venous return improves; therefore the cardiac output increases within a few seconds. However, the arteriolar bed remains constricted temporarily, and there is a transient overshoot of arterial pressure.

Figure 32.9, *B*, shows the abnormal 'square wave' pattern that occurs with raised end-diastolic pressure or left ventricular failure or both. The initial increase in arterial pressure (phase 1) occurs normally, but the decline in pressure in phase 2 is missing because the output of the congested heart is not usually limited by end-diastolic pressure. Because the cardiac output is unchanged, there is no increase in pulse rate or systemic vascular resistance, and there is no overshoot of pressure when the intrathoracic pressure is restored to normal.

Figure 32.9, *C*, shows a different abnormal pattern, which may be seen with defective systemic vasoconstriction (e.g., autonomic neuropathy or a spinal anaesthetic). Phase 1 is normal, but in phase 2 the decreased cardiac output is not accompanied by an increase in systemic vascular resistance, and the arterial pressure therefore continues to decline. The normal overshoot is replaced by a slow recovery of arterial pressure as the cardiac output returns to control values.

Cardiovascular Effects of Positive Pressure Ventilation[35]

Initially there was great reluctance to use PEEP, partly because of the well-known Valsalva effect and partly because of the circulatory hazard that had been described in the classic paper by Cournand and his colleagues published in 1948.[36] The cardiovascular effects of IPPV and PEEP continue to cause problems in clinical practice, and after another half-century of investigation, the effects remain incompletely elucidated.

Cardiac Output

Bindslev et al.[37] reported a progressive decrease in cardiac output with IPPV and PEEP in anaesthetized patients without pulmonary pathology. Compared with when

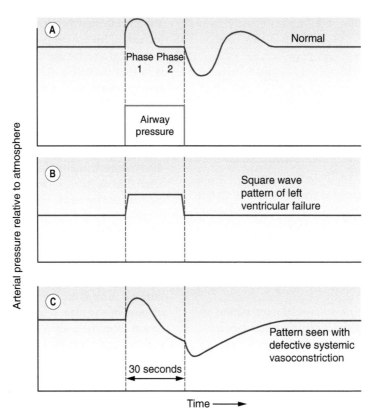

• **Fig. 32.9** Qualitative changes in mean arterial blood pressure during a Valsalva manoeuvre as seen in the normal subject **(A)** and for two abnormal responses, including left ventricular failure **(B)** and defective systemic vasoconstriction **(C)**. See text for explanation of the changes.

anaesthetized and breathing spontaneously, cardiac output was reduced by 10% with IPPV and ZEEP, 18% with 9 cmH$_2$O of PEEP and 36% with 16 cmH$_2$O of PEEP. Another study, this time in patients with severe ALI, also demonstrated a progressive reduction in cardiac output for PEEP in the range of 5 to 30 cmH$_2$O, but the effect was partially reversed by blood volume expansion (Fig. 32.10).

There is general agreement that the main cause of reduction in cardiac output is obstruction of filling of the right atrium caused by elevated intrathoracic pressure.[38] With spontaneous respiration, the negative intrathoracic pressure during inspiration draws blood into the chest from the major veins, known as the *thoracic pump*. Positive intrathoracic pressure abolishes this effect and also imposes a further reduction in driving pressure for flow between extrathoracic and intrathoracic vessels. Reduced right ventricle (RV) filling pressures quickly lead to reduced left ventricle (LV) filling, and cardiac output falls. These changes will clearly be more pronounced with hypovolaemia, and this phenomenon forms the basis of current clinical techniques to assess circulatory volume, such as pulse pressure variation and stroke volume variation.[35] Paradoxically, the same physiological response may be used to treat hypovolaemia by imposing an inspiratory resistance to further reduce the negative inspiratory pressure and improve venous return.[39]

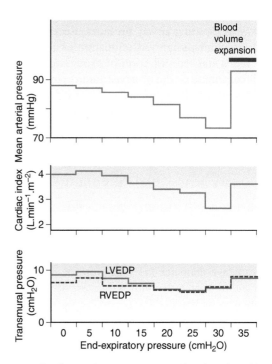

• **Fig. 32.10** Cardiovascular responses as a function of positive end-expiratory pressure in patients with acute lung injury. Left and right ventricular end-diastolic pressure (*LVEDP* and *RVEDP*) were measured relative to intrapleural pressure. (Drawn from data of reference 32 and reproduced from Nunn JF. Positive end-expiratory pressure. *Int Anesthesiol Clin.* 1984;22:149-164, by permission of the publishers of *International Anesthesiology Clinics*.)

A second cause for reduced cardiac output may come into play with high airway pressures, moderate PEEP or lung hyperinflation, such as occurs with PEEPi. As previously described, increasing lung volume leads to elevated pulmonary vascular resistance, which will cause an increase in RV volume. There is now good evidence that dilation of the RV has profound effects on LV function, preventing adequate LV filling and reducing LV compliance, both of which lead to a fall in cardiac output.[35] Contractility of the LV is not thought to change with positive intrathoracic pressure. Interactions of some of the factors by which PEEP may influence cardiac output and systemic arterial pressure are shown in Figure 32.11.

Oxygen Delivery

In many patients with pulmonary disease, PEEP tends to improve the arterial Po_2 while decreasing the cardiac output. As PEEP is increased the oxygen delivery (the product of cardiac output and arterial oxygen content; page 154) tends to rise to a maximum and then fall. Assuming that a normal or high oxygen delivery is desirable, use of IPPV or PEEP therefore requires optimization of cardiac output with fluid replacement (Fig. 32.10) or with positive inotropes, and this is now routine practice in critical care units.

Arterial Blood Pressure

Figure 32.10 shows the decline in mean arterial pressure closely following the change in cardiac output with increasing PEEP. Although there was some increase in systemic vascular resistance, this was only about half that required for maintenance of the arterial pressure in the face of the declining cardiac output.

Interpretation of Vascular Pressures

Atrial pressures are normally measured relative to atmospheric pressure. With positive pressure ventilation, atrial pressures tend to be increased relative to atmospheric. However, relative to intrathoracic pressure, they are reduced at higher levels of PEEP (Fig. 32.10). It is the transmural pressure gradient, and not the level relative to atmosphere, that is relevant to cardiac filling.

Transmission of Airway Pressure to Other Intrathoracic Structures

Intrathoracic pressures are protected from the airway pressure by the transmural pressure gradient of the lungs, such that in humans with healthy lungs the intrapleural pressure increase is around two-thirds that seen in the airway, and the increased pressure in the pericardium about one-third.[38] Animal studies have shown that reduced pulmonary compliance is the main factor governing the transmission of airway pressure to other thoracic structures. With reduced compliance the effect of raised intrathoracic pressure on cardiac output is reduced. Patients with diseased lungs tend to have reduced pulmonary compliance which limits the rise in intrapleural pressure (Fig. 32.12). Therefore their cardiovascular systems are better protected against the adverse effects of IPPV and PEEP.

Haemodynamic Response in Heart Failure

The cardiovascular responses described thus far apply only to patients with normal cardiac function, and, like the Valsalva

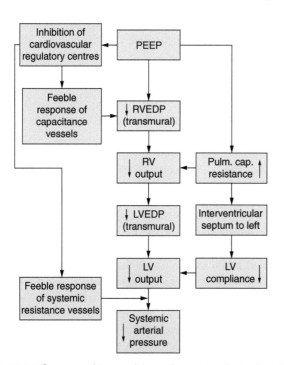

• **Fig. 32.11** Summary of the possible cardiovascular effects of positive end-expiratory pressure (*PEEP*). See text for full explanation. *RVEDP* and *LVEDP*, Right and left ventricular end-diastolic pressure; *RV* and *LV*, right and left ventricle.

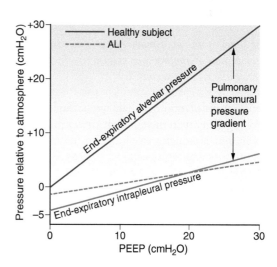

• **Fig. 32.12** End-expiratory alveolar and intrapleural pressures as a function of positive end-expiratory pressure (*PEEP*). The lower unbroken line shows intrapleural pressure in the relaxed healthy subject. The broken line shows values of intrapleural pressure in patients with acute lung injury taken from reference 32. Absolute values of pressure probably reflect experimental technique, and cannot be compared between studies. (Reproduced from Nunn JF. Positive end-expiratory pressure. *Int Anesthesiol Clin.* 1984;22:149-164, by permission of the publishers of *International Anesthesiology Clinics.*)

response, are very different in patients with raised ventricular end-diastolic pressure with or without ventricular failure. Reduction of venous return to an overloaded and failing right heart will return the RV to a more favourable section of its Frank–Starling curve (see Fig. 29.3), improving its function. Reducing RV end-diastolic volume will overcome some of the adverse ventricular interactions that occur in heart failure, and also improve LV function. These factors almost certainly contribute to the success of CPAP in the treatment of cardiogenic pulmonary oedema.

Renal Effects[40]

The cardiovascular effects of artificial ventilation described so far inevitably affect renal function. Arterial pressure tends to be reduced, whereas central venous pressure is raised, and so the pressure gradient between renal artery and vein is reduced, which has a direct effect on renal blood flow and glomerular filtration rate. In addition, positive pressure ventilation activates the sympathetic and renin–angiotensin systems, which suppresses atrial natriuretic peptide activity. Finally, tissue hypoxia in critically ill patients will also impair renal function, and the systemic inflammation that accompanies any critical illness can lead to kidney damage. This combination of effects on renal function mean oliguria and acute kidney injury are almost inevitable with prolonged artificial ventilation.

Ventilator-Induced Lung Injury[41,42]

The first description of the potential harm that artificial ventilation may cause to the lungs was published in 1745 by John Fothergill.[43] Following the successful resuscitation of a patient using expired air respiration rather than bellows, which were fashionable at the time, Fothergill wrote that:

> The lungs of one man may bear, without injury, as great a force as those of another man can exert; which by the bellows cannot always be determin'd.

Artificial ventilation may damage normal lungs only after prolonged ventilation with high airway pressures or large tidal volumes, although a role for IPPV in initiating postoperative pulmonary complications is becoming more recognized (page 263). In abnormal lungs, such as during ALI (Chapter 31), ventilator-induced lung injury (VILI) may contribute not only to further lung damage, but also to multisystem organ failure affecting other body systems.

Barotrauma

A sustained increase in the transmural pressure gradient can damage the lung. The commonest forms of barotrauma attributable to artificial ventilation with or without PEEP are subcutaneous emphysema, pneumomediastinum and pneumothorax. Pulmonary barotrauma probably starts as a disruption of the alveolar membrane, with air entering the interstitial space and tracking along the bronchovascular

bundles into the mediastinum, from which it can reach the peritoneum, the pleural cavity or the subcutaneous tissues. Radiological demonstration of pulmonary interstitial gas may provide an early warning of barotrauma.

Volutrauma

Many animal studies have demonstrated pulmonary oedema following artificial ventilation with high inflation pressures. In one of these studies, lung damage with high inflation pressures was attenuated by restricting chest movement to prevent overdistension of the lungs, indicating that alveolar size rather than pressure was responsible for lung injury. Termed *volutrauma*, this is now believed to contribute significantly to lung damage in patients with ALI, in whom only a small proportion of alveoli may receive the entire tidal volume (page 370). This form of VILI most commonly manifests itself as interstitial or alveolar pulmonary oedema. There are several possible underlying mechanisms, all of which are closely interrelated.

Alveolar distension causes permeability pulmonary oedema (page 343). With extreme lung distension in animal studies this occurs quickly, and probably results from direct trauma to alveolar structures. Studies using lung cell cultures in vitro reveal some of the mechanisms of this cellular trauma.[44] Severe stretching of the cells can induce apoptosis, provoke the release of inflammatory cytokines[45] or damage tight junctions between cells or the plasma membrane. Stretch frequency is also an important determinant of the damage done, supporting the inclination towards slower respiratory rates in injured lungs. In larger animals and humans, the permeability changes occur slowly (several hours), and are likely to result from the alterations in surfactant and inflammatory mediators described later rather than widespread cellular damage.

Atelectrauma

Airway trauma occurs with repeated closure and reopening of small airways with each breath and has been termed *atelectrauma*. In vitro studies show that physical stresses on epithelial cells as lung reopens are considerable and sufficient to damage tight junction proteins, increasing paracellular permeability.[46] In vivo, mucosal oedema will develop, and the airways will become progressively more difficult to open until collapse occurs. Recruitment of lung units with positive pressure ventilation has beneficial effects on gas exchange, and thus encourages the use of higher pressures and volumes to recruit more airways, leading to further VILI.

Surfactant function is affected by artificial ventilation, exacerbating atelectrauma.[47] Animal studies have demonstrated that surfactant *release* is increased by artificial ventilation, but that function is soon reduced, possibly because de novo synthesis of surfactant in the lamellar bodies cannot keep pace with the increased amount being released.[48] Cyclical closure of airways during expiration causes surfactant to be drawn from the alveoli into the airway, and alveolar proteins seen with permeability oedema inactivate surfactant. The resultant increase in alveolar surface forces will not only affect lung compliance but will also increase local microvascular permeability and encourage alveolar collapse.

Biotrauma

Lung inflammation occurs with VILI. Termed *biotrauma*, this includes a proinflammatory response to the mechanical damage to lung tissue already described.[49] Biotrauma is independent of any infection present, and includes activation of immune and coagulation systems, and cellular growth and apoptotic pathways.[45] Pulmonary neutrophils are implicated in biotrauma, and their migration into lung tissue was described earlier. Once activated—for example, by stretching as described previously or by exposure to the alveolar basement membrane—inflammatory mediators will contribute to permeability oedema and further loss of surfactant function.

Prevention of Ventilator-Induced Lung Injury[41]

In spite of its contribution to mean airway pressure, animal studies show that modest amounts of PEEP are helpful in reducing VILI. Reduction of interstitial oedema, prevention of cyclical airway closure and preservation of surfactant function are all possible mechanisms for this effect. Determination of an acceptable level of PEEP in injured lungs is discussed on page 370.

Tidal volume and airway pressure should be minimized as far as possible. Plateau pressure or driving pressure are the ventilator measurements that equate most closely to the degree of alveolar distension. Both are associated with adverse outcomes such as mortality, but evidence of causation linking ventilator variables and clinical effects are lacking.[50] It is currently recommended that, in patients with normal chest wall compliance, the plateau pressure should not be allowed to exceed 30 cmH$_2$O.

A 'protective' ventilation strategy that combines these requirements is described on page 371, and its use in the clinical setting to reduce VILI is now widely accepted.

Artificial Ventilation for Resuscitation

Until about 1960, artificial ventilation was usually attempted by application of mechanical forces directly to the trunk. Methods were based on the rescuer manipulating the trunk and arms of the victim to achieve changes in lung volume which, when performed in sequence, could produce some degree of pulmonary ventilation.

Expired Air Ventilation

Recognition of the inadequacy of the manual methods of artificial ventilation led directly to a radical new approach to artificial ventilation in an emergency. Around 1960 there

TABLE 32.3	Alveolar Gas Concentrations During Expired Air Resuscitation		
	Normal Spontaneous Respiration	Expired Air Resuscitation with Doubled Ventilation	
		Rescuer	Victim
Alveolar CO$_2$	6%	3%	6%
Alveolar O$_2$	15%	18%	15%

Doubling the rescuer's ventilation increases his or her alveolar oxygen concentration to a value midway between the normal alveolar oxygen concentration and that of room air.

was vigorous reexamination of the concept of the rescuer's expired air being used for inflation of the victim's lungs.

At first sight, it might appear that expired air would not be a suitable inspired air for the victim. However, if the rescuer doubles his ventilation he is able to breathe for two. If neither party had any respiratory dead space, the simple relationship shown in Table 32.3 would apply. In fact, the rescuer's dead space improves the situation. At the start of inflation the rescuer's dead space is filled with fresh air, and this is the first gas to enter the victim's lungs. If the rescuer's dead space is artificially increased by apparatus dead space, this will improve the freshness of the air that the victim receives and also reduce the likelihood of hypocapnia in the rescuer.

Expired air ventilation has now displaced the manual methods in all except the most unusual circumstances, and its success depends on the following factors:

1. It is normally possible to achieve adequate ventilation for long periods of time without fatigue, although symptomatic hypocapnia can occur.[51]
2. The hands of the rescuer are free to control the patency of the victim's airway.
3. The rescuer can monitor the victim's chest expansion visually and can also hear any airway obstruction and sense the tidal exchange from the proprioceptive receptors in his own chest wall.
4. The method is extremely adaptable, and has been used, for example, before drowning victims have been removed from the water and on linesmen electrocuted while working on pylons. No manual method would have any hope of success in such situations.
5. The method seems to come naturally, and many rescuers have achieved success with the minimum of instruction.

In 'out-of-hospital' cardiac arrest situations bystanders are often reluctant to attempt cardiopulmonary resuscitation (CPR), particularly mouth-to-mouth ventilation, to such an extent that CPR is attempted only in about one-third of victims. This has led to extensive study of the contribution made by ventilation, comparing standard CPR with chest compressions alone. Oxygen consumption and carbon dioxide production during cardiac arrest are low, and the oxygen stored in blood may suffice for more than 10 minutes, obviating the need for ventilation during this time following a witnessed cardiac arrest.[52] The results of observational studies thus far have been mixed, with the most recent study finding no difference in outcomes with or without interruptions for ventilation.[53] Some CPR is always better than none in out-of-hospital cardiac arrest, and chest compressions should always be initiated promptly, and, for now, artificial ventilation should be attempted by rescuers prepared to do so. There are also concerns that airway interventions during CPR, even with skilled personnel in hospital, still interrupt the provision of effective chest compressions. A recent study found worse clinical outcomes from in-hospital ardiac arrest when intubation was performed in the first 15 minutes.[54]

Extrapulmonary Gas Exchange

The development of an artificial lung remains only a distant possibility, but techniques for short-term replacement of lung function or more prolonged partial respiratory support have existed for many years. Extracorporeal gas exchangers were first developed for cardiac surgery to facilitate cardiopulmonary bypass, allowing surgery on a motionless heart. Subsequently the use of extracorporeal and intracorporeal gas exchange was extended into the treatment of respiratory failure.

Factors in Design

The lungs of an adult have an interface between blood and gas of the order of 126 m^2. It is not possible to achieve this in an artificial substitute, and artificial lungs can be considered to have a very low 'diffusing capacity'. Nevertheless, they function satisfactorily within limits for many reasons.

Factors Favouring Performance

- The real lung is adapted for maximal exercise, whereas patients requiring extrapulmonary gas exchange are usually close to basal metabolic rate, or less if hypothermia is used, for example, during cardiac surgery.
- Under resting conditions at sea level, there is an enormous reserve in the capacity of the lung to achieve equilibrium between pulmonary capillary blood and alveolar gas (see Fig. 8.2). Therefore a subnormal diffusing capacity does not necessarily result in arterial hypoxaemia.
- It is possible to operate an artificial lung with an 'alveolar' oxygen concentration in excess of 90%, compared with 14% for real alveolar gas under normal circumstances. This greatly increases the oxygen transfer for a given diffusing capacity of the artificial lung.
- The 'capillary transit time' of an artificial lung can be increased beyond the 0.75 seconds in the real lung. This facilitates the approach of blood P_{O_2} to 'alveolar' P_{O_2} (see Fig. 8.2).
- It is possible to use countercurrent flow between gas and blood. This does not occur in the lungs of mammals,

although it is used extensively elsewhere in the animal kingdom (Chapter 26).

Carbon dioxide exchanges much more readily than oxygen because of its greater blood and lipid solubility. Therefore, in general, elimination of carbon dioxide does not present a major problem, and the limiting factor of an artificial lung is oxygenation.

Unfavourable Factors

Against these favourable design considerations, there are certain advantages of the real lung—apart from its very large surface area—that are difficult to emulate in an artificial lung.

- The pulmonary capillaries have a diameter close to that of a red blood cell (RBC). Therefore each RBC is brought into very close contact with the alveolar gas (see Fig. 1.8). The diffusion distance for artificial lungs is considerably greater.
- The vascular endothelium is specially adapted to prevent undesirable changes in the formed elements of blood, particularly neutrophils and platelets. Most artificial surfaces cause blood clotting and platelet activation.
- The lung is an extremely efficient filter with an effective pore size of about 10 μm for flow rates of blood up to about 25 L.min^{-1}. This is difficult to achieve with any man-made filter.

Bubble Oxygenators

By breaking up the gas stream into small bubbles, it is possible to achieve a large surface area of interface. However, the smaller the bubbles, the greater the tendency for them to remain in suspension when the blood is returned to the patient. This is dangerous during cardiopulmonary bypass because of the direct access of the blood to the systemic circulation. With a mean RBC transit time of 1 to 2 seconds and an oxygen concentration of more than 90%, bubble oxygenators achieve an acceptable outflow blood P_{O_2} with blood flow rates up to about 6 L.min^{-1}.

Cellular and protein damage (see later) at the blood–gas interface occurs in bubble oxygenators. This is not considered to have significant clinical effects during short-term use, as, for example, with cardiac surgery, but may become significant when used for prolonged periods in the treatment of respiratory failure.

Membrane Oxygenators

Diffusion properties. Unlike their predecessors, currently available membranes offer little resistance to the diffusion of oxygen and carbon dioxide. At 25- to 50-μm thick, artificial membranes are several times thicker than the active side of the alveolar/capillary membrane (Fig. 1.8), but they contain small (<1 μm) pores, which increase gas transfer substantially. The hydrophobic nature of the membrane material prevents water entering the pores, and in normal use membranes can withstand a hydrostatic pressure gradient of the order of normal arterial blood pressure. Over time the pores tend to fill with protein, which slowly reduces the membrane efficiency.

Gas diffusion within the blood presents a considerable barrier to efficiency of membrane oxygenators. Slow diffusion of gases through plasma is now thought to limit gas transfer in normal lung, in which the RBC is almost in contact with the capillary wall (page 114). Streamline flow through much wider channels in a membrane oxygenator tends to result in a stream of RBCs remaining at a distance from the interface. It has been estimated that in membrane oxygenators the diffusion path for oxygen is about 25 times further than in lung. Much thought has been devoted to the creation of turbulent flow to counteract this effect by 'mixing' the blood. Unfortunately, this inevitably leads to a greater degree of cell damage (see later) and increased resistance to flow through the oxygenator.

Biocompatibility. Adsorption of proteins, particularly albumin, onto the membrane reduces platelet, neutrophil and complement activation (see later), and this technique may be used to 'prime' oxygenators before use. Attempts to mimic endothelial cell properties have led to the production of membranes with heparin bonded to the surface, which also reduces activation of most of the processes described later.

Damage to Blood

During prolonged extracorporeal oxygenation for respiratory failure, the type of oxygenator and pump becomes important, and membrane oxygenators are superior to bubble oxygenators.

Protein denaturation. Contact between blood and either gas bubbles or synthetic surfaces results in protein denaturation, and synthetic surfaces become coated with a layer of protein. With membrane oxygenators this tends to be self-limiting, and the protein products remain bound to the membrane. Bubble oxygenators cause a continuous and progressive loss of protein, including the release of denatured proteins into the circulation where they may have biological effects.

Complement activation. Complement activation occurs when blood comes into contact with any artificial surface and complement C5a is known to be formed after cardiopulmonary bypass surgery.

RBCs. Shear forces, resulting from turbulence or foaming, may cause shortened survival or actual destruction of RBCs. Haemolysis is a common occurrence with extracorporeal membrane oxygenation (ECMO), and increases with greater blood flows through the oxygenator.[55]

Leukocytes and platelets. Counts of these elements are usually reduced by an amount in excess of the changes attributable to haemodilution. Platelets are lost by adhesion and aggregation, and neutrophil activation may occur within the extracorporeal circuit, leading to pathological effects in distant organs.

Coagulation. No oxygenator can function without causing coagulation of the blood. Anticoagulation is therefore a sine qua non of the technique, and heparin is usually used for this purpose. Heparin-bonded components have significantly reduced the systemic anticoagulant requirement and allowed more prolonged use of circuits, but coagulopathy remains the most common complication of extracorporeal circulation.

Systems for Extrapulmonary Gas Exchange

Cardiopulmonary bypass for cardiac surgery remains the most common situation in which patients are exposed to extrapulmonary gas exchange. The duration of such exposure is normally very short and causes few physiological disturbances postoperatively. Providing longer term respiratory support is much less common and also considerably more difficult, but three techniques exist.

Extracorporeal Membrane Oxygenation[56]

A traditional ECMO system requires continuous blood flow from the patient to a reservoir system, from which a pump propels blood through an oxygenator and a heat exchanger back to the patient. Venovenous ECMO is acceptable for treatment of respiratory failure and may be instituted via percutaneous venous catheters. If circulatory support is also required, then venoarterial ECMO is used, which normally requires surgical access to the vessels. A typical adult ECMO circuit provides 7 m^2 of membrane for oxygenation using 100% oxygen, with blood flows of approximately 2 to 4 L.min^{-1}. The technique is only available in specialized centres, so portable ECMO systems are used to facilitate transporting the patient to the ECMO centre.

Extracorporeal Carbon Dioxide Removal[57]

Extracorporeal carbon dioxide removal (ECCO$_2$R), a different approach to artificial gas exchange, was first attempted by Gattinoni et al.[58] An ECMO system was used only to remove carbon dioxide, and oxygenation maintained by a modification of apnoeic mass movement oxygenation (page 133). The lungs were either kept motionless or were ventilated two to three times per minute. The technique depends on two important differences between the exchange of carbon dioxide and oxygen. First, membrane oxygenators remove carbon dioxide about 10 to 20 times more effectively than they take up oxygen. Second, the normal arterial oxygen content (20 mL.dL^{-1}) is very close to the maximum oxygen capacity, even with 100% oxygen in the gas phase (22 mL.dL^{-1}). Therefore there is little scope for superoxygenation of a fraction of the cardiac output to compensate for a larger fraction of the cardiac output in which oxygenation does not take place. In contrast, the normal mixed venous carbon dioxide content is 52 mL.dL^{-1} compared with an arterial carbon dioxide content of 48 mL.dL^{-1}. Therefore there is ample scope for removing a larger than normal fraction of carbon dioxide from a part of the cardiac output to compensate for the remaining fraction that does not undergo any removal of carbon dioxide. Thus it is possible to maintain carbon dioxide homoeostasis by diversion of only a small fraction of the cardiac output through an extracorporeal membrane oxygenator.

Intravascular Oxygenators

Siting the gas exchange membrane within the patient's own circulation obviates the need for any extracorporeal circulation. In return, the size of the gas exchange surface is severely limited, and the blood flow around the membrane no longer controlled. The device is inserted surgically via the femoral vein until it lies throughout the length of both inferior and superior vena cavae, through the right atrium. A typical intravascular oxygenator device is 40 to 50 cm long, with 600 to 1100 fibres through which oxygen flows, providing a surface area of 0.21 to 0.52 m^2 for gas exchange. This small membrane surface area is such that total extrapulmonary gas exchange is impossible, and the technique is suitable only for partial respiratory support. These devices are rarely used in clinical practice because of problems with clot formation around the device.

Clinical Applications[59]

Neonates and Infants

Acute respiratory failure in neonates and infants results from a variety of causes such as meconium aspiration syndrome, congenital diaphragmatic hernia, acute respiratory distress syndrome and a variety of infections. ECMO is indicated for treatment of acute respiratory failure of such severity that predicted survival is less than 20%. Although survival varies with the aetiology, there is general agreement that ECMO improves outcome substantially in infants, with some centres achieving survival figures of almost 80%. Complications of ECMO are, however, numerous. Vascular access in infants is difficult, and venoarterial ECMO using the carotid and jugular vessels is often required, although venovenous ECMO with a double lumen cannula is now widely used. In either case, cerebral blood flow may be affected during ECMO, and as a result, a significant number of ECMO-treated infants develop cerebral damage, which in some infants causes long-term disability.[60] Improvements in other therapies, including artificial ventilation, for these very sick patients have led to a progressive reduction in the number treated with ECMO.

Adults

Extrapulmonary gas exchange is used as a therapeutic 'bridge' in patients waiting for lung transplantation,[61] but its main indication is for management of severe ALI (Chapter 31). VILI as a result of artificial ventilation (page 392) contributes to respiratory failure in severe ALI, and the prospect of using extrapulmonary gas exchange to facilitate 'lung rest' is attractive.

Unfortunately, the clinical benefits of ECMO use in infants have been harder to find in adults, and its place in treatment remains poorly defined.[62–64] The invasive nature of extrapulmonary gas exchange and the serious potential complications mean that ECMO is used only in the most severely ill patients. There have now been four randomized controlled trials, all with methodological weaknesses, suggesting no major survival benefit for patients receiving ECMO.[63]

Current interest in extracorporeal gas exchange is focused more on $ECCO_2R$, with ongoing research currently exploring its feasibility[65] and potential uses.[66]

References

1. Stiller K. Physiotherapy in intensive care. An updated systematic review. *Chest.* 2013;144:825-847.
2. Hough A. *Physiotherapy in Respiratory and Critical Care.* 4th ed. Andover: Cengage Learning; 2014.
3. Agostini P, Singh S. Incentive spirometry following thoracic surgery: what should we be doing? *Physiotherapy.* 2009;95:76-82.
*4. **Slutsky AS. History of mechanical ventilation. From Vesalius to ventilator-induced lung injury. *Am J Respir Crit Care Med.* 2015;191:1106-1115.**
5. Grasso F, Engelberts D, Helm E, et al. Negative-pressure ventilation: better oxygenation and less lung injury. *Am J Respir Crit Care Med.* 2008;177:412-418.
6. Hess DR, Branson RD. Know your ventilator to beat the leak. *Chest.* 2012;142:274-275.
7. Chiumello D. Is the helmet different than the face mask in delivering noninvasive ventilation? *Chest.* 2006;129:1402-1403.
8. Bourke SC, Piraino T, Pisani L, et al. Beyond the guidelines for non-invasive ventilation in acute respiratory failure: implications for practice. *Lancet Respir Med.* 2018;6: 935-947.
9. Rochwerg B, Brochard L, Elliott MW, et al. Official ERS/ATS clinical practice guidelines: noninvasive ventilation for acute respiratory failure. *Eur Respir J.* 2017;50:1602426.
10. Patel BK, Wolfe KS, MacKenzie EL, et al. One-year outcomes in patients with acute respiratory distress syndrome enrolled in a randomized clinical trial of helmet versus facemask noninvasive ventilation. *Crit Care Med.* 2018;46:1078-1084.
11. Schnell D, Timsit J-F, Darmon M, et al. Noninvasive mechanical ventilation in acute respiratory failure: trends in use and outcomes. *Intensive Care Med.* 2014;40:582-591.
12. Yeung J, Couper K, Ryan EG, et al. Non-invasive ventilation as a strategy for weaning from invasive mechanical ventilation: a systematic review and Bayesian mata-analysis. *Intensive Care Med.* 2018.44:2192-2204.
13. Gordo-Vidal F, Lobo-Valbuena B. SOS asynchronies: do we need help? *Crit Care Med.* 2018;46:1549-1550.
14. Akoumianaki E, Prinianakis G, Kondili E, et al. Physiologic comparison of neurally adjusted ventilator assist, proportional assist and pressure support ventilation in critically ill patients. *Respir Physiol Neurobiol.* 2014;203:82-89.
*15. **Blanch L, Villagra A, Sales B, et al. Asynchronies during mechanical ventilation are associated with mortality. *Intensive Care Med.* 2015;41:633-641.**
16. Demoule A, Clavel M, Rolland-Debord C, et al. Neurally adjusted ventilatory assist as an alternative to pressure support ventilation in adults: a French multicentre randomized trial. *Intensive Care Med.* 2016;42:1723-1732.
17. Kirakli C, Naz I, Ediboglu O, et al. A randomized controlled trial comparing the ventilation duration between adaptive support ventilation and pressure assist/control ventilation in medical patients in the ICU. *Chest.* 2015;147:1503-1509.
*18. **Bagchi A, Rudolph MI, Ng PY, et al. The association of postoperative pulmonary complications in 109,360 patients with pressure-controlled or volume-controlled ventilation. *Anaesthesia.* 2017;72:1334-1343.**
19. Venkataraman S, Kinsella J. Airway pressure release ventilation: A therapy in search of a disease? *Am J Respir Crit Care Med.* 2018;198:1118-1119.
20. Bouchut J-C, Godard J, Claris O. High-frequency oscillatory ventilation. *Anesthesiology.* 2004;100:1007-1012.
21. Pillow JJ. High-frequency oscillatory ventilation: Mechanisms of gas exchange and lung mechanics. *Crit Care Med.* 2005; 33(suppl):S135-S141.
22. Wise MP, Saayman AG, Gillies MA. High-frequency oscillatory ventilation and acute respiratory distress syndrome: at the crossroads? *Thorax.* 2013;68:406-408.
*23. **McConville JF, Kress JP. Weaning patients from the ventilator. *N Engl J Med.* 2012;367:2233-2239.**

24. MacIntyre N. Another look at outcomes from mechanical ventilation. *Am J Respir Crit Care Med.* 2017;195:710-711.

25. Criner GJ. Measuring diaphragm shortening using ultrasonography to predict extubation success. *Thorax.* 2014;69:402-404.

26. Russell JA. Biomarker (BNP)-guided weaning from mechanical ventilation. Time for a paradigm shift? *Am J Respir Crit Care Med.* 2012;186:1202-1204.

27. Brown SM. Toward an integrative approach to liberation from mechanical ventilation. *Crit Care Med.* 2016;44:1792-1793.

28. Frutos-Vivar F, Esteban A. Our paper 20 years later: how has withdrawal from mechanical ventilation changed? *Intensive Care Med.* 2014;40:1449-1459.

29. Schmidt GA, Girard TD, Kress JP, et al. Official executive summary of an American Thoracic Society/American College of Chest Physicians clinical practice guideline: liberation from mechanical ventilation in critically ill adults. *Am J Respir Crit Care Med.* 2017;195:115-119.

30. Maggiore SM, Battilana M, Serano L, et al. Ventilatory support after extubation in critically ill patients. *Lancet Respir Med.* 2018;6:948-962.

31. Simonds AK. Streamlining weaning: protocols and weaning units. *Thorax.* 2005;60:175-177.

32. Marini JJ. Dynamic hyperinflation and auto–positive end-expiratory pressure. Lessons learned over 30 years. *Am J Respir Crit Care Med.* 2011;184:756-762.

*33. Soni N, Williams P. Positive pressure ventilation: what is the real cost? *Br J Anaesth.* 2008;101:446-457.

34. Loick HM, Wendt M, Rötker J, et al. Ventilation with positive end-expiratory airway pressure causes leukocyte retention in human lung. *J Appl Physiol.* 1993;75:301-306.

35. Pinsky MR. Why knowing the effects of positive-pressure ventilation on venous, pleural, and pericardial pressures is important to the bedside clinician? *Crit Care Med.* 2014;42:2129-2131.

36. Cournand A, Motley HL, Werko L, et al. Physiological studies of the effects of intermittent positive pressure breathing on cardiac output in man. *Am J Physiol.* 1948;152:162-174.

37. Bindslev LG, Hedenstierna G, Santesson J, et al. Ventilation-perfusion distribution during inhalational anaesthesia. *Acta Anaesthesiol Scand.* 1981;25:360-371.

*38. Lansdorp B, Hofhuizen C, van Lavieren M, et al. Mechanical ventilation–induced intrathoracic pressure distribution and heart-lung interactions. *Crit Care Med.* 2014;42:1983-1990.

39. Ryan KL, Cooke WH, Rickards CA, et al. Breathing through an inspiratory threshold device improves stroke volume during central hypovolemia in humans. *J Appl Physiol.* 2008;104:1402-1409.

40. Darmon M, Legrand M, Terzi N. Understanding the kidney during acute respiratory failure. *Intensive Care Med.* 2017;43:1144-1147.

41. Slutsky AS, Ranieri VM. Ventilator-induced lung injury. *N Engl J Med.* 2013;369:2126-2136.

*42. Nieman GF, Satalin J, Kollisch-Singule M, et al. Physiology in medicine: understanding dynamic alveolar physiology to minimize ventilator-induced lung injury. *J Appl Physiol.* 2017;122:1516-1522.

43. Fothergill J. Observations on a case published in the last volume of the medical essays, & c. of recovering a man dead in appearance, by distending the lungs with air. *Philos Trans R Soc Lond.* 1745;43:275-281.

44. Trepat X, Farré R. Alveolar permeability and stretch: too far, too fast. *Eur Respir J.* 2008;32:826-828.

45. dos Santos CC. The role of the inflammasome in ventilator-induced lung injury. *Am J Respir Crit Care Med.* 2012;185:1141-1144.

46. Jacob AM, Gaver DP III. Atelectrauma disrupts pulmonary epithelial barrier integrity and alters the distribution of tight junction proteins ZO-1 and claudin 4. *J Appl Physiol.* 2012;113:1377-1387.

47. Albert RK. The role of ventilation-induced surfactant dysfunction and atelectasis in causing acute respiratory distress syndrome. *Am J Respir Crit Care Med.* 2012;185:702-708.

48. Milos S, Khazaee R, McCaig LA, et al. Impact of ventilation-induced lung injury on the structure and function of lamellar bodies. *Am J Physiol Lung Cell Mol Physiol.* 2017;313:L524-L533.

49. Curley GF, Laffey JG, Zhang H, et al. Biotrauma and ventilator-induced lung injury clinical implications. *Chest.* 2016;150:1109-1117.

50. Fan E, Rubenfeld GD. Driving pressure—the emperor's new clothes. *Crit Care Med.* 2017;45:919-920.

51. Thierbach AR, Wolcke BB, Krummenauer F, et al. Artificial ventilation for basic life support leads to hyperventilation in first aid providers. *Resuscitation.* 2003;57:269-277.

52. Nassar BS, Kerber R. Improving CPR Performance. *Chest.* 2017;152:1061-1069.

*53. Nichol G, Leroux B, Wang H, et al. Trial of continuous or interrupted chest compressions during CPR. *N Engl J Med.* 2015;373:2203-2214.

54. Angus DC. Whether to intubate during cardiopulmonary resuscitation. Conventional wisdom vs big data. *JAMA.* 2017;317:477-478.

55. Schwartz SM. Tattered and torn: the life of a RBC on the extracorporeal membrane oxygenation circuit. *Crit Care Med.* 2014;42:1314-1315.

56. Abrams D, Brodie D. Extracorporeal membrane oxygenation for adult respiratory failure 2017 Update. *Chest.* 2017;152:639-649.

57. Morelli A, Del Sorbo L, Pesenti A, et al. Extracorporeal carbon dioxide removal (ECCO2R) in patients with acute respiratory failure. *Intensive Care Med.* 2017;43:519-530.

58. Gattinoni L, Pesenti A, Rossi GP, et al. Treatment of acute respiratory failure with low-frequency positive-pressure ventilation and extracorporeal removal of CO_2. *Lancet.* 1980;2:292-294.

59. Gaffney AM, Wildhirt SM, Griffin MJ, et al. Extracorporeal life support. *BMJ.* 2010;341:c5317.

60. Field D, Davis C, Elbourne D, et al. UK laborative randomised trial of neonatal extracorporeal membrane oxygenation. *Lancet.* 1996;348:75-82.

61. Munshi L, Fan E. Lung transplant and extracorporeal membrane oxygenation more is better and better together? *Am J Respir Crit Care Med.* 2016;194:255-256.

62. Parhar K, Vuylsteke A. What's new in ECMO: scoring the bad indications. *Intensive Care Med.* 2014;40:1734-1737.

63. Derwall M, Rossaint R. ECMO in severe acute respiratory distress syndrome: a light at the end of the tunnel? *Lancet Respir Med.* 2018;6:661-662.

64. Karagiannidis C, Brodie D, Strassmann S, et al. Extracorporeal membrane oxygenation: evolving epidemiology and mortality. *Intensive Care Med.* 2016;42:889-896.

65. Combes A, Fanelli V, Pham T, et al. Feasibility and safety of extracorporeal CO_2 removal to enhance protective ventilation in acute respiratory distress syndrome: the SUPERNOVA study. *Intensive Care Med.* 2019;45:592-600.

66. Boyle AJ, Sklar M, McNamee J, et al. Extracorporeal carbon dioxide removal for lowering the risk of mechanical ventilation: research questions and clinical potential for the future. *Lancet Respir Med.* 2018;6:874-884.

33

Pulmonary Surgery

KEY POINTS

- Surgical resection of lung tissue via thoracotomy is a routine procedure, used mostly for treating lung cancer, which requires careful assessment of the patient's physiological reserve.
- Less invasive surgical techniques such as video-assisted thoracic surgery are increasing rapidly and associated with less physiological disturbance and clinical complications.
- One-lung ventilation is required for many pulmonary surgery procedures, and understanding of the physiology involved is vital for its safe use.

- Lung transplantation is an established technique for treating advanced lung disease, with chronic obstructive pulmonary disease currently being the most common indication.
- Lung transplant results in completely denervated lungs, which leaves the respiratory pattern unaffected but impairs the cough reflex.

In current clinical practice surgery of the lungs, mediastinum and chest wall is routinely performed, and although still high risk by modern surgical standards, the outcome for most patients is favourable. The physiological disturbances caused during and after pulmonary surgery are immense, and in this chapter the effects of the more common pulmonary surgical procedures are outlined.

Physiological Aspects of Common Interventions

Bronchoscopy

Bronchoscopy allows direct visualization of the airway and, if necessary, the collection of washings and biopsies of airway, lung and mediastinal tissue. It may also be used therapeutically to, for example, remove inhaled foreign bodies, resect tumours or place stents to overcome airway obstruction. Two types of bronchoscopy are performed, flexible and rigid.

Flexible Bronchoscopy[1]

The flexibility of fibreoptic bronchoscopes allows a view of all the major branches of the tracheobronchial tree with minimal risk of trauma and discomfort for the patient. The procedure can therefore be performed without general anaesthesia, although extensive topical anaesthesia to the airway is

required, and most clinicians also provide sedation to relieve the anxiety associated with having a bronchoscopy. Hypoxia during a flexible bronchoscopy is common, occurring in 17% of patients from one study,[2] and supplemental oxygen is therefore normally used. Lung function during bronchoscopy is significantly impaired. While the bronchoscope is in place the functional residual capacity (FRC) is increased by about one-fifth, and forced vital capacity (FVC), forced expiratory volume in one second (FEV_1) and peak expiratory flow are all decreased, indicating expiratory air flow obstruction. These observations are not explained simply by the presence of the bronchoscope in the airway, as the observed airway flow limitation begins after the airway local anaesthetic is applied (before insertion of the bronchoscope) and continues for several minutes after the bronchoscope has been removed, suggesting that a bronchoconstrictor action of the topical anaesthesia is responsible. Respiratory depression may also occur during or soon after bronchoscopy, and the causes of this are uncertain but likely to relate either to the sedative drugs or the topical anaesthesia in the airway. The major limitation of flexible bronchoscopy is the size of the instruments that may be passed down the bronchoscope. They are suitable for visualization and biopsies of the airway, and the development of endobronchial ultrasound has allowed flexible bronchoscopes to also be used for biopsies of mediastinal lymph nodes and tumours, revolutionizing the diagnosis and staging of lung cancer.[3] However, for removal of foreign bodies or airway surgery a larger portal for access to the tracheobronchial tree is required.

Rigid Bronchoscopy

Straight, rigid bronchoscopes are available with internal diameters up to 8 mm that may be passed into the trachea, and a variety of instruments can then be used through the bronchoscope. To see around corners in the bronchial tree 30- and 90-degree angled telescopes are used. With rigid bronchoscopy foreign bodies that are wedged in the airway can be removed, tracheal tumours resected, airway haemorrhage treated and stents deployed in the trachea or main bronchi to overcome stenosing tumours or airway leaks. The major disadvantage of the technique is the requirement for general anaesthesia, often in a patient with significant respiratory disease.

Ventilation during a rigid bronchoscopy is challenging, and four main techniques may be used:

1. *Spontaneous ventilation.* A ventilating bronchoscope allows the normal anaesthetic breathing system to be attached to a side port of the bronchoscope, which also must have a glass window to occlude its proximal lumen to prevent escape of the anaesthetic gases. Spontaneous breathing may be continued during the procedure, with anaesthesia maintained by inhalational or intravenous agents. Leaks around the bronchoscope are a problem, particularly if the surgeon wishes to pass instruments through the bronchoscope, so this technique is now used only rarely and usually in children in whom the small size of the cricoid cartilage minimizes leakage of inhaled gases from around the bronchoscope.

2. *Positive pressure ventilation.* This form of ventilation may be achieved via a ventilating bronchoscope, as described earlier, but once again the lack of a seal between the airway and bronchoscope makes the technique problematic. The most common technique used for ventilation is the Sanders injector, which is a high-pressure oxygen supply (4 atm) intermittently applied to the proximal end of the rigid bronchoscope through a small diameter 'injector'. As a result of the Venturi effect, the high-velocity jet of oxygen entrains room air and increases the pressure along the bronchoscope, causing lung inflation. Anaesthesia must be maintained by intravenous agents, and adequacy of ventilation can only be assessed by observation of the chest rather than the usual capnography (page 134), but this technique does allow the surgeon to operate down the bronchoscope whilst the patient is being ventilated. The Sanders injector system for ventilation is problematic in patients with lung disease, as the inspired oxygen concentration and pulmonary inflation pressure are variable, influenced not only by the bronchoscope dimensions and side ports but also by the mechanics of the patient's lungs.

3. *High-frequency jet ventilation* (page 384). This may be used during bronchoscopy, and the ability of the technique to ventilate the lungs with minimal increase in airway pressure makes it particularly useful in patients with airway leaks such as bronchopleural fistulae.

4. *Apnoeic oxygenation.* This may be used during rigid bronchoscopy, but normally only as a last resort and for a short period of time—that is, until hypercapnia develops (page 133).

Thoracoscopy

Insertion of a telescope through the chest wall into the pleural space allows direct inspection of the pleura, lungs, mediastinum and diaphragm to facilitate diagnosis or therapeutic interventions. Three types of thoracoscopy exist:

1. *Medical thoracoscopy.*[4] This technique may be used to investigate pleural effusions or pneumothorax when less invasive interventions such as thoracocentesis have failed to reach a diagnosis. One or two ports are inserted into the chest in an awake or sedated patient using local anaesthesia, similar to inserting a chest drain. In most cases the thoracoscope is inserted into an existing pleural space, that is, a pleural effusion or pneumothorax, so the physiological insult is less than may be imagined. Minor interventions such as biopsies, breaking down of pleural adhesions or talc pleurodesis (page 402) may be performed if accompanied by suitable analgesia.

2. *Thoracoscopy using gas insufflation.* This technique is usually performed under general anaesthesia and involves insertion of multiple ports and insufflation of carbon dioxide into the pleural space to create a compartment in which the operation can be performed. Increasing the intrapleural pressure above atmospheric in this way effectively causes a tension pneumothorax (page 361); therefore it is vital that the pressure used is both well-controlled and kept as low as possible (usually <10 mmHg). Intermittent positive pressure ventilation of the lung on the operative side may be continued, minimizing the effect of the capnothorax on gas exchange, and close monitoring allows any cardiovascular changes to be quickly corrected by releasing carbon dioxide from the chest cavity. Any carbon dioxide left in the pleura at the conclusion of surgery will be quickly reabsorbed (page 363).

3. *Video-assisted thoracic surgery (VATS).* This term describes any operation that is facilitated by insertion of a video camera into the chest cavity. Usually a small thoracotomy is made, and the camera and operating instruments all pass through this small opening, although other ports may be inserted elsewhere in the chest wall. This procedure differs from a thoracoscopy, as described earlier, in that the chest cavity is open to the atmosphere, so a positive intrathoracic pressure cannot occur. One-lung ventilation (OLV) is therefore needed, and the lung on the operative side collapses under its own elastic recoil or has to be retracted by the surgeon. The small breach of the chest cavity required for VATS has numerous advantages compared with the effects of a thoracotomy (see later) and the technique is widely used for pleural surgery such as pleurodesis (page 402) and for

intervention after a pneumothorax. Minor lung surgery such as wedge resection and lung biopsy are particularly suitable for a VATS approach, and this has now become the standard approach for lobectomy in many centres, and even pneumonectomy in some.[5]

Thoracotomy

A surgical opening in the chest cavity was first used more than 100 years ago, usually for the treatment of empyema (page 363) and tuberculosis. In current surgical practice the indications for thoracotomy have widened to include surgery of the lungs, major vessels, oesophagus and thoracic spine. In most cases, thoracotomy is performed in the lateral position, which has significant effects on respiratory physiology (see later), and through a posterolateral incision.

The effects of thoracotomy on postoperative respiratory function are profound, with significant reductions in chest wall compliance and respiratory muscle activity resulting from chest wall oedema, pain, disruption of muscle anatomy and, later in the recovery phase, scarring of chest wall tissues. In the first 24 hours following surgery, FVC and FEV_1 are only 30% to 50% of the preoperative volumes, with some evidence that the type of thoracotomy incision used may affect these values. Chest wall compliance falls to around 60% of the preoperative value by the third postoperative day before slowly improving. At 1 week after surgery, FVC and FEV_1 are around 70% to 80% of preoperative values, and by this stage the different incisions seem to have little effect on recovery.[6]

Other measures of respiratory muscle strength such as maximum inspiratory and expiratory mouth pressures are also reduced to about one-half the preoperative values following thoracotomy, and in one study had not returned to normal 12 weeks after surgery.[7] The same study showed a rapid return to normal of both measures of muscle function following VATS procedures. Older patients, who have poor respiratory muscle strength relative to younger patients, took longer to recover muscle function following surgery, possibly explaining the greater incidence of pulmonary complications with increasing age.[8] Therefore thoracotomy alone impairs respiratory muscle function to such an extent that ventilation may not be able to keep pace with the extra ventilatory requirements associated with having major surgery, and alveolar hypoventilation can occur along with regional pulmonary collapse and impaired oxygenation. Even in less severely affected patients the ability to cough is always weakened, with an increased risk of chest complications. For patients who have a lung resection through their thoracotomy, lung compliance is also decreased to about half their preoperative value, compounding these problems.

Lung Resection

Assessing Patient Fitness for Lung Resection[9]

Lung function is assessed using either the FEV_1 or, if the patient has parenchymal lung disease, the diffusing capacity for carbon monoxide (D_{LCO}; page 117). If these are less than 80% of normal predicted values for that patient, an attempt is made to calculate predicted postoperative values based on which anatomical sections of lung need to be removed. Radionucleotide ventilation or perfusion scans or quantitative computed tomography scans may all be used to measure functional lung units; these are useful techniques as they also show which pathological lung units are already not contributing to overall function. Less invasive is the anatomical method in which the lungs are divided into 19 anatomical segments of equal value, and knowing which segments are to be removed enables estimation of postoperative predicted lung function. For many years a general rule of lung resection was that a predicted postoperative FEV_1 of less than 0.8 to 1.0 L precluded resection, although evidence for this rule is poor. Using an absolute value for FEV_1 or D_{LCO} is fraught with difficulties because sex, age and height all affect the normal values, and decisions should now always be based on the values as a percentage of the predicted normal for that patient (page 24).

Different studies have produced varied results on the association between percentage predicted postoperative FEV_1 or D_{LCO} and outcome, but a value of less than 40% of predicted normal is now accepted as being associated with an increased mortality and complication rate. For patients in this situation, measurement of preoperative exercise tolerance has the advantage of also including a cardiovascular component to the assessment and may help to further define risks and outcomes. The most objective way of quantifying exercise activity is by measuring $\dot{V}O_{2peak}$ (page 184). Values of less than 15 mL.min^{-1}.kg^{-1} are again associated with poor outcome. Clinical measures of exercise tolerance have some value, but these must be performed under supervision, as patients' own reported exercise tolerance is normally greatly exaggerated. Tests which have some limited use in predicting outcome after lung resection include the shuttle test and 6-minute walk test (page 189) and stair climbing (the number of stairs or height of stairs the patient is able to climb[10]).

Partial Lung Resection

The magnitude of lung resection operations varies from removal of a small tumour in the lung periphery to a complete pneumonectomy, with the more minor procedures performed via VATS and the more major via a thoracotomy. Wherever possible, dissection is made between lobes or in intersegmental planes. Care is required when operating on pulmonary vessels, particularly pulmonary arteries because they have thin walls and are easy to damage, which can result in significant haemorrhage that may be difficult to control.

Following lung resection, the remaining lung in the hemithorax quickly expands to fill the available space. One or two chest drains are usually placed in the chest cavity and connected to underwater seal systems to allow any air or blood to drain. If the remaining lung does not fully expand, a negative pressure of up to 20 cmH$_2$O may be applied to the drains to encourage expansion.

Pneumonectomy

Resection of an entire lung is usually performed for removal of large, central lung tumours (Fig. 33.1, *A*). Following pneumonectomy correct management of the empty hemithorax is crucial. If air is drained from the cavity too quickly mediastinal shift will occur, which impairs venous drainage to the heart and can cause cardiovascular collapse. One option is to not leave a drain in the chest cavity and to monitor the position of the mediastinum daily with a chest radiograph. Alternatively, a chest drain can be placed (Fig. 33.1, *B*), but be clamped for most of the time and only released briefly and intermittently to ensure the pressure in the cavity is approximately atmospheric. A more interventional approach is to measure the pressure in the chest cavity and instil or remove air to maintain a pressure of -2 to -4 cmH$_2$O on inspiration and $+2$ to $+4$ cmH$_2$O on expiration. Within a few weeks of pneumonectomy the volume of the hemithorax decreases because of a combination of mediastinal shift, elevation of the diaphragm and contraction of the chest wall, and pleural fluid replaces the air in the chest cavity (Fig. 33.1, *C*). Over the ensuing months or years, the fluid volume decreases as the mediastinal shift continues, and the other lung herniates anteriorly or posteriorly across the midline to partially fill the vacated hemithorax.

Studies in animals have demonstrated the intriguing phenomenon of 'neoalveolarization' following lung resection.[11] Within 20 days of lung resection in mice the number of alveoli in the remaining lung increased by 50%, completely restoring the gas-exchanging surface area.[12] Neoalveolarization probably occurs by new alveoli forming in the walls of existing alveolar ducts and respiratory bronchioles, and is thus far only described in young animals, as would be expected from the observation that in mammals formation of alveoli is a postnatal process (page 176).

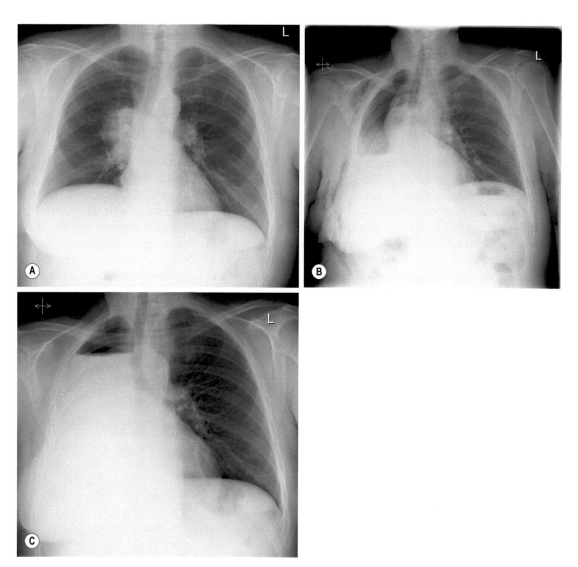

• **Fig. 33.1** **(A)** Chest radiograph showing large lung cancer at the right hilum. **(B)** The same patient 24 hours after a right pneumonectomy. Note the shifted trachea and mediastinum, contracted right thoracic cage and early accumulation of fluid in the empty hemithorax. **(C)** One month later, with the empty hemithorax already almost completely filled with fluid and a hyperexpanded left lung.

Surgery for Emphysema

Surgical treatment is reserved for patients with severe chronic obstructive pulmonary disease (COPD) in whom emphysematous changes predominate. When the airspaces created in emphysema become larger than 1 cm in diameter they are referred to as a *bulla*. Nearby bullae can merge and result in extremely large air spaces, occupying up to one-third of the lung volume. Like emphysema, bullae have little effect on gas exchange because both tidal ventilation and blood flow to the bulla are negligible (page 332). However, with giant bullae the airspace acts in a similar fashion to a pneumothorax (page 361) and compresses surrounding lung tissue, causing further worsening of airway collapse and subsequent disturbance of gas exchange. In these cases surgical treatment involves 'bullectomy', and with careful patient selection this can be a useful operation. Improved surgical techniques led to a resurgence of interest in surgery for COPD and extended the indications to include patients who do not have bullae.

Lung volume reduction surgery (LVRS) involves removing 20% to 30% of lung volume, to include the most emphysematous areas, and can have impressive results. Improved long-term survival compared with the best medical therapy has only been proven in patients with poor exercise capacity and upper lobe emphysema;[13] conversely, patients with high exercise capacity and emphysema elsewhere in the lung have a higher mortality following surgery compared with medical treatment. Despite these mixed survival results, in appropriately selected groups of patients LVRS can improve exercise capacity, lung volumes, quality of life, arterial Po_2 and cardiovascular function.[13,15]

The high risks of surgical LVRS led to the development of other techniques to try and achieve the same effect in a less invasive way. The most widely used is bronchoscopic insertion of endobronchial valves (EBVs) which only allow air out of a lung lobe, causing the lobe to collapse (Fig. 33.2).[16] Similar results can be achieved as for surgical LVRS, but careful selection is needed to identify patients who do not have collateral ventilation between lung lobes, which prevents the EBV from causing collapse.[17] Trials are also now underway of emphysematous lung sealant therapy which involves occluding upper lobe bronchi to collapse affected lung regions.[18]

Understanding of the physiological mechanisms leading to clinical improvements following LVRS by whatever method remains incomplete. Potential benefits of LVRS include reduced pulmonary collapse adjacent to emphysematous areas, improved elastic recoil of the remaining lung tissue and better respiratory muscle function secondary to reduced hyperinflation (see Fig. 5.1).[19]

Pleurodesis

Pleurodesis describes a variety of procedures, all of which aim to induce adhesions between the visceral and parietal pleura. The two most common indications are pneumothorax that has failed to respond to conservative management (page 361) or palliation of malignant pleural effusion. Although the preferred technique varies with the indication, the success of any pleurodesis depends on inducing inflammation in the pleura while simultaneously ensuring the two pleural layers are closely apposed, allowing the normal inflammation and tissue repair processes to cause scarring in the pleural space. Apposition of the pleura is usually achieved by using a pleural drain, but if required an inflammatory reaction in the pleura can be initiated by various means. A pleurectomy may be performed, with the parietal pleura stripped from the inside of the chest wall, or a less traumatic technique is pleural abrasion in which the pleura is rubbed with a dry gauze or other abrasive surface. Alternatively, sclerosants can be instilled into the pleural cavity, including antibiotics (e.g., doxycycline), antiseptics (e.g., iodopovidone), anticancer drugs or minerals such as talc. Talc pleurodesis is the most common technique, and the talc may either be instilled as a slurry through a small pleural catheter to avoid surgical intervention or as a dry

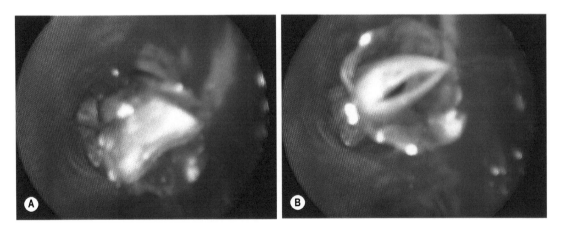

• **Fig. 33.2** A 4-mm endobronchial valve in an upper lobe segmental bronchus. The 'duck-billed' valve is contained within a metal stent, held in place by radial forces from its expansion within the rigid airway. These images were captured immediately after valve insertion, and the valve can be seen to be closed during inspiration **(A)** and open during expiration **(B)**.

powder (poudrage) via a surgical approach. The particle size of talc is important in the development of adverse effects from talc pleurodesis. Talc particles have been found to enter the lung parenchyma or systemic circulation following pleurodesis, risking the development of pulmonary fibrosis or systemic inflammation, respectively. Use of particle sizes greater than 5 μm reduces the complication rate, presumably because the talc particles are unable to pass through the similarly sized stoma in the pleura (page 360) to gain access to the lymphatics and circulation.

Obliterating the pleura by these techniques may be expected to cause long-term impairment to lung function, but after an initial decline immediately after the procedure, total lung capacity returns to normal approximately 6 months later.[20] This is in keeping with the bizarre observation, first made in the 1700s, that elephants have no pleural space, with connective tissue binding their lungs tightly to the inside of the chest wall, with no apparent long-term ill effects for the species.[21]

One-Lung Ventilation

Many of the surgical procedures already described will be facilitated by apnoea of the operative lung during surgery. These, and other indications for OLV, are shown in Table 33.1. Indications are divided into absolute, where without OLV the patient's life is at risk, and relative, when OLV will help manage the patient's condition but is not mandatory.

Lung Isolation Techniques

Isolation of one lung requires knowledge of some anatomical features of the large airways. First, the angle at which the right and left main bronchi branch from the trachea is highly variable: on average it is 25 degrees from the vertical for the right main bronchus and 45 degrees for the left. There is, however, wide individual variation in these angles both in health and disease, although the right main bronchus is almost always at the less acute angle. Second, the

distance between the carina and the first segmental bronchus is normally 5 cm in the left main bronchus and only 2.5 cm in the right, making occlusion of the right upper lobe a possibility when a cuffed tube is in the right main bronchus.

There are three options available to isolate one lung:
1. *Endobronchial tube.* This involves placement of a small-diameter single-lumen cuffed endotracheal tube into the main bronchus of the lung that needs to remain ventilated (Fig. 33.3, *A*). Deliberate endobronchial intubation is rarely used, because of the difficulties of positioning the tube in the correct side and because the technique does not allow ventilation of the other lung without repositioning the tube.
2. *Bronchial blockers.* A bronchial blocker is a narrow catheter with a balloon at the tip which is inserted through a standard singe-lumen tracheal tube into the main bronchus of the lung requiring isolation, and the cuff intermittently inflated to block gas flow into that lung (Fig. 33.3, *B*). Bronchial blockers have the advantage of being placed through a standard tracheal tube; the cuff is small compared with a double-lumen tube (DLT) and is less likely to occlude segmental bronchi. Bronchial blockers also have several disadvantages, mostly arising from the small lumen of the device, such as an inability to suction the nonventilated

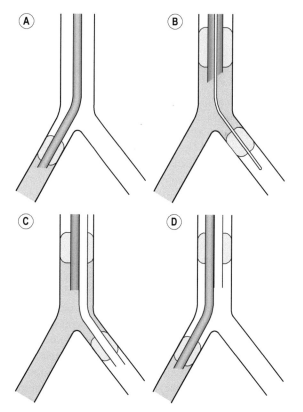

• **Fig. 33.3** Four methods of achieving one-lung ventilation of the right lung. **(A)** Single-lumen endobronchial tube in the right main bronchus. **(B)** Bronchial blocker passed through a standard tracheal tube into the left main bronchus. **(C)** Left-sided double-lumen tube with ventilation via the tracheal lumen. **(D)** Right-sided double-lumen tube with ventilation via the bronchial lumen. In each case the pink area shows where ventilation is occurring.

TABLE 33.1	Indications for One-Lung Ventilation
Absolute Indications	**Relative Indications**
Isolation of lung to avoid cross contamination:	Surgical exposure:
Lung abscess	Thoracic aortic surgery
Massive haemorrhage	Lung resection
Unilateral ventilation:	Video-assisted thoracic surgery
Bronchopleural fistula	Oesophagectomy
Giant lung cyst or bulla	Thoracic spine surgery
Bronchial tree disruption	
Pneumonectomy	
Intensive care:	Intensive care:
Life-threatening hypoxia from unilateral lung disease	Severe hypoxia from unilateral lung disease

lung and slow collapse of the nonventilated lung, although this can be accelerated by use of 100% oxygen or a nitrous oxide/oxygen mixture[22] immediately before lung isolation (page 406).

3. *Double-lumen tubes.* This is the most common technique for lung isolation, and the correct position for both left and right DLTs is shown in Figure 33.3, *C* and *D*, respectively. The advantageous angle of the right main bronchus means right-sided DLTs are more likely to enter the correct bronchus, but the close proximity of the right upper lobe bronchus means these tubes usually have modified bronchial cuff shapes to minimize the chances of occlusion of the right upper lobe. Use of a left-sided DLT avoids this problem, but then the risk of the tube entering the incorrect bronchus is increased. Once correctly sited, irrespective of whether a right- or left-sided DLT has been used, both lungs can be ventilated or suction catheters passed independently, and the two lungs are isolated from each other to prevent cross-contamination with blood or infectious secretions.

Physiology of One-Lung Ventilation

Despite OLV now being a routine technique in many situations, hypoxia still occurs in 5% to 10% of patients.[23] A detailed understanding of the physiology of OLV is therefore vital if a logical approach to management is to be adopted. First, the factors that influence lung function during OLV will be considered.

Patient Position

Although OLV may be required in a supine patient, the lateral position is most commonly used for thoracic surgery, and this position significantly affects ventilation and perfusion of the lungs. The loss of muscle tone in the chest wall and diaphragm associated with general anaesthesia (page 247) causes gravity to affect the volumes of the left and right hemithoraces. The volume of the dependent lung is decreased by the weight of the mediastinum above and by cephalad movement of the diaphragm from the weight of the abdominal contents. Table 7.1 (page 89) shows the distribution of FRC and ventilation in the left and right lungs in both lateral positions when anaesthetized. FRC in the dependent lung is approximately 1 L less than the nondependent lung, and inevitably, under general anaesthesia, atelectasis forms in the dependent lung (see Fig. 21.9, *B*). 'Breaking' the operating table to open the intercostal space on the operative side of the chest will further compress the dependent lung.

These changes in lung volume affect the position of each lung on a regional compliance curve. In a spontaneously breathing awake patient in the lateral position, the lower lung is on a steeper part of the compliance curve than the nondependent lung, and therefore receives more ventilation (Fig. 33.4, *A*). Dependent lung ventilation is also enhanced by the cephalad movement of the lower diaphragm, increasing its efficiency. When the patient is anaesthetized, paralysed and ventilated in the lateral position, the effect

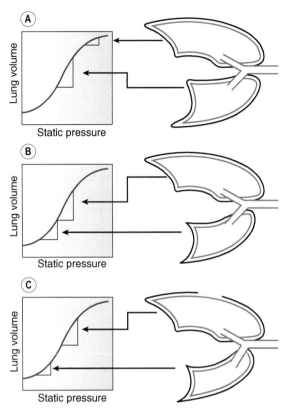

• **Fig. 33.4** Schematic representation of lung volumes and regional compliance in the right lateral position. **(A)** Awake patient, spontaneously breathing. The nondependent *(left)* lung has a higher functional residual capacity (FRC) than in the supine position, so is at a less favourable part of the compliance curve, and the dependent *(right)* lung will receive relatively more ventilation. **(B)** Anaesthetized and paralysed patient in the same position. The loss of muscle activity in the diaphragm and chest wall reduces FRC in both lungs, and the weight of the mediastinum compresses the dependent lung. This changes their position on the compliance curve, and the nondependent *(left)* lung is now the better ventilated. **(C)** Same situation with the chest open. Loss of the negative pleural pressure of the nondependent lung causes further mediastinal shift, further compromising the function of the dependent lung. In the left lateral position the same physiological changes occur, but the impact is greater when the smaller left lung is the dependent one.

of the diaphragm position is lost, and the reduction of FRC for both lungs causes the nondependent lung to reside in the steep middle part of a compliance curve, and it is this lung that now receives approximately 60% of ventilation (Fig. 33.4, *B*). Because of the larger volume of the right lung, these considerations are affected by which side the patient is on, with a larger differential FRC and ventilation when the left lung is dependent. Perfusion of the dependent lung is always greater than the nondependent lung in the lateral position, and this differential is mostly uninfluenced by anaesthesia and paralysis. Thus the ventilation/perfusion ($\dot{V}/\dot{Q}$) ratios of the lung are well matched when the patient is in the lateral position and awake, but anaesthesia and artificial ventilation in this position results in significant mismatch, with greater ventilation of the nondependent lung associated with greater perfusion of the dependent lung.

Ceasing ventilation of the nondependent lung therefore removes the better ventilated lung, leaving the challenge of ventilating the low-volume, low-compliance dependent lung, but also removing the larger part of the $\dot{V}/\dot{Q}$ mismatch.

Open Chest

Allowing air to enter the pleural space of the nondependent lung will exacerbate the changes described thus far. The negative intrapleural pressure of the upper hemithorax helps to hold up the mediastinum, and when this is lost the full weight of the heart and other mediastinal structures further compresses the dependent lung (Fig. 33.4, C). With a thoracotomy, the compliance of the chest wall is in effect removed, and only lung compliance (page 14) will determine ventilation of the nondependent lung, which will be free to expand to a large volume if ventilation of both lungs continues.

Perfusion of the Nonventilated Lung

Once ventilation of the nondependent lung ceases, matching of ventilation to perfusion becomes almost entirely dependent on the amount of blood flowing through the apnoeic nondependent lung. Factors affecting pulmonary vascular resistance (PVR) are described in detail in Chapter 6, and include passive factors such as gravity and lung volume and active control of pulmonary blood vessel size. During OLV the effect of gravity depends on patient position: in the lateral position perfusion of the upper lung will be reduced, but this will not be the case if OLV is used in the supine position. As a result of this, relatively high blood flow in the supine position oxygenation is more often impaired than during OLV in the lateral position.[24] PVR is minimal at FRC (see Fig. 6.4), so a small reduction in pulmonary blood flow will occur when the nonventilated lung collapses towards residual volume. Surgical manipulation of the lung is also likely to reduce its blood flow, either by distorting and thus occluding pulmonary vasculature or by directly clamping pulmonary vessels as part of the surgical procedure.

Of the many mechanisms involved in active control of PVR (see Table 6.2), it is hypoxic pulmonary vasoconstriction (HPV; page 80) that is believed to be the most important determinant of pulmonary blood flow in the nonventilated lung.[25] The 40% to 50% of cardiac output that would be expected to flow through the nonventilated lung is believed to be reduced to 20% to 25% by HPV. The passive increase in PVR as a result of reduced lung volume is thought to be small compared with the effect of HPV—if during OLV the nonventilated lung is reinflated and ventilated with nitrogen, the blood flow to the lung is unaffected, but performing the same manoeuvre with oxygen increases the blood flow to normal.[26] How much HPV occurs is influenced by both alveolar and mixed venous P_{O_2} (see Fig. 6.7), thus changes in cardiac output or oxygen consumption that will affect venous P_{O_2} may influence blood flow to the nonventilated lung. A fall in mixed venous P_{O_2} enhances the HPV response, and an abnormally high mixed venous P_{O_2}

may have the opposite effect as oxygen diffuses from the alveolar capillary blood into the nonventilated alveoli.

The effect of general anaesthesia on HPV has been controversial for some years. Results from in vitro or animal studies have shown that all inhalational anaesthetic agents, including nitrous oxide, cause some inhibition of HPV whereas propofol and fentanyl have been shown to have no effect. Translating these observations into clinical practice is problematic because of the numerous other factors that may affect HPV such as:[25]

- *Cardiac output.* This is reduced by most general anaesthetic drugs. A fall in cardiac output reduces blood flow through both shunt and normal regions of lung (page 102) and decreases the mixed venous P_{O_2}, which will affect HPV, as described earlier.
- *Individual variation in the HPV response.* This is large and difficult to predict. Evidence for this is seen at high altitude, where varying degrees of HPV between individuals affects their likelihood of developing pulmonary oedema (page 213).
- *Nonanaesthetic drugs, particularly vasoactive drugs.* Commonly used vasodilators such as calcium channel blockers are known to attenuate the HPV response. Conversely, routinely used vasoconstrictors such as phenylephrine may preferentially constrict pulmonary vessels in normoxic lung regions.
- Pa_{CO_2} *and alkalosis.* Hypocapnia or metabolic alkalosis may attenuate HPV, whereas hypercapnia and acidosis have the opposite effect. Thus any abnormality of Pa_{CO_2} or acid–base balance may adversely affect relative blood flow between the two lungs during OLV.
- *Epidural analgesia.* This is widely used during thoracic surgery and may affect the HPV response by changes in the systemic circulation affecting mixed venous oxygen saturation. Thoracic epidural anaesthesia has also been shown to have little effect on oxygenation during OLV unless high doses of local anaesthetic are used; this latter situation possibly occurs because of inhibition of sympathetic nerves leading to pulmonary vasodilation.[27]
- *Temperature.* This affects HPV, with animal studies showing an attenuated response during hypothermia and vice versa.

Clinical studies of OLV using various anaesthetic agents have failed to show any consistent differences between anaesthetic techniques. Inhalational anaesthetic agents used at clinically appropriate doses of around 1 minimum alveolar concentration produce similar degrees of impaired oxygenation as intravenous anaesthetic techniques,[23] particularly if depth of anaesthesia with the two techniques is equivalent.[28] Use of inhalational anaesthesia during OLV for lung resection is associated with improved long-term clinical outcomes, but the reasons underlying this observation are unclear.[29]

Pharmacological enhancement of HPV can be used to improve oxygenation during OLV. Inhaled nitric oxide (page 84) may be used to improve blood flow to the ventilated lung, although the expected improvement in oxygenation only seems to occur in patients who are already hypoxic or who have existing pulmonary hypertension. Almitrine is a systemically administered peripheral chemoreceptor agonist that can enhance HPV and thus improve oxygenation during OLV.[30] Its effects are dose dependent, and if the dose is too high then generalized pulmonary vasoconstriction occurs, rather than only in hypoxic regions, and pulmonary hypertension and a greater shunt fraction occur. These two potential therapeutic techniques are therefore not yet in routine clinical use.

Management of One-Lung Ventilation

The aim of ventilation during OLV is to maintain arterial P_{O_2} and P_{CO_2} as near normal as possible, and this is achieved by maintaining adequate alveolar ventilation while minimizing the amount of shunt through the nonventilated lung. Understanding of the physiology already described allows a logical approach to management.

Ventilation

If alveolar minute volume during OLV is maintained at similar values as when ventilating two lungs, then carbon dioxide elimination is also maintained, although achieving adequate alveolar ventilation, particularly in diseased lungs, may be a significant challenge. The traditional technique is to use smaller tidal volumes than two-lung ventilation at a faster respiratory rate, with the latter adjusted to achieve normal end-tidal or arterial P_{CO_2} values. Reducing tidal volume increases the anatomical dead space (page 98), so significant increases in respiratory rate may be needed to maintain alveolar ventilation. If respiratory rate is too fast, intrinsic positive end-expiratory pressure (PEEP; page 386) may occur and cause overexpansion of the dependent lung, increasing airway pressures and reducing blood flow through the dependent lung, leading to a worsening of shunt and oxygenation. This is a particular risk in patients with increased airway resistance of any cause. The optimum size of tidal volume to use for OLV remains uncertain.[31] Use of a standard two-lung ventilation value of 10 to 15 mL.kg^{-1} will commonly lead to unacceptably high airway pressures, may overdistend alveoli (potentially damaging the lung), cause increased pulmonary vascular resistance (so increasing shunt) and contribute to postoperative lung injury.[32] If small tidal volumes are used, such as 5 to 8 mL.kg^{-1}, then alveolar ventilation will be difficult to maintain and atelectasis more likely to occur. Finally, the addition of PEEP to the ventilated lung during OLV seems like a logical response to its reduced lung volume and propensity to develop atelectasis, but PEEP will also increase the pulmonary vascular resistance of the dependent lung and potentially worsen the shunt. Numerous studies have reported conflicting results concerning the benefit of dependent-lung PEEP on oxygenation during OLV, with the most recent suggesting that a level of 10 cmH$_2$O is optimal.[33,34]

Tidal volume, respiratory rate and PEEP each have opposing and undesirable effects at extreme values, risking either inadequate alveolar ventilation with hypoxia or hypercapnia at one extreme, or lung damage that may result in acute lung injury of the ventilated lung at the other. Suggested optimal ventilator settings for OLV have followed the debate regarding ventilation in patients with acute lung injury (page 371) and during general anaesthesia (page 263), who share the challenge of having only a small functional lung. The suggested 'protective ventilation' strategy requires pressure-controlled ventilation, low tidal volume (6 mL.kg^{-1} predicted body weight) and moderate levels of PEEP (5–10 cmH$_2$O). This strategy has been shown to improve oxygenation during OLV, reduce the systemic inflammatory response associated with OLV[35] and reduce major postoperative complications in some, but not all, studies.[36,37]

Use of a high inspired oxygen fraction (F_{IO_2}) during OLV is routine to maximize oxygenation of blood in areas of lung with low, but greater than zero, $\dot{V}/\dot{Q}$ ratios. Use of 100% oxygen may risk encouraging atelectasis formation in a lung with an already reduced lung volume (page 251). Conversely, as previously described, achievement of a high mixed venous P_{O_2} may reduce pulmonary vascular resistance in the ventilated lung, thus reducing shunt fraction.

As for two-lung ventilation (page 251) a recruitment manoeuvre can be performed before or during OLV to reexpand atelectasis in the dependent lung, a strategy that has been shown to decrease dead space and improve oxygenation.[38] The recruitment manoeuvre described for OLV involves volume-controlled ventilation with a respiratory rate of 12 breaths per minute and an inspiratory time of 50%. Every five breaths the tidal volume and PEEP are then increased to achieve peak inspiratory pressures and PEEP values (respectively) of 30/10, 35/15 and 40/20; these last settings are maintained for 10 breaths before reducing the settings in the same stepwise manner.

Management of the Nonventilated Lung

In some patients no action needs to be taken with the nonventilated lung, which can be allowed to collapse, following which the gas exchange will remain acceptable. Sadly this is often not the case. Given that the most likely cause of hypoxia during OLV is shunt through the nonventilated lung, the first approach should be to minimize this blood flow. Ventilation with 100% oxygen before isolating the lung causes it to collapse more quickly, and although in theory this will delay the onset of HPV there were no adverse effects on oxygenation 10 minutes after lung isolation in a clinical study.[39] As described earlier, manipulating the lung or, if appropriate, clamping the pulmonary vessels, are direct ways of reducing nonventilated lung perfusion. Facilitating effective HPV by avoiding the various factors already described that attenuate the response should be routine practice. The second approach is to accept that shunt through the nonventilated lung is inevitable, and to oxygenate this blood by apnoeic oxygenation. Insufflation of a few litres per minute of oxygen at zero end-expiratory pressure (ZEEP) may be effective, but care must be taken to ensure there is a route for gas to flow back out of the non-ventilated lung to avoid lung expansion or even baro-trauma.

Using ZEEP, the lung will continue to collapse, and the oxygen therefore will not gain access to those areas of lung where the shunt is occurring. A more effective technique is to apply continuous positive airway pressure (CPAP) to the nonventilated lung, which delivers 100% oxygen, limits the maximum pressure that can be attained in the lung and reduces the amount of lung collapse that occurs. Applying 5 to 10 cmH$_2$O of CPAP has been shown to not inflate the lung to such an extent that it interferes with surgery and to be very effective at improving oxygenation. The timing of the application of CPAP may be important, as it will be less effective if lung collapse has already occurred, in which case, provided the surgery permits, the lung may be briefly rein-flated and CPAP applied during the deflation phase.

Summary of the Clinical Management of One-Lung Ventilation

Before commencing OLV, initial ventilator settings should be:
- F_{IO_2} of 0.6 to 1.0;
- Respiratory rate 15;
- Pressure-controlled ventilation, with inflation pressure adjusted to achieve tidal volume of 6 mL.kg^{-1} predicted body weight; and
- PEEP of 5 to 10 cmH$_2$O.
  If hypoxia occurs:
- Establish that the DLT position is still correct and that ventilation of the nonventilated lung is still occurring with the required gas mixture; and
- Administer 100% oxygen and 5 to 10 cmH$_2$O of CPAP to the nonventilated lung, after a single inflation of the lung if surgery permits.
  If hypoxia continues:
- Perform a recruitment manoeuvre of the dependent lung as described earlier;
- Ensure cardiac output is not reduced; and
- Consider whether the blood flow to the nonventilated lung can be clamped, or the surgery performed with in-termittent two-lung ventilation.

Lung Injury Following One-Lung Ventilation[40]

Acute lung injury (Chapter 31) is a serious complication that occurs in the postoperative period in between 2.5% and 9% of pneumonectomies, and more rarely follows smaller lung resections such as lobectomy.[41] Mortality is high, with a quarter of patients dying. The pathophysiology of postpneumonectomy acute lung injury is controversial, with perioperative fluid overload viewed by many clinicians as the main cause, although the pathophysiology is now better elucidated and far more complex than simply administer-ing excessive volumes of intravenous fluid. High-protein pulmonary oedema develops approximately 24 hours post-operatively, and is believed to result from endothelial cell injury in the pulmonary capillaries. How this initial injury

occurs is less clear, although its origins almost certainly involve intraoperative OLV. Factors leading to potential damage of the ventilated lung during OLV include:
1. Overdistension of the lung during surgery with inap-propriately large tidal volumes[32] or use of PEEP leading to disruption of the alveolar–capillary barrier.[41]
2. Reduced FRC and atelectasis during anaesthesia.
3. Oxidative damage from the requirement for a high in-spired PO_2 during OLV.
4. Hyperperfusion resulting from the lateral positioning and reduction of blood flow through the operative lung. Increased capillary blood flow in the remaining lung is likely to cause stretching of endothelial cells or excessive shear forces in the vessels, both of which may disrupt the intercellular junctions leading to capillary stress failure.
5. Release of inflammatory cytokines in response to surgi-cal trauma, leading to increased capillary permeability for several days.

Once this initial lung injury has occurred, many other factors will then affect the severity of the clinical picture and its management, including fluid administration, inspired oxygen levels and the ventilation strategy, all of which should follow the same principles as for the management of acute lung injury whatever the cause (Chapter 31).

Lung Transplantation

Transplantation of a human lung was first performed in 1963, but in the years following this few patients survived for longer than a month. In the early 1980s improved immuno-suppression led to a resurgence of interest, and the technique has now become an established form of treatment. The func-tion of a transplanted lung is important for the well-being of the recipient, but also furthers our understanding of certain fundamental issues of pulmonary physiology.

Clinical Aspects[42,43]

Indications

Patients who are considered for transplant have severe re-spiratory disease and are receiving optimal therapy, but still have a life expectancy of less than 2 to 3 years. Uncon-trolled respiratory infection, significant disease of other organs, continued smoking or an age in excess of 55 to 65 years are normally contraindications. Precise selection cri-teria for recipients vary between transplant centres and with the respiratory disease, but in general patients referred for transplant have a FEV$_1$ of less than 30% predicted, rest-ing hypoxia, hypercapnia and, commonly, pulmonary hy-pertension. The main indications for lung transplant are shown in Table 33.2, where it can be seen that interstitial lung disease and COPD account for the vast majority of transplants performed.[44]

The number of patients awaiting transplant exceeds the number of donors. In recent years the number of donor or-gans available has remained static, whereas the number of candidates for lung transplants has risen rapidly. As a result,

TABLE 33.2 **Major Indications for Lung Transplantation and the Usual Type of Operation Performed**

Indication	Total Number	Operation Performed for Each Indication	
		Bilateral (%)	Single (%)
Interstitial lung disease	18 440	55.7	44.3
Chronic obstructive pulmonary disease	18 030	58.3	41.7
Cystic fibrosis	9096	97.5	2.5
α_1-Antitrypsin deficiency	2862	71.8	28.2
Pulmonary arterial hypertension	2605	91.2	8.8
Sarcoidosis	1454	77.4	22.6

Bilateral lung transplant includes double-lung and bilateral single-lung procedures.
(Data are from the Registry of the International Society for Heart and Lung Transplantation,[44] and include transplants performed worldwide between 1995 and June 2017 for the indications shown.)

the median waiting time for an organ to become available has increased, and many patients die while waiting. Cadaveric donor lungs are taken from patients with limited smoking history and no evidence of lung disease. Using current selection criteria only 15% to 20% of organ donors are suitable for lung donation, with some suggestion that this figure is falling as donor comorbidity increases. Strategies to improve the number of lung transplants performed include living-related lobar transplants (see the next section), extending donor selection criteria using more objective tests of lung function, donation after circulatory death or ex vivo lung ventilation and perfusion. This last approach potentially offers unique advantages for lung donation, as oxygenation of the donor lung after cessation of circulation by ex vivo ventilation and perfusion can conserve lung function for up to 5 hours.[45] A portable system is now available that ventilates the donor lung at normothermia with a nitrogen, oxygen and carbon dioxide mixture and also perfuses it with a high oncotic solution and red blood cells. Use of this technique is reported to lead to a lower incidence of severe early graft dysfunction, but studies of longer-term outcomes are awaited.[46]

Types of Transplant

Donor and recipient chest sizes are matched. With current organ preservation solutions, lung transplants must be performed within 8 hours of organ removal.

Single-lung transplant is the simplest procedure. The recipient's pneumonectomy is undertaken via a thoracotomy using OLV (page 403), which presents a significant challenge in these patients. The donor lung is implanted, with anastomoses of the main bronchus, the left or right pulmonary artery and a ring of left atrium containing both pulmonary veins of one side. Cardiopulmonary bypass is required in some cases, particularly those patients with preoperative pulmonary hypertension who are at risk of right-sided heart failure during OLV.

Bilateral lung transplant comes in two forms. Double-lung transplant performed at a single operation is a more complex procedure for which sternotomy and cardiopulmonary bypass are required. The donor lungs are implanted with

anastomoses of either the trachea or both bronchi, the main pulmonary artery and the posterior part of the left atrium containing all four pulmonary veins. A simpler alternative is to transplant two lungs sequentially (termed a *double single-lung transplant*) through bilateral thoracotomies, and this has now almost completely replaced double-lung transplant.

Heart–lung transplant was originally used for patients with primary pulmonary hypertension and Eisenmenger's syndrome and continues to be the operation of choice for congenital heart disease. Total cardiopulmonary bypass is, of course, essential, and the anastomoses involve the right atrium, the aorta and the trachea. The complexity and complication rates of heart–lung transplantation are high, and, wherever possible, alternative procedures are now used.

Choice of operation depends on the indication for the transplant (Table 33.2). Single-lung transplantation is favoured, partly because mortality may be lower following this operation, but also because each suitable donor can be used to transplant two recipients. Congenital heart disease commonly requires heart–lung transplant, whereas diseases associated with pulmonary hypertension ideally need either heart–lung transplant or bilateral lung transplant to normalize pulmonary arterial pressure. Lung disease alone is satisfactorily treated with single-lung transplant.

Living-related lung transplants are performed at several centres in the world. Left or right lower lobes of the donor relative are transplanted into the whole hemithorax of the recipient, so the technique is only suitable for children or small adults. The same selection criteria apply as for cadaveric transplantation, thus patients with cystic fibrosis must have bilateral transplants and therefore two related donors. Survival figures are at least comparable with other forms of lung transplantation, and possibly better in paediatric lung transplants when living-related, rather than cadaveric, organs are used.

Outcome Following Transplant

Given the nature of the surgery, it is not surprising that there is significant perioperative and early postoperative mortality. Thereafter, mortality rates are low when consideration is given to the 2-year predicted survival of recipients before transplant, with a median survival of 6.5 years in the most recent report of clinical outcomes.[44]

After lung transplantation, FEV_1 is initially poor attributed to the effects of the surgery, but then shows a gradual improvement, reaching a peak 3 to 6 months after surgery. From pretransplant values of 20% to 30% of predicted normal, recipients of a single-lung transplant achieve values of 50% to 60% and patients receiving bilateral-lung transplant typically have normal values. These improvements in ventilatory performance contribute to the huge improvement in quality of life following lung transplant.

Exercise performance depends on many factors, which, in addition to pulmonary function, include circulation, condition of the voluntary muscles, motivation and freedom from pain on exertion. Improvement in performance does occur following lung transplantation, but exercise limitation remains common, with maximal oxygen uptake (page 184) of about one-half of normal. There is no evidence that this limitation results from poor pulmonary function, and a muscular origin is more likely,[47] possibly related to myopathy induced by immunosuppressant drugs.

Rejection

Acute rejection occurs following activation of cytotoxic T-lymphocytes by helper T-cells which 'recognize' the foreign tissue. This form of rejection occurs in about 15% of patients, and presents as acute lung injury (Chapter 31) within 72 hours of the transplant. Treatment involves escalation of immunosuppressive therapy and supportive management, as for other forms of lung injury. Recovery of the transplanted lung may occur, but mortality from acute rejection is high.

Chronic rejection in the lung manifests itself as bronchiolitis obliterans syndrome, the origin of which is not clear, but which occurs in up to half of patients by 5 years posttransplant.[48] Detection of chronic rejection is problematic, because in the early stages of acute rejection it is difficult to distinguish rejection from infection. Both conditions feature arterial hypoxaemia, pyrexia, leucocytosis, dyspnoea and reduced exercise capacity. These changes are followed by a decrease in diffusing capacity and FEV_1, and later by perihilar infiltration or graft opacification on the chest radiograph. Bronchiolitis obliterans, as the name suggests, causes significant air-flow limitation; the FEV_1 is used as a screening test and also to stage the degree of rejection.

Physiological Effects of Lung Transplant

Transplantation inevitably disrupts the nerve supply, lymphatics and the bronchial circulation. The condition of the recipient is further compromised by immunosuppressive therapy.

Denervated Lung

The transplanted lung has no afferent or efferent innervation, and there is no evidence that reinnervation occurs in humans. However, in dogs vagal stimulation has been observed to cause bronchoconstriction 3 to 6 months after lung reimplantation, and sympathetic reinnervation has been demonstrated after 45 months.[49]

In Chapter 4, attention was paid to the weakness of the Hering–Breuer reflex in humans. It was therefore expected that denervation of the lung, with block of pulmonary baroreceptor input to the medulla, would have minimal effect on the respiratory rhythm. This is in contrast to the dog and most other laboratory animals, in which vagal block is known to cause slow deep breathing. Bilateral vagal block in human volunteers was already known to leave the respiratory rhythm virtually unchanged, and it was therefore no great surprise when it was shown that bilateral lung transplant had no significant effect on the respiratory rate and rhythm in patients when awake or asleep.

The cough reflex, in response to afferents arising from below the level of the tracheal or bronchial anastomosis, is permanently lost after lung transplantation.[50] Following single-lung transplant, the remaining diseased lung will continue to stimulate coughing, which will facilitate clearance of secretions from the transplanted lung. Similarly, a bilateral single-lung transplant will be preferable to a double-lung transplant, because the potent carinal cough reflex remains intact. The abnormality in cough reflex is a major contributor to lung infection following transplant, along with altered mucous clearance, as described later.

Ventilation/Perfusion Relationships

Bilateral lung or heart–lung transplants usually result in normal $\dot{V}/\dot{Q}$ relationships, but after a single-lung transplant the situation is more complex. For most indications, including COPD, the single transplanted lung receives the majority of pulmonary ventilation (60%–80% of the total) and a similar proportion of pulmonary blood flow, thus $\dot{V}/\dot{Q}$ relationships are acceptable, although not normal. However, following single-lung transplant for primary pulmonary hypertension, ventilation to the two lungs remains approximately equal, whereas the majority of blood flow (often >80%) is to the transplanted lung. This $\dot{V}/\dot{Q}$ mismatch fortunately has little effect on arterial oxygenation at rest.

HPV seems to be an entirely local mechanism, and, as might be expected, has been shown to persist in the human transplanted lung,[51] although some studies have demonstrated abnormalities, particularly in patients with pulmonary hypertension.

Mucociliary Clearance

Mucociliary clearance is abnormal after lung transplantation.[52] The cause seems to be defective production of mucus, rather than changes in the function of the cilia. This, together with the absent cough reflex below the line of the airway anastomosis, means that the patient is at a disadvantage in clearing secretions. Side effects of immunosuppression compound these changes and lead to enhanced susceptibility to infection of the transplanted lung. Although these factors clearly do not preclude long-term survival of the graft, one-quarter of deaths following lung transplantation result from infection.

References

1. Du Rand IA, Blaikley J, Booton R, et al. British Thoracic Society guideline for diagnostic flexible bronchoscopy in adults. *Thorax.* 2013;68:i1-i44.

2. Putinati S, Ballerin L, Corbetta L, et al. Patient satisfaction with conscious sedation for bronchoscopy. *Chest.* 1999;115:1437-1440.

3. Kinsey M, Arenberg DA. Endobronchial ultrasound–guided transbronchial needle aspiration for non–small cell lung cancer staging. *Am J Respir Crit Care Med.* 2014;189:640-649.

4. Froudarakis ME. Medical thoracoscopy. The green shapes of grey. *Chest.* 2015;147:869-871.

5. Battoo A, Jahan A, Yang Z, et al. Thoracoscopic pneumonectomy. An 11-year experience. *Chest.* 2014;146:1300-1309.

6. Akçali Y, Demir H, Tezcan B. The effect of standard posterolateral versus muscle-sparing thoracotomy on multiple parameters. *Ann Thorac Surg.* 2003;76:1050-1054.

7. Nomori H, Horio H, Fuyuno G, et al. Respiratory muscle strength after lung resection with special reference to age and procedures of thoracotomy. *Eur J Cardiothorac Surg.* 1996;10:352-358.

8. Aldrich JM, Gropper MA. Can we predict pulmonary complications after thoracic surgery? *Anesth Analg.* 2010;110:1261-1263.

9. van Tilburg PMB, Stam H, Hoogsteden HC, et al. Pre-operative pulmonary evaluation of lung cancer patients: a review of the literature. *Eur Respir J.* 2009;33:1206-1215.

10. Brunelli A, Al Refai M, Monteverde M, et al. Stair climbing test predicts cardiopulmonary complications after lung resection. *Chest.* 2002;121:1106-1110.

*11. **Weibel ER. How to make an alveolus. *Eur Respir J.* 2008;31: 483-485.**

12. Fehrenbach H, Voswinckel R, Michl V, et al. Neoalveolarisation contributes to compensatory lung growth following pneumonectomy in mice. *Eur Respir J.* 2008;31:515-522.

13. Criner GJ, Cordova F, Sternberg AL, et al. The National Emphysema Treatment Trial (NETT). Part II: lessons learned about lung volume reduction surgery. *Am J Respir Crit Care Med.* 2011;184:881-893.

14. Kaplan RM, Sun Q, Ries AL. Quality of well-being outcomes in the National Emphysema Treatment Trial. *Chest.* 2015; 147:377-387.

15. Clarenbach CF, Sievi NA, Brock M, et al. Lung volume reduction surgery and improvement of endothelial function and blood pressure in patients with chronic obstructive pulmonary disease: a randomized controlled trial. *Am J Respir Crit Care Med.* 2015;192:307-314.

16. Mather NL, Padmakumar AD, Milton R, et al. Emphysema, lung volume reduction and anaesthesia. *Trend Anaesth Crit Care.* 2012;2:166-173.

17. Kemp SV, Slebos DJ, Kirk A, et al. A multicenter randomized controlled trial of Zephyr endobronchial valve treatment in heterogeneous emphysema (TRANSFORM). *Am J Respir Crit Care Med.* 2017;196:1535-1543.

18. Come CE, Kramer MR, Dransfield MT, et al. A randomised trial of lung sealant versus medical therapy for advanced emphysema. *Eur Respir J.* 2015;46:651-662.

19. Fessler HE, Scharf SM, Ingenito EP, et al. Physiologic basis for improved pulmonary function after lung volume reduction. *Proc Am Thorac Soc.* 2008;5:416-420.

20. Tschopp JM, Brutsche M, Frey JG. Treatment of complicated spontaneous pneumothorax by simple talc pleurodesis under thoracoscopy and local anaesthesia. *Thorax.* 1997;52: 329-332.

21. West JB. Snorkel breathing in the elephant explains the unique anatomy of its pleura. *Respir Physiol.* 2001;126:1-8.

22. Yoshimura T, Ueda K, Kakinuma A, et al. Bronchial blocker lung collapse technique: nitrous oxide for facilitating lung collapse during one-lung ventilation with a bronchial blocker. *Anesth Analg.* 2014;118:666-670.

23. Ng A, Swanevelder J. Hypoxaemia associated with one-lung anaesthesia: new discoveries in ventilation and perfusion. *Br J Anaesth.* 2011;106:761-763.

24. Karzai W, Schwarzkopf K. Hypoxemia during one-lung ventilation. Prediction, prevention, and treatment. *Anesthesiol.* 2009; 110:1402-1411.

25. Lumb AB, Slinger PS. Hypoxic pulmonary vasoconstriction: physiology and anesthetic implications. *Anesthesiol.* 2015; 122:932-946.

26. Benumof JL. Mechanism of decreased blood flow to atelectactic lung. *J Appl Physiol.* 1979;46:1047-1048.

27. Xu Y, Tan Z, Wang S, et al. Effect of thoracic epidural anesthesia with different concentrations of ropivacaine on arterial oxygenation during one-lung ventilation. *Anesthesiol.* 2010;112:1146-1154.

28. Pruszkowski O, Dalibon N, Moutafis M, et al. Effects of propofol vs sevoflurane on arterial oxygenation during one-lung ventilation. *Br J Anaesth.* 2007;98:539-544.

29. de la Gala F, Piñeiro P, Reyes A, et al. Postoperative pulmonary complications, pulmonary and systemic inflammatory responses after lung resection surgery with prolonged one-lung ventilation. Randomized controlled trial comparing intravenous and inhalational anaesthesia. *Br J Anaesth.* 2017;119:655-663.

30. Dalibon N, Moutafis M, Liu N, et al. Treatment of hypoxemia during one-lung ventilation using intravenous almitrine. *Anesth Analg.* 2004;98:590-594.

31. Rozé H, Lafargue M, Perez P, et al. Reducing tidal volume and increasing positive end-expiratory pressure with constant plateau pressure during one-lung ventilation: effect on oxygenation. *Br J Anaesth.* 2012;108:1022-1027.

32. Fernández-Pérez ER, Keegan MT, Brown DR, et al. Intraoperative tidal volume as a risk factor for respiratory failure after pneumonectomy. *Anesthesiology.* 2006;105:14-18.

33. Ferrando C, Mugarra A, Gutierrez A, et al. Setting individualized positive end-expiratory pressure level with a positive end-expiratory pressure decrement trial after a recruitment maneuver improves oxygenation and lung mechanics during one-lung ventilation. *Anesth Analg.* 2014;118:657-665.

34. Spadaro S, Grasso S, Karbing DS, et al. Physiologic evaluation of ventilation perfusion mismatch and respiratory mechanics at different positive end-expiratory pressure in patients undergoing protective one-lung ventilation. *Anesthesiology.* 2018;128:531-538.

35. Michelet P, XB, Roch A, et al. Protective ventilation influences systemic inflammation after esophagectomy. *Anesthesiology.* 2006;105:911-919.

36. Amar D, Zhang H, Pedoto A, et al. Protective lung ventilation and morbidity after pulmonary resection: a propensity score–matched analysis. *Anesth Analg.* 2017;125:190-199.

37. Marret E, Cinotti R, Berard L, et al. Protective ventilation during anaesthesia reduces major postoperative complications after lung cancer surgery A double-blind randomised controlled trial. *Eur J Anaesthesiol.* 2018;35:727-735.

38. Unzueta C, Tusman G, Suarez-Sipmann F, et al. Alveolar recruitment improves ventilation during thoracic surgery: a randomized controlled trial. *Br J Anaesth.* 2012;108:517-524.

39. Ko R, McRae K, Darling G, et al. The use of air in the inspired gas mixture during two-lung ventilation delays lung collapse during one-lung ventilation. *Anesth Analg.* 2009;108:1092-1096.

*40. **Lohser J, Slinger P. Lung injury after one-lung ventilation: a review of the pathophysiologic mechanisms affecting the ventilated and the collapsed lung. *Anesth Analg.* 2015;121:302-318.**

41. Slinger PD. Postpneumonectomy pulmonary edema. Good news and bad news. *Anesthesiol.* 2006;105:2-5.

*42. **Young KA, Dilling DF. The future of lung transplantation. *Chest.* 2019;155:465-473.**

43. Adegunsoye A, Strek ME, Garrity E, et al. Comprehensive care of the lung transplant patient. *Chest.* 2017;152:150-164.

44. Chambers DC, Cherikh WS, Goldfarb SB, et al. The international thoracic organ transplant registry of the international society for

heart and lung transplantation: thirty-fifth adult lung and heart-lung transplant report—2018; focus theme: multiorgan transplantation. *J Heart Lung Transplant.* 2018;37:1169-1183.

45. Warnecke G, Moradiellos J, Tudorache I, et al. Normothermic perfusion of donor lungs for preservation and assessment with the Organ Care System Lung before bilateral transplantation: a pilot study of 12 patients. *Lancet.* 2012;380:1851-1858.

46. Warnecke G, Van Raemdonck D, Smith MA, et al. Normothermic ex-vivo preservation with the portable Organ Care System Lung device for bilateral lung transplantation (INSPIRE): a randomised, open-label, non-inferiority, phase 3 study. *Lancet Respir Med.* 2018;6:357-367.

47. Reinsma GD, ten Hacken NHT, Grevink RG, et al. Limiting factors of exercise performance 1 year after lung transplantation. *J Heart Lung Transplant.* 2006;25:1310-1316.

48. Verleden SE, Sacreas A, Vos R, et al. Advances in understanding bronchiolitis obliterans after lung transplantation. *Chest.* 2016:150:219-225.

49. Lall A, Graf PD, Nadel JA, et al. Adrenergic reinnervation of the reimplanted dog lung. *J Appl Physiol.* 1973;35:439-442.

50. Higenbottam T, Jackson M, Woolman P, et al. The cough response to ultrasonically nebulized distilled water in heart-lung transplantation patients. *Am Rev Respir Dis.* 1989;140:58-61.

51. Robin ED, Theodore J, Burke CM, et al. Hypoxic pulmonary vasoconstriction persists in the human transplanted lung. *Clin Sci.* 1987;72:283-287.

52. Herve P, Silbert D, Cerrina J, et al. Impairment of bronchial mucociliary clearance in long- term survivors of heart/lung and double-lung transplantation. *Chest.* 1993;103:59-63.

34

The Atmosphere

JOHN F NUNN

KEY POINTS

- The mass of the Earth and its distance from the sun provide optimal conditions of gravity and temperature for the long-term existence of liquid surface water and the retention in its atmosphere of oxygen, nitrogen and carbon dioxide.
- Primitive life-forms generated energy by photosynthetic reactions, producing oxygen and so facilitating the development of an oxygen-containing atmosphere and aerobic organisms.

- Carbon dioxide was initially the main component of the Earth's atmosphere, but by 300 million years ago rock weathering and photosynthesis had reduced its concentration to the current low levels.
- There is now an acceptance that human activity is causing an increase in atmospheric carbon dioxide, unprecedented in the last 40 million years.

The atmosphere of Earth is radically different from that of any other planet in the solar system (Table 34.1), and may well be rare on planets of other stars in the universe as a whole. The character of our atmosphere is unique for two main reasons. First, temperature has permitted the existence of liquid surface water for at least 3800 million years (Ma), and this has resulted in weathering of silicate rocks, reducing the concentration of carbon dioxide far below the levels still present on the rocky planets Venus and Mars. Secondly, the existence of liquid surface water enabled living organisms to appear at a very early stage: life forms then evolved to undertake oxygenic photosynthesis. When oxygen sinks were saturated, oxygen appeared in the atmosphere, and some organisms began to use highly efficient oxidative metabolic pathways. An atmosphere containing oxygen is in inorganic chemical disequilibrium, and is an indication of the existence of life.

Evolution of the Atmosphere

Formation of the Earth and the Prebiotic Atmosphere

The Earth was formed by a relatively short-lived but intense gravitational accretion of rather large planetesimals orbiting the newly formed sun some 4560 Ma ago. The kinetic energy of the impacting bodies was sufficient to raise the temperature to a few thousand degrees Celsius. This would have melted the entire Earth, resulting in loss of the primary atmosphere.

Earth cooled rapidly by radiation when the initial bombardment abated, and the very high-temperature (Hadean)

phase is not thought to have lasted longer than a few hundred Ma. The crust solidified, but massive outgassing from volcanoes continued, resulting in an atmosphere mainly comprising carbon dioxide and steam (Table 34.2), as probably also occurred on Venus and Mars.[1,2] In the case of Earth, the water vapour condensed to surface water, and there is good evidence that oceans existed about 3800 Ma ago and perhaps even earlier.[4] Once Earth's crust was cool, and surface water was in existence, it was possible for comets and meteorites to leave a secondary veneer of their contents, including water and a wide range of organic compounds.[5]

Important physicochemical changes occurred in the early secondary atmosphere. Helium and hydrogen tended to be lost from the Earth's gravitational field. Ammonia dissociated to nitrogen and hydrogen, the former retained and the latter lost from the atmosphere. Some carbon dioxide might have been reduced by hydrogen to form traces of methane, but very large quantities slowly reacted with surface silicates to become trapped as carbonates, while forming silica (weathering). Traces of water vapour underwent photodissociation to hydrogen and oxygen. However, oxygen from this source was present in only minimal quantities, and the early atmosphere is no longer thought to have been as strongly reducing as was formerly believed.[6]

The initial very high partial pressure of carbon dioxide, and probably some methane, would have provided a powerful greenhouse effect to offset the early minimal weak solar radiation, which was some 30% less than today (Figure 34.1). However, the Sun commenced its main sequence of thermonuclear fusion of hydrogen to helium about 3000 Ma ago. Since then solar radiation has been increasing steadily as the Sun proceeds remorselessly towards becoming a red giant,

TABLE 34.1	Composition of the Atmosphere of Earth and the Nearer Planets			
Planet	**Atmosphere**			
Mercury	Extremely tenuous			
Venus	Carbon dioxide	96.5%	+ Traces: Argon, Helium, Neon, Krypton (all <20 ppmv)	
	Nitrogen	3.5%		
Earth	Nitrogen	78.08%	Water vapour—variable	
	Oxygen	20.95%	Neon	18.2 ppmv
	Argon	0.93%	Helium	5.2 ppmv
	Carbon dioxide	0.039%	Methane	1.8 ppmv
Mars	Carbon dioxide	95.3%	Oxygen	0.13 %
	Nitrogen	2.7%	Carbon monoxide	0.27 %
	Argon	1.6%	+ Traces: Neon, Krypton, Xenon	
Jupiter	Hydrogen	89%	Methane	1750 ppmv
	Helium	11%	+ Traces: Ammonia, Water vapour, etc.	
Saturn	Hydrogen	94%	Methane	4500 ppmv
	Helium	6%	+ Traces: Ethylene, Phosphine	

ppmv, Parts per million volume.
Earth's data for carbon dioxide have been updated (see text).
(Planetary data are from Taylor, reference 1 reproduced from Nunn, reference 2 by permission of the Geologists' Association.)

TABLE 34.2	Average Composition of Gas Evolved from Hawaiian Volcanoes
Constituent	**Percent**
Water vapour	70.75
Carbon dioxide	14.07
Sulphur dioxide	6.40
Nitrogen	5.45
Sulphur trioxide	1.92
Carbon monoxide	0.40
Hydrogen	0.33
Argon	0.18
Sulphur	0.10
Chlorine	0.05

(Data are from reference 5, reproduced from reference 2 by permission of the Geologists' Association.)

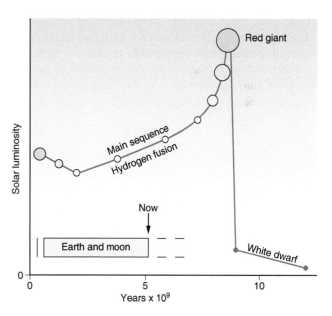

• **Fig. 34.1** Solar luminosity plotted against the age of the Sun, with the open circles giving a qualitative impression of the diameter of the Sun. Superimposed is an indication of the life of the Earth and Moon, which is now about halfway through the main sequence of the Sun deriving its energy from hydrogen fusion to helium. The times can only be very approximate. (From reference 7, with kind permission of Springer Link and Business Media.)

which will ultimately envelop the inner planets. It is fortunate that increasing solar radiation has been approximately offset by a diminishing greenhouse effect, caused mainly by decreasing levels of carbon dioxide (see later). As a result, Earth's temperature has remained relatively stable, permitting the existence of surface water for the last 3800 Ma.

Significance of the Mass of Earth and its Distance from Sun

Small bodies, such as Mercury and most planetary satellites, have a gravitational field which is too weak for the retention of any significant atmosphere (Fig. 34.2). The gas giants (Jupiter, Saturn, Uranus and Neptune) have gravitational fields which are sufficiently strong to retain all gases, including helium and hydrogen, thereby ensuring the retention of a reducing atmosphere. The gravitational field of the Earth is intermediate, resulting in a differential retention of the heavier gases (oxygen, carbon dioxide and nitrogen), while permitting the escape of hydrogen and helium. This is essential for the development of an oxidizing atmosphere and life as we know it. Water vapour (with a molecular weight of only 18) would be lost from the atmosphere were it not for the 'cold trap' at the tropopause, where the temperature falls sufficiently low to turn water vapour into ice.

Surface temperature of a planetary body is crucial for the existence of liquid water, which is essential for life and therefore the composition of our atmosphere. To a first approximation, temperature is dependent on the distance of a planet from the Sun and the intensity of solar radiation (Fig. 34.2). The major secondary factor is the greenhouse effect of any atmosphere which the planet may possess. Mercury and Venus have surface temperatures far above the boiling point of water. All planets (and their satellites) which are further away from the Sun than Earth have a surface temperature too cold for liquid water to exist today. However, there is now evidence that Mars had liquid surface water in the past,[8] now present only as ice.[9]

Earth is the only planet in the solar system which has both a mass permitting retention of an oxidizing atmosphere and a distance from the Sun at which the temperature permits liquid water to exist on its surface. It is difficult to see how there could be life as we know it anywhere in the solar system outside the small parallelogram shown in Figure 34.2. However, an environment similar to that of Earth may well exist on some planets of the 10^{22} other sun-like stars in the universe.

Origin of Life and the Development of Photosynthesis

Amino acids and a wide range of organic compounds are found in a type of meteorite known as carbonaceous chondrites.[3] Therefore, whether or not such compounds were actually synthesized on the early Earth, as Stanley Miller had proposed,[6] it is highly likely that a wide range of organic compounds were available on the pre-biotic Earth when liquid oceans were formed.

It is less easy to explain the next stage in the evolution of life. An essential feature of all life is the synthesis of proteins using a ribonucleic acid (RNA) template, usually transcribed from the genetic code carried on deoxyribonucleic acid (DNA). There would appear to have been a classical 'chicken and egg' situation. Useful proteins could not be formed without the appropriate sequences of RNA or DNA: RNA and DNA could not be polymerized without appropriate enzymes, which are normally proteins. Nevertheless, life did appear, perhaps in the first instance with the genetic code carried only on RNA, or even the much simpler peptide nucleic acid.[10]

An essential requirement for life is the availability of bio-usable forms of energy. The forms of available energy and their location at the dawn of life remain a mystery.

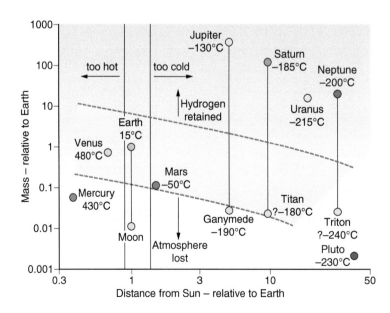

• **Fig. 34.2** The planets and some of their larger satellites, plotted according to distance from the Sun (abscissa), and mass (ordinate), both scales being logarithmic and relative to Earth. Mean surface temperatures are shown. Potential for life as we know it exists only within the parallelogram surrounding the Earth.

However, one cannot ignore the possibility of hydrothermal vents, such as the black smokers along the midocean ridges at great depths, which still support very simple life forms whose biochemistry is based on chemoautotrophy. They are totally independent of sunlight, and exploit the profound chemical disequilibrium between the emerging hot, reducing and acid water, containing hydrogen sulphide, methane, ammonia, phosphorus and a range of metals, and the surrounding sea water.[11] It is likely that there have been hydrothermal vents on Earth for as long as surface water has coexisted with volcanic activity. Chemoautotrophs might, therefore, have appeared as early as 3800 Ma ago.

Hydrothermal vents provide an extremely constrained and hazardous environment for life, dependent on the continued existence of the energy supply. A much more attractive alternative was to utilize the limitless availability of energy in the form of solar visible light. The most familiar of such reactions is the oxygenic photosynthesis of glucose, summarized as follows:

$$6CO_2 + 6H_2O + energy = C_6H_{12}O_6 + 6O_2$$

The biochemical adaptation from thermal detection in hydrothermal vents to photosynthesis does not seem to have been insuperable,[12] and it was thought that photosynthesizing cyanobacteria (blue-green algae) may have existed 2700 Ma ago.[13] However, it has recently been suggested that this crucial development may have occurred later, closer to 2400 Ma ago when oxygen first appeared in the atmosphere.[14] At a later date, cyanobacteria underwent symbiotic incorporation into the cells of certain eukaryotes to become chloroplasts, which then conferred the biochemical benefits of photosynthesis on their hosts, which include all plants.

The Appearance of Oxygen in the Atmosphere

Oxygenic photosynthesis releases oxygen, apparently as a waste product. Initially it accumulated in the surface waters of the oceans, where it oxidized soluble ferrous iron (Fe^{2+}), leached from basalt, which was then deposited as insoluble ferric iron oxide (Fe^{3+}) in the vast so-called banded iron formations. This process prevented concentrations of oxygen in the atmosphere reaching 10^{-5} bar until about 2320 Ma ago.[15] After the atmosphere attained a higher but critical level of oxygen about 1800 Ma ago, banded iron formations seldom appeared, and iron was thereafter deposited in red (ferric) beds.[2]

Oxygen continued to accumulate in the oceans and atmosphere, probably reaching a peak of 25% to 35% of an atmosphere 300 Ma ago[16] (Fig. 34.3). It then decreased to about 14%, contributing to the end-Permian mass extinction at the end of the Palaeozoic Era, about 250 Ma ago.[2] Thereafter it rose slightly above the present atmospheric level for about 100 Ma.

Biological Consequences of an Oxidizing Environment

It seems likely that the appearance of molecular oxygen in their environment would have been unwelcome to anaerobic organisms. Chapter 25 describes the toxicity of oxygen and its derived reactive oxygen species, against which primitive anaerobes would probably have had no defences. Three lines of response can be identified. Some anaerobes sought an anaerobic microenvironment in which to remain and survive. Others developed in-depth defences against oxygen and its derived reactive species (page 289). The best response was the development of aerobic metabolism, which gave enormous energetic advantages over organisms relying on anaerobic metabolism (page 153). This required the symbiotic incorporation of purple bacteria which became mitochondria, and the increased availability of biological energy was essential for the evolution of all forms of life more complex than microorganisms.

Photosynthesis and aerobic metabolism eventually established a cycle of energy exchange between plants and animals, with its ultimate energy input in the form of solar visible light, which was interrupted only under exceptional circumstances. Such circumstances included major meteor strikes and exceptional volcanic activity, both of which can throw vast quantities of persistent dust into the atmosphere and cause extinctions by blocking photosynthesis.

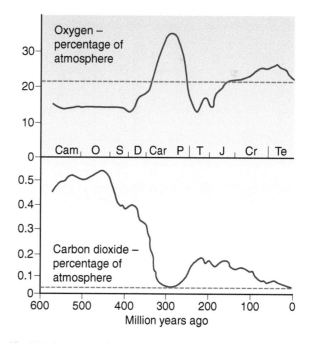

• **Fig. 34.3** Long-term changes in oxygen and carbon dioxide concentrations during the last 600 Ma. Broken horizontal lines show present atmospheric levels of oxygen and carbon dioxide. Geological periods shown by their capital letters are: Cambrian, Ordovician, Silurian, Devonian, Carboniferous and Permian (Palaeozoic Era), and Triassic, Jurassic, Cretaceous (Mesozoic Era) and Tertiary. Recent research suggests levels of carbon dioxide may be slightly less than shown, but the nature of the changes is not in doubt. (From Nunn, reference 2 reproduced by permission of the Geologists' Association).

Changes in Carbon Dioxide Levels

After the major outgassing phase of the newly formed Earth, the concentration of carbon dioxide in the atmosphere probably exceeded 90% of an atmosphere.[17] It declined rapidly, because of weathering (CO_2 + $CaSiO_3$ → SiO_2 + $CaCO_3$) and photosynthesis, falling to about 0.5% at the time that the overt fossil record begins, the Palaeozoic Era, 570 Ma ago (Fig. 34.3). A secondary major decline to near the present atmospheric level occurred during the Carboniferous Period, when the coal-forming forests involved photosynthesis and carbon burial on a massive scale. A sharp increase occurred at the end of the Permian Period (the last Period of the Palaeozoic Era) about 250 Ma ago, and carbon dioxide may have contributed to the end-Permian mass extinction. This coincided with the decrease in oxygen concentration mentioned above. Carbon dioxide concentrations rose to about 0.2% of an atmosphere just before 200 Ma ago, and then declined until about 20 Ma ago, when it entered a range of the order of 180 to 300 parts per million, volume (ppmv), which was not seriously exceeded until the last few decades.[18]

Carbon Dioxide and the Ice Ages

Carbon dioxide is a greenhouse gas, with a doubling of atmospheric concentration causing an increase in global average surface temperature '… likely to be in the range 2°C to 4.5°C … values substantially higher than 4.5°C cannot be excluded'.[19] DeConto cites the carbon dioxide threshold for Antarctic glaciation as 750 ppmv and for the northern hemisphere as 280 ppmv.[18] However, there is also a periodicity in solar insolation (Milankovitch cycles) which initiates glacial and interglacial cycles. For the last 500 ka, the dominant cycle has been the degree of ellipticity of the Earth's orbit, with a periodicity of about 100 ka, and its effect is very clear in the mean global temperature record for the last 420 ka derived from Antarctic ice cores (Fig. 34.4).[20]

Figure 34.4 also shows a remarkably close correlation between temperature and the atmospheric concentration of carbon dioxide. Detailed analysis of time relations shows that the start of end-glacial warming usually preceded the start of the increase in carbon dioxide by a few thousand years. The initial warming released carbon dioxide from stores, and then the increased carbon dioxide concentration provided powerful positive feedback to temperature. The resultant warming is far greater than can be accounted for simply by the change in insolation.

Casual inspection of Figure 34.4 suggests that the next glacial period is overdue. However, it appears that the rhythmic changes in global mean temperature shown for the last 420 ka will not continue, as we now enter a long phase when the Earth's orbit will remain almost circular. The 100 ka cycle will be in virtual abeyance for about 50 ka, during which there will be a prolonged interglacial.[22]

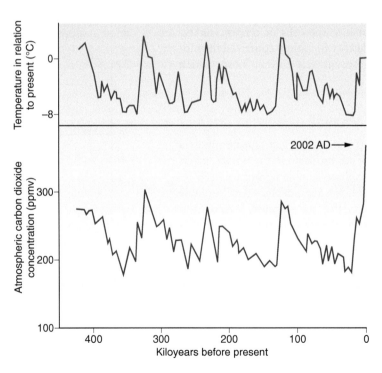

• **Fig. 34.4** General trends for temperature and atmospheric carbon dioxide concentration, obtained from ice cores from Vostok, Antarctica, for the last 420 000 years. (Data from Petit et al., reference 20, and reproduced in part from reference 21, with the permission of the Editor of the Optimum Population Trust Journal.)

However, it is highly unlikely that mean global temperature will remain constant, because of the current increase in the atmospheric carbon dioxide concentration, unprecedented in the last 20 Ma.

Recent Changes in Carbon Dioxide Levels

Atmospheric carbon dioxide remained close to 280 ppmv from the beginning of the current interglacial until the start of the industrial revolution (AD 1750). In the next 200 years it increased to 310 ppmv, which averaged 0.155 ppmv.yr^{-1} (Table 34.3). The annual rate of increase rose progressively and, from AD 2000 to 2009, reached 1.89 ppmv.yr^{-1}, which is nearly 200 times the rate during the rapid rewarming after the last glacial period (Fig. 34.4).

On this basis, extrapolation of trends from AD 1750 to the present suggests that the concentration might reach 1000 ppmv by the year AD 2100. This prediction is similar to computed predictions based on analysis of the many primary factors governing atmospheric carbon dioxide concentrations. Thus, we may expect to reach the highest concentration since 24 Ma ago, and above the threshold for Antarctic glaciations.[18] Whether the rate of change continues its present exponential course is critically dependent on the continued efficiency of the global carbon sinks and attempts to control emissions, with all the associated political uncertainty at present. The only certain limitation on emissions would seem to be exhaustion of the world's fossil fuels. Global warming may have disturbing short-term effects on ocean currents, particularly a weakening of the north Atlantic conveyor (including the Gulf Stream).[23] This could result in a substantial cooling of north-western Europe.

TABLE 34.3	Recent Changes in Atmospheric Carbon Dioxide Concentrations		
	Atmospheric Carbon Dioxide		Rate of Change
Date	Mass in Gt	ppmv	ppmv per Year
18 ka ago	426	200	
10 ka ago	597	280	0.01
1750 AD	597	280	0
1950 AD	661	310	0.15
2000 AD	789	370	1.20
2006 AD	810	380	1.74
2013 AD	842	395	2.54

Gt, Gigatonne; ka, thousand years; ppmv, parts per million volume. Data are from various sources. (Reproduced from Nunn[2] by permission of the Geologists' Association)

The Greenhouse Effect

The balance of heat gain from solar radiation is the difference between incoming radiation, mainly in the visible wavelengths, and outgoing radiation, which is largely infrared. The latter is partially trapped in the troposphere, mainly by water vapour (60%) and carbon dioxide (25%). Atmospheric water vapour concentration increases with rising global temperature, and therefore provides positive feedback to global warming. It is estimated that the present greenhouse effect raises the mean surface temperature of the Earth by some 30°C. Carbon dioxide makes a major contribution to the very high surface temperature of Venus (480°C), hotter than Mercury but further from the Sun.

Other Greenhouse Gases

There are no infrared absorption bands for water vapour and carbon dioxide between 7 and 13 μm wavelength, and heat loss in this band is considerable. It follows that any gas or vapour with strong infrared absorption in this range will have a disproportionate greenhouse effect. Such a gas could be considered not so much as thickening the panes in the greenhouse as replacing a missing pane.

After water and carbon dioxide, the most important greenhouse gases are ozone (8% of total effect) and methane (3% of total effect), which are present in the atmosphere at a concentration of only 2 ppmv but rapidly increasing: it absorbs infrared some 25 times as effectively as carbon dioxide. Dissolved methane is currently escaping from lakes in the melting tundra, but of greater concern is the vast quantity of buried methane held at high pressure and low temperature in cages of water molecules, known as hydrates or clathrates. Massive escape from hydrates is thought to have been a major factor in the Palaeocene/Eocene Thermal Maximum, 55 Ma before present, with temperature rises of 5°C to 6°C.[24] Fortunately the half-life of methane in the atmosphere is only about six years. The chlorofluorocarbons (2% of total effect) absorb infrared some 10 000 times as effectively as carbon dioxide, but present atmospheric concentrations are only of the order of 0.003 ppmv. However, with their long half-life, they cannot be ignored. Nitrous oxide, mainly of biological origin, also makes a small contribution.

With Earth in an approximately circular orbit for the next 50 ka and solar gain likely to remain reasonably constant,[22] greenhouse gases are now the major factors governing global temperature. Carbon dioxide is rising rapidly towards the highest levels in the last 24 Ma, and water vapour will increase with rising temperature. The mean global temperature is predicted to increase to within 90% confidence limits of 1.5°C to 4.5°C by AD 2100. Temperature has already increased by 0.6°C in the last century, mostly since 1950.[25] Not the least serious consequence will be melting of polar ice, which has the ultimate potential to raise sea level by 67 m. Sea level has been rising at about 1.8 mm.yr^{-1} since AD 1850, but, since 2004, there have been several reports of increased sea level rise up to 3.0 mm.yr^{-1}, and predictions for 2100 indicate a total sea level rise for this century of 0.35 to 0.5 m.[26]

Turnover Rates of Atmospheric Gases

Biological and geological turnover rates of carbon dioxide are quantitatively totally different.[2] Living organisms, the atmosphere and ocean surface waters contain about 2200 gigatonnes (Gt) of carbon. The annual exchange between photosynthesis and aerobic metabolism is approximately 100 Gt annually, as shown in Figure 34.5. The total release of carbon from burning of fossil fuels and release from cement containing carbonates from rocks has risen from 5 Gt.yr^{-1} in 1983 to 9.8 Gt.yr^{-1} in 2014.

In stark contrast, geological stores (ocean depths, organic biomass and limestone) have a carbon content in excess of 30 000 000 Gt, but with an annual turnover (volcanoes, weathering, etc.) of less than 0.1 Gt per year. Thus long-term changes are governed by the geological stores, whereas very rapid atmospheric changes can occur as a result of anthropogenic activity. Fossil fuels were buried over the course of 350 Ma, and probably all that is recoverable will be burned in 300 years.

Atmospheric stores of oxygen are almost 600 times greater than those for carbon dioxide. If oxygen decreases at the same rate as the current increase in carbon dioxide, it would take 40 000 years for sea level $P\text{O}_2$ to fall to the level found in Denver today.

Oxygen, Ozone and Ultraviolet Screening

In addition to its toxicity and potential for more efficient metabolism, oxygen had a profound effect on evolution by ultraviolet screening. Oxygen itself absorbs ultraviolet radiation to a certain extent, but ozone is far more effective. It is formed in the stratosphere from oxygen, which undergoes photodissociation, producing free oxygen atoms. The oxygen atoms then rapidly combine with oxygen molecules to form ozone thus:

$$O_2 \rightleftharpoons 2O$$
$$\downarrow$$
$$O + O_2 \rightleftharpoons O_3$$

The absolute quantity is very small, being the equivalent of a layer of pure ozone only a few millimetres thick. A Dobson unit of ozone is defined as the equivalent of a layer of pure ozone 0.01 mm thick. About 10% of the total atmospheric ozone is in the troposphere, mainly as a pollutant. This also acts as an ultraviolet screen and may become relatively more important in the years to come.

Life evolved in water, which provided adequate screening from ultraviolet radiation. The first colonization of dry land by plants and animals was in the late Silurian Period about 400 Ma years ago, and it has been suggested that this coincided with oxygen and ozone reaching concentrations at which the degree of ultraviolet shielding first permitted organisms to leave the shelter of an aqueous environment.

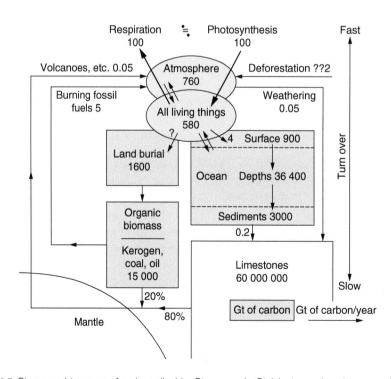

• **Fig. 34.5** Stores and turnover of carbon dioxide. Stores are in Gt (gigatonnes) and turnover in Gt per year. For recent increases in the burning of fossil fuels see text. (After reference 2, where sources are cited. Reproduced by permission of the Geologists' Association.)

Ozone is in a state of dynamic equilibrium in the stratosphere, and its concentration varies markedly from year to year, in addition to displaying a pronounced annual cycle. Ozone can be removed by the action of many free radicals, including chlorine and nitric oxide. Highly reactive chlorine radicals cannot normally pass through the troposphere to reach the stratosphere, but the situation was disturbed by the manufacture of chlorofluorocarbons (e.g., CF_2Cl_2) for use as propellants and refrigerants. These compounds are highly stable in the troposphere, with a half-life of the order of 100 years. This permits their diffusion through the troposphere to reach the stratosphere, where they undergo photodissociation to release chlorine radicals, which then react with ozone as follows:

$$Cl + O_3 \rightarrow ClO + O_2$$
$$\uparrow \qquad\qquad \downarrow$$
$$Cl + O_2 \leftarrow ClO + O$$

Chlorine is recycled, and it has been estimated that a single chlorine radical will destroy 10 000 molecules of ozone before it combines with hydrogen to form the relatively harmless hydrochloric acid. The Antarctic 'hole' in the ozone layer forms in October of each year, when spring sunlight initiates photochemical reactions. Minimal levels fell from 300 Dobson Units in 1960 to a lowest point (88) in 1995,[27] with levels recovering since, being greater than 110 since 2012, along with a gradually reducing hole area.

Evolution and Adaptation

This chapter has outlined the environmental conditions and biological factors under which the atmosphere has evolved to its present composition. In the past, nothing has been permanent, and we can expect a continuation of the interaction between organisms and their environment. What is new is that one species now has the power to cause major changes in the environment, and the atmosphere in particular. These changes are already impacting on the respiratory health of humans,[28] an effect which is expected to worsen very soon because of heatwaves causing exacerbations of airways disease, increased air pollution and even long-term damage from smoke inhalation from wildfires.[29,30]

References

1. Taylor SR. *Solar System Evolution*. Cambridge: Cambridge University Press; 1992.
*2. **Nunn JF. Evolution of the atmosphere. *Proc Geol Assoc*. 1998;109:**1-13.
3. MacDonald GA, Hubbard DH. *Volcanoes of the National Parks in Hawaii*. 6th ed. Honolulu: Hawaii Natural History Association; 1972.
4. Nisbet EG, Sleep NH. The habitat and nature of early life. *Nature*. 2001;409:1083-1091.
5. Oró J. Early chemical stages in the origin of life. In: Bengston S, ed. *Early Life on Earth. Nobel Symposium No. 84*. New York: Columbia University Press; 1994:48-59.
6. Miller SL. A production of amino acids under possible primitive earth conditions. *Science*. 1953;117:528-529.
7. Chapman CR, Morrison D. *Cosmic Catastrophes*. London: Plenum Press; 1989;97.
8. Malin MC, Edgett KS. Evidence of persistent flow and aqueous sedimentation on early Mars. *Science*. 2003;302:1931-1934.
9. Schorghofer N. Dynamics of ice ages on Mars. *Nature*. 2007; 449:192-194.
10. Böhler C, Nielsen PE, Orgel LE. Template switching between PNA and RNA oligonucleotides. *Nature*. 1995;376:578-581.
11. Nisbet EG. Archaean ecology. In: Coward MP, Reis AC, eds. *Early Precambrian Processes*. London: Geological Society; 1995:27-51.
12. Nisbet EG. Origins of photosynthesis. *Nature*. 1995;373: 479-480.
13. Kasting JF. The rise of atmospheric oxygen. *Science*. 2001;293: 819-820.
*14. **Rasmussen B, Fletcher IR, Brocks JJ, et al. Reassessing the first appearance of eukaryotes and cyanobacteria. *Nature*. 2008;455:**1101-1104.
15. Bekker A, Holland HD, Wang PL, et al. Dating the rise of atmospheric oxygen. *Nature*. 2004;427:117-120.
*16. **Berner RA, Van den Brooks JM, Ward PD. Oxygen and evolution. *Science*. 2007;316:**557-558.
17. Kaufman AJ, Xiao S. High CO_2 levels in the Proterozoic atmosphere estimated from analyses of individual microfossils. *Nature*. 2003;425:279-282.
18. DeConto RM, Pollard D, Wilson PA, et al. Thresholds for Cenozoic bipolar glaciation. *Nature*. 2008;455:652-656.
19. Christensen JH, Hewitson B, Busuioc A, et al. *Regional climate projections, Climate Change, 2007*: **The Physical Science Basis. Contribution of Working group I to the Fourth Assessment Report of the Intergovernmental Panel on Climate Change**. Cambridge: Cambridge University Press 2007.
20. Petit JR, Jouzel J, Raynaud D, et al. Climate and atmospheric history of the past 420,000 years from the Vostok ice core, Antarctica. *Nature*. 1999;399:429-436.
21. Nunn JF. Climate change and sea level in relation to overpopulation. *J Optim Popul Trust*. 2004;4:3-9.
22. Loutre MF, Berger A. Future climatic changes: are we entering an exceptionally long interglacial? *Clim Change*. 2000;46:61-90.
23. Broecker WS. Thermohaline circulation, the Achilles heel of our climate system: will man-made CO_2 upset the current balance? *Science*. 1997;278:1582-1588.
24. Story M, Duncan RA, Swisher CC. Paleocene-Eocene thermal maximum and opening of the northeast Atlantic. *Science*. 2007;316:587-589.
25. Karl TR, Trenberth KE. Modern global climate change. *Science*. 2003;302:1719-1723.
26. Nunn JF. Climate change and rising sea level. *Optim Popul Trust J*. 2006;6:14-19.
27. Jones AE, Shanklin JD. Continued decline of total ozone over Halley, Antarctica, since 1985. *Nature*. 1995;376:409-411.
28. Bayram H, Bauer AK, Abdalati W, et al. Environment, global climate change, and cardiopulmonary Health. *Am J Respir Crit Care Med*. 2017;195:718-724.
29. Bernstein AS, Rice MB. Lungs in a warming world. Climate change and respiratory health. Chest 2013;143:1455-1459.
*30. **Anonymous. Breathing on a hot planet. *Lancet Respir Med*. 2018;6:**647.

35

The History of Respiratory Physiology

KEY POINTS

- That breathing was essential for life was clear to the ancient Egyptian civilizations 5000 years ago, but the reasons for this were unknown.
- Early explanations for the function of breathing involved the air drawn into the lungs fuelling combustion in the heart and removing 'sooty and fuliginous spirits' from the body.
- In the Renaissance, advances in knowledge of anatomy led to the discovery of the pulmonary circulation and the

- observation that blood changed colour on passing through the lungs.
- Physiology in the 17th century involved more rigorous scientific experimentation and led to several discoveries about the mechanics and function of breathing.
- Developments in fundamental sciences, particularly chemistry and physics, facilitated the elucidation of current knowledge of breathing and respiration.

The historical path along which we have gained our current knowledge of respiratory physiology is long and varied. There are periods when our understanding leapt forward in just a few years, interspersed by prolonged periods when progress was negligible, and even some periods when progress was reversed. That breathing is essential for life was clear from the beginnings of history, but the mechanism of breathing and the reasons for it remained elusive for many centuries. Progress usually occurred in parallel with understanding in other scientific disciplines, particularly chemistry, physics and anatomy. Innovative ideas on the physiology of breathing led, in more than one instance, to the premature death of the physiologist, and the history of respiratory physiology includes some of the most famous controversies seen in medical science.

This chapter is of necessity only a brief overview of the subject, and ends around 100 years ago, when the explosion of scientific progress makes the subject too large for such a short account. Significant advances in respiratory physiology in the last 100 years are reported in the other chapters of this book, and the reader interested in the history of this period is referred to more authoritative accounts.[1,3] For more general information on the history of respiratory physiology, numerous recent sources (by historical standards) are available.[4,6]

Ancient Civilizations

Egyptian Physiology[7]

Ancient Egyptian civilizations existed from around 3100 to 332 BCE, when the Graeco-Roman period began. The most remarkable contribution made to history by ancient Egyptians is their writings, although knowledge of their language was mostly lost after CE 500. Approximately 1300 years later, 19th century scholars were able to use the Coptic language to assist in translating the ancient Egyptian writings. This has allowed an insight into medical knowledge from as early as 1820 BCE, the date of the earliest known medical writings in the Kahun papyrus.

Medical Papyri

Many Egyptian papyri are concerned with medical topics, mostly descriptions of pragmatic 'recipes' for the treatment of a multitude of specific conditions.[7]

The longest and best known of the medical papyri is the Ebers Papyrus,[8,9] which dates from about 1534 BCE, and is accepted as being a compilation of various earlier works. The Ebers Papyrus is unique in containing a section on physiology, including comments on respiration. The overall purpose of respiration is described thus:

As to the air that penetrates into the nose. It enters into the heart and the lung. They are those which give air to the entire body.[9]

Further sections include detailed descriptions of specific numbers of *metu* conducting 'moisture and air' to many parts of the body. These *metu* seem to mostly relate to blood vessels, but also probably included such structures as tendons, muscles and the ureters. At first, this primitive view of anatomy is surprising, considering the embalming abilities of ancient Egyptians, although in practice embalming was carried out using very small inconspicuous incisions that would have revealed very little internal anatomy. Two *metu* are described in each ear, through which '*the breath of life enters into the right ear and the breath of death enters into the left*',[9] illustrating the 'magical' aspect of medicine at the time.

Ancient Greece

Greek writers were primarily philosophers, but they were also outstanding physicians, with one of their number, Hippocrates, forming a school that is now widely attributed with the foundation of modern medical conduct. Early Greek philosophers such as Anaximenes (570 BCE–?) clearly stated that 'pneuma', or air, was essential to life,[6] but in contrast to this correct observation, Alcmaeon reportedly claimed that goats breathed through their ears, and that some air passed from the nose directly to the brain.[4] Empedocles (495–435 BCE) disputed many of Alcmaeon's writings, suggesting instead that breathing occurred through the skin, and that blood flow from the heart was tidal in nature, ebbing and flowing to and from the heart. Empedocles successfully combined physiology and philosophy in his description of the 'innate heat' in the heart, which was closely related to the soul, and which was distributed throughout the body by the heart. This concept of heat generation within the heart gained acceptance throughout the ancient Greek period and was to remain at the centre of respiratory physiological ideas for about 1000 years.

The writings of Plato, Aristotle and the Hippocratic school only rarely directed their attention to respiration, but their contribution to scientific method and thinking was enormous. Subsequent philosopher-physicians adopted a more scientific approach to investigating physiology. At this time, dissection became widely practised, sometimes in public, and on both animals and humans. Animal vivisection also took place, and there are even disputed reports of human vivisection of criminals.[4] Herophilus (circa 325 BCE) distinguished between arteries and veins, and, along with Aristotle, asserted that they contained air. Erasistratus (304–250 BCE), more widely renowned as the father of philosophy, was the first to apply scientific principles to explain breathing. His view was that air was taken into the lungs and passed to the heart along the pulmonary artery. In the heart, air was converted into a 'vital spirit' that was distributed to all parts of the body by the arteries, whilst the brain further converted the vital spirit into 'animal spirit' which travelled down the hollow nerves to activate muscles. Erasistratus seemed to understand that heart valves only allowed flow to occur in one direction but failed to apply this knowledge to elucidate the transport of vital spirit around the body. After Erasistratus, Greek interest moved away from medicine to philosophy and the physical sciences, and the progression of physiological knowledge halted for about 400 years.

Roman Medicine and Galen (129–199 BCE)

By the age of 28 years Claudius Galen was physician to the gladiators of Pergamun, and 12 years later became physician to the Roman emperor Marcus Aurelius. He wrote numerous works on anatomy and physiology, many of which still exist in modern form, including two with much material on respiration: *On the usefulness of the parts of the body* and *On the use of breathing*.[10,11] Galen's work provides the first direct evidence of experimentation and the application of clinical observations to explain physiology.

Galen's System of Physiology and Anatomy

In Galen's descriptions, food was processed in the gut before being used by the liver to produce blood, which passed to the right heart. Much of this blood flowed into the pulmonary artery to nourish the lung, whilst the remainder passed across invisible pores in the interventricular septum, to be combined with 'pneuma' brought from the lung via the pulmonary vein (Fig. 35.1). In the left heart, the pneuma instilled the blood with vital spirit that was circulated to the body and brain, as described by Erasistratus.

Anatomically Galen regarded the lungs as having three types of intertwining vessels, the pulmonary artery, pulmonary vein and the 'rough artery' (trachea). On respiratory mechanics, Galen regards the ribs as primarily providing protection for the intrathoracic organs, particularly the heart, but he also clearly describes the role of the intercostal muscles and diaphragm in effecting both inspiratory and expiratory movements. He understood the potential problems of diaphragmatic splinting, describing respiration as 'little and fast' in such conditions as pregnancy and 'water or phlegm in the liver'.

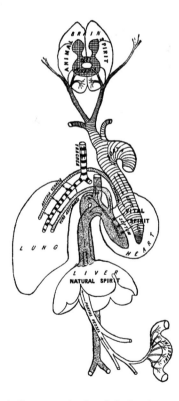

• **Fig. 35.1** Illustration reconstructing Galen's scheme of cardiovascular and respiratory physiology as described in the text. Galen did not use illustrations in his writings; this diagram is taken from reference 12.

Experiments on Respiration

Galen's experiments provided mixed results:

1. For the first time he proved that arteries contained no air, but only blood, by ligating an animal's artery in two places before opening the vessel under water. He wrote at length about blood flow, realizing that tidal blood flow to and from the lungs with each breath was '*in no way suitable for the blood*'.[10] He suggested the existence of capillaries 1500 years before they were discovered by stating:

   All over the body the arteries and veins communicate with one another by common openings and exchange blood and pneuma through certain invisible and extremely narrow passages.

2. Galen ligated both carotid arteries of a dog, an intervention that he observed caused the animal no detectable harm. He concluded that the brain could therefore derive pneuma directly from the nose, to make the animal spirit earlier described by the Greeks (termed 'psychic pneuma' by Galen).

3. During his time in the gladiator arena he observed that the level of neck injury sustained by gladiators affected their breathing,[6] so proving that respiration originated in the brain. He did many animal experiments to ascertain more precisely the spinal level at which the nerves responsible for respiration originated and went on to describe the nerve roots and destination of the phrenic nerves.[11]

4. On the necessity for breathing via the mouth and nose Galen was unclear, writing in earlier works that pneuma could enter arteries via the pharynx, heart or skin as well as the lungs. An experiment to attempt to demonstrate this was carried out:

   Covering the mouth and nostrils of a boy with a large ox-bladder, or any such vessel, so that he was unable to draw breath at all outside it, we saw him breathing unhindered through a whole day.

   Galen's conclusion from this study is contradictory: '*Hence it is clear that the arteries all through the animal draw in the outer air very little or not at all*'. Modern views of this experiment are that the ox-bladder was unlikely to be airtight, or that Galen's assistants must have removed the bladder to allow the boy to breathe easily when their master was not directly supervising the experiment.[11]

The Functions of Breathing

Apart from providing pneuma to the heart, Galen described other functions for breathing:

1. *Regulation of heat.* Galen's writings strengthened the analogy between the heart and a flame, and several pages of *On the use of breathing* are concerned with the similarities between the two. For example, the observation that flames were extinguished when deprived of air or that an oil lamp burns out when its sustenance, the oil, is used up, were seen as analogous to humans seen '*perishing when deprived of air*' or who lacked sufficient nourishment. Galen was concerned about the contradictory requirements for the idea of the heart and lungs generating innate heat, realizing that a fine balance must be drawn between '*fanning the source of the innate heat and from cooling in due proportion*', citing examples such as fever, with increased breathing, when the balance was disturbed.

2. *Voice.* Galen described in detail the anatomy of the laryngeal cartilages and muscles, and wrote a whole treatise on the voice, clearly recognizing the importance of the lungs. The rough artery (trachea) provided preliminary regulation of the voice, which was produced in the larynx and amplified off the roof of the mouth with the uvula acting as a plectrum. The purpose of having such a large volume of air in the lung was to allow continuous use of the voice.

3. *Removal of sooty and fuliginous spirits.* Waste products from the blood were discharged from the lung, and this was the function of expiration. Without doing so, the heart would have become stifled by its own '*smoky vapours*', once again like a burning flame. Explanations by Galen as to how the body separated the fuliginous spirits from the pneuma have become uncertain with the passage of time, one explanation being that the fuliginous spirits were regurgitated through the incompetent mitral valve and passed back along the pulmonary vein to the lung.[6]

4. *Physical protection of the heart.* The spongy nature of lung tissue, and the position of the heart in the centre of the chest, led Galen to suggest that the lung served to cushion the heart from the effects of body movements.

Galen's Legacy

Galen was the first physician to apply the Hippocratic method of scientific thinking to physiology, and he ingeniously combined the knowledge of his predecessors with his own thinking to produce an impressive treatise on the workings of the human body. Also, it is from the writings of Galen that we have obtained our knowledge of many of his predecessors: most of what is known of Erasistratus's views on physiology is derived from Galen's comments on it. Galen's work also deserves a place in history as the longest unchallenged scientific work. The physiology described in this section was taught in medical schools throughout the world, and scientifically mostly unchallenged, for around 1400 years.

There was also a darker and more controversial side to Galen. He is widely believed to have been conceited, dogmatic and abusive of those criticising him.[6] *On the usefulness of the parts of the body* contains several prolonged and personal refutations of the ideas of his predecessors, for example, accusing '*Asclepiades, wisest of men*' of making errors '*no child would fail to recognise, not to mention a man so full of his own importance*'.

After Galen

When Galen died, the study of physiology and anatomy effectively ceased. The Roman Empire was in decline, and in CE 389 Christian fanatics burned down the library in Alexandria, which contained many writings by the Greek philosopher-physicians.

Preservation of knowledge now fell to scholars of the Byzantine and Arabic empires. The latter embraced Galen's ideas with enthusiasm and translated many Greek works into Arabic, almost certainly adding their own refinements as they did so. The greatest of these Arabic scholars was Avicenna (circa 980–1037), whose canon was an impressive document pulling together and classifying all the available medical knowledge of the time, creating what has been described as a popular medical encyclopaedia of the medieval period. Some years later, Ibn Al Nafis[13] (1210–1288), a prolific Arabic writer on many subjects, studied Avicenna's writings and wrote his own treatise *Sharh Tashirh Al-Qanun* (Commentary on the Anatomy of the Canon of Avicenna). In this he challenged Galen's scheme of pores in the interventricular septum through which blood passed, and instead suggested that blood passed through the lung substance where it permeated with the air.[5,13] This was an early breakthrough in explaining the true nature of the pulmonary circulation, but Ibn Al Nafis' work did not become well known for many more centuries.

The Renaissance

In the 12th and 13th centuries, scholastic pursuits began again with the foundation of many European universities, firstly Oxford, Cambridge and Bologna, closely followed by Paris, Naples and Padua. Soon, many of the ancient documents were translated from Greek or Arabic into Latin, and human dissection began to be performed after many centuries of interdiction by the Pope. Knowledge of anatomy again began to advance, although interest in the function of the body only began again with Leonardo da Vinci in the 15th century.

Leonardo da Vinci (1452–1519)[4,14]

Leonardo da Vinci exemplified the Renaissance trend for combining art with science. His anatomical drawings are both extensive and ingenious, being mostly surrounded by extensive explanatory notes.[15,16] These notes are written in Latin and in mirror writing, possibly simply because da Vinci was left-handed and received no formal schooling to correct this, or possibly to make his notes harder to read by uneducated persons described by him as '*bad company*'.[4]

Although da Vinci is known to have dissected over 30 human cadavers, most of his drawings of the respiratory system are based on dissections of animals, including Figure 35.2, showing in beautiful detail the structure of the pig lung. In the commentary on this drawing, da Vinci

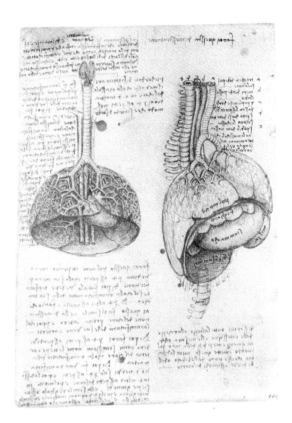

• **Fig. 35.2** da Vinci's drawing of the thoracic organs of a pig (*c.* 1508). The organs are labelled in mirror writing in Latin: *polmone*, lung; *feghato*, liver; *milza*, spleen; *stommacco*, stomach; *djaflamma*, diaphragm; *spina*, spine. See text for an explanation of labels a–e above the drawing on the right. (Royal Collection Trust © 2019, Her Majesty Queen Elizabeth II.)

considers the use of the '*substance*' of the lung and extends Galen's protective function of the lung parenchyma when he states that '*the substance is interposed between these ramifications* [of the trachea] *and the ribs of the chest to act as a soft covering*'. Structures entering the chest cavity are labelled a–e, and their functions described:

a. trachea, whence the voice passes
b. oesophagus, whence the food passes
c. apoplectic [carotid] arteries, whence the vital spirit passes
d. dorsal spine, whence the ribs arise
e. spondyles [spinous processes of the vertebrae], whence the muscles arise which end in the nape of the neck and elevate the face towards the sky.

da Vinci adhered to other Galenic ideas such as the presence of air in the pleural space but was unsure how the air entered or left this space, and in his later drawings he was clearly beginning to doubt that air was always present. da Vinci's adherence to Galen's ideas was in some areas unshakable, in particular his depiction of the nonexistent interventricular pores in several drawings of the cardiovascular system.

He did however challenge some Galenic ideas by applying his engineering expertise. For example, he did not accept that the heart generated innate heat, instead writing that heat generation in the heart resulted from mechanical friction between the blood and the walls of the heart.[4] Similarly, his engineering knowledge made him intrigued by the actions of the chest wall and respiratory muscles, including the complexities of defining the different function of internal and external intercostal muscles. For the diaphragm, da Vinci described four functions—dilating the lung for inspiration; pressing the stomach to drive food into the intestine; contracting with the abdominal muscles to drive out abdominal superfluities; and separating the spiritual (thoracic) organs from the natural (abdominal) ones. Finally, he considered in detail the movements of the trachea and bronchi on breathing, showing them to dilate and open wider at branches on inspiration as shown to the right of Figure 35.3.

da Vinci and the Bronchial Circulation

In Figure 35.3, da Vinci depicts in detail the relationship of the pulmonary circulation to a bronchus. Much of the commentary in the drawing is concerned with the superiority of drawings rather than words to describe such anatomical configurations. The figure clearly shows a dual blood supply to the lung, and suggests that the smaller of these two

supplies is to '*nourish and vivify the trachea*'. From this drawing, many writers have credited da Vinci with discovering the bronchial circulation, although this claim is disputed.[17,18] The drawing is believed to be based on an ox, a species recently shown to have distinct small pulmonary veins draining directly into the left atrium, which may be those found by da Vinci.

The possibility of artistic license in his drawings has caused disputes that will never be resolved, such as that of the bronchial circulation. For example, in Figure 35.2 the perfectly branching pattern of the bronchi on the lung surface is clearly not based on true observation of pig lungs. In Figure 35.3 of ox lungs, the right upper lobe bronchus that arises directly from the trachea in this species is absent. However, in spite of these misgivings regarding his drawings, da Vinci's genius in combining art, science and engineering in the study of physiology is undisputed.

Anatomy in the Renaissance

After da Vinci, the pursuit of medical knowledge in the universities continued, with anatomy in particular aided by the continuing resurgence of dissection and vivisection. Andreas Vesalius (1514–1564) is primarily remembered as the founder of modern anatomy, his dissections culminating in the publication in 1543 of *De Humanis Corporis Fabrica*, a book of seven volumes including over 250 anatomical illustrations (Fig. 35.4).[19] His ideas met with

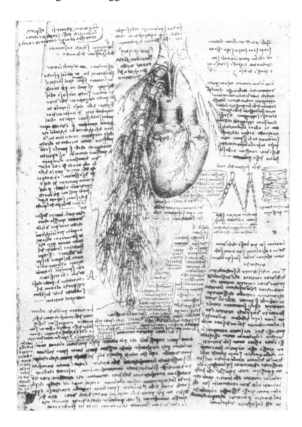

• **Fig. 35.3** da Vinci's drawing of the pulmonary circulation in relation to the bronchi (c. 1513). Pulmonary vessels arise from several parts of the heart, leading da Vinci to propose a dual blood supply to the lung. Coronary arteries and veins can be clearly seen on the heart. At the lower end of the main drawing, da Vinci has drawn a small circle containing the letter N. The notes describe the structure as having '*a crust, like a nutshell*' containing a '*dust and watery humour*', possibly representing his discovery of a lung cyst[17] or a tuberculous cavity.[15] (Royal Collection Trust ©2019, Her Majesty Queen Elizabeth II.)

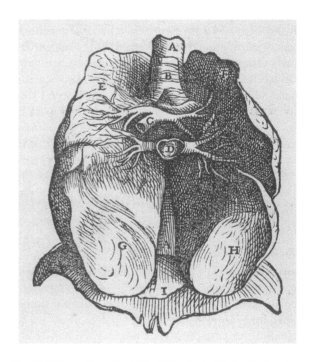

• **Fig. 35.4** Figure from Book VI of Vesalius's *Fabrica*,[19] showing an anterior view of the lungs after removal of the heart. A, Oesophagus; B, trachea; C, pulmonary artery; D, pulmonary vein; I, diaphragm. E–H refer to the lobes of the lun—Vesalius's illustrations always showed each lung to have four lobes. (Reproduced by permission of the Special Collections, Leeds University Library.)

resistance from his contemporaries whenever his views were at odds with those of Galen, and this eventually forced Vesalius to cease his study of anatomy and to return to work as a physician. Nevertheless, the *Fabrica* continued to gain acceptance, and became the foundation for future anatomy texts. Vesalius was also a skilled physiologist.[20] He was the first to describe an experiment reproduced much later, in which a section of the chest wall of an animal was carefully removed without breaching the pleura beneath, so enabling direct observation of lung movements through the transparent pleura.[6]

Pulmonary Circulation[21]

Unaware of the earlier writings of Ibn Al Nafis, Servetus (1509–1553), in his religious treatise *Christianismi restitutio*,[22] again challenged the existence of Galen's interventricular pores. He wrote that, rather than passing through the middle wall of the heart, '*blood is urged forward by a long course through the lung … and is poured from the pulmonary artery to the pulmonary vein*'.[23] He also commented that, on passing through the lung, the blood changed colour, becoming '*reddish-yellow*', although an explanation for this observation was still two centuries away. Tragically, *Christianismi restitutio* was deemed to be heretical by the Christian church of the time, and the book, along with its author, was burned at the stake in 1553. Only three copies of *Christianismi restitutio* are believed to exist today,[23] although more recent reprints are available.[24]

Just a few years later, Realdus Colombo (1516–1559) became the third physiologist to independently describe the pulmonary circulation. Colombo, a pupil of Vesalius, posthumously published his account of anatomy, *De Re Anatomicae*, in which he clearly describes blood flowing through the lung whilst mixing with air.[25] There is a suspicion that Colombo had previously had access to Servetus's *Christianismi restitutio*, or that he knew of the writings of Ibn Al Nafis from 300 years earlier, causing confusion as to which of these eminent physiologists should be credited with the discovery of pulmonary blood flow.[5,21]

Experimental Physiology in the 17th Century

At the start of the 17th century the dominance of Italian universities with respect to medicine and anatomy subsided, and progress in the understanding of respiration moved to England, where a new approach of experimental philosophy was developing.[4]

Discoveries to Assist the Respiratory Physiologists

Circulation

William Harvey (1578–1657) studied at Cambridge and Padua Universities, so was well-placed to combine the Italian methods and knowledge of anatomy with the English approach of physiological experimentation engendered by Francis Bacon. The most notable of Harvey's teachers in Padua was Hieronymus Fabricius, who is credited with the discovery of the venous valves, including the simple demonstration in arm veins that valves prevent blood from flowing distally. In 1616 Harvey first presented his ideas of the blood circulating continuously in a lecture to the College of Physicians in London. After a further 12 years of experimentation, Harvey published *De Motu Cordis*, in which he describes the circular motion of the blood in both the lesser (pulmonary) and greater (systemic) circulations.[26,27] Harvey's comments on respiration in *De Motu Cordis* are sparse, and although he refers in several places to a future separate treatise on respiration, it seems this was never written.

Atmospheric Pressure[4]

The Italian physicists Berti and Torricelli both accidentally discovered air pressure in their search to create a vacuum. First Berti, with a water barometer built of lead pipe attached to his house in Rome, measured the height of the water column at 27 feet. Torricelli and a mathematician colleague Vivianni then made the first mercury barometer using mercury in a glass tube inverted over a bowl of mercury, and so allowed the height of the column to be visualized.

The Microscope

Harvey and his numerous predecessors who described blood flowing through the lung tissue were not able to determine by what route this occurred or how the blood and air were mixed. Harvey thought it most likely that the blood and air came into contact through pores in the lung structures. Marcelus Malpighi (1628–1694) used a primitive microscope to observe lung tissue. His original communication in 1661, *De Pulmonibus*,[28,29] consisted of two letters to his friend Borrelli, who was a professor of science in Pisa.[5] Malpighi used frogs for his studies, and describes in detail the lung preparations used, remarking that he had '*destroyed almost the whole race of frogs*' in the course of his work.[29] He described lung tissue to be '*an aggregate of very light and very thin membranes, which, tense and sinuous, form an almost infinite number of orbicular vesicles and cavities, such as we see in the honeycomb of bees*'. This first description of the alveoli was accompanied by a drawing of his preparation (Fig. 35.5), and he went on to describe how the vesicles were all terminations of branches of the bronchi, and that under normal circumstances the blood and air were separated by them.

The mystery of the structure of lung tissue was now solved. Blood flowed from the right heart to the lung, through Malpighi's 'smallest of vessels' past the air containing vesicles and returned to the left heart. However, scientists were still no closer to discovering the purpose of this elaborate arrangement.

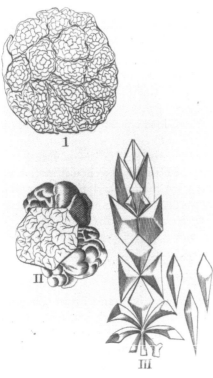

De Pulmon: pag. 144 to. 2.

• **Fig. 35.5** Drawing of Malpighi's preparation of frog lungs.[28] I, Seen from the surface of the lungs; II, showing the cut surface of the lung (including blood vessels on the surface of the vesicles [alveoli]); III, a schematic representation of the branching of the bronchi into vesicles. (Reproduced by permission of the Special Collections, Leeds University Library.)

The Oxford Physiologists and the 'Use of Breathing'[1,5,6]

In the mid-17th century a remarkable group of scientists happened upon each other in London, where they held meetings to exchange ideas and discuss scientific topics, often in their lodgings. The group was initially referred to by its members in London as the 'Invisible College', but later, in Oxford, became the 'Experimental Philosophy Club'. After around 15 years in existence the club was granted a royal charter by the King and formed the Royal Society of London. Of the numerous notable club members, four are worthy of particular mention here in view of their contribution to knowledge of respiration.

Robert Boyle (1627–1691)[30]

Assisted by Hooke, Boyle constructed a 'new pneumatical engine' that was capable of pumping air out of closed containers to produce a vacuum. He soon demonstrated that flames were extinguished, and animals died in the vacuum, and so began to believe there was some vital component present in air that was necessary for both combustion and animal life. Other experiments led Boyle

away from the truth about the purpose of respiration. Enclosing a candle and a chick together, he observed that the chick survived much longer than the flame, indicating that combustion and respiration were different. Similarly, using a mercury gauge, observations that the pressure within closed vessels did not change when animals expired led Boyle to believe that the vital component was present in only tiny amounts. For a scientist so dedicated to experimentation, Boyle was considered poor at interpreting their results,[4] often leaving this important task to his close friend Robert Hooke.

Robert Hooke (1635–1702)[31]

A crucial partnership between Hooke and Boyle brought about the studies described in the previous paragraph. However, Hooke is best known in the area of respiration for a dramatic demonstration to the Royal Society in 1667.[32] Keeping animals alive by artificial ventilation with bellows had been demonstrated many times before by both da Vinci and Vesalius. However, in Hooke's demonstration, he used two pairs of bellows to provide a constant stream of air and ventilated a dog with part of the chest wall removed, and with '*numerous small holes pricked in the outer coat of the lungs*' (pleura). With this experiment he achieved successful apnoeic ventilation for well over an hour, and so conclusively demonstrated that '*bare motion of the lungs without fresh air contributes nothing to the life of the animal*'.

Richard Lower (1631–1691)

Lower performed many animal experiments to investigate the known colour change of blood on exposure to air. Firstly he proved that the colour change occurred within the lungs, rather than in the heart, by demonstrating the colour difference between blood from the pulmonary artery and vein. He then proceeded to show that the colour change occurred only when air was present within the lung, by, for example, ceasing artificial respiration of an animal and observing that blood in the pulmonary vein quickly turned blue.

John Mayow (1641–1679)[4]

Mayow was the youngest of the Oxford physiologists, having studied with Lower and worked as Boyle's laboratory assistant. His major work on respiration, *Tractatus Quinque Medico-Physici*,[33] was published in 1674, a few years after Boyle, Lower and Hooke had moved on from their studies of respiration. *Tractatus Quinque* was an impressive treatise, bringing together in a single book the ideas of Mayow's eminent colleagues, supplemented with his own experimental work and ideas on chemistry and the physiology of respiration. His many experiments were illustrated with a single-page drawing containing six figures (Fig. 35.6). Mayow again showed that animal respiration and combustion had similar effects on the volume of air within the enclosed glasses. By good fortune,

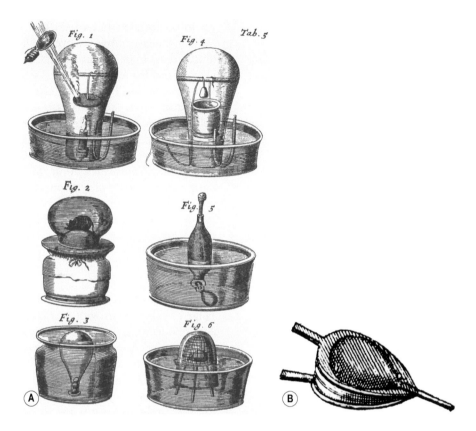

• **Fig. 35.6** Illustration of Mayow's experiments on respiration.[33] **(A)** Combustible materials, ignited by a magnifying glass and the sun's heat (Fig. 1) or animal respiration (Fig. 6) cause the water to rise within the enclosed glass, or a moistened bladder to be drawn into the glass (Fig. 2). Chemical reactions were instituted within the closed glasses by, for example, adding iron to spirit of nitre (Fig. 4) directly or leaving globules of iron in the base of a glass in contact with diluted spirit of nitre. Fig. 5 shows Mayow's system for transferring air from one glass to another. **(B)** drawing of the bladder in the bellows to demonstrate the passive expansion and contraction of the lungs by the chest wall.

Mayow found a much greater change in volume than Boyle's pressure changes. Mayow's use of water, and observations over a longer time period, allowed the carbon dioxide to be absorbed into the water and the temperature within the vessel to return to ambient. This led him to extend Boyle's ideas that air contained a vital component, which he named nitro-aerial spirit. When breathed in by animals nitro-aerial spirit combined with salino-sulfureous particles in the blood to produce a 'fermentation', which ultimately gave rise to muscular contraction. This last observation occurred from Mayow's appreciation of increased breathing during exercise.

Tractatus Quinque also contains excellent sections on respiratory mechanics. Mayow clearly understood that lung movement was brought about only by expansion and contraction of the chest wall. He demonstrated this by placing a bladder within a pair of bellows fitted with a glass window to allow observation of the bladder inflating and deflating as the bellows were worked (Fig. 35.6, *B*). Mayow then applied his knowledge of physiology to pathology by explaining that difficulty in breathing occurs if the abdominal contents resist the descent of the diaphragm, a situation seen with overeating, enlarged abdominal viscera, orthopnoea and even in the 'hysteric passion'. He fully understood the problems of pneumothorax, giving advice to his surgical colleagues:

Here, by the way, surgeons should be warned not to close the wound if the chest has been perforated except when the thorax is contracted to the utmost; for, otherwise, if the opening made by the wound is closed when the chest cavity is expanded it will be impossible for the chest to contract on account of the resistance of the air inside, or for the lungs to expand, except partially, and, in consequence, suffocation will occur.

Tractatus Quinque was controversial soon after it was written, with Mayow being accused of failing to properly acknowledge his use of other people's ideas and '*clogging the work with absurd additions of his own*'. The work was rarely referred to by his peers, and remained obscure for over a century. In particular, it is likely that the chemists of the following century (see later) who discovered oxygen were completely unaware of Mayow's work.

Physiology Hibernates

After the death of Mayow, the study of respiratory physiology again halted, this time for about 100 years. The other Oxford scientists had already moved on to different pursuits such as physical chemistry (Boyle), architecture (Hooke) and lucrative private medicine (Lower). The other great centres of learning in Europe did not take up the mantle of respiratory research. The cause of this stagnancy is uncertain:[4] this was another politically turbulent period of history in Europe, and conditions may not have been conducive to academic study. There may even have been a sense that respiration was now effectively explained, considering that knowledge of other closely related scientific disciplines, particularly chemistry, was still at a very primitive stage.

Chemistry and Respiration

Different Types of Air

Phlogiston[6]

George Ernst Stahl (1660–1734) had begun to investigate the chemistry of combustion in the early 18th century, and provided the scientific community with a completely erroneous explanation, which was nevertheless widely accepted. Stahl proposed that all combustible substances were made up of two components: calx, combined with a fiery principle named phlogiston. On burning, the phlogiston was driven off from the substance, leaving just the calx, or ash. Substances such as charcoal, which left very little ash, must have contained a greater proportion of phlogiston. Combustion in an enclosed space was extinguished when the air contained within became saturated with phlogiston. Calcination of metals (intense heating in air until oxidation occurs) was explained as driving off the phlogiston contained in the metal, whereas conversion of the metal oxide back to metal by heating with charcoal was achieved by the charcoal donating its phlogiston to recreate the metal. A powerful piece of evidence contradicted the phlogiston theory for metal calcination. Boyle, Mayow and others had all demonstrated that when metals were calcined, they gained weight, so could not have lost phlogiston. Stahl provided a very dubious explanation of this by explaining that, on calcination, the metal also lost some of its 'negative weight'.

Although the phlogiston theory was a complete inversion of what we now know to be true, it fitted with almost all known observations of combustion in the 18th century, with only the single exception already described. Stahl's views therefore became very enduring, and are believed to have impeded progress in understanding the chemistry of gases for many decades.

Fixed Air and Vitiated Air

Joseph Black (1728–1799) was a Scottish chemist whose work focussed on the chemistry of alkalis, a group of substances widely used at the time for the treatment of kidney complaints. He demonstrated that heating chalk caused a gas to be liberated and a reduction in weight to occur. To explain the large observed weight loss, Black believed the liberated gas to be air, rather than phlogiston. After further experiments Black found that the same gas was produced by fermentation and by burning charcoal and was present in expired air. From these observations he named it 'fixed air', believing that the gas made up all the nonrespirable portion of air. Only a few years later in 1772, the discovery of 'vitiated air' (nitrogen) demonstrated that fixed air was present in only small quantities in air. Black's explanation of the chemical reactions of carbon dioxide did not involve phlogiston at all, which must have been surprising considering the fundamental place phlogiston held in the chemistry of the time, but the phlogiston theory continued unchallenged.

Dephlogisticated Air

Joseph Priestley[34] (1733–1804) in England carried out a range of experiments with respiratory gases to characterize a component we now know to be oxygen. His work was published in *Experiments and observations on different kinds of air*,[35] which included an illustration of the equipment used (Fig. 35.7). Initially described by Priestley as 'pure air', the gas produced by heating mercuric oxide was found to cause a candle to burn with '*a remarkably vigorous flame*' and allow a mouse to survive much longer than in 'common air'. Priestley tried breathing the pure air himself with no apparent ill effects. His experiments on plants led to the major discovery that vegetation, in particular fast-growing species such as spinach, reversed the gaseous changes caused by respiration, burning candles or putrefaction within his closed vessels. He fully appreciated the import of this discovery on a global scale by commenting that air in the common atmosphere that has been reduced to a noxious state

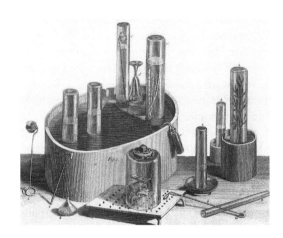

• **Fig. 35.7** Frontispiece from Priestley's '*Experiments and observations on different kinds of air*',[35] showing the variety of apparatus used in his experiments. Mice can be seen contained within a beer glass (d) which allowed them to breathe for 20 to 30 minutes in 'common air', whilst others are held in receivers open at the top and bottom for use in later experiments (at the front of the illustration). Plants can be seen growing in the jar on the far right. (Reproduced by permission of the Special Collections, Leeds University Library.)

by respiration or combustion '*has never failed to be perfectly restored by vegetation, so that the growing vegetables with which the surface of the Earth is overspread, may be a cause of the purification of the atmosphere*'. An advocate of phlogiston, Priestley soon renamed his 'pure air' as 'dephlogisticated air'. He believed his experiments confirmed the phlogiston theory, that is, the mercuric oxide removed phlogiston from the air, so allowing candles to burn longer, or animals to respire longer, before the air became saturated with phlogiston.

Fire Air

Carl Scheele[34] (1742–1786) studied chemistry and pharmacy in Sweden. Unaware of Priestley's work, Scheele, using a variety of methods, also produced oxygen, which he named 'fire air'. He too demonstrated its effect on burning candles and animal respiration, but he also failed to use his results to challenge the phlogiston theory.

Oxygen

Antoine-Laurent Lavoisier[36] (1743–1794) was born in Paris and graduated in science before the age of 20, specializing in chemistry soon after. In a very productive few years commencing around 1772 Lavoisier studied combustion and respiration, during which time he was visited by Priestley, who discussed his own experiments with 'pure air'. Lavoisier approached chemistry differently, in effect introducing quantitative studies to the qualitative ones of his predecessors.[6] He showed that, when metals were calcined in a closed jar, the combined weight of apparatus, air and jar remained unchanged, so proving that it was air combining with the metal that increased their weight. In experiments with animals breathing nearly pure oxygen, he observed that the animals expired before all the oxygen was used up, and this led him to investigate the harmful effects of carbon dioxide in the atmosphere.

Respiratory experiments over acidified water allowed the carbon dioxide produced by respiration to be absorbed, and allowed quantification of oxygen consumption, which in a resting subject was measured by Lavoisier as 1200 cubic inches per hour ($\approx$330 mL.min^{-1}), a result very close to the modern value (page 155). However, it is Lavoisier's discovery that 'eminently respirable air' was a chemical element, and his naming of the element as oxygen, for which he is most remembered. Once again, the contribution made by the scientists of the time to this seminal discovery is controversial; for example, Priestley was later irritated at Lavoisier's use of the ideas they had discussed in 1774, and Mayow's work is never referred to in Lavoisier's writings, in spite of him being aware of it at the time.[4] Lavoisier's interests were wider than his study of science, and he was closely involved in a French financial institution responsible for generating tax revenues, the Ferme Generale. Income from this clearly provided the resources for Lavoisier's extensive experiments, but also resulted in accusations of financial impropriety which

led to his untimely death at the guillotine in 1794.[6] After Lavoisier's death, his friend Lagrange commented that '*It took but a second to cut off his head; a hundred years will not suffice to produce one like it*'.[37]

Early Development of Current Ideas of Respiratory Physiology

Tissue Respiration

Ancient ideas of some type of combustion in the heart to generate heat gave way in the 16th century to the suggestion that heat was generated by friction within the ever-moving blood. As chemistry developed, the similarities between combustion and respiration became progressively more compelling, but where this oxidation reaction took place eluded even Lavoisier, who believed it occurred in the bronchi. The impetus to look beyond the lungs and heart to find the site of combustion in the body came from the discovery of calorimetry by Adair Crawford (1748–1795).[36] Measurements made by Crawford and Lavoisier of the heat generated by the body made it clear to Lavoisier's mathematician friend Lagrange that if all the heat were produced in the lungs their temperature '*would necessarily be raised so much that one would have reason to fear they would be destroyed*'.[38]

In Italy, further experiments investigating where in the body combustion took place were performed by Lazzaro Spallanzani (1729–1799), although his work was only published posthumously in 1803.[39] He studied respiration in a huge variety of creatures, including insects, reptiles, amphibians and mammals, and described how those creatures without lungs exchanged oxygen and carbon dioxide via their integument (page 306). That respiration still occurred in the absence of lungs led Spallanzani to his most important respiratory discovery, when he showed that a variety of tissues from recently deceased creatures (including humans) continued to respire for some time, so showing that the tissues were the site of oxygen consumption.

In the 19th century, advances in science led to improved techniques for gas and temperature measurement. Heat production was measured in animals and humans and found to correlate with the specific heat capacity of the oxygen consumed and carbon dioxide produced. The respiratory quotient was measured at between 0.6 and 1.0, and found to depend on diet. Finally, with the birth of organic chemistry, and the foundation of the laws of conservation of energy, the modern account of energy metabolism was elucidated.[6]

Blood Gases[40,41]

Once it was clear that oxygen metabolism occurred in the tissues, the search was on to find how the blood carried oxygen to, and returned carbon dioxide from, the tissues in sufficient quantities. However, other fundamental discoveries were needed before this question could be addressed in detail.

Partial Pressure

John Dalton (1766–1844), whose law on partial pressures (page 415) is widely used today, first developed the concept that mixtures of gases could exist together irrespective of the pressure and temperature of the mixture. His description stated that the particles of each component gas had no interaction with those of the other gases and so '*arranged themselves just the same as in a void space*' whilst paradoxically occupying the whole space allotted to the mixture of gases. He illustrated this as shown in Figure 35.8.[42]

Paul Bert (1833–1886), most famous for his studies of altitude physiology and medicine, also made a significant contribution to fundamental respiratory physiology by discovering that it was the partial pressure, rather than concentration, of respiratory gases that affected biological systems.[43,44] In an elegant series of experiments, he exposed animals to a variety of atmospheric pressures whilst maintaining the partial pressure of oxygen constant, with no ill effect on the animals. Whenever inspired Po_2 was reduced below that of air at atmospheric pressure, irrespective of the total pressure, the animal suffered the consequences of hypoxia. He repeated the experiments on humans in a large, specially constructed chamber (Fig. 35.9) and showed that, by breathing supplementary oxygen, the harmful effects of low ambient pressure could be entirely alleviated.

Bert applied his knowledge to the recently discovered pastime of ballooning, and assisted his friend Gaston Tissandier to use oxygen to ascend to record new heights in his balloon. However, in his quest for higher altitude, M. Tissandier and two friends undertook a balloon flight with the specific aim of reaching 8000 m (26 200 feet) altitude, but in their enthusiasm they did not have time to consult Bert on the likely oxygen requirement. An unusually rapid ascent (Fig. 35.10) resulted in confusion in all three balloonists,

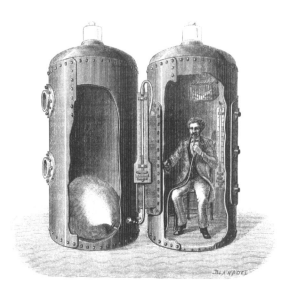

• **Fig. 35.9** Figure from *La pression barométrique*[43] showing Paul Bert breathing oxygen while sitting in the chamber at progressively subatmospheric pressure. Note the sparrow in the cage above the subject—the bird falls in its cage when the pressure reaches 450 mmHg, but Bert persists with the experiment down to 410 mmHg, maintained conscious by intermittently breathing oxygen. (Reproduced by permission of the Wellcome Library, London.)

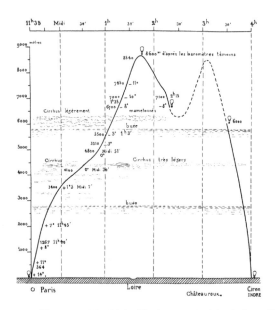

• **Fig. 35.10** Diagram of the high-altitude ascent of the balloon *Zenith* on April 15th 1875.[43] The dashed line indicates estimated altitude, as the only survivor of the flight Gaston Tissandier, was too hypoxic to make recordings of the altitude. (Reproduced by permission of the Wellcome Library, London.)

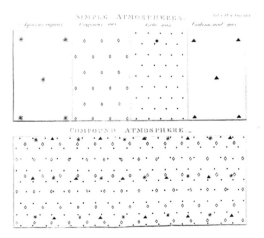

• **Fig. 35.8** Dalton's drawing to illustrate a compound atmosphere, made up of a mixture of simple atmospheres.[42] Two centuries after it was drawn, this diagram would be helpful to today's physiology students when first learning of Dalton's law of partial pressures. Aqueous vapour, water vapour; oxygenous gas, oxygen; azotic gas, nitrogen; carbonic acid gas, carbon dioxide. (Reproduced by permission of the Wellcome Library, London.)

who were unable to breathe the oxygen and lost consciousness (page 206). Only Tissandier recovered sufficiently to record their altitude at 8600 m (28 200 feet), before battling with hypoxia to intermittently breathe oxygen and facilitate a controlled descent, during which the full tragedy of the flight unfolded, and he discovered that his two friends had died some time earlier in the flight.

Haemoglobin and its Dissociation Curve

Boyle and Mayow had both used a vacuum to extract gases from blood and surmised that these gases may have been air or nitro-aerial spirit (oxygen). In the 19th century the excellence of German chemists led them to dominate this field of research. Gustav Magnus (1802–1870) extracted oxygen and carbon dioxide from blood, showing that the former was more abundant in arterial blood and vice versa.[45] Lothar Meyer did similar experiments in 1857, but showed that the liberation of oxygen as pressure was reduced was not linear, so demonstrating that the oxygen was not simply dissolved in the blood.[46] Meanwhile, the red compound in blood was identified and soon chemically found to be a combination of globulin proteins and an iron containing haematin. The affinity of this new 'haemoglobin' for oxygen was soon understood, and Hüfner quantified this binding by showing that 1.34 mL of oxygen combined with 1 g of crystallized haemoglobin, a remarkably accurate measurement (page 144).[47] By 1888, Hüfner had used haemoglobin solutions to record the relationship between the partial pressure of oxygen and haemoglobin saturation, and obtained a rectangular hyperbola.[5] Finally, in 1904 Christian Bohr and colleagues showed that, when fresh whole blood was used to measure the haemoglobin dissociation, an S-shaped curve was found, and that the curve altered with varying partial pressures of carbon dioxide (Fig. 35.11).[48,49]

The Oxygen Secretion Controversy[1,41,50]

Measurement of the partial pressure of oxygen in arterial blood in the 19th century provoked a huge scientific controversy. In 1870, Bohr and colleagues developed a primitive aerotonometer and found arterial Po_2 to be around 80 mmHg (10.7 kPa), although in some measurements the arterial Po_2 was found to be slightly higher than the alveolar Po_2. At around this time, physiologists studying other body systems were discovering numerous active membrane transport systems in such places as the kidney and bowel. This

led Bohr to suggest that active transport of oxygen may occur in the lung, and he soon had the support for this hypothesis from the eminent respiratory physiologist John Scott Haldane. In his laboratories in Oxford, Haldane devised a new technique for measuring arterial Po_2. His technique involved the subject breathing small concentrations of carbon monoxide, and then using direct colour-matching of the subject's blood with standard samples to ascertain the carboxy-haemoglobin concentration from which the Po_2 could be calculated.[51] To standardize the light used for comparing colours, experiments had to be done during daylight, and by today's standards several aspects of the technique seem remarkably subjective, but nevertheless Haldane was an excellent scientist who applied rigorous methodology. Using his technique Haldane found the average arterial Po_2 to be 200 mmHg (26.7 kPa), so claiming to have proved that oxygen secretion was occurring in the lung.

A Danish husband and wife team, August and Marie Krogh,[52] became Haldane's adversaries over oxygen secretion. August Krogh, a former pupil of Bohr, continued to refine the technique of aerotonometry, using analysis of smaller volumes of gas from continuously flowing blood samples. His results always showed arterial Po_2 to be slightly less than alveolar Po_2, even when tested across a variety of inspired oxygen concentrations. Meanwhile his wife performed extensive investigations of the diffusing capacity of the lung for carbon monoxide to show that, in theory, the lung was easily able to passively absorb sufficient oxygen without the need for active secretion.

Following a bitter exchange of contradictory scientific papers over a period of 20 years, the Kroghs did begin to win the argument. By 1911, Haldane and his team seemed to accept that oxygen secretion may only be occurring when inspired oxygen levels were low. They demonstrated this, using their usual methodology, in an adventurous study of Po_2 measurements on the summit of Pikes Peak at an altitude of 4300 m (14 100 feet), where they again found arterial Po_2 to be higher than alveolar Po_2.[53]

Haldane never abandoned his faith in oxygen secretion, despite subsequent investigations in his lifetime by Barcroft, who also found the phenomenon did not exist. Why a physiologist as brilliant as Haldane had such an unshakeable believe in an erroneous hypothesis remains unexplained, and for this reason the controversy continues. When a review of these events was published in the *Lancet* in 1985,[50] the dispute over Haldane's contribution was reignited.[54,55]

Lung Mechanics[56]

Galen knew that inflation of the lungs was a passive phenomenon and occurred as a result of chest movement brought about by the respiratory muscles. However, the way in which this occurred was not understood for many centuries until the discovery of air pressure, when it soon became clear that chest expansion would draw air into the lungs. Even then there were those who would not accept the

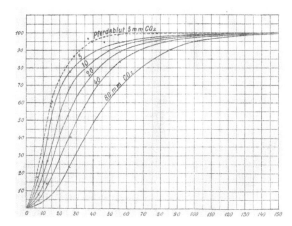

• **Fig. 35.11** The first publication (from 1904) showing the shape of the oxyhaemoglobin dissociation curve.[48] Note the effect of blood Pco_2 on the position and shape of the curve (page 146). Pferdeblut, horse blood. (Reproduced by permission of the Special Collections, Leeds University Library.)

scientific explanation; Rene Descartes proposed in 1662 that, when the chest expanded, the air outside was pushed away from the chest, compressing adjacent air until the air near the mouth was forced into the lungs.[6] Mayow's elegant demonstration with the bladder within the bellows, described above, provided clear confirmation of the scientific theory.

Around 1500 years after Galen, Vesalius' experiments demonstrated that, on puncturing the pleura, the lung retracted into the chest cavity. Many of his successors repeated this observation, Mayow commenting that *'the lungs, as if shrinking from observation, cease their movement and collapse at once on the first entrance of light and self-revelation'*.[33] It was another 160 years before further investigation of lung elasticity occurred. In 1820 Carson measured the pressure in the trachea (with a closed airway) when the chest was opened, and so made the first measurement of lung recoil pressure.[57] A short time later, Ludwig recorded a subatmospheric pressure in the pleura, leading to the proposal by Donders in 1849 that in the intact subject the recoil outwards by the chest wall is equal to the lung recoil inwards[4] (Chapter 2). Finally, John Hutchinson, whose work on lung volumes is described below, produced the first lung compliance curves in a human, obtained shortly after the subject's death.

Elasticity and Surfactant

For some time lung recoil seems to have been adequately explained as simply resulting from the inherent elasticity of lung tissue. At the start of the 20th century the geometry and size of the alveoli was well known, and around 100 years had elapsed since Laplace had described the relationship between pressure, surface tension and the radii of curved surfaces (page 15). Yet the inherent instability of lung tissue based on these laws was not recognized until 1929, when Kurt von Neergard first questioned whether tissue elasticity alone was sufficient explanation for the properties of lung tissue.[58] von Neergard's experiments demonstrated that surface tension in alveoli was indeed lower than expected by Laplace's law, and just a few years later Richard Pattle demonstrated that lung tissue contained an insoluble protein layer that reduced the surface tension of alveoli to almost zero,[59] and surfactant (page 16) was discovered.

Lung Volumes

The first measurements of the volume of air contained in the lung were made in the 17th century by Borelli, who also raised the concept of a residual volume.[6] Following this, numerous scientists measured a confusing variety of lung volumes by various methods, such as estimating total lung capacity from plaster casts made in the chest cavity of cadavers. Measurement of lung volumes similar to those in modern use was first made by John Hutchinson in 1846, alongside his description of the first pulmonary spirometer.[60] Hutchinson's spirometer (Fig. 35.12) differs little from the water spirometers used until very recently, with a

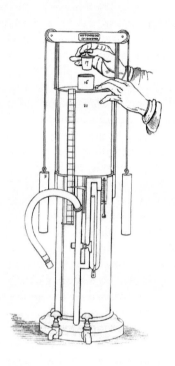

• **Fig. 35.12** The Hutchinson spirometer (1846).[60] This figure shows the operator removing the bung to reset the level of the spirometer before making another measurement. (Reproduced by permission of the Special Collections, Leeds University Library.)

volume-measuring chamber over water counterbalanced with weights to offer minimal resistance to the subject's breathing. Hutchinson described the following divisions of the air in the chest, with the modern equivalents in parentheses:

Residual air – *the quantity of air that remains in the lungs after the most violent muscular effort, and over which we have no control* (residual volume)

Reserve air – *the air in the lungs after a gentle respiratory movement, which may be thrown out if required* (expiratory reserve volume)

Breathing air – *the portion required to perform ordinary gentle inspiration and expiration* (tidal volume)

Complemental air – *the volume that can at will be drawn into the lungs by a violent exertion* (inspiratory reserve volume)

Vital capacity – *the last three divisions combined.*

In the same paper,[60] Hutchinson reported his measurements of vital capacity in 1970 healthy subjects to establish normal values. He showed with great accuracy that vital capacity was directly related to subject height and age, and obtained measurements comparable with today, for example, 188 in³ at 60°F for a 55-year-old male subject 5 ft 4 in tall (188 in³ equals 3.31 L body temperature and pressure saturated [BTPS], compared with a modern predicted normal value of 3.64 L). He then measured vital capacity in

60 patients with phthisis (cough) from a variety of causes, and compared the results obtained with predicted normal values based on height, weight, and so on, and was able to use his results to demonstrate declining lung volumes as respiratory disease progressed.

Control of Ventilation

Galen's observations of gladiator injuries had shown that the brain was responsible for respiratory activity, and that the phrenic nerves were involved in bringing about this action.

More specific localization of the respiratory centre did not begin until the 18th century, when the French physiologist Antoine Lorry (1725–1783) showed that, in animals, all parts of the brain above the brainstem could be removed before respiration ceased.[4] In 1812, the French physiologist Antoine Legallois published reports of similar, but more precise, experiments showing that rhythmic inspiratory movements ceased only when the medulla was removed.[61] During the next 150 years a long series of distinguished investigators carried out more detailed localization of the neurones concerned in the control of respiration and studied their interaction.[4] These experiments resulted in the description of anatomical regions which, when isolated in animals, caused a specific respiratory pattern, for example, the apneustic and pneumotaxic centres. The complexity of respiratory control in the intact animal is such that this crude anatomical approach to unravelling the various interactions was limited, and human studies of function were mostly impossible until recent imaging techniques were developed (page 42).

The origin of rhythmicity in the respiratory centre received much attention from 19th century physiologists.[62] The role of afferent neural inputs into the respiratory centre, particularly those from the vagus nerve, were clearly demonstrated. In particular, Hering and Breuer described how lung inflation led to inhibition of inspiratory activity, and a 'deflation' reflex was also described (page 48). These observations gave rise to the basis of the *Selbsteuerung* (self-steering) hypothesis where rhythm generation was simply two alternating inhibitory reflexes.

Chemical Control of Breathing[63]

Rapid breathing followed by gasping and death had been observed by the Oxford physiologists in the 17th century in their experiments on animals in closed atmospheres. As the analysis of gases in blood improved, so the chemical control of breathing could be elucidated. In 1868, Pflüger performed a comprehensive study in dogs showing that both oxygen lack and carbon dioxide excess stimulated respiration, and that the former was the stronger stimulant.[64] Soon after, a fellow German physiologist Miescher-Rusch investigated the carbon dioxide response in humans to show that the respiratory system exerted very tight control over carbon dioxide concentrations, and concluded that this, rather than oxygen, was the predominant chemical stimulus to

breathing.[65] Leon Fredericq demonstrated in a series of very elegant experiments that the chemical control of breathing predominated over the vagal reflex control described in the previous paragraph.[66] He managed to crossconnect the blood supply to and from the heads of two animals, and, for example, produce apnoea in one dog by hyperventilating the other, the apnoea occurring even though the dog's lungs were not inflated to induce the Hering–Breuer reflex (page 48). Finally, at the start of the 20th century, further improvements in analytical chemistry led to the work of Haldane and Priestley, published in 1905, which involved meticulous quantitative analysis of the chemical control of breathing and the interactions between oxygen, carbon dioxide and exercise.[67]

References

*1. West JB. *Respiratory Physiology: People and Ideas.* Oxford: American Physiology Society & Oxford University Press; 1996.
2. West JB. A century of pulmonary gas exchange. *Am J Respir Crit Care Med.* 2004;169:897-902.
3. Macklem PT. A century of the mechanics of breathing. *Am J Respir Crit Care Med.* 2004;170:10-15.
4. Proctor DF. *A History of Breathing Physiology.* New York: Marcel Dekker; 1995.
5. Gottlieb LS. *A History of Respiration.* Springfield, Illinois: Charles C Thomas; 1964.
6. Perkins JF. Historical development of respiratory physiology. In: Fenn WO, Rahn H, eds. *Handbook of Physiology. Section 3: Respiration.* Washington: American Physiological Society; 1964.
*7. Nunn JF. *Ancient Egyptian Medicine.* London: British Museum Press; 1996.
8. Bryan CP. *Ancient Egyptian Medicine The Papyrus:* Ebers. Chicago: Ares; 1974.
9. Ghalioungui P. *The Ebers Papyrus. A New English Translation, Commentaries and Glossaries.* Cairo: Academy of Scientific Research and Technology; 1987.
*10. May MT. *Galen – On the Usefulness of the Parts of the Body.* New York: Cornell University Press; 1968.
11. Furley DJ, Wilkie JS. *Galen on Respiration and the Arteries.* Princeton: Princeton University Press; 1984.
12. Singer C. *A Short History of Anatomy & Physiology from the Greeks to Harvey.* New York: Dover Publications; 1957.
*13. West JB. Ibn al-Nafis, the pulmonary circulation, and the Islamic Golden Age. *J Appl Physiol.* 2008;105:1877-1880.
14. West JB. Leonardo da Vinci: engineer, bioengineer, anatomist, and artist. *Am J Physiol Lung Cell Mol Physiol.* 2017;312: L392-L397.
15. Leonardo da Vinci. *Anatomical Drawings from the Royal Collection.* London: Royal Academy of Arts; 1977.
16. Clark K. *The Drawings of Leonardo da Vinci in the Collection of Her Majesty the Queen at Windsor Castle (Volume 3).* London: Phaidon Press; 1969.
17. Mitzner W, Wagner E. On the purported discovery of the bronchial circulation by Leonardo da Vinci. *J Appl Physiol.* 1992;73:1196-1201.
18. Charan NB, Carvalho P. On the purported discovery of the bronchial circulation by Leonardo da Vinci: a rebuttal. *J Appl Physiol.* 1994;76:1836-1838.
19. Vesalius A. *De Humani Corporis Fabrica Libri Septem.* Venice: Basel; 1543.
20. Hage JJ, Brinkman RJ. Andreas Vesalius' understanding of pulmonary ventilation. *Respir Physiol Neurobiol.* 2016;231:37-44.

21. Coppola ED. The discovery of the pulmonary circulation: a new approach. *Bull Hist Med.* 1957;31:44-77.
22. Servetus M. *Christianismi restitutio.* 1553.
23. O'Malley CD. *Michael Servetus*: A translation of his geographical, medical and astrological writings with introductions and notes. Philadelphia: American Philosophical Society; 1953.
24. Servetus M. *Christianismi Restitutio.* Frankfurt: Minerva; 1966.
25. Colombo R. *De Re Anatomica libri XV.* Paris: Andreum Wechelum; 1572.
26. Harvey W. *De Motu Cordis.* Frankfurt: Wm Fitzeri; 1628.
27. Harvey W. *Movement of the Heart and Blood in Animals.* Oxford: Blackwell Science; 1957.
28. Malpighi M. *De Pulmonibus.* Bologna; 1661.
29. Young J. Malpighi's 'De Pulmonibus'. *Proc R Soc Med Lond.* 1929;23:1-11.
30. West JB. Robert Boyle's landmark book of 1660 with the first experiments on rarified air. *J Appl Physiol.* 2005;98:31-39.
31. Harsch V. Robert Hooke, inventor of the vacuum pump and the first altitude chamber (1671). *Aviat Space Environ Med.* 2006;77:867-869.
32. Hooke R. An account of an experiment made by Mr Hook of preserving animals alive by blowing through their lungs with bellows. *Phil Trans R Soc Lond.* 1667;2:539-540.
33. Mayow J. *Medico-Physical Works: Being a Translation of Tractatus Quinque Medici-Physici.* Edinburgh: The Alembic Club; 1907.
*34. **Severinghaus JW. Priestley, the furious free thinker of the enlightenment, and Scheele, the taciturn apothecary of Uppsala. *Acta Anesthesiol Scand.* 2002;46:2-9.**
35. Priestley J. *Experiments and Observations on Different Kinds of Air.* London: J. Johnson; 1775.
36. Crawford A. *Experiments and Observations on Animal heat, and the Inflammation of Combustible Bodies: Being an Attempt to Resolve These Phenomena into a General Law of Nature.* London: J. Johnson; 1788.
37. Lusk G. Nutrition. *Clio Medica: A Series of Primers on the History of Medicine* Vol 10. New York: Hoeber Inc.; 1933.
38. Hassenfratz JH. Mémoire sur la combinaison de l'oxygèn dans le sang et sur la manière dont la calorique se degage. *Ann Chim Paris.* 1791;9:261-274.
39. Spallanzani L. *Mémoire sur la respiration.* Geneva: Paschoud; 1803.
40. Severinghaus JW. Monitoring oxygenation. *J Clin Monit Comput.* 2011;25:155-161.
41. Severinghaus JW, Astrup P, Murray JF. Blood gas analysis and critical care medicine. *Am J Respir Crit Care Med* 1998;157:S114-S122.
42. Dalton J. Experimental essays on the constitution of mixed gases; on the force of steam or vapour from water and other liquids in different temperatures, both in a Torricellean vacuum and in air; on evaporation; and on the expansion of gases by heat. *Mem Lit Phil Soc, Manchester.* 1802;5:535-602.
43. Bert P. *La pression barométrique.* Paris: Masson; 1878.
44. Hitchcock MA, Hitchcock FA. *Paul Bert. Barometric Pressure. Researches in Experimental Physiology.* Columbus Ohio: College Book Company; 1943.
45. Magnus H. Ueber die im blute enthalten gase, sauerstoff stickstoff und kohlensaure. *Ann Phys Chem.* 1837;40:583-606.
46. Meyer L. Die gase des blutes. *Z Rat Med.* 1857;8:256.
47. Hüfner G. Ueber die quantität sauerstoff, welche 1 gramm hämoglobin zu binden vermag. *Z Phys Chem.* 1877;1:317-329.
48. Bohr C, Hasselbalch K, Krogh A. Ueber einen in biologischer beziehung wichtigen einfluss, den die kohlensäurespannung des blutes auf dessen sauerstoffbindung übt. *Skand Arch Physiol.* 1904;16:402-412.
*49. **West JB. Three classical papers in respiratory physiology by Christian Bohr (1855–1911) whose work is frequently cited but seldom read. *Am J Physiol Lung Cell Mol Physiol.* 2019;316:L585-L588.**
*50. **Milledge JS. The great oxygen secretion controversy. *Lancet.* 1985;2:1408-1411.**
51. Haldane JS, Lorrain Smith J. The oxygen tension of arterial blood. *J Physiol.* 1891;20:497-520.
52. Schmidt-Nielsen B. August and Marie Krogh and respiratory physiology. *J Appl Physiol.* 1984;57:293-303.
53. Douglas CG, Haldane JS, Henderson Y, et al. Physiological observations made on Pike's Peak, Colorado, with special reference to adaptation to low barometric pressures. *Phil Trans R Soc Lond.* 1913;203:185-318.
54. Passmore R. Haldane and Barcroft. *Lancet.* 1986;1:443.
55. Cunningham DJC. The oxygen secretion controversy. *Lancet.* 1986;1:683.
56. Otis AB. History of respiratory mechanics. In: Fishman AP, Macklem PT, Mead JT, Geiger SR, eds. *Handbook of Physiology. Section 3: The Respiratory System.* Bethesda: American Physiological Society; 1986.
57. Carson J. On the elasticity of the lungs. *Phil Trans R Soc Lond.* 1820;110:29-44.
58. von Neergard K. Neue auffassungen über einen grundbegriff der atemmechanik. Die retraktionkraft der lunge, abhängig von der oberflächenspannung in den alveolen. *Z Ges Exp Med.* 1929;66:1-22.
59. Pattle RE. Properties, function and origin of the alveolar lining layer. *Nature.* 1955;175:1125-1126.
60. Hutchinson J. On the capacity of the lungs, and on the respiratory functions, with a view of establishing a precise and easy method of detecting disease by the spirometer. *Med Chir Trans (Series 2).* 1846;29:137-252.
61. Legallois C. *Experiences sur le principe de la vie.* Paris: d'Hautel; 1812.
62. Widdicombe J. Reflexes from the lungs and airways: historical perspective. *J Appl Physiol.* 2006;101:628-634.
63. Remmers JE. A century of control of breathing. *Am J Respir Crit Care Med.* 2005;172:6-11.
64. Pflüger E. Ueber die ursache der athembewegungen, sowie der dyspnoë und apnoë. *Arch Ges Physiol.* 1868;1:61-106.
65. Miescher-Rüsch F. Bemerkungen zur lehre von den atembewegungen. *Arch Anat u Physiol Leipzig.* 1885;6:355-380.
66. Fredericq L. Sur la cause de l'apnée. *Archiv Biol Liége.* 1900;17:561-576.
67. Haldane JS, Priestley JG. The regulation of lung ventilation. *J Physiol.* 1905;32:225-266.

Appendix A

Physical Quantities and Units of Measurement

International System of Units

A clean transition from the old to the new metric units failed to occur. The old system was based on the centimetre-gram-second (CGS), and was supplemented with many noncoherent derived units such as the millimetre of mercury (mmHg) for pressure and the calorie for work, which could not be related to the basic units by factors, which were powers of ten. The new system, the Système Internationale (SI), is based on the metre-kilogram-second (MKS) and comprises base and derived units which are obtained simply by multiplication or division without the introduction of numbers, not even powers of ten.

Base units are metre (length), kilogram (mass), second (time), ampere (electric current), kelvin (thermodynamic temperature), mole (amount of substance) and candela (luminous intensity).

Derived units include newton (force: kilograms metre second^{-2}), pascal (pressure: newton metre^{-2}), joule (work: newton metre) and hertz (periodic frequency: second^{-1}).

Special non-SI units are recognized as having sufficient practical importance to warrant retention for general or specialized use. These include litre, day, hour, minute and the standard atmosphere.

Nonrecommended units include the dyne, bar and calorie and gravity-dependent units such as the kilogram-force, centimetre of water (cmH$_2$O) and mmHg, but many remain in use today.

The use of SI units in respiratory physiology and clinical practice remains incomplete. The kilopascal has replaced the mmHg for blood gas partial pressures in Europe, but the old units continue to be used in the US and Australasia. The introduction of the kilopascal for fluid pressures in the medical field has failed to occur. In the clinical setting we continue to record arterial pressure in mmHg and venous pressure in cmH$_2$O.

As in previous editions of this book, it has proved necessary to make text and figures bilingual, with both SI and CGS units for the benefit of readers who are unfamiliar with one or other of the systems. Some useful conversion factors are listed in Table A.1. There are still some areas of physiology

and medicine where non-SI units continue to be extensively used, such as mmHg for most vascular pressures and cmH$_2$O for airway pressure, so these units are retained throughout this book to aid clarity.

Physical quantities relevant to respiratory physiology are defined below, together with their mass/length/time (MLT) units. These units provide a most useful check of the validity of equations and other expressions which are derived in the course of studies of respiratory function. Only quantities with identical MLT units can be added or subtracted, and the units must be the same on both sides of an equation.

Volume (Dimensions: L^3)

In this book we are concerned with volumes of blood and gas. Strict SI units would be cubic metres and submultiples. However, the litre (L) and millilitre (mL) are recognized as special non-SI units, and will remain in use. For practical purposes, we may ignore changes in the volume of liquids which are caused by changes of temperature. However, the changes in volume of gases caused by changes of temperature or pressure are by no means negligible, and constitute an important source of error if they are ignored. These are described in Appendix C.

Fluid Flow Rate (Dimensions: L^3/T, OR L^3.T^{-1})

In the case of liquids, flow rate is the physical quantity of cardiac output, regional blood flow, and so on. The strict SI units would be metre^3.second^{-1}, but litres per minute (L.min^{-1}) and millilitres per minute (mL.min^{-1}) are special non-SI units which may be retained. For gases, the dimension is applied to minute volume of respiration, alveolar ventilation, peak expiratory flow rate, oxygen consumption, and so on. The units are the same as those for liquids, except that litres per second are used for the high instantaneous flow rates that occur during the course of inspiration and expiration.

In the case of gas flow rates, just as much attention should be paid to the matter of temperature and pressure as when volumes are being measured (Appendix C).

TABLE A.1 Conversion Factors for Units of Measurement

Force

1 N (newton)	$= 10^5$ dyn

Pressure

1 kPa (kilopascal)	$= 7.50$ mmHg
	$= 10.2$ cmH$_2$O
	$= 0.00987$ standard atmospheres
	$= 10\,000$ dyn.cm^{-2}
1 standard atmosphere	$= 101.3$ kPa
	$= 760$ mmHg
	$= 1033$ cmH$_2$O
	$= 10$ m of sea water (S.G. 1.033)
1 mmHg	$= 1.36$ cmH$_2$O
	$= 1$ torr (approx)

Compliance

1 L.kPa^{-1}	$= 0.098$ L.cmH$_2$O^{-1}

Flow resistance

1 kPa.L^{-1}.s	$= 10.2$ cmH$_2$O.L^{-1}.sec

Work

1 J (joule)	$= 0.102$ kilopond-metres
	$= 0.239$ calories

Power

1 W (watt)	$= 1$ J.s^{-1}
	$= 6.12$ kp.m.min^{-1}

Surface tension

1 N.m^{-1} (Newton/metre or pascal metre)	$= 1000$ dyn.cm^{-1}

In the Figures, Tables and text of this book 1 kPa has been taken to equal 7.5 mmHg or 10 cmH$_2$O.

Force (Dimensions: MLT^{-2})

Force is defined as mass times acceleration. An understanding of the units of force is essential to an understanding of the units of pressure. Force, when applied to a free body, causes it to change either the magnitude or the direction of its velocity.

The units of force are of two types. The first is the force resulting from the action of gravity on a mass, and is synonymous with weight. It includes the kilogram-force and the pound-force. All such units are nonrecommended under the SI, and have almost disappeared. The second type of unit of force is absolute and does not depend on the magnitude of the gravitational field. In the CGS system, the absolute unit of force was the dyne, and this has been replaced under the MKS system and the SI by the newton (N), which is defined as the force which will give a mass of 1 kilogram an acceleration of 1 metre per second per second.

$$1N = 1kg.m.s^{-2}$$

Pressure (Dimensions: MLT^{-2}/L^2, Or ML^{-1}T^{-2})

Pressure is defined as force per unit area. The SI unit is the pascal (Pa), which is 1 newton per square metre.

$$1Pa = 1N.m^{-2}$$

The pascal is inconveniently small (one hundred-thousandth of an atmosphere), and the kilopascal (kPa) has been adopted for general use in the medical field. Its introduction is simplified by the fact that the kPa is very close to 1% of an atmosphere. Thus a standard atmosphere is 101.3 kPa, and the P_{O_2} of dry air is therefore very close to 21 kPa.

The standard atmosphere may continue to be used under the SI. It is defined as $1.013\,25 \times 10^5$ pascals.

The torr came into use only shortly before the move towards SI units. This is unfortunate for the memory of Torricelli, as the torr will disappear from use. The torr is defined as exactly equal to 1/760 of a standard atmosphere, and it is therefore very close to the millimetre of mercury, the two units being considered identical for practical purposes. The only distinction is that the torr is absolute, whereas the millimetre of mercury is gravity-based.

The bar is the absolute unit of pressure in the old CGS system and is defined as 10^6 dyn.cm^{-2}. The unit was convenient because the bar is close to 1 atmosphere (1.013 bars), and a millibar is close to 1 centimetre of water (0.9806 millibars).

Compliance (Dimensions: M^{-1}L^{4}T^2)

The term 'compliance' is used in respiratory physiology to denote the volume change of the lungs in response to a change of pressure. The dimensions are therefore volume divided by pressure, and the commonest units have been litres (or millilitres) per centimetre of water. This continues to slowly change over to litres per kilopascal (L.kPa^{-1}).

Resistance to Fluid Flow (Dimensions: ML^{-4}T^{-1})

Under conditions of laminar flow (see Fig. 3.2) it is possible to express resistance to gas flow as the ratio of pressure difference to gas flow rate. This is analogous to electrical resistance, which is expressed as the ratio of potential difference to current flow. The dimensions of resistance to gas flow are pressure difference divided by gas flow rate, and typical units in the respiratory field have been cmH$_2$O per litre per second (cmH$_2$O.L^{-1}.s) or dynes.sec.cm^{-5} in absolute units.

Work (Dimensions: ML^{2}T^{-2}, Derived from MLT^{-2} × L OR ML^{-1}T^{-2} × L^3)

Work is done when a force moves its point of application or gas is moved in response to a pressure gradient. The dimensions are therefore either force times distance or pressure times volume, in each case simplifying to ML^{2}T^{-2}. The multiplicity of units of work has caused confusion in the past. Under the SI, the erg, calorie and kilopond-metre have disappeared in favour of the joule, which is defined as the work done when a force of 1 N moves its point of application 1 metre. It is also the work done when 1 litre of gas moves in response to a pressure gradient of 1 kilopascal. This represents a welcome simplification.

1 joule = 1 newton metre = 1 litre kilopascal

Power (Dimensions: ML^2T^{-2}/T OR ML^2T^{-3})

Power is the rate at which work is done, and so has the dimensions of work divided by time. The SI unit is the watt, which equals 1 joule per second. Power is the correct dimension for the rate of continuous expenditure of biological energy, although one talks loosely about the 'work of breathing.' This is incorrect, and 'power of breathing' is the correct term.

Appendix B

The Gas Laws

Certain physical attributes of gases are customarily presented under the general heading of the gas laws. These are of fundamental importance in respiratory physiology.

Boyle's law describes the inverse relationship between the volume and absolute pressure of a perfect gas at constant temperature:

$$PV = K \qquad \text{(Eq. A.1)}$$

where P represents pressure and V represents volume. At temperatures near their boiling point, gases deviate from Boyle's law. At room temperature, the deviation is negligible for oxygen and nitrogen and of little practical importance for carbon dioxide or nitrous oxide.

Charles' law describes the direct relationship between the volume and absolute temperature of a perfect gas at constant pressure:

$$V = KT \qquad \text{(Eq. A.2)}$$

where T represents the absolute temperature. There are appreciable deviations at temperatures immediately above the boiling point of gases. Equations A.1 and A.2 may be combined as:

$$PV = RT \qquad \text{(Eq. A.3)}$$

where R is the universal gas constant, which is the same for all perfect gases and has the value of 8.1314 joules.degrees kelvin^{-1}.moles^{-1}. From this it may be derived that the mole volume of all perfect gases is 22.4 L at standard temperature and pressure, dry (STPD). Carbon dioxide and nitrous oxide deviate from the behaviour of perfect gases to the extent of having mole volumes of about 22.2 L at STPD.

Henry's law describes the solution of gases in liquids with which they do not react. The general principle of Henry's law is simple enough. The number of molecules of gas dissolving in the solvent is directly proportional to the partial pressure of the gas at the surface of the liquid, and the constant of proportionality is an expression of the solubility of the gas in the liquid. This is a constant for a particular gas and a particular liquid at a particular temperature, but usually falls with rising temperature.

Physicists are more inclined to express solubility in terms of the *Bunsen coefficient*. For this, the amount of gas in solution is expressed in terms of volume of gas (standard temperature and pressure dry [STPD]) per unit volume of solvent (i.e., one-hundredth of the amount, expressed as vols%), and the pressure is expressed in atmospheres.

Biologists, on the other hand, prefer to use the *Ostwald coefficient*. This is the volume of gas dissolved, expressed as its volume under the conditions of temperature and pressure at which solution took place. It might be thought that this would vary with the pressure in the gas phase, but this is not so. If the pressure is doubled, according to Henry's law, twice as many molecules of gas dissolve. However, according to Boyle's law, they would occupy half the volume at double the pressure. Therefore, if Henry's and Boyle's laws are obeyed, the Ostwald coefficient will be independent of changes in pressure at which solution occurs. It will differ from the Bunsen coefficient only because the gas volume is expressed as the volume it would occupy at the temperature of the experiment rather than at 0°C. Conversion is thus in accord with Charles' law, and the two coefficients will be identical at 0°C. This should not be confused with the fact that, like the Bunsen coefficient, the Ostwald coefficient falls with rising temperature.

The partition coefficient is the ratio of the number of molecules of gas in one phase to the number of molecules of gas in another phase when equilibrium between the two has been attained. If one phase is gas and the other liquid, the liquid/gas partition coefficient will be identical to the Ostwald coefficient. Partition coefficients are also used to describe partitioning between two media (e.g., oil/water, brain/blood, etc.).

Graham's law of diffusion governs the influence of molecular weight on the diffusion of a gas through a gas mixture. Diffusion rates through orifices or through porous plates are inversely proportional to the square root of the molecular weight. This factor is only of importance in the gaseous part of the pathway between ambient air and the tissues, and is, in general, only of importance when the molecular weight is greater than that of oxygen or carbon dioxide. Graham's law is not relevant to the process of 'diffusion' through the alveolar/capillary membrane (page 113).

Dalton's law of partial pressure states that, in a mixture of gases, each gas exerts the pressure that it would exert if it occupied the volume alone (see Fig. 35.8). This pressure is known as the partial pressure, and the sum of the partial pressures equals the total pressure of the mixture. Thus, in a mixture of 5% carbon dioxide in oxygen at a total pressure of 101 kPa (760 mmHg), the carbon dioxide exerts a partial pressure of $5/100 \times 101 = 5.05$ kPa (38 mmHg). In general terms:

$$P_{CO_2} = F_{CO_2} \times P_B$$

In the alveolar gas at sea level, there is about 6.2% water vapour, which exerts a partial pressure of 6.3 kPa (47 mmHg). The available pressure for other gases is therefore $(P_B - 6.3)$ kPa or $(P_B - 47)$ mmHg. Gas concentrations are usually measured in the dry gas phase, and therefore it is necessary to apply this correction for water vapour in the lungs.

Appendix C

Conversion Factors for Gas Volumes

Gas volumes are usually measured at ambient (or environmental) temperature and pressure, either dry (e.g., from a cylinder passing through a rotameter) or saturated with water vapour at ambient temperature (e.g., an expired gas sample). Customary abbreviations are ATPD (ambient temperature and pressure, dry) and ATPS (ambient temperature and pressure, saturated).

Conversion of Gas Volume—ATPS to BTPS

Gas volumes measured by spirometry and other methods usually indicate the volume at ATPS. Tidal volume, minute volume, dead space, lung volumes, ventilatory gas flow rates, and so on should be converted to the volumes they would occupy in the lungs of the patient at body temperature and pressure, saturated (BTPS).

Conversion from ATPS to BTPS is based on Charles' and Boyle's laws (Appendix B), and conversion factors are listed in Table C.1.

Derivation of Conversion Factors

$$\text{Volume}_{(BTPS)} = \text{volume}_{(ATPS)} \left(\frac{273 + 37}{273 + t} \right) \left(\frac{P_B - P_{H_2O}}{P_B - 6.3} \right)$$

where P_B is barometric pressure (kPa), and Table C.1 has been prepared for a barometric pressure of 100 kPa (750 mmHg): variations in the range 99 to 101 kPa (740–760 mmHg) have a negligible effect on the factors. t is ambient temperature (°C). Table C.1 has been prepared for a body temperature of 37°C: variations in the range 35° to 39°C are of little importance.

P_{H_2O} is the water vapour pressure of the sample (kPa) at ambient temperature (see Table C.1).

Conversion of Gas Volume—ATPS to STPD

In measurement of absolute amounts of gases such as oxygen uptake, carbon dioxide output and the exchange of 'inert' gases, we need to know the actual quantity (i.e., number of molecules) of gas exchanged, and this is most conveniently expressed by stating the gas volume as it would be under standard conditions; that is, 0°C, 101.3 kPa (760 mmHg)

| TABLE C.1 | Factors for Conversion of Gas Volumes Measured Under Conditions of Ambient Temperature and Pressure, Saturated (ATPS) to Volumes that Would be Occupied Under Conditions of Body Temperature and Pressure, Saturated (BTPS) |

Ambient Temperature °C	Conversion Factor	Saturated Water Vapour Pressure	
		kPa	mmHg
15	1.129	1.71	12.8
16	1.124	1.81	13.6
17	1.119	1.93	14.5
18	1.113	2.07	15.5
19	1.108	2.20	16.5
20	1.103	2.33	17.5
21	1.097	2.48	18.6
22	1.092	2.64	19.8
23	1.086	2.80	21.0
24	1.081	2.99	22.4
25	1.075	3.16	23.7
26	1.069	3.66	25.2

pressure and dry (STPD). Under these conditions, one mole of an ideal gas occupies 22.4 l.

Conversion from ATPS to STPD is again by application of Charles' and Boyle's laws, as follows:

$$\text{Volume}_{(STPD)} = \text{volume}_{(ATPS)} \left(\frac{273}{273 + t} \right) \left(\frac{P_B - P_{H_2O}}{101} \right)$$

P_B is barometric pressure (kPa).

t is ambient temperature (°C).

P_{H_2O} is the saturated water vapour pressure of the sample (kPa) at ambient temperature (see Table C.1).

Appendix D

Symbols and Abbreviations

Symbols used in this book are in accord with recommendations for editors of medical and scientific publications in the United Kingdom.[1] There continues to be variation between journals, particularly between Europe and the USA. The use of these symbols is very helpful for an understanding of the quantitative relationships that are so important in respiratory physiology.

Primary symbols (large italic capitals) denoting physical quantities.

- F fractional concentration of gas
- P pressure, tension or partial pressure of a gas
- V volume of a gas
- Q volume of blood
- C content of a gas in blood
- S saturation of haemoglobin with oxygen
- R respiratory exchange ratio
- D diffusing capacity
- B binding capacity
- • denotes a time derivative; for example, $\dot{V}$, ventilation; $\dot{Q}$, perfusion

Secondary symbols denoting location of quantity.

In Gas Phase	In Blood
(small capitals)	**(lower case)**
I inspired gas	a arterial blood
E expired gas	v venous blood
A alveolar gas	c capillary
D dead space	t total
T tidal	s shunt
B barometric (usually pressure)	

⁻ denotes mixed or mean; for example, v̄, mixed venous blood; Ē, mixed expired gas
′ denotes end; for example, e′, end-expiratory gas; c′, end-capillary blood

Tertiary symbols indicating particular gases.

- O_2 oxygen
- CO_2 carbon dioxide
- N_2O nitrous oxide
- and so on
- f denotes the respiratory frequency
- BTPS, ATPS and STPD—see Appendix C.

Examples of respiratory symbols

- $P_{A_{O_2}}$ alveolar oxygen tension
- $C\bar{v}_{O_2}$ oxygen content of mixed venous blood
- $\dot{V}_{O_2}$ oxygen consumption

Reference

1. Baron DN, McKenzie Clarke H. Units, symbols, and abbreviations. *A guide for Authors and Editors in Medicine and Related Sciences.* 6th ed. London: Royal Society of Medicine Press; 2008.

Mathematical Functions Relevant to Respiratory Physiology

This book contains many examples of mathematical statements which relate respiratory variables under specified conditions. Appendix E is intended to refresh the memory of those readers whose knowledge of mathematics has been attenuated under the relentless pressure of new information acquired in the course of study of the biological sciences.

The most basic study of respiratory physiology requires familiarity with at least four types of mathematical relationship. These are:

a. The linear function.
b. The rectangular hyperbola or inverse function.
c. The parabola or squared function.
d. Exponential functions.

These four types of function will now be considered separately, with reference to examples drawn from this book.

Linear Function

Examples

1. Pressure gradient against flow rate with laminar flow (page 28). There is no constant factor, and the pressure gradient is zero when flow rate is zero.
2. Respiratory minute volume against $P\mathrm{CO_2}$ (page 49). In this case there is a constant factor corresponding to a 'negative' respiratory minute volume when $P\mathrm{CO_2}$ is zero.
3. Over a limited range, lung volume is proportional to inflating pressure (page 18). The slope of the line is then the compliance.

Mathematical Statement

A linear function describes a change in one variable (dependent or y variable) that is directly proportional to another variable (independent or x variable). There may or may not be a constant factor which is equal to y when x is zero. Thus:

$$y = ax + b$$

where a is the slope of the line and b is the constant factor. In any one particular relationship a and b are assumed to be constant, but both may have different values under other circumstances. They are not therefore true constants (like π, for example), and are more precisely termed parameters, whereas y and x are variables.

Graphical Representation

Figure E.1 shows a plot of a linear function following the convention that the independent variable (x) is plotted on the abscissa and the dependent variable (y) on the ordinate. Note that the relationship is a straight line, and simple regression analysis is based on the assumption that the relationship is of this type. If the slope (a) is positive, the line goes upwards and to the right. If the slope is negative, the line goes upwards and to the left.

The Rectangular Hyperbola or Inverse Function

Examples

1. The ventilatory response to hypoxia (expressed in terms of $P\mathrm{O_2}$) approximates to a rectangular hyperbola, asymptotic on the horizontal axis to the respiratory minute volume at high $P\mathrm{O_2}$ and, on the vertical axis, to the $P\mathrm{O_2}$ at which it is assumed ventilation increases towards infinity.
2. The relationships of alveolar gas tensions to alveolar ventilation are conveniently described by rectangular hyperbolas (for carbon dioxide see page 130, and for oxygen see page 138). The curves are concave upwards for gases that are eliminated (e.g., carbon dioxide) and concave downwards for gases that are taken up from the lungs (e.g., oxygen). Curvature is governed by gas output (or uptake), and the asymptotes in each case are zero ventilation and partial pressure of the gas under consideration in the inspired gas.
3. Airway resistance approximates to an inverse function of lung volume (page 31).

Mathematical Statement

A rectangular hyperbola describes a relationship when the dependent variable y is inversely proportional to the independent variable x, thus:

$$y = a/x + b$$

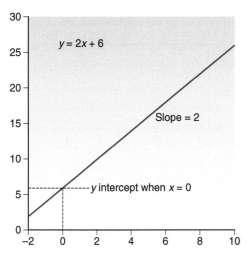

• **Fig. E.1** A linear function plotted on linear coordinates. Examples include pressure/flow rate relationships with laminar flow (see Fig. 3.2) and P_{CO_2}/ventilation response curves (see Fig. 4.6).

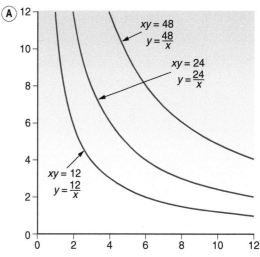

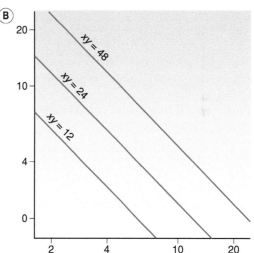

• **Fig. E.2** Rectangular hyperbolas plotted on (**A**) linear coordinates and (**B**) logarithmic coordinates. Examples include the relationships between alveolar gas tensions and alveolar ventilation (see Figs 9.9 and 10.2), P_{O_2}/ventilation response curves (see Fig. 4.8) and the relationship between airway resistance and lung volume (see Figs 3.5 and 21.12).

The asymptote of x is its value when y is infinity, and the asymptote of y is its value when x is infinity. If b is zero, then the relationship may be simply represented as follows:

$$xy = a$$

Graphical Representation

Figure E.2A shows rectangular hyperbolas with and without constant factors. Changes in the value of a alter the curvature but not the asymptotes. Figure E.2B shows the same relationships plotted on logarithmic coordinates. The relationship is now linear, but with a negative slope of unity, because if:

$$xy = a$$

then:

$$\log y = -\log x + \log a$$

The Parabola or Squared Function

Example

With fully turbulent gas flow, pressure gradient changes according to the square of gas flow, and the plot is a typical parabola (Chapter 3).

Mathematical Statement

A parabola is described when the dependent variable (y) changes in proportion to the square of the independent variable (x), thus:

$$y = ax^2$$

Graphical Representation

On linear coordinates, a parabola, with positive values of the abscissa, shows a steeply rising curve (Fig. E.3A), which may be confused with an exponential function (see below),

although it is fundamentally different. On logarithmic coordinates for both abscissa and ordinate, a parabola becomes a straight line with a slope of two (Fig. E.3B) because $\log y = \log a + 2 \log x$ (a and $\log a$ are parameters).

Exponential Functions

General Statement

An exponential function describes a change in which the rate of change of the dependent variable is proportional to the magnitude of the independent variable at that time. Thus, the rate of change of y with respect to x (i.e., dy/dx)[a]

---

[a]dy/dx is the mathematical shorthand for the rate of change of y with respect to x. The 'd' means 'a very small bit of'; therefore dy/dx means a very small bit of y divided by the corresponding very small bit of x. This is equal to the slope of the graph of y against x at that point. In the case of a curve, it is the slope of a tangent drawn to the curve at that point.

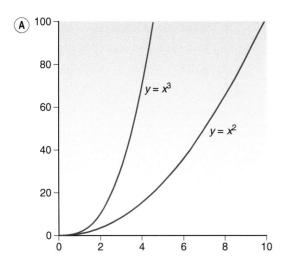

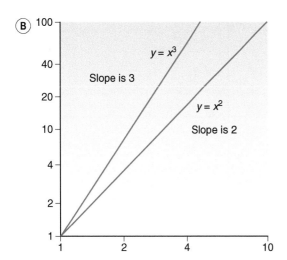

• **Fig. E.3** Parabolas plotted on (**A**) linear coordinates and (**B**) logarithmic coordinates. An example is the pressure/volume relationship with turbulent flow (see Fig. 3.3, B).

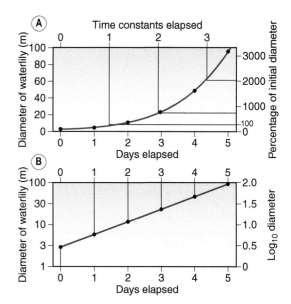

• **Fig. E.4** The growth of a waterlily that doubles its diameter every day, a typical tear-away exponential function. Initial diameter, 3 m; size doubled every day (i.e., doubling time = 1 day).

varies in proportion to the value of y at that instant. That is to say:

$$\frac{\mathrm{d}y}{\mathrm{d}x} = ky$$

where k is a constant or a parameter.

This general equation appears with minor modifications in three main forms. To the biological worker they may be conveniently described as the tear-away, the wash-out and the wash-in.

The Tear-Away Exponential Function

This must be described first, as it is the simplest form of the exponential function. It is, however, the least important of the three in relation to respiratory function.

Simple Statement

In a tear-away exponential function, the quantity under consideration increases at a rate which is in direct proportion

to its actual value—the richer one is, the faster one makes money.

Examples

Classic examples are compound interest, and the mythical waterlily that doubles its diameter every day (Fig. E.4). A typical biological example is the free spread of a bacterial colony in which (for example) each bacterium divides every 20 minutes. The doubling time of this example would be 20 minutes.

Mathematical Statement

In the case of exponential functions relevant to respiratory function, the independent variable x almost invariably represents time, and so we shall take the liberty of replacing x with t throughout. The tear-away function may thus be represented as follows:

$$\frac{\mathrm{d}y}{\mathrm{d}t} = ky$$

A little mathematical processing will convert this equation into a more useful form, which will indicate the instantaneous value of y at any time, t.

First multiply both sides by $\mathrm{d}t/y$:

$$\frac{1}{y}\mathrm{d}y = k\mathrm{d}t$$

Next integrate both sides with respect to t:

$$\log_e y + C_1 = kt + C_2$$

where (C_1 and C_2 are constants of integration and may be collected on the right-hand side.)

$$\log_e y = (C_2 - C_1) + kt$$

Finally, take antilogs of each side to the base e:

$$y = e^{(C_2 - C_1)} \times e^{kt}$$

At zero time, $t = 0$ and $e^{kt} = 1$. Therefore the constant $e^{(C_2 - C_1)}$ equals the initial value of y, which we may call y_0. Our final equation is thus:

$$y = y_0 e^{kt}$$

k is a constant that defines the speed of the particular function. For example, it will differ by a factor of two if our mythical waterlily doubles its size every 12 hours instead of every day. In the case of the wash-out and wash-in, we shall see that k is directly related to certain important physiological quantities, from which we may predict the speed of certain biological changes.

Instead of using e, it is possible to take logs to the more familiar base 10, thus:

$$y = y_0 10^{k_1 t}$$

This is a perfectly valid way of expressing a tear-away exponential function, but you will notice that the constant k has changed to k_1. This new constant does not have the simple relationships of physiological variables mentioned above. It does, however, bear a constant relationship to k, as follows:

$$k_1 = 0.4343k \text{ (approx.)}$$

Graphical Representation

On linear graph paper, a tear-away exponential function rapidly disappears off the top of the paper (Fig. E.4). If plotted on semilogarithmic paper (time on a linear axis and y on a logarithmic axis), the plot becomes a straight line, and this is a most convenient method of presenting such a function. The logarithmic plots in Figures E.4 to E.6 are all plotted on semilogarithmic paper.

The Wash-Out or Die-Away Exponential Function

The account of the tear-away exponential function has really been an essential introduction to the wash-out or die-away exponential function, which is of great importance to the biologist in general, and the respiratory physiologist in particular.

Simple Statement

In a wash-out exponential function, the quantity under consideration falls at a rate which decreases progressively in proportion to the distance it still has to fall. It approaches but, in theory, never reaches zero.

Examples

Familiar examples are cooling curves, radioactive decay and water running out of the bath. In the last example the rate of flow of bath water to waste is proportional to the pressure of water, which is proportional to the depth of water in the

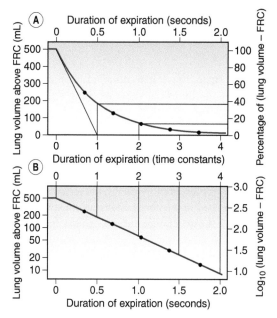

• **Fig. E.5** Passive expiration—a typical wash-out exponential function. Tidal volume, 500 mL; compliance, 0.5 L.kPa^{-1}(50 mL.cmH$_2$O^{-1}); airway resistance, 1 kPa.L^{-1}.s (10 cmH$_2$O.L^{-1}.s); time constant, 0.5 seconds; half-life, 0.35 seconds. The point on the curve indicate the passage of successive half-lives. Note that the logarithmic coordinate has no zero. This accords with the lung volume approaching, but never actually equalling, the functional residual capacity (FRC).

bath, which in turn is proportional to the quantity of water in the bath (assuming that the sides are vertical). Therefore the flow rate of water to waste is proportional to the amount of water left in the bath and decreases as the bath empties. The last molecule of bath water takes an infinitely long time to drain away.

In the field of respiratory physiology, examples include:
1. Passive expiration (Fig. E.5).
2. The elimination of inhalational anaesthetics.
3. The fall of arterial $P\text{CO}_2$ to its new level after a step increase in ventilation.
4. The fall of arterial $P\text{CO}_2$ to its new level after a step decrease in ventilation.
5. The fall of blood $P\text{CO}_2$ towards the alveolar level as it progresses along the pulmonary capillary.
6. The fall of blood $P\text{O}_2$ towards the tissue level as blood progresses through the tissue capillaries.

Mathematical Statement

When a quantity *decreases* with time, the rate of change is *negative*. Therefore, the wash-out exponential function is written thus:

$$\frac{\mathrm{d}y}{\mathrm{d}t} = -ky$$

from which we may derive the following equations, which give the value of y at any time t:

$$y = y_0 e^{-kt}$$

which is simply another way of saying:

$$y = \frac{y_0}{e^{kt}}$$

where y_0 is again the initial value of y at zero time. In Figure E.5, y_0 is the initial value of (lung volume – functional residual capacity [FRC]) at the start of expiration; that is to say, the tidal volume inspired;

e is again the base of natural logarithms (2.718 28…).

k is the constant that defines the rate of decay and is the reciprocal of a most important quantity known as the *time constant*, represented by the Greek letter tau (τ). Three things should be known about the time constant:

1. Figure E.5 shows a tangent drawn to the first part of the curve. This shows the course events would take if the initial rate were maintained instead of slowing down in the manner characteristic of the wash-out curve. The time that would then be required for completion would be the time constant (τ) or $1/k$. The wash-out exponential function may thus be written:

$$y = y_0 e^{-t/\tau}$$

2. After 1 time constant, y will have fallen to $1/e$ of its initial value, or approximately 37% of its initial value.
   After 2 time constants, y will have fallen to $1/e^2$ of its initial value, or approximately 13.5% of its initial value.
   After 3 time constants, y will have fallen to $1/e^3$ of its initial value, or approximately 5% of its initial value.
   After 5 time constants, y will have fallen to $1/e^5$ of its initial value, or approximately 1% of its initial value.

3. The time constant is often determined by physiological factors. When air escapes passively from a distended lung, the time constant is governed by two variables, compliance and resistance (see Chapters 2, 3 and 32).
   We may now consider the example of passive expiration. Let V represent the lung volume (above FRC), then $-\mathrm{d}V/\mathrm{d}t$ is the instantaneous expiratory gas flow rate. Assuming Poiseuille's law is obeyed:

$$-\frac{\mathrm{d}V}{\mathrm{d}t} = \frac{P}{R}$$

where P is the instantaneous alveolar-to-mouth pressure gradient and R is the airway resistance. However, compliance (C) = V/P. Therefore:

$$-\frac{\mathrm{d}V}{\mathrm{d}t} = \frac{1}{CR}V$$

or:

$$\frac{\mathrm{d}V}{\mathrm{d}t} = -\frac{1}{CR}V$$

Then by integration and taking antilogs as described previously:

$$V = V_0 e^{-(t/CR)}$$

By analogy with the general equation of the wash-out exponential function, it is clear that $CR = 1/k = \tau$ (the time constant). Thus the time constant equals the product of

compliance and resistance.[b] This is analogous to the discharge of an electrical capacitor through a resistance, when the time constant of discharge equals the product of the capacitance and the resistance.

Half-Life

It is often convenient to use the half-life instead of the time constant. This is the time required for y to change to half of its previous value. The special attraction of the half-life is its ease of measurement. The half-life of a radioactive element may be determined quite simply. First of all the degree of activity is measured and the time noted. Its activity is then followed, and the time noted at which its activity is exactly half the initial value. The difference between the two times is the half-life, and is constant at all levels of activity. Half-lives are shown in Figures E.4 to E.6 as dots on the curves. For a particular exponential function there is a constant relationship between the time constant and the half-life.

$$\text{Half-life} = 0.69 \times \text{time constant}$$
$$\text{Time constant} = 1.44 = \text{half-life.}$$

Graphical Representation

Plotting a wash-out exponential function is similar to the tear-away function (Fig. E.5). A semilogarithmic plot is particularly convenient as the curve (being straight) may then be defined by far fewer observations. It is also easy to extrapolate backwards to zero time if the initial value is required but could not be measured directly for some reason. It is, for example, an essential step in the measurement of cardiac output with a dye that is rapidly lost from the circulation (page 86).

The Wash-In Exponential Function

The wash-in function is also of special importance to the respiratory physiologist and is the mirror image of the wash-out function.

Simple Statement

In a wash-in exponential function, the quantity under consideration rises towards a limiting value, at a rate that decreases progressively in proportion to the distance it still has to rise.

Examples

A typical example would be a mountaineer who each day manages to climb half the remaining distance between his overnight camp and the summit of the mountain. His rate of ascent declines exponentially, and he will never reach the

---

[b]It is strange at first sight that two quantities as complex as compliance and resistance should have a product as simple as time. In fact, the mass/length/time (MLT) units (Appendix A) check perfectly well:

$$\text{Compliance} \times \text{resistance} = \text{time}$$
$$M^{-1}L^4T^2 \times ML^{-4}T^{-1} = T$$

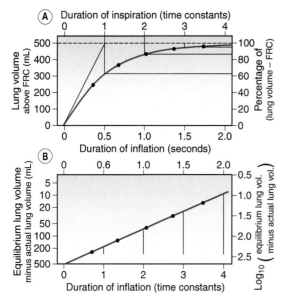

• **Fig. E.6** Passive inflation of the lungs with a sustained mouth pressure – a typical wash-in exponential function. Final tidal volume, 500 mL; compliance, 0.5 L.kPa^{-1}(50 mL.cmH$_2$O^{-1}); airway resistance, 1 kPa.L^{-1}.s (10 cmH$_2$O.L^{-1}.s); time constant, 0.5 seconds; half-life, 0.35 seconds. The points on the curves indicate the passage of successive half-lives. Note that, for the semilogarithmic plot, the log scale (ordinate) is from above downwards and indicates the difference between the equilibrium lung volume (inflation pressure maintained indefinitely) and the actual lung volume.

summit. A graph of his altitude plotted against time would resemble a 'wash-in' curve.

Biological examples include the reverse of those listed for the wash-out function:

1. Inflation of the lungs of a paralysed patient by a sustained increase of mouth pressure (Fig. E.6).
2. The uptake of inhalational anaesthetics.
3. The rise of arterial $P\text{CO}_2$ to its new level after a step decrease of ventilation.
4. The rise of arterial $P\text{O}_2$ to its new level after a step increase of ventilation.
5. The rise of blood $P\text{O}_2$ to the alveolar level as it progresses along the pulmonary capillary.
6. The rise of blood $P\text{CO}_2$ to the venous level as blood progresses through the tissue capillaries.

Mathematical Statement

With a wash-in exponential function, y increases with time, and therefore the rate of change is positive. As time advances, the rate of change falls towards zero. The initial value of y is often zero, and y approaches a final limiting value that we may designate y_∞ – that is, the value of y when time is infinity (∞). A change of this type is indicated thus:

$$\frac{\mathrm{d}y}{\mathrm{d}t} = k\left(y_\infty - y\right)$$

As y approaches y_∞, so the quantity within the parentheses approaches zero, and the rate of change slows down. The corresponding equation that indicates the instantaneous value of y is:

$$y = y_\infty(1 - e^{-kt})$$

where y_∞ is the limiting value of y (attained only at infinite time).

e is again the base of natural logarithms.

k is a constant defining the rate of build-up and, as is the case of the wash-out function, it is the reciprocal of the *time constant* the significance of which is described above. It is the time that would be required to reach completion, if the initial rate of change were maintained without slowing down.

After 1 time constant, y will have risen to approximately $100 - 37 = 63\%$ of its final value.

After 2 time constants, y will have risen to approximately $100 - 13.5 = 86.5\%$ of its final value.

After 3 time constants, y will have risen to approximately $100 - 5 = 95\%$ of its final value.

After 5 time constants, y will have risen to approximately $100 - 1 = 99\%$ of its final value.

As in the wash-out function representing passive exhalation, the time constant for the corresponding wash-in exponential function (passive inflation of the lungs) equals the product of compliance and resistance. For the wash-in of a substance into an organ, the time constant equals tissue volume divided by blood flow or FRC divided by alveolar ventilation, as the case may be. As previously, the time constant is approximately 1.5 times the half-life.

There are many situations in which the same parameters apply to both wash-in and wash-out functions of the same system. The time constant for each function will then be the same. A classic example is the charging of an electrical capacitor through a resistance, and then allowing it to discharge to earth through the same resistor. The time constant is the same for each process and equals the product of capacitance and resistance. This is approximately true for passive deflation and inflation of the lungs (Figs E.5 and E.6), on the assumption that compliance and airway resistance remain the same.

Graphical Representation

The wash-in function may be represented on linear paper as for the other types of exponential function. However, for the semilogarithmic plot, the paper must be turned upside down and the plot made as indicated in Figure E.6. The curve will then be a straight line.

Index

Page numbers followed by '*f*' indicate figures, '*t*' indicate tables, and '*e*' indicate online content.